Spine
Trauma

Spine Trauma

Alan M. Levine, M.D.

Associate Chief of Orthopaedic Surgery
Professor of Orthopaedic Surgery and Oncology
Division of Orthopaedic Surgery
University of Maryland School of Medicine
Consultant in Spinal Injury
Maryland Shock Trauma Unit
Baltimore, Maryland

Frank J. Eismont, M.D.

Professor and Vice Chairman
Department of Orthopaedics and Rehabilitation
University of Miami School of Medicine
Miami, Florida

Steven R. Garfin, M.D.

Professor and Chair, Department of Orthopaedics
University of California, San Diego
San Diego, California

Jack E. Zigler, M.D.

Texas Back Institute
Plano, Texas
Former Chief, Spinal Injury Service
Rancho Los Amigos Medical Center
Downey, California
Clinical Professor of Orthopaedic Surgery
University of Southern California School of Medicine
Los Angeles, California

W.B. SAUNDERS COMPANY
A Division of Harcourt Brace & Company
Philadelphia   London   Toronto   Montreal   Sydney   Tokyo

W.B. SAUNDERS COMPANY
A Division of Harcourt Brace & Company

The Curtis Center
Independence Square West
Philadelphia, Pennsylvania 19106

Library of Congress Cataloging-in-Publication Data

Spine trauma / Alan M. Levine . . . [et al.].

p.   cm.

ISBN 0–7216–2957–1

1. Spinal cord—Wounds and injuries.   I. Levine, Alan M.   [DNLM: 1. Spinal
Cord Injuries.   2. Spinal Injuries.   3. Cervical Vertebrae—injuries.
4. Lumbar Vertebrae—injuries.   WL 400 S7595 1998]

RD594.3.S694 1998   617.4′82044—dc21

DNLM/DLC   97–39760

SPINE TRAUMA ISBN 0–7216–2957–1

Printed in the United States of America.

Last digit is the print number: 9   8   7   6   5   4   3   2   1

Dedication

I would like to express my deepest appreciation to my wife, Barbara, and to my children, Dana, Lissy, and Ahnie, for being understanding and supportive in spite of the time commitment involved in caring for victims of spine trauma and in producing this text.

ALAN M. LEVINE

I would like to thank my wife, Emily, and my children, Adam, April, Allison, and Andy, for their understanding and for encouraging me to pursue my medical interests.

FRANK J. EISMONT

Helping others through direct patient care, through education of physicians who provide care, and by doing research that improves lives encompasses unique opportunities and responsibilities. I have been able to provide time and energy in these pursuits because of the devotion, love, and support of my wonderful wife, Susan, my children, Jessica and Cory, and my parents. I cannot thank them enough. A book dedication is only a small statement for a lifetime's commitment.

STEVEN R. GARFIN

Dedicated to Henry H. Bohlman, M.D., who helped me become a good spine surgeon; to my wife, Wendy, and my children, Jeffrey and Jennifer, who helped me become a good husband and father; and to my parents, Florence and Irving Zigler, and Edith and Nat Drutman, who helped me become a good person.

JACK E. ZIGLER

Contributors

Jean-Jacques Abitbol, M.D.
Clinical Instructor, State University of New York at Syracuse, Syracuse; Long Island Spine Specialists, Commack, New York.

Odontoid Fractures; Cervical Burst Fractures; Teardrop Fractures of the Cervical Spine

Sohail S. Ahmad, M.D.
Department of Orthopaedic Surgery, Albert Einstein University, Bronx, New York.

Anatomy and Pathophysiology of the Spinal Cord

Glenn Amundson, M.D.
Assistant Professor of Orthopaedics, University of Kansas Medical Center, Kansas City, Kansas.

Vascular Anatomy of the Spine

Michal S. Atkins, M.A., O.T.R.
Occupational Therapy Clinical Specialist, Rancho Los Amigos Medical Center, Downey, California.

Rehabilitation

Robert Benz, M.D.
Clinical Instructor, UCSD Medical Center, University of California, San Diego, San Diego, California.

Cervical Burst Fractures

Kel Bergmann, C.P.O.
Southern California Orthotics and Prosthetics, San Diego, California.

Spinal Orthoses in the Management of Spine Trauma

Benjamin Blair, M.D.
Affiliated Faculty Member, Idaho State University; Affiliated Faculty Member, Bannock Regional Medical Center and Pocatello Regional Medical Center, Pocatello, Idaho.

Thoracolumbar Compression Fractures

Michael Botte, M.D.
Section of Hand and Foot Surgery, Division of Orthopaedic Surgery, Scripps Clinic, La Jolla; Clinical Professor, Department of Orthopaedics, University of California, San Diego, School of Medicine, San Diego, California.

Spinal Orthoses in the Management of Spine Trauma; Complications of the Musculoskeletal System Following Spinal Cord Injury

Brian C. Bowen, M.D., Ph.D.
Associate Professor of Radiology and Neurologic Surgery, Department of Radiology, Section of Neuroradiology, University of Miami School of Medicine, Miami, Florida.

Post-traumatic Syringomyelia

Frank P. Cammisa, Jr., M.D.
Assistant Professor, Department of Surgery, Chief, Spinal Surgical Service, Cornell University Medical College, New York, New York.

Hyperextension Injuries of the Cervical Spine

Daniel A. Capen, M.D.
Associate Professor of Orthopaedic Surgery, USC Medical Center, University of Southern California, Los Angeles, California.

Epidemiology of Spinal Cord Injury: A Perspective on the Problem

Gregory D. Carlson, M.D.
Assistant Professor, Case Western Reserve University School of Medicine; Orthopaedic Surgeon, University Hospital, Cleveland, Ohio.

Odontoid Fractures

Mark S. Cohen, M.D.
Assistant Professor and Director, Orthopaedic Education, Director, Hand and Elbow Program, Department of Orthopaedic Surgery, Rush–Presbyterian–St. Luke's Medical Center, Chicago, Illinois.

Thoracolumbar Compression Fractures

Aleksandar Curcin, M.D.
Assistant Professor of Orthopaedic Surgery, University of Maryland Medical System, Baltimore, Maryland.

Fractures of the Sacrum

Joel K. Curé, M.D.
Associate Professor of Radiology, Director of Magnetic Resonance Imaging, Medical University of South Carolina, Charleston, South Carolina.

Radiologic Evaluation of the Spine-Injured Patient

Bradford L. Currier, M.D.
Assistant Professor, Department of Orthopaedics, Mayo Medical School; Head, Mayo Clinic Spine Group; Director, Mayo Clinic Spine Fellowship, Rochester, Minnesota.

Atlantoaxial Rotatory Deformities; Thoracolumbar Burst Fractures

John C. Drummond, M.D.
Chairman, Department of Anesthesiology, UCSD Medical Center, University of California, San Diego, San Diego, California.

Intraoperative Evaluation: Somatosensory Evoked Potentials and Motor Evoked Potentials

Frank J. Eismont, M.D.
Professor and Vice Chairman, Department of Orthopaedics and Rehabilitation, University of Miami School of Medicine, Miami, Florida.

Craniocervical Trauma; Hyperextension Injuries of the Cervical Spine; Flexion-Distraction Injuries of the Thoracic and Lumbar Spine; Gunshot Wounds of the Spine

Steven Falcone, M.D.
Assistant Professor of Clinical Radiology and Neurologic Surgery, Director of MR Services, University of Miami School of Medicine, Miami, Florida.

Post-traumatic Syringomyelia

Daveed Frazier, M.D.
Department of Orthopedic Surgery, St. Luke's–Roosevelt Hospital, New York, New York.

Craniocervical Trauma

Steven R. Garfin, M.D.
Professor and Chair, Department of Orthopaedics, University of California, San Diego, San Diego, California.

Vascular Anatomy of the Spine; Anatomy and Pathophysiology of Spinal Cord Injury; Spinal Orthoses in the Management of Spine Trauma; Odontoid Fractures; Cervical Burst Fractures; Teardrop Fractures of the Cervical Spine; Thoracolumbar Compression Fractures; Complex Instability of the Thoracic and Lumbar Spine

Barth A. Green, M.D.
Professor and Chairman, Department of Neurosurgery, University of Miami School of

Medicine; Chief of Service, Neurosurgery, Jackson Memorial Hospital Medical Center, Miami, Florida.

Experimental Spinal Cord Injury; Post-traumatic Syringomyelia

Daniel A. Green, M.D.
Clinical Instructor, Department of Orthopaedic Surgery, UCSD Medical Center, University of California, San Diego, San Diego; San Dieguito Orthopaedic Medical Group, La Jolla, California.

Complex Instability of the Thoracic and Lumbar Spine

Harry Herkowitz, M.D.
Chairman, Department of Orthopaedic Surgery, William Beaumont Hospital, Royal Oak, Michigan.

Insufficiency of the Transverse Ligament

John G. Heller, M.D.
Associate Professor of Orthopaedic Surgery, Emory University School of Medicine; Director of Education, The Emory Spine Center, Atlanta, Georgia.

Odontoid Fractures

Zaki G. Ibrahim, M.D.
Northland Orthopaedic Group, Inc., Florissant, Maryland.

Teardrop Fractures of the Cervical Spine

Cor J. Kalkman, M.D., Ph.D.
Associate Professor of Anesthesiology, Department of Anesthesiology, Academic Medical Center, Amsterdam, The Netherlands.

Intraoperative Evaluation: Somatosensory Evoked Potentials and Motor Evoked Potentials

Scott H. Kitchel, M.D.
Clinical Assistant Professor, Department of Orthopaedic Surgery, Oregon Health Sciences University, Portland, Oregon.

Surgical Approaches to the Cervical Spine; Surgical Approaches to the Thoracic and Lumbar Spine

Lawrence T. Kurz, M.D.
Department of Orthopaedics, William Beaumont Hospital, Royal Oak, Michigan.

Insufficiency of the Transverse Ligament

Michael K. Kwan, Ph.D.
Formerly Department of Orthopaedics, University of California, San Diego, San Diego, California.

Biomechanics of Spinal Cord and Nerve Root Injury

Carlos J. Lavernia, M.D.
Associate Professor of Orthopaedic Surgery and Biomedical Engineering, Director, Division of Arthritis Surgery, University of Miami School of Medicine, Miami, Florida.

Spinal Orthoses in the Management of Spine Trauma

Alan M. Levine, M.D.
Associate Chief of Orthopaedic Surgery, Professor of Orthopaedic Surgery and Oncology, Division of Orthopaedic Surgery, University of Maryland School of Medicine; Consultant in Spinal Injury, Maryland Shock Trauma Unit, Baltimore, Maryland.

Classification of Spinal Injury; Fractures of the Atlas; Traumatic Spondylolisthesis of the Axis (Hangman's Fracture); Facet Fractures and Dislocations; Facet Fractures and Dislocations of the Thoracolumbar Spine; Low Lumbar Spine Trauma; Fractures of the Sacrum

Parley W. Madsen III, M.D., Ph.D.
Assistant Clinical Professor of Anatomy and Neurobiology, St. Louis University School of Medicine; Member, Board of Directors, Practical Anatomy and Surgical Technique Workshop of St. Louis, St. Louis, Missouri.

Post-traumatic Syringomyelia

Alberto Martinez-Arizala, M.D.
Associate Professor, University of Miami School of Medicine; Principal Investigator, The Miami Project to Cure Paralysis, Miami, Florida.

Experimental Spinal Cord Injury

Gregory S. McDowell, M.D.
Chief of Orthopaedic Surgery, St. Vincent's Hospital and Health Center; Co-Director, Northern Rockies Regional Spine Injury Center, Billings, Montana.

Hyperextension Injuries of the Cervical Spine

Edward J. McGuire, M.D.
Director and Professor, Division of Urology, University of Texas, Houston, Texas.

Urologic Complications of Spinal Cord Injury

Robert A. McGuire, Jr., M.D.
Professor of Orthopaedics, Associate Professor of Neurosurgery, University of Mississippi Medical Center, Jackson, Mississippi.

Physical Examination in Spinal Trauma

Friedhelm Noll, M.D.
Chief of Urology, Division of Urology, Knappschaftskrankenhaus, Bardenberg, Wuerselen, Germany.

Urologic Complications of Spinal Cord Injury

Dana Ohl, M.D.
Associate Professor, Section of Urology, University of Michigan, Ann Arbor, Michigan.

Urologic Complications of Spinal Cord Injury

Kjell Olmarker, M.D., Ph.D.
Associate Research Professor, Department of Orthopaedics, University of Gothenburg, Sahlgrenska University Hospital, Gothenburg, Sweden.

Biomechanics of Spinal Cord and Nerve Root Injury

Stephen Ozanne, M.D.
Metroplex Orthopaedics, Dallas, Texas.

Cervical Burst Fractures

Wesley W. Parke, Ph.D.
Professor and Chairman Emeritus, Anatomy Department, University of South Dakota School of Medicine, Vermillion, South Dakota.

Vascular Anatomy of the Spine

Peter D. Pizzutillo, M.D.
Professor, Department of Orthopaedics and Pediatrics, MCP ◆ Hahnemann School of Medicine; Director, Orthopaedic Center for Children, St. Christopher's Hospital for Children, Philadelphia, Pennsylvania.

Management of Pediatric Spinal Cord Injury Patients

Wolfgang Rauschning, M.D., Ph.D.
Research Professor in Clinical Anatomy, Department of Orthopaedic Surgery, Academic University Hospital, Uppsala, Sweden.

Anatomy and Pathophysiology of the Spinal Cord

Cheryl D. Resnik, M.S., D.P.T.
Assistant Professor of Clinical Physical Therapy, University of Southern California, Los Angeles; Director, Physical Therapy, USC University Hospital, Los Angeles, California.

Rehabilitation

Reynold L. Rimoldi, M.D.
Assistant Professor, University Medical Center, University of Nevada Medical School, Las Vegas, Nevada.

Immediate Postoperative Care

Björn L. Rydevik, M.D., Ph.D.
Professor and Chairman, Department of Orthopaedics, University of Gothenburg, Sahlgrenska University Hospital, Gothenburg, Sweden.

Biomechanics of Spinal Cord and Nerve Root Injury

Mark M. Scheffer, M.D.
Orthopaedic Surgeon, U.S. Air Force Academy
Hospital, U.S.A.F., Colorado.

Thoracolumbar Burst Fractures

Steven R. Shackford, M.D.
Professor and Chairman, Department of Surgery,
University of Vermont; Surgeon-in-Chief, Fletcher
Allen Health Care, Burlington, Vermont.

Spine Injury in the Polytrauma Patient: General Surgical and Orthopaedic Considerations

Richard Skalak, Ph.D., M.D. (Hon.)†
Formerly Professor, Department of Bioengineering,
Director, Institute for Mechanics and Materials,
University of California, San Diego, San Diego,
California.

Biomechanics of Spinal Cord and Nerve Root Injury

Lilli Thompson, P.T.
Physical Therapy Clinical Specialist, Rancho Los
Amigos Medical Center, Downey, California.

Rehabilitation

Alexander R. Vaccaro, M.D.
Associate Professor, Department of Orthopaedic
Surgery, Thomas Jefferson University and the

Rothman Institute, Philadelphia, Pennsylvania.

Anatomy and Pathophysiology of Spinal Cord Injury; Spinal Orthoses in the Management of Spine Trauma; Management of Pediatric Spinal Cord Injury Patients

Elizabeth Vasher, B.S., R.N.
Formerly Nurse-Clinician, Urology Section, University
of Michigan, Ann Arbor, Michigan.

Urologic Complications of Spinal Cord Injury

Steven Wang, M.D.
Urological Services, Flint, Michigan.

Urologic Complications of Spinal Cord Injury

Jeremy W.R. Young, B.M., B.Ch., F.R.C.R.
Professor and Chairman, Department of Radiology,
Medical University of South Carolina, Charleston,
South Carolina.

Radiologic Evaluation of the Spine-Injured Patient

Jack E. Zigler, M.D.
Texas Back Institute, Plano, Texas; Former Chief,
Spinal Injury Service, Rancho Los Amigos Medical
Center, Downey, California; Clinical Professor of
Orthopaedic Surgery, University of Southern
California School of Medicine, Los Angeles,
California.

Epidemiology of Spinal Cord Injury: A Perspective on the Problem; Immediate Postoperative Care; Rehabilitation

---

†Deceased.

Foreword

Contributions in the medical literature relating to spine trauma, including sprains, subluxations, dislocations, and paralysis of various types, have been found dating from 4000 to 5000 years ago. These reported works of antiquity were attributed to Imhotep, vizir of Djosei, who lived in the era of the second pharaoh of the Third Dynasty. Reports of this surgical work were found in the papyrus of Edwin Smith, which he acquired in 1862, and which was translated by J.H. Breasted in 1930. Countless subsequent contributions to the spine literature have been offered since the translation of the papyrus of Edwin Smith. The 20th century appears to represent an era of proliferation of specialty centers of care in many areas of medicine, including trauma centers with subdivisions for spinal injury. As a result of the existence of these specialty centers, many valuable contributions to the literature have been made detailing the experience garnered from the high volume of patients in these centers.

Emergency medical service systems provide innovative methods resulting in improved care offered to trauma victims. The French began transport of wounded soldiers for care by physicians away from the scene of battle in the 1790s. Similar services were offered during the Civil War by Clara Barton, a nurse, who later founded the American Red Cross. Military (and, later, nonmilitary) ambulance services were developed in American cities in the later 1800s. In 1966, the National Highway Safety Act of the Department of Transportation upgraded the services and developed EMS (emergency medical services) standards. In 1970 the National Registry of emergency medical technicians (EMTs) started and developed standards ranging among levels of education and expertise from EMT-basic to intermediate and paramedic.

In the early 1940s, small, new spinal care facilities were developed in both Mandeville in Aylesbury, England, and in Boston. In 1968 in the United States, the Rehabilitation Services Administration (RSA) set a federal initiative in motion for unmet needs for rehabilitation in patients with spinal cord injuries. By 1970 the RSA awarded the Good Samaritan Hospital in Phoenix the first national model spinal cord injury (SCI) system, which is a system for comprehensive care of the spine-injured patient. These model system SCI centers have grown to a present number of 17, strategically positioned around the United States. Thus the stage was set by a combination of level 1 trauma units and SCI systems for total and comprehensive care of the spine-injured patient. Through these centers, care for the

spinal fracture has advanced exponentially from both a clinical standpoint and that of data collection. Thus, the editors of this text have taken the opportunity, utilizing the experience of those who have gone before, to describe the state of the art in spinal surgery care in the twilight of the 20th century. Areas of peripheral support for the trauma patient include first responders, transport, and specialty centers in addition to the myriad of specialty nurses and physicians involved with the care of trauma.

The four editors of this comprehensive tome on spinal trauma are eminently qualified for their position, as each has served as a leader in an SCI center and/or trauma unit at a different site in this country. In turn, the editors have selected freely from national and international experts for contributions in the basic science and clinical areas. The text subdivides the material appropriately into four sections. Section I, General Principles, includes epidemiology of injury and general assessment of the patient, including physical examination and radiographic evaluation relating to osseous, connective, and neural tissue damage. There is also a chapter on experimental SCI and biomechanics of cord and root injury. This section also includes surgical approaches to specific areas, intraoperative neurologic monitoring techniques, and postoperative orthoses. In Sections II and III (one each for cervical and thoracolumbar spine, respectively) the evaluation and treatment of each specific type of injury is discussed in depth. Section IV addresses postoperative care and rehabilitation and includes such subjects as urologic complications and post-traumatic syringomyelia, as well as generally recognized sequelae of musculoskeletal injury.

This text deals specifically with each of the many facets of spinal trauma and will serve as an excellent clinical guide to all who are interested in the continuum of care necessary for patients with these complex injuries. The authors have included the most current concepts and techniques, making this information readily available to any reader with an interest in or need to care for spine trauma patients. The publisher, contributors, and editors are to be congratulated for offering assistance to patients and caregivers at all levels in the treatment of spinal injuries from occurrence through rehabilitation. This text also supports the concept of the ability of centers of specialty care to collect their experience and data and to provide contributions to the spine trauma literature to minimize the incidence and the potential devastating progression of disability for these patients. For all their efforts, the editors are to be congratulated for the breadth and quality of the contributors and their material. The text should stand the test of time as a major contribution in the care of such a potentially devastated patient population.

The text is well presented with 37 chapters, myriad illustrations and images, and a complete current bibliography in each area. This offering should represent a wonderful guideline to aid the student as well as the practitioner in the management of the spine-injured patient.

The practice of medicine is an art, based on science.[1]
Sir William Osler, 1849–1914

As no two faces, so no two cases are alike in all respects, and unfortunately it is not only the disease itself which is so varied, but the subjects themselves have peculiarities which modify its action.[2]

Sir William Osler

JEROME M. COTLER, M.D.
The Everett J. and Marian Gordon Professor of
Orthopaedic Surgery
Department of Orthopaedic Surgery
Jefferson Medical College of Thomas Jefferson University
Philadelphia, Pennsylvania

1. Osler W: Teacher and student. *In* Aequanimitas, with Other Addresses to Medical Students, Nurses and Practitioners of Medicine, ed 34. Philadelphia, Blakiston, 1943, p 34.
2. Osler W: Teaching and thinking. *In* Aequanimitas, with Other Addresses to Medical Students, Nurses and Practitioners of Medicine, ed 34. Philadelphia, Blakiston, 1943, p 123.

Preface

The preface in many of the books dealing with spinal injury has usually emphasized the importance of the team approach to treating patients with this devastating problem. Beginning with George Bedbrook in his text, *The Care and Management of Spinal Cord Injuries,* the emphasis has been on addressing all of the health professionals involved in the complex care of spinal injury patients from admission through the completion of rehabilitation. "My purpose in writing this book is to describe the practical, day-to-day care and medical management of individuals with spinal paralysis. Emphasis is placed on the team approach."[1] However, as the care of the spine injured patient has evolved, certain elements of the care have become more and more complex. Therefore, the editors and authors of *Spine Trauma* have, in this text, both broken with and adhered closely to the tradition of the care of the spinal cord–injured patient. The team approach continues to remain the major hallmark of spinal injury care. If anything, the importance of this concept is stronger than it was with the establishment of spinal cord injury centers in the 1950s. Thus, it was planned that the text would address many of the elements of the care of spinal injury, such as epidemiology, emergency evaluation, and spine injury in the polytrauma patient. In addition, significant attention has been directed to the rehabilitation aspects of the care of the spine-injured patient. It was evident, however, that the evolution of the acute care of the spine-injured patient has progressed rapidly over the last 10 years. For example, many more options are currently available for radiologic imaging. Advances in pharmacologic management of the spinal cord injury as well as in the surgical treatment of spinal injuries are the result of the better understanding of the etiology of spinal cord injury.

This text was conceived as a departure from many of the previous texts on spinal injury in that it delves more intensively and specifically into the acute management of specific types of spinal trauma in both the non–cord-injured and cord-injured patient. The editors, as well as the publisher, were in agreement that the existing texts did not deal specifically enough with individual types of spine injuries and their evaluation and treatment. It was also thought that a number of types of presentations of spine trauma had not been extensively examined in other texts. Of all patients sustaining injuries to the spine, only 10% develop significant neurologic deficit; even in injuries to the cervical region, only 40% of patients sustaining trauma to the spine have neural deficit. A large proportion of the patients are therefore not spinal cord injury patients, but rather are spinal trauma patients without neurologic injury. It was thought to be important to address spine injury in this population. Likewise, it is also evident that both spine trauma and spinal cord–injury victims can suffer either isolated injuries or polytrauma. As a result of the advent of both trauma centers and spinal-injury centers, patients with polytrauma (spinal injury and other musculoskeletal and visceral injuries) are surviving. These patients may require modification of the approach to the spinal injury or to other musculoskeletal or visceral injuries based on the presence of the spinal cord injury. A distinction is made between patients with cord and non-cord injuries as well between those with isolated spinal trauma and polytrauma.

A broad spectrum of professionals attends to these patients. The text was intended to serve the needs of those initially involved in evaluating and treating the spine trauma victim by specifically addressing these areas while providing a background on the etiology of spinal injury and the rationale for the remaining specific treatment pathways. Surgical traumatologists, critical care specialists, and rehabilitation professionals were thought to be able to benefit from the text. It was one of our primary intentions, however, to provide a resource for spinal surgeons by delineating how to evaluate a specific injury as well as how to treat the injury both nonoperatively and operatively. In addition, specific illustrations are provided to outline the anatomic dissection as well as the technical aspects of operative procedures. Instead of being a general reference on spinal cord injury, this book provides both general knowledge about the spine and spinal cord injury and specific information about each particular type of spine trauma.

Although this text may, at first glance, appear to be most relevant to surgeons who see spine trauma on a daily basis in major trauma centers, it has actually been constructed to have a wider application for practitioners who treat patients with isolated spine trauma in emergency rooms and trauma centers. Because residents, practicing neurosurgeons, and orthopaedic surgeons are currently seeing a significant volume of both high- and low-energy trauma injuries to the spine, this text can serve as a specific reference to treating the types of injuries that may be encountered on almost a daily basis. The first section provides a general educational resource, addressing the anatomy and pathophysiology of spinal trauma and spinal cord injury. This section also contains detailed initial evaluation of the patient who has a potential spinal injury. Within this section is a chapter on the classification of spine trauma. The absence of a universally agreed on, comprehensive classification system has been a major nemesis to those who treat spinal injury. However, the limitations and strengths of the various existing classifications are outlined, and the rationale for adopting the method of subdivision of spinal injury used in this book is discussed as a transition to the second and third sections of the book. The second section of this book deals with both upper and lower cervical spine injuries. Each specific injury is detailed in a consistent fashion. The specific anatomy of the injured area of the spine is defined with reference to its influence on both evaluation and care. Evaluation of each type of injury is delineated and followed by discussion of the appropriate methods of operative and nonoperative care, concluding with the expected results of treatment as well as any potential complications of treatment. The third section is devoted to the major thoracic, lumbar, and sacral injuries, which are discussed in the same consistent fashion as are cervical injuries. The final section of the book addresses the rehabilitation of the spinal cord injury patient, with emphasis on some of the more frequently encountered long-term complications.

In selecting the editors of the book, a conscious effort was made to include physicians who are currently involved in the day-to-day management of these injuries from four different major centers around the country. This, I hoped, would instill a breadth of opinion to the text, rather than narrowing its scope, as regards decision making and treatment. In addition, I sought to incorporate the work of noted authors in specific areas, and am clearly indebted to those contributors for their efforts. The final evaluation of a text of this type is not dependent as much on the conception of the text as on the execution of the plan in each chapter. Thus, the more in-depth the understanding of the injury by the contributor, the more likely that the reader will be able to grasp the nuances of evaluation, treatment, and outcome of these injuries. I hope that the text will be of lasting value to all of the professionals treating these injuries, and most specifically to those making the decisions and executing the treatment plans.

ALAN M. LEVINE, M.D.

1. Bedbrook GM: The Care and Management of Spinal Cord Injuries. New York, Springer-Verlag, 1981, p xiii.

Acknowledgments

We would initially like to pay tribute to our mentors. They have inspired us and introduced us to the fascinating and complicated area of spinal injury. We hope that they are proud of our contributions and especially what we have conveyed in this text. We also need to acknowledge and thank the many residents and fellows who have played an integral part in the management of these patients, which has allowed us to garner the experience necessary to produce this text. We hope that they have learned from us and, in fact, that we have passed some of the enthusiasm and excitement that we have gotten from our mentors on to them.

In addition, we would like to acknowledge the staff at W.B. Saunders. This project was originally conceived with the help of Ed Wickland, who was the senior editor at that time, but it would not have come to fruition without the guidance of the current senior editor, Richard Lampert. We are most indebted to Beth Hatter, our developmental editor, who in her kind yet strong way has inspired us to complete this long-delayed task. A special thank you is also due the members of the production team for all of their hard work: Laurie Sander, production manager; Deborah Thorp, supervising copy editor; Rita Martello, illustrations specialist; Jonel Sofian, designer; and Bob Keller, marketing manager. One of the things that we hope will make this text useful to its readers is the strong emphasis on illustrations. Tedd Huff has taken our sketches and transformed them into a critical element of the book.

Each of the editors has relied heavily on his personal staff, whose members have gone a step beyond in helping to produce this book. Thus, each of us would like to acknowledge his own staff.

Alan Levine acknowledges the work of his secretary, Bobbi Quinn, who has handled the many telephone calls and communications back and forth between W.B. Saunders and our office. Managing the transfer of documents has been a formidable task. In addition, Martha Keltz has helped with much of the research, as well as the proofreading of the various manuscripts. However, a large debt of appreciation is owed to the residents, fellows, and attending staff at the Maryland Shock Trauma unit who have, over the last 18 years, provided the opportunity to learn about these patients and to develop a level of expertise, which hopefully is conveyed in this text.

Frank Eismont would like to acknowledge the extra effort put forth by his secretary, JoAnn Moyer, and his nurse-clinician, Laurie Roberts, without whose help his part of this book could not have been completed.

Steve Garfin respects, appreciates, and thanks Bonnie Carren, administrator, Liz Stimson, nurse practitioner, and Jennifer Massie, research coordinator, for their time and effort, which provided him the time and energy to complete the task.

Jack Zigler would like to thank Beverly Riggins, Scott Riggins, and Susan J. Buchanan, the transcriptionists who worked on the drafts and revisions over the years.

Contents

GENERAL PRINCIPLES

CHAPTER 1

Epidemiology of Spinal Cord Injury: A Perspective on the Problem

Jack E. Zigler ‖ *Daniel A. Capen*

Spinal cord injury with neurologic function loss represents the single most devastating survivable injury the physician will treat and the patient will suffer. The practitioner will have to deal with true multisystem injury. Most of the injury factors have an effect on long-term survival.

Because spinal cord injury results from differing types of trauma and disease, there is a variable geographic occurrence. Rural areas do not experience spinal cord injury as frequently as urban areas. In fact, many practitioners rarely see this injury. Physicians who work at rehabilitation centers may look on spinal injury as epidemic. In these organized centers, up to 95% of acute spinal cord injury patients will survive the initial hospitalization.[7]

INCIDENCE

Traumatic spinal cord injury occurs at a yearly rate of 30 cases per million population.[8] Thus approximately 8000 new cases per year in the United States may be anticipated with this incidence, but this figure may be too low. The patient with spinal column injury but with little neurologic deficit or a rapidly resolving deficit may not be reported, leading to a lower reported incidence. Death due to multiple trauma and head injury in the early stage of injury may also lead to underreporting. There are believed to be 200,000 patients in the United States living with a spinal cord injury.

Recent statistical information gathered by the Model Spinal Cord Injury Care Systems indicates that there are 906 chronic patients per million.[5] This expanding population of spinal cord injury patients is a result of improved emergency and long-term care.

ETIOLOGY

Figure 1–1 demonstrates the more traditional causes of spinal cord injury.[13] These data have recently

changed due to increases in the incidence of urban violence,[12] as well as a clear reduction in the incidence of vehicular trauma that has occurred nationwide (Table 1–1).

Legislation against alcohol use and laws requiring seat belt use have reduced the incidence of vehicle-related spinal trauma. Safety programs for water sports and contact sports have also been geared toward reducing the risk of cord injury. Neurologic involvement in sports injuries is shown in Figure 1–2. Table 1–2 demonstrates the distribution of sports-related injuries compiled at the University of Alabama, Birmingham.[16]

DEMOGRAPHICS

Spinal cord injury is predominantly a disease of young men. The average age at injury is 29.7 years and the median age is 25 years. An overwhelming (82%) male majority is consistently noted. Risk-related activities are associated with young males.

The occurrence of spinal cord injury increases with increased daylight hours, and with increased temperature. Summer seasonal activities and outdoor sports activity increase during June, July, and August when 31.9% of injuries occur. Weekend days (Friday through Sunday) account for 53.1% of all injuries.

Table 1–1 ▬ **ETIOLOGY OF SPINAL CORD INJURY**

	UNIVERSITY OF ALABAMA, BIRMINGHAM	RANCHO LOS AMIGOS MEDICAL CENTER, DOWNEY, CALIF.
Vehicle trauma	47.7%	39.4%
Violence	14.6%	36.6%
Sports	14.2%	15.2%
Falls	20.8%	7.5%
Other	2.7%	1.3%

Data from Stover SL, Fine PR (eds): Spinal Cord Injury: The Facts and Figures. Birmingham, University of Alabama; and Kane T, Capen DA, Waters R, et al: Spinal cord injury from civilian gunshot wounds: The Rancho experience 1980–1988. J Spinal Disord 4:306–311, 1991.

Supported in part by the National Institute for Disability and Rehabilitation Research Grant No. G008535134.

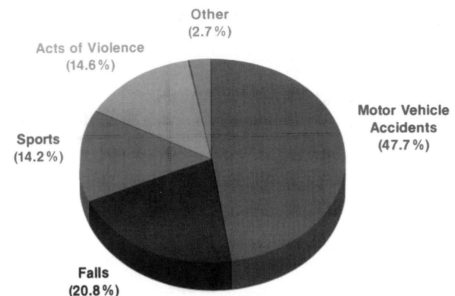

Figure 1–1 = Distribution by etiology. (From Stover SL, Fine PR (eds): Spinal Cord Injury: The Facts and Figures. Birmingham, The National Spinal Cord Injury Statistical Center, University of Alabama, 1986, p 15.)

NEUROLOGIC LEVEL AND SKELETAL LEVEL

Although frequently anatomically consistent, there is not always exact correlation between neurologic level and bony level of injury. Additionally, the severity of neurologic injury is variable. In general, upper spinal levels tend to be more severe, but partial neurologic loss may be seen at all levels of trauma (Fig. 1–3).

Neurologic level is uniformly described by examination to determine the most caudal segment of the spinal cord in which normal motor and sensory function exists. Quadriplegia is defined by total or partial loss of any of the upper eight cervical segments. Paraplegia is confined to functional loss in the thoracic, lumbar, or sacral segments.

Neurologic trauma is total (complete) in some cases, and partial (incomplete) in others. Half of all spinal injuries cause quadriplegia, with the percentage remaining relatively stable over the past 20 years (51.7% in 1973, 54.6% in 1984, and 47% in 1995). However, improvements in emergency care and early stabilization techniques can be cited in the change from 38.1% incomplete cord injuries noted in 1973 to 52% incomplete injuries noted in 1995.[6] The distribution of neurologic involvement in the 16- to 30-year-old age group is shown in Figure 1–4.

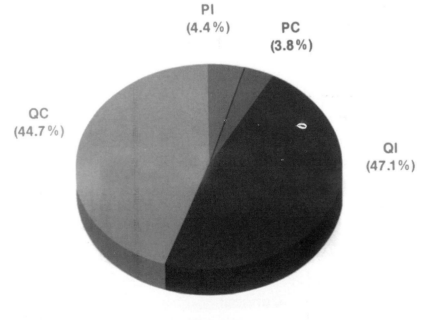

Figure 1–2 = Distribution of neuro-category in sports injuries. *PI*, neurologically incomplete paraplegia; *PC*, neurologically complete paraplegia; *QI*, neurologically incomplete quadriplegia; *QC*, neurologically complete quadriplegia. (From Stover SL, Fine PR (eds): Spinal Cord Injury: The Facts and Figures. Birmingham, The National Spinal Cord Injury Statistical Center, University of Alabama, 1986, p 35.)

Table 1–2 = **SPORTS IN SPINAL CORD INJURY**

Diving and surfing	69.1%
Football	6.1%
Snow skiing and other winter sports	6.1%
Gymnastics	4.8%
Wrestling	2.3%
Horseback riding	2.0%

Table 1–3 = **ASSOCIATED TRAUMA WITH SPINAL CORD INJURY**

No injury	55.8%
Fractures of the trunk	17.2%
Long bone fractures	13.9%
Head and facial trauma	13.8%
Pneumothorax and chest injury	8.8%
Abdominal injury	8.6%

ASSOCIATED TRAUMA

Spinal cord trauma occasionally results in isolated spinal injury. However, other medically significant injuries occur in slightly less than 50% of all spinal cord injuries.[14] Table 1–3 lists the associated trauma breakdown. The most frequent injuries are to the trunk, which most likely is related to high-energy trauma and gunshot injuries.[12]

The management of these associated injuries frequently supersedes the management of the cord injury. Emergency surgery for thoracic, abdominal, and head trauma often delays the diagnosis and surgical management of the spine injury.[2] Shock and hypoperfusion are clearly detrimental to the neurocirculation and must be managed to facilitate optimal cord recovery.

The long bone injuries also require attention early, as rehabilitation of the spinal cord injury patient requires stability and appropriate joint function. Late internal fixation is often compromised by pressure sores, osteopenia, and heterotopic bone. Internal fixation of long bone fractures in the acute phases of spinal injury generally allows for satisfactory stabilization.[9, 17]

Multiple trauma and associated injuries frequently delay the start of rehabilitation. The average length of rehabilitation is decreased in many cases because of improved emergency and early management techniques. The mean time in days from injury to Model Systems rehabilitation center admission has decreased from 20 days in 1973, to 15 days in 1984, to 6 days in 1992. Presently, approximately 33% of patients are admitted within 48 hours after injury.

MEDICAL PROBLEMS IN SPINAL CORD INJURY

The presence of complete spinal cord injury implies loss of motor and sensory function. System loss extends far beyond the impairment of ambulation and upper extremity function. The total care of the cord-injured patient requires a great deal of attention to pulmonary, genitourinary, and skin systems. Injuries to these systems have a profound effect on survival, rehabilitation, and daily living.

One of the more devastating associated injuries is to the pulmonary system. Loss of innervation of intercos-

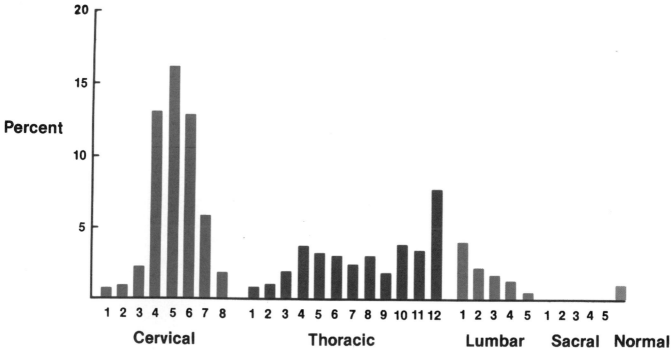

Figure 1–3 = Distribution of neurologic level of lesion at discharge. (From Stover SL, Fine PR (eds): Spinal Cord Injury: The Facts and Figures. Birmingham, The National Spinal Cord Injury Statistical Center, University of Alabama, 1986, p 36.)

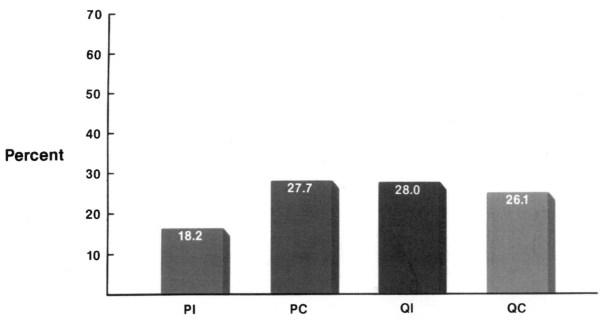

Figure 1–4 = Distribution of neuro-category in patients age 16 to 30 years. For abbreviations, see legend, Figure 1–2. (From Stover SL, Fine PR (eds): Spinal Cord Injury: The Facts and Figures. Birmingham, The National Spinal Cord Injury Statistical Center, University of Alabama, 1986, p 31.)

tal musculature and the diaphragm depletes respiratory reserve, and in some upper cervical injuries can render the patient respirator dependent, either temporarily or permanently. Early outcomes can be further compromised by chest and rib injury and by premorbid lung disease.

A recent review of a large number of C1–T12 injuries categorized respiratory complications.[11] In this group of 261 patients, atelectasis was the most common complication (36.4%), followed by pneumonia (31.4%) and ventilatory failure (22.6%). Preventing and treating these complications requires an acute respiratory therapy program, as well as aggressive involvement by pulmonary specialists.

Despite the best efforts, respiratory failure and pneumonia remain the leading cause of death in the acute phase of spinal cord injury. Pulmonary problems also remain a leading cause of readmission in the first year following initial discharge from the rehabilitation center.

Alterations in voluntary motor and sensory function have a profound effect on the genitourinary system. Loss of bladder and sexual function requires immediate and ongoing involvement by the urology team. The primary focus requires attention to adequate bladder drainage, prevention of infection, and management of sexual dysfunction.

Urologic management begins with emergency room insertion of a Foley catheter. When the acute injuries have been stabilized and transfer to the spinal cord center has been made, intermittent catheterization begins. Bladder drainage on a long-term basis can be accomplished by permanent intermittent self-catheterization or periodic reflex voiding, depending upon bladder reflex innervation.

Owing to bacterial colonization of the urinary tract, which is associated with significant residual bladder urine, there is a high incidence of urinary sepsis. Repeat sepsis also predisposes the patient to renal calculi. Management improvements have resulted in a decreased mortality and incidence of infection.[15] Improved catheter techniques and prophylactic medication have been shown to significantly lower the incidence of urinary sepsis.[1]

Table 1–4 shows the distribution of methods of bladder management over a 10-year period. Reeducation of the patient can lead to a significant reduction in external manipulation of the urinary tract. However, some home failures of treatment lead to an increased use of suprapubic catheters, especially in women.

Table 1–4 = **BLADDER MANAGEMENT METHODS**

	% OF PATIENTS				
	Intermittent Catheterization	*Condom Catheter*	*Suprapubic Catheter*	*Indwelling Catheter*	*Other*
At discharge	30.1	21.7	7.7	16.6	23.9
Year 5	8.1	36.8	17.6	14.4	23.9
Year 10	6.3	38.3	17.9	15.9	21.6

Table 1–5 = **LOCATION OF PRESSURE SORES**

Sacrum	38.6%
Heel	13.8%
Ischium	8.9%
Foot and ankle	7.3%
Genitals	5.5%
Scapula	4.1%
Trochanter	3.8%
Occiput	2.4%

Table 1–6 = **LEADING CAUSES OF DEATH IN SPINAL CORD INJURY PATIENTS**

Cardiac disease	20.9%
Diseases of the respiratory system	20.5%
Accidents, poisonings, violence	9.7%
Circulatory disease	8.8%
Infections	8.8%
Genitourinary disease	4.0%
Neoplasm	3.9%

Probably the single most debilitating and costly problem in spinal cord injury remains the pressure sore. Attention to all other system injuries frequently results in overlooking the fact that sensory loss prohibits sensory feedback. Positioning and turning is overlooked, and decubitus ulcers result.

From the acute setting to long-term living in a seated position there is continuous weight bearing on areas other than the feet. Table 1–5 outlines the most frequently seen pressure sore areas. While bed and cushion advances have reduced the severity of many sores, 32% of patients admitted within 48 hours of injury to a spinal cord center already have a decubitus ulcer.

Chronic infected sores occur in a small but significant patient population.[3] These individuals require attention from plastic, surgical, and orthopaedic specialists to eradicate infection, release contractures, and provide myocutaneous flap coverage. The cost of treatment of a significant decubitus ulcer averages $78,000 and requires up to 90 days of inpatient treatment.

SUICIDE IN SPINAL CORD INJURY

Many of those involved in the treatment of spinal cord–injured patients may consider death a more palatable alternative to a life of quadriplegia or paraplegia. This thought is clearly shared by a number of victims of cord injury at certain times following injury.

One study revealed an incidence of suicide of 50 patients in a group of 9135 cases from regional centers.[4] This is a fivefold increase compared with the able-bodied population. The presence of suicidal ideation on admission is also alarmingly high at 30%.[13] Psychological counseling, rehabilitation therapy, and surgery all help to reduce the actual incidence of suicide. For many, however, the loss of job, sexual function, self-esteem, and limb function remains too great to endure.

SURVIVABILITY IN SPINAL CORD INJURY

Statistical analysis of survival rates in spinal cord injury provides an excellent barometer of the progress and advances made in treatment techniques. From emergency field management of trauma, to spinal surgery, to rehabilitation techniques, the last 20 years has demonstrated a substantial improvement in survival.

The causes of death in cord injury are shown in Table 1–6. Clearly, some natural age-related conditions are noted in this population. Rather than succumbing to spinal cord–related system failure, other cerebrovascular, cardiovascular, and respiratory diseases may supervene. Also, many rehabilitated cord injury patients develop neoplasms or become victims of accidents and violence.

The severity of trauma obviously has a significant impact on long-term survival. The survivability in quadriplegia compared with that in paraplegia is shown in Table 1–7. The prognosis for life expectancy in the older patient who suffers a spinal injury is severely compromised. The age-related compromise of all systems together with spinal cord injury results in substantial shortening of life expectancy.

The most gratifying result of improved care in the spinal cord–injured patient is the presence of increased survivability. Longevity was once determined by 5-year survival in the early stages of cord injury treatment, whereas modern statistics deal in percentage of normal life expectancy. Actuarial tables now clearly show that younger patients with paraplegia approach 90% of normal life expectancy. Quadriplegia, with appropriate care, has a near 80% of normal life expectancy[10] (Fig. 1–5).

EMPLOYMENT AFTER CORD INJURY

If one assumes 100% employability prior to spinal cord trauma, the results of postrehabilitation employment may appear disappointing (Fig. 1–6). However,

Table 1–7 = **SURVIVABILITY IN SPINAL CORD INJURY (YEARS)**

	TYPE OF INJURY			
AGE AT INJURY (YR)	*Paraplegic, Incomplete*	*Paraplegic, Complete*	*Quadriplegic, Incomplete*	*Quadriplegic, Complete*
20	33.2%	32.1%	27.4%	20.1%
40	18.0%	17.0%	13.8%	9.3%
60	6.5%	5.9%	4.2%	1.9%

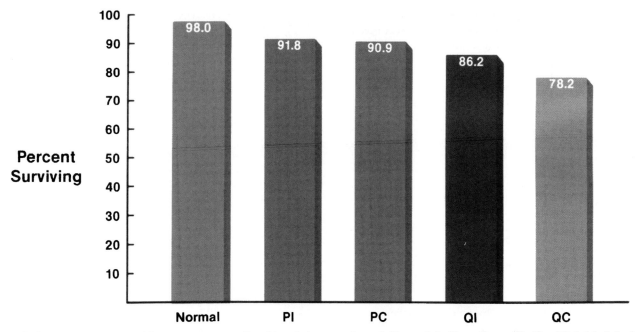

Figure 1–5 = Ten-year survival by neuro-category. For abbreviations, see legend, Figure 1–2. (From Stover SL, Fine PR (eds): Spinal Cord Injury: The Facts and Figures. Birmingham, The National Spinal Cord Injury Statistical Center, University of Alabama, 1986, p 58.)

considering the magnitude of loss, there have been substantial advances. Programs to encourage employment of partially disabled individuals, together with the goal of returning to as normal a life as possible, have helped to provide an environment conducive to employment. The American Disabilities Act (ADA) of 1992 addressed issues of handicapped access as well as hiring practices to ensure the handicapped a fairer opportunity in the marketplace.

Vocational rehabilitation programs target all spinal cord centers and their patients. The percentage of pa-tients employed is highest for incomplete paraplegics and is lowest for neurologically complete patients. At 5 years postinjury, there is a 27.6% employment rate among incomplete paraplegics, and a 13.8% rate for complete quadriplegics. Improvement can be antici-pated as programs continue their development.

CONCLUSION

An obvious benefit to studying the epidemiology of spinal cord injury is enabling the treating physician to

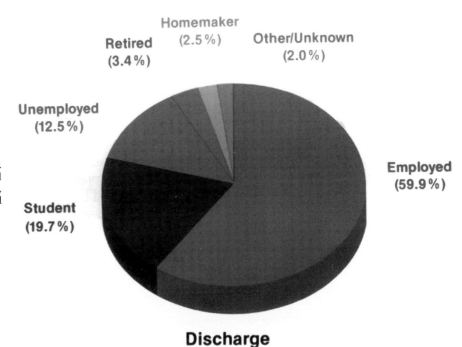

Figure 1–6 = Occupational status at injury. (From Stover SL, Fine PR (eds): Spinal Cord Injury: The Facts and Figures. Birmingham, The National Spinal Cord Injury Statistical Center, University of Alabama, 1986, p 56.)

make predictive assumptions. Information gathered by the Regional Model Spinal Cord Injury Systems can also direct efforts toward prevention, not only of cord injury itself but also of many of the secondary problems seen in these patients.

From 1970 to the present, there have been great advances made, as demonstrated by the reduction in vehicular injuries and the substantial improvements in survival statistics. The goals should remain to continue to improve services so that patients may resume near-normal postinjury and postrehabilitation lives.

REFERENCES

1. Banovac K, Wade N, Gonzalez F, et al: Decreased incidence of urinary tract infections in patients with spinal cord injury. Effect of methenamine. J Am Paraplegia Soc 14(April):52–52, 1991.
2. Bohlman HH: Acute fractures and dislocations of the cervical spine. J Bone Joint Surg Am 61:1119, 1979.
3. Capen D: Treatment of pressure sores. *In* Lee BY (ed): Chronic Ulcers of the Skin. Philadelphia, JB Lippincott, 1984.
4. DeVivo MJ, Black KJ, Richards JS, et al: Suicide following spinal cord injury. J Am Paraplegia Soc 14(April):620–627, 1991.
5. DeVivo MJ, Fine PR, Maetz HM, et al: Prevalence of spinal cord injury. Arch Neurol 37:707–708, 1980.
6. DeVivo MJ, Kartus PO, Fine PR: Benefits of early admission to an organized spinal cord injury care system. Arch Phys Med Rehabil 66:533, 1985.
7. DeVivo MJ, Kartus PL, Stover SL, et al: Benefits of early admission to an organized spinal cord injury care system. Paraplegia 28:545–555, 1990.
8. Fine PR, Kuhlemeir KV, DeVivo MJ, et al: Spinal cord injury. An epidemiologic perspective. Paraplegia 17:237–250, 1979.
9. Garland DE, Rieser TV, Singer DI: Treatment of femoral shaft fractures associated with acute spinal cord injuries. Clin Orthop 197:191, 1985.
10. Geisler WO, Jousse AT, Wynne-Jones M, et al: Survival in traumatic spinal cord injury. Paraplegia 21:364–373, 1983.
11. Jackson AB, Groomes TE: Incidence of respiratory complications following spinal cord injury. J Am Paraplegia Soc 14(April):87, 1991.
12. Kane T, Capen DA, Waters R, et al: Spinal cord injury from civilian gunshot wounds: The Rancho experience 1980–1988. J Spinal Disord 4:306–311, 1991.
13. Kettl P: Prevalence of suicidal ideation after spinal cord injury. J Am Paraplegia Soc 14(April):62, 1991.
14. Key AG, Retief PJM: Spinal cord injuries: An analysis of 300 new lesions. Paraplegia 8:243–249, 1970.
15. Perkash I: Intermittent catheterization and bladder rehabilitation in spinal cord injury patients. J Urol 114:230–233, 1975.
16. Stover SL, Fine PR (eds): Spinal Cord Injury: The Facts & Figures. Birmingham, University of Alabama, 1986.
17. Zigler JE, Field BT: Surgical procedures for spinal cord injury. Phys Med Rehabil Clin North Am 3:711–723, 1992.

CHAPTER 2

Spine Injury in the Polytrauma Patient: General Surgical and Orthopaedic Considerations

Steven R. Shackford

Trauma, a disease that kills 140,000 Americans annually, is the leading cause of death during the first four decades of life. For every person who dies, two are permanently disabled. The cost of trauma to American society has been estimated to be $100 billion annually.[9]

For many trauma victims the outcome is determined within milliseconds of the injury. These patients are "dead at scene" and usually have suffered severe injuries to the head or cardiovascular system. With the best medical management existing in the best trauma system, these patients would not survive.[26] Of those transported to hospitals, 30% die in the early or initial phases of care, whereas 20% survive for weeks or months, eventually to succumb to infection or infection-related organ failure.[2] Early trauma deaths, those occurring within hours of admission at the hospital, are primarily due to head injury, hemorrhagic shock, or the physiologic derangements associated with hemorrhage and massive resuscitation.[2, 26] A consideration of the initial management of patients sustaining multiple severe injuries must, therefore, include the evaluation and treatment of hemorrhagic hypovolemia and those metabolic and physiologic derangements associated with shock and resuscitation that have a negative impact on outcome. A discussion of the initial evaluation of polytrauma patients emphasizing management of the head injury may be found elsewhere.[8]

This chapter addresses the initial evaluation and management of patients who have sustained spine trauma in association with blunt multisystem trauma. The primary considerations discussed here are airway access, maintenance of gas exchange, treatment of hypovolemic and neurogenic shock, evaluation of injuries that may be considered to be immediately life-threatening, and the early evaluation of the injured spine.

AIRWAY ACCESS

When evaluating the airway there are two major concerns: airway patency to allow gas exchange, and airway protection from aspiration of gastric contents. Any patient who can respond appropriately to a simple question such as, What is your name? or, How are you? has a patent airway and can protect it from aspiration. Patients who do not respond must be suspected of needing airway control for gas exchange, for protection from aspiration, or for hyperventilation to control intracranial pressure.

Every physician who evaluates patients with multiple trauma is concerned about the need to urgently control the airway of the severely injured patient. During the initial management phase, there are several indications for intubating a trauma patient:

1. The patient has suffered a cardiac or respiratory arrest.
2. The patient is in obvious respiratory distress, as manifested by tachypnea or dyspnea, after the relief of mechanical impediments to ventilation such as a pneumothorax or hemothorax.
3. The patient has suffered a brain injury, has a depressed sensorium, and may not be able to protect the airway. In addition, there may be increased intracranial pressure. Airway control will permit hyperventilation, which will reduce arterial carbon dioxide tension (Pa_{CO_2}). Hypocarbia will induce cerebral vasoconstriction which in turn will reduce cerebral blood volume and thereby decrease intracranial pressure.
4. The patient may have suffered a spinal cord injury and may have insufficient innervation of the respiratory muscles to maintain gas exchange.

There are three acceptable methods to intubate the trachea in the polytrauma patient: (1) nasotracheal, (2) orotracheal, and (3) surgical.

Nasotracheal intubation has several advantages. It does not require hyperextension of the neck and this makes it a logical choice in patients who are suspected of having a cervical spine injury. If the trachea must be intubated for a prolonged period of time, a nasotracheal tube is more comfortable than a tube placed orally and is less traumatic to the airway because it is fixed at several points and moves less freely within the larynx, the subglottic area, and the trachea.[3] On the other hand, a nasotracheal tube is technically more difficult to place and is inflammatory to the nasal and maxillary sinuses, occasionally producing a sinusitis when maintained for long-term intubation (> 1 week). The option of using a nasotracheal tube does not exist in the patient who has suffered respiratory arrest since placement of the tube requires that the patient be breathing in order for the person placing the tube to localize the airway during the process of intubation.

Orotracheal intubation should be utilized in those patients who have midface injuries, such as severe maxillary or nasal fractures. Since the fracture may communicate with the anterior cranial vault, nasotracheal intubation is much less desirable because the potential exists for inserting the tube into the forebrain through the unstable fracture. Orotracheal intubation in the trauma patient is a *two*-person procedure since in-line cervical traction must be applied during intubation to avoid hyperextension of the neck and the possibility of an injury to the cervical spinal cord in a patient who might have a cervical spine fracture.[1, p. 155]

Surgical access to the airway should be considered for those patients who have severe midface and mandibular injuries and for whom oral or nasotracheal intubation is difficult, hazardous, or impossible. Further, the surgical option should be exercised whenever airway access cannot be established by nonsurgical means in a patient who is clinically deteriorating, as evidenced by tachycardia, cardiac arrhythmias, hypotension, or progressive neurologic signs. Surgical access to the airway can be obtained by either tracheostomy or cricothyrotomy. Cricothyrotomy is the preferred method because it is easier to perform in the emergent situation.[22] The cricothyroid membrane, a subcutaneous structure in the neck, is easily located by palpation. Tracheostomy, a more technically demanding procedure, is usually performed between the second and third tracheal rings which lie deep in the neck where the trachea descends more dorsally behind the sternum. Access to this area frequently requires division of the isthmus of the thyroid gland, a surgical maneuver which can be associated with significant hemorrhage. Until recently, it had been suggested that a cricothyrotomy performed for emergency airway access should be replaced by a conventional tracheostomy within 48 hours because of the risk of subglottic stenosis.[10] However, it has subsequently been shown that the incidence of subglottic stenosis is very low after cricothyrotomy used for long-term airway access.[22] Therefore, it is entirely reasonable to maintain a cricothyrotomy placed during the initial resuscitation for the duration of tracheal intubation, especially if one anticipates that the need for airway access will only be required for a week to 10 days.

After placement of an airway, the chest should be auscultated to assure that bilateral breath sounds are present. In a noisy resuscitation area it may be difficult to hear the breath sounds and to confirm appropriate tube placement. In this situation, one may attempt to palpate the tracheal balloon in the sternal notch or listen over the epigastrium during ventilation. A radiograph of the chest should always be taken to document tube placement and to ensure that a main stem intubation has not occurred. If a chest film is not readily

Table 2–1 = **GLASGOW COMA SCALE**	
Eye opening	
Spontaneous	4
To voice	3
To pain	2
None	1
Verbal response	
Oriented	5
Confused	4
Inappropriate	3
Incomprehensible	2
None	1
Motor response	
Obeys commands	6
Localizes pain	5
Withdrawal (pain)	4
Flexion (pain)	3
Extension (pain)	2
None	1

From Teasdale G, Jannett B: Assessment of coma and impaired consciousness: A practical scale. Lancet 2:81, 1974.

available, end-tidal CO_2 should be monitored. In cases of esophageal intubation the end-tidal CO_2 will be less than 0.5%.[18]

Airway control and hyperventilation can be lifesaving in the patient with a severe head injury and elevated intracranial pressure.[7, 8, 20] It has become our practice to control the airway in all patients who present to our trauma resuscitation room with a Glasgow coma score of 8 or less[25] (Table 2–1). The option we most frequently exercise is nasotracheal intubation. Once we recognize the need for intubation, we perform a very quick neurologic examination and then perform the intubation. If the patient is hemodynamically stable, as evidenced by blood pressure, pulse, and arterial blood gas analysis (see later), the patient is paralyzed with pancuronium (0.1 mg/kg), and given morphine (0.1 mg/kg) for sedation. Recently, we have used vecuronium (0.1 mg/kg) because it has a shorter duration of action and will allow neurologic evaluation at more frequent intervals if so desired. In those patients who are hemodynamically stable, we administer a tidal volume of 15 mL/kg combined with a ventilator rate of 10 per minute. We adjust the ventilator rate to maintain a P_{CO_2} between 25 and 30 torr. In those patients who are hemodynamically unstable, no morphine or relaxant is administered because of the potential for exaggerating hypotension.

MAINTENANCE OF GAS EXCHANGE

Pulmonary tidal exchange is evaluated by auscultation of the chest. Immediately after auscultation, a radiograph of the chest is taken. This allows identification of any mechanical impediments to ventilation, such as a hemopneumothorax. Simultaneous with auscultation, arterial blood gas values are obtained. This quantifies abnormalities in gas exchange and helps to direct the resuscitation effort, not only with respect to oxygenation and ventilation but also with respect to the patient's blood volume status. Knowledge of the arterial pH and P_{CO_2} allows estimates of the base deficit and the severity of the metabolic acidosis which accompanies hypovolemic shock.[5, 21, 23] In general, a deficit of greater than 5 mEq/L is abnormal. The greater the base deficit, the greater the volume loss and the greater the requirement for intravenous (IV) fluid and blood.[5]

Management of blood gas abnormalities by manipulation of the ventilator should only be done after one has obtained sufficient information on the patient's blood volume status and hemodynamic stability. Initially, deficiencies in oxygenation should be treated with increases in inspired oxygen concentration in those patients who are hemodynamically unstable. The application of positive end-expiratory pressure (PEEP) in hemodynamically unstable patients can be disastrous, since PEEP increases the mean intrathoracic pressure and will reduce venous return resulting in a decrease in cardiac output and a further deterioration in the blood pressure. High ventilator rates (12 to 16 per minute) will also increase the mean intrathoracic pressure and diminish the cardiac output. Therefore, before abnormalities in gas exchange are managed by the addition of PEEP or increased ventilator rate, it is important to treat hypoxemia with oxygen enrichment while assessing blood volume status and assuring that adequate IV access is available to support the blood volume.

TREATMENT OF HYPOVOLEMIC SHOCK

After the airway and gas exchange are established, attention should be turned to the circulatory status. External hemorrhage should be controlled. This should be done with digital pressure and not with hemostats. Even if one is lucky enough to apply the hemostat precisely to the bleeding vessel, the trauma induced by the hemostat on the vessel wall will increase the severity of the arterial or venous injury. More frequently, hemostats are blindly placed into a bleeding wound and result in damage to adjacent structures such as nerves or tendons. Such iatrogenic trauma increases, by an order of magnitude, the severity of any given injury. The use of hemostats is therefore to be condemned. The application of tourniquets should also be avoided as they are often applied with insufficient pressure to occlude major arteries but with sufficient pressure to occlude major veins, thereby increasing the rate and volume of hemorrhage from the wound. Further, tourniquets will occlude collateral blood flow, thereby exposing the injured extremity to an increase in warm ischemia time. As demonstrated by the Korean War experience, the use of tourniquets can result in an increase in the amputation rate.[11] There are situations, however, especially in the prehospital setting, in which an appropriately applied tourniquet can be lifesaving. This is particularly true of patients who have suffered a traumatic amputation for whom the tourniquet can be applied above the amputation site. In all other cases, external hemorrhage can be controlled with a well-placed gloved finger.

Once hemorrhage is controlled, circulating blood volume must be restored. This requires appropriate access to a suitable vein for infusion of an asanguinous solution or type O negative, low-titer blood. Large-bore (14- or 16-gauge) IV cannulas inserted into the basilic or cephalic vein in the upper extremity will provide adequate access for the majority of major trauma victims. If hemodynamic instability continues after the infusion of 2 L of Ringer's lactate, a moderate blood volume deficit exists indicating the need for additional access sites and for blood infusion, if blood has not already been started. Options for additional venous access include a saphenous vein cutdown (either at the ankle or the groin) with insertion of the IV tubing directly into the vein, percutaneous femoral vein cannulation, or subclavian vein cannulation with insertion of a large (8-F) catheter. The selection of additional IV infusion sites should be based upon the perceived blood volume deficit, the location and type of associated injuries, and the accessibility of additional sites. For example, massive lower extremity injuries may contraindicate the use of the ankle cutdown. Similarly, a suspected iliac vein injury would contraindicate use of the ipsilateral femoral or saphenous vein for venous access. Finally, an inflated MAST (military antishock trousers) can be an impediment to groin access. However, MAST application does not contraindicate use of the ankle cutdown site since fluid can be satisfactorily infused through the saphenous vein, even with the suit inflated.

At the time the IV line is started blood should be obtained for laboratory studies. Blood can be drawn from the venous lines, but it is much easier to draw all laboratory samples from an artery at the time the initial arterial blood gases are sampled. The only routine laboratory tests we perform are blood type determination, arterial blood gas analysis, and blood toxicology screen (including alcohol). A sample of blood is centrifuged in the resuscitation room for a baseline hematocrit. Clotting studies, serum electrolytes, serum amylase, liver enzymes, white blood cell count, and so forth, are not performed routinely because they rarely direct or affect treatment or evaluation in the early stage. In fact, a scattershot approach to laboratory assessment may hinder or delay the performance of tests that directly affect care, such as the arterial blood gas analysis and blood typing. If, however, there is concern about a potential abnormality and one feels compelled to obtain a specific test, it is best to draw the sample and hold it until the more important tests can be performed.

Administration of blood and other fluids should be titrated to physiologic end points such as diastolic or mean arterial blood pressure, central venous pressure, urine output, or base deficit. We administer fluid and blood to evaluate the mean arterial pressure (>60 torr), to increase the urine output (>0.5 ml/kg), and to normalize the base deficit (±2 mEq/L).

Our choice of asanguinous fluid is Ringer's lactate. When blood is needed our first choice is type-specific packed red blood cells. Less than 2% of patients receiving transfusions at our institution require O negative blood. Type-specific cells can be ready in 5 minutes and most patients can be sustained with asanguinous crystalloid for that time interval. While there are distinct advantages to the immediate availability of O negative blood, there are some disadvantages. Type O negative is in scant supply; only 8% of donors are O negative. In addition, once a patient has received sufficient quantities of O negative blood (more than 50% to 75% of the estimated blood volume), it must continue to be administered. If transfusion is initiated with blood that is type-specific for the recipient after a large volume of O negative blood has been infused, there is a possibility of a crossmatch reaction. Even though O negative blood is low titer, it may still contain antibodies to the A or B antigens.

The polytrauma patient with a spinal cord injury who is hypotensive may present a diagnostic and therapeutic problem. The hypotension could be due to either neurogenic or hypovolemic shock. Neurogenic shock is caused by loss of vascular tone with a subsequent increase in vascular capacitance. It is usually associated with bradycardia rather than tachycardia. As demonstrated by Soderstrom et al.[24] in a review of 228 cervical spine injury patients, 40 of 58 (69%) patients with a systolic blood pressure less than 100 mm Hg at presentation had neurogenic shock. The other 18 patients had other causes of shock. The treatment of neurogenic shock is limited volume replacement followed by vasopressors if shock continues, since the overinfusion of the hypotensive spinal cord injury patient can result in fatal pulmonary edema.[6] The severity of spinal cord injury, as indicated by the Frankel grade, has a direct relationship to the degree of hypotension, bradycardia, and incidence of cardiac arrest. In a series of 45 cervical spinal cord injury patients with high-grade lesions, 87% of the Frankel A patients had a pulse rate less than 55 beats/minute, 21% had cardiac arrest, and 39% required pressors. However, of the Frankel B patients, only 62% had a pulse less than 55 beats/minute and none had cardiac arrest or needed pressors.[17] Hypovolemic shock, on the other hand, is caused by a decrease in circulating blood volume and is characterized by an increase in vascular tone, usually with accompanying tachycardia. Treating a hypovolemic patient with an α-adrenergic agonist, or any vasopressor for that matter, will further increase vascular tone and may interrupt essential nutrient flow, resulting in ischemia, necrosis, or tissue loss. Conversely, administering a large volume of fluid to "fill up" the enlarged atonic vascular compartment of the patient in neurogenic shock can result in congestive heart failure when vascular tone normalizes. Therefore, the cause of hypotension should be expeditiously determined. Intravascular volume status should be assessed with a central venous catheter and urine output monitored. All potential sites of hemorrhage should be investigated (see later). If there are no major fractures and no evidence of major blood loss and the patient remains hypotensive, vasopressors may be used judiciously. If the patient is hypotensive and has bradycardia (pulse less than 60 beats/minute), the blood pressure may be dependent upon the heart rate, and atropine may be effective in evaluating blood pressure without the use of vasopressors.

FURTHER EVALUATION AND TREATMENT

Once the airway is assured, gas exchange maintained, hemorrhage controlled, and blood volume restored, it is necessary to rapidly determine if life-threatening or limb-threatening injuries are present and to deal with their management appropriately. The first priority is to determine the source of any hemorrhage which might not be readily apparent. In general terms, hemorrhage can be considered to be cavitary (bleeding into the thoracic or abdominal cavity) or noncavitary (bleeding from lacerations or fractures).[16] Thoracic cavitary hemorrhage can be ruled out with a chest radiograph. Cavitary hemorrhage into the abdomen can be ruled out with a diagnostic peritoneal lavage[4] or a computed tomography (CT) scan.[27] Our preference is the diagnostic peritoneal lavage because it is safe, rapid, and simple to interpret. A CT scan is time-consuming, occasionally difficult to interpret, and contraindicated in the hemodynamically unstable patient. A negative chest film and a negative diagnostic peritoneal lavage generally will rule out major cavitary hemorrhage. If these two tests are grossly negative, persistent hypotension is due to noncavitary hemorrhage[16] or to spinal shock. In our experience, in 1 year, noncavitary hemorrhage was either primarily responsible for, or contributed significantly to, the volume loss in 56% of the patients admitted with shock to our institution who had suffered blunt trauma and who did not have a spinal cord injury.[16] The most frequent sources of noncavitary hemorrhage were scalp lacerations and open fractures, emphasizing the importance of early control of external hemorrhage. Another potential source of often fatal noncavitary hemorrhage is the pelvic fracture.

Proceeding from the top of the head to the tip of the foot, the following should be done: careful palpation of the head and scalp for cephalohematoma, fractures (crepitus), and lacerations; examination of the ears for hemotympanum; examination of the pupils and documentation of pupillary size and reactivity; determination of level of consciousness by application of the Glasgow coma scale[25] (see Table 2–1); examination of the mouth and oropharynx for foreign bodies (e.g., broken teeth); palpation of the midface and jaw for fractures; determination of cervical spine tenderness; palpation of the chest for tenderness or crepitus from subcutaneous emphysema or rib fractures; auscultation of the abdomen for the presence of bowel sounds; palpation of the abdomen for tenderness; palpation of the iliac wings and pubic symphysis for tenderness and pelvic stability; examination and palpation of the lower extremities for fracture deformities; palpation and documentation of all peripheral pulses; and palpation and examination of the back with the patient logrolled while maintaining spinal alignment.[13] As stated, the neurologic examination includes documentation of

patient. Asanguinous resuscitative fluids may ...assed through a blood warmer. However, at ...sion rates (<60 mL/minute), fluid passed ...e IV tubing between the warmer and the ...equilibrate with ambient temperature. That ...e blood warmer is set at the maximum (37 ...the flow rate is 4 L/hour, the fluid will ...room temperature (approximately 21°C). ...nce, fluid warmed in a convection oven ...nfused faster and at a higher tempera- ...warmed in a conventional blood

...rt of a patient with fractures, all ...hould be splinted. After splints ...vascular status should be re- ...f fractures will cushion them ...reduce hemorrhage into the ...soft tissue injury. ...al cord surgery patients the ...cher should be maintained ...can be implemented. The ...s uncontrolled motion ...e thoracic and lumbar ...s are currently available ...fractures during trans-

gas-
gastric
placed
gastric de-
...tients with
d gastrointes-

...y injured patients
...ent. There is no
...ially stable will
...uate the mental
...signs and uri-
...ently. The ab-
...is negative.
...even if the
...emity must
...e develop-
...with spi-
...e spinal
...begin
...ard

a rectal examina-
...nation is extremely
...ment in males with
...injury to the membra-
...ethral transection and a
...be a "high-riding" prostate
...ertion of a bladder catheter
...nazardous since it can worsen
...dings that may indicate a mem-
...ury include blood at the penile
...rotal or perineal hematoma. Suspi-
...njury mandates a retrograde urethro-
...gic consultation.
...nitial evaluation, all radiographs should
...able type. Some trauma units have x-ray
...into each evaluation bay. This will avoid
...sport a potentially unstable patient to
...epartment. If an untoward event were
...radiology department, resuscitation
...a major problem since the necessary

...ersonnel may not be immediately avail-
...our resuscitation area are equipped
...machines, allowing us to take the
...e acute care environment. The
...frequently in the patient
...lateral cervical, lateral
...nd lateral lumbar
...hese are required
...hs to diagnose
...rast studies, can
...artment after life-
...led out. However,
...ment all major trauma
...d to the radiology de-
...d nurse in the event that
...eriorates as the result of an
...ing injury (Table 2–2).
...logic survey in the polytrauma
...sed level of consciousness (Glas-
...ess than 10) often poses a diagnos-
...g the initial evaluation. Major skele-
...equently overlooked in these patients
...creased pain response to physical exam-
...because the central nervous system injury
...ediate precedence over less severe injuries.
...ound a 31% incidence of major skeletal injury
...as one or more fractures of the axial spine,
..., hip, or long bones of the lower extremity) in
...nded patients suffering blunt trauma.[12] Injuries to
...e axial spine were present in 14% of the patients,
...0% sustained pelvic fractures or hip dislocations, and
15% sustained femur or tibia-fibula fractures. Patients
who were pedestrians struck by a motor vehicle had a
57% incidence of major skeletal injury, and injured
motorcyclists had an incidence of 40%. Based on these
data, we recommend a routine radiologic survey that
includes the axial spine, pelvis, and long bones of the
lower extremity in *obtunded* patients sustaining multiple trauma, especially if they have been struck by a
motor vehicle or have been in a motorcycle accident.
The timing of such a radiologic evaluation depends on
the nature and severity of associated injuries and the
overall condition of the patient.

The knowledge of combined injury patterns also aids

Table 2–2 = **EXAMPLES OF LIFE-THREATENING COMPLICATIONS OF COMMON INJURIES**

INJURY	COMPLICATION	CONTRIBUTING FACTOR
Pneumothorax	Tension pneumothorax	Positive pressure ventilation
Blunt chest trauma	Arrhythmia	Myocardial contusion
Tracheal fracture	Airway obstruction	Hemorrhage, edema
Blunt chest trauma	Pericardial tamponade	Atrial rupture
Subcapsular hematoma (spleen, liver)	Massive hemorrhage	Delay in diagnosis

incidence of sacral fractures, often with neurologic deficit. Thus, recognition of the patterns allows proper evaluation.

OTHER CONSIDERATIONS

Organization

Most trauma centers utilize a team concept. This implies the presence of a team leader who directs the team members and who establishes the order of importance of management and evaluation protocols. The team leader should be a general surgeon. Other members of the resuscitation team usually include an emergency physician and an anesthesiologist. Coordination of team effort is achieved through the use of standard protocols based on advanced trauma life support[1] guidelines established by the American College of Surgeons. Neurosurgeons, orthopaedic surgeons, urologists, plastic surgeons, and ophthalmologists are called on frequently in a consultative capacity. Because the team leader is the person who must assume the ultimate responsibility for the management of multiple injuries, he or she is obligated to direct the consultants. The team leader must adjudicate treatment priority when consultants disagree.

Appropriate protocols should be worked out beforehand with various consultants to determine which particular service handles specific injuries. For example, facial fractures can be treated by the otolaryngology service, the oral surgery service, or the plastic surgery service. Similarly, deep tendon lacerations of the hand and forearm could be handled by a reimplantation team, a plastic surgery team, or by the orthopaedic service. Prior agreement regarding these issues will greatly facilitate and streamline early management. This is particularly true in dealing with spine injuries, which can be managed by the orthopaedic or neurosurgical service.

HYPOTHERMIA

The temperature of the resuscitation area should be kept at the maximum considered bearable by the medical staff. It is important to remember that hypothermia poses a great risk to the polytrauma patient. Maintaining a high but comfortable ambient temperature, covering the patient with warm blankets, and removing wet or damp clothing will reduce radiant heat loss, which is the primary cause of hypothermia in trauma patients.[14] All fluid infusions should be warmed. Blood from the blood bank is stored at 4°C and should be passed through blood warmers before being infused

be infused at
In our experie
to 40°C can be
ture than fluid
warmer.[19]

TRANSPORT

During the transpo
obvious fracture sites
are applied, the neurc
checked. The splinting
during transfer. This wil
fracture site and diminish

In the transport of spin
backboard or a scoop stret
until definite immobilizatio
logrolling maneuver allow
through fracture sites in tl
spine.[13] Inboard traction device
for immobilized cervical spine
port.

REASSESSMENT

Continual reassessment of severel
is mandatory during initial managen
guarantee that a patient who is init
remain so. One must continually reeval
status and level of consciousness. Vital
nary output should be monitored frequ
dominal examination should be repeated
CT scan or diagnostic peritoneal lavage
The neurovascular status of the injured extr
be assessed frequently for loss of pulses or th
ment of a compartment syndrome.[15] Patients
nal cord injuries should be moved from t
board as soon as feasible. Pressure necrosis
within 2 to 4 hours if the patient is kept o
surface.

During the continual reassessment one m
vigilant for complications of injuries that
immediately life-threatening (see Table 2
most of these complications arise from c
we routinely monitor the central venous
the electrocardiogram in all patients w
chest injury (sternal fracture, multiple r
flail chest). Patients with a history of lo
ness or who have any neurologic ab
physical examination are admitted for
that the neurologic status can be eval

SUMMARY

The essence of initial management of patients with multiple system injury is close attention to the airway and blood volume status, bearing in mind those injuries and complications that can be immediately life-threatening. The evaluation and management must be timely and efficient. This is best accomplished by a team of physicians and nurses with a specified team leader who directs the resuscitation and who is ultimately responsible for decision making. Evaluation and early treatment are best governed by a protocol utilizing a judicious sufficiency of intellectual flexibility and surgical judgment.

REFERENCES

1. American College of Surgeons: Advanced Trauma Life Support Course for Physicians, Instructor Manual. 1985.
2. Baker CC, Oppenheimer L, Stephens B, et al: Epidemiology of trauma deaths. Am J Surg 140:144, 1980.
3. Colice GL: Prolonged intubation versus tracheostomy in the adult. J Intern Care Med 2:85, 1987.
4. Danto LA: Paracentesis and diagnostic peritoneal lavage. *In* Blaisdell FW, Trunkey DD (eds): Trauma Management, vol 1: Abdominal Trauma. New York, Thieme-Stratton, 1982, pp 45–58.
5. Davis JW, Shackford SR, Mackersie RC, et al: Base deficit as a guide to volume resuscitation. J Trauma 28:1464–1467, 1988.
6. Grundy D, Swain A, Russell J: ABC of spinal cord injury. Early management and complications. Br Med J 292:44–47, 1986.
7. Guss DA: The head-injured patient: Prehospital care. Trauma Q 2:1, 1985.
8. Hoyt DB, Shackford SR, Marshall LF: Initial resuscitation: The trauma surgeon and neurosurgeons—a combined perspective. Trauma Q 2:8, 1985.
9. Injury in America, a Continuing Public Health Problem. Washington, DC, National Academy Press, 1985, p 18.
10. Jackson C: High tracheostomy and other errors the chief causes of chronic laryngeal stenosis. Surg Gynecol Obstet 32:392, 1921.
11. Jahnke EJ, Seeley SF: Acute vascular injuries in the Korean War: An analysis of 77 consecutive cases. Ann Surg 138:158, 1953.
12. Mackersie RC, Shackford SR, Garfin SR, et al: Major skeletal injuries in the obtunded blunt trauma patient: A case for routine radiologic surgery. J Trauma 28:1450, 1988.
13. McGuire RA, Neville S, Green BA, et al: Spinal instability and the logrolling maneuver. J Trauma 27:525–531, 1987.
14. Moss J: Accidental severe hypothermia. Surg Gynecol Obstet 162:501, 1986.
15. Mubarak SJ: Recognition and treatment of compartment syndromes. *In* Meyers MH (ed): The Multiply Injured Patient with Complex Fractures. Philadelphia, Lea & Febiger, 1984, pp 71–89.
16. Pedowitz R, Shackford SR, Hansborough JF, et al: The incidence and severity of noncavitary hemorrhage in hypovolemic trauma patients. J Trauma 25:709, 1985.
17. Pepmeier JM, Lehrmon KB, Lane JG: Cardiovascular instability following acute cervical spinal cord trauma. Cent Nerv Syst Trauma 2:153–160, 1985.
18. Shackford SR: Personal observation, 1988.
19. Shackford SR, Fortlage DF, Hoyt DB, et al: Warming of asanguinous fluids for massive resuscitation: A comparison of techniques. J Trauma 25:715, 1985.
20. Shackford SR, Mackersie RC, Hoyt DB, et al: Impact of a trauma system on outcome of the severely injured patient. Arch Surg 122:523–527, 1987.
21. Siggard-Anderson O: Blood acid-base alignment normogram. Scand J Clin Lab Invest 15:211, 1963.
22. Sise MJ, Shackford SR, Cruickshank JC, et al: Cricothyroidotomy for long-term tracheal access: A prospective analysis of morbidity and mortality in 76 patients. Ann Surg 200:13, 1984.
23. Sladen A: Acid-base balance. *In* McIntyre KM, Lewis AJ (eds): Advanced Cardiac Life Support. Dallas, American Heart Association, 1983, pp 135–140.
24. Soderstrom CA, McCordle DQ, Duder TB, et al: The diagnosis of intro-abdominal injury in patients with cervical cord trauma. J Trauma 23:1061–1065, 1983.
25. Teasdale G, Jannett B: Assessment of coma and impaired consciousness: A practical scale. Lancet 2:81, 1974.
26. Trunkey DD: Trauma. Sci Amer 249:28, 1983.
27. Trunkey DD, Federle M, Cello J: Special diagnostic procedures. *In* Blaisdell FW, Trunkey DD (eds): Trauma Management, vol 1: Abdominal Trauma. Thieme-Stratton, 1982, pp 19–43.

CHAPTER 3

Physical Examination in Spinal Trauma

Robert A. McGuire, Jr.

Every year spinal injuries occur as a result of motor vehicle accidents, falls, gunshot wounds, and recreational accidents. Many of these injuries are missed in the initial emergency evaluation because of other, distracting factors such as a head injury, acute intoxication secondary to drugs or alcohol, and multiple trauma. Critical factors such as spinal stability and neurologic compromise become important issues in planning treatment regimens and counseling the patient and family members regarding the prognosis. It is paramount to have an accurate, documented physical examination when treating patients with spinal injuries.

The physical examination begins by obtaining a history from the patient, investigating officer, and paramedical personnel involved in treating the patient. This inquiry should include the circumstances of the accident, the position in which the patient was found, whether or not the patient was wearing a seat belt or shoulder harness, and the type of treatment provided at the accident scene. It is important to ask for specific information regarding transient motor or sensory loss or the presence of Lhermitte's sign. This information provides insight into the forces involved and the possible mechanisms of injury. A high correlation has been reported between head injury and resulting neck injury.[1, 3, 4] These patients must also be thoroughly evaluated for multiple spinal fractures.[10] In patients with multiple trauma, strict adherence to principles of airway maintenance, breathing, and circulation take precedence over bony injury.

INSPECTION

The physical examination begins with inspection of the patient. All clothing should be carefully removed, allowing a systematic visual evaluation to be performed, and all areas of tissue abrasions, contusions, lacerations, and limb asymmetry should be noted. Chest expansion is observed for abnormal motion or paradoxical movement of the thoracic cage signifying possible pulmonary or cardiac injury.

PALPATION

Palpation is then undertaken in a systematic manner. The extremities and joints are evaluated for crepitus, abnormal motion, and malalignment. Careful attention to the peripheral pulse is mandatory because vessel lacerations, transections, and intimal tears often produce either absent or asymmetrical pulsations. Low pulse rate with low blood pressure can be indicative of a sympathectomy from a spinal cord injury rather than hypovolemic shock. The abdomen is then evaluated for possible peritoneal signs indicating damaged viscera. Seat belt injuries causing lumbar fractures have been associated with bowel rupture and major vessel, liver, spleen, and urologic injury.[6] In evaluating the chest, each rib is carefully palpated for continuity or crepitus. Soft tissue crepitus is indicative of major pulmonary trauma with probable pneumothorax. The pelvis is evaluated for widening of the symphysis pubis or any asymmetry of the iliac wings. The spine is then palpated in a systematic manner.

The cervical collar is carefully removed and the anterior aspect of the neck is evaluated. Evidence of venous congestion such as distended jugular veins should be noted. The carotid pulses are palpated carefully for any evidence of hematoma formation or thrills. The position of the trachea is evaluated for any deviation from the midline and the anterior aspect of the cervical spine is carefully palpated for malalignment or tenderness. Attention is next directed to the head, occipitocervical junction, and posterior aspect of the cervical spine. If tenderness is encountered, the collar is replaced and the patient carefully rolled to allow palpation of the thoracic and lumbar spine. Great care must be used with the logroll maneuver as an unstable spine can become displaced and potentially lead to neural compromise.[7] In a comatose patient, the cervical spine must be radiographically evaluated before removal of the collar as 3% to 5% of these patients will have an associated neck injury. Each spinous process should be palpated noting tenderness, alignment, asymmetry, or interspinous widening. The sacroiliac joints are evaluated for instability in lateral compression or longitudinal migration. The patient is then carefully rolled back to the supine position and a thorough neurologic examination is performed.

NEUROLOGIC EVALUATION

The neurologic examination consists of evaluation of the motor, sensory, and reflex portion of the nervous system. Strict attention must be directed to sharp vs. dull discrimination, temperature, and the ability to distinguish between light and deep pressure. Evaluation of motor function must include not only the presence or absence of function but grades of strength.

Muscle grading is important to allow consistency of evaluation between different examiners as well as monitoring improvement or deterioration of function with time. The grading system for muscle strength is as follows: grade 0, no function, grade 1 or trace, palpable contraction without joint motion; grade 2 or poor, complete joint range of motion (ROM) with gravity eliminated; grade 3 or fair, full joint ROM against gravity; grade 4 or good, complete ROM against gravity with slight resistance; grade 5, normal, full ROM against gravity and resistance. Using this grading scheme the motor index score serves as a numeric system to document improvement or deterioration of function (Fig. 3–1).

The Frankel classification also provides a standardized method of evaluation of both motor and sensory function in spinal injury patients.[5] It is as follows: Frankel A, no motor or sensory function; Frankel B, no motor function, sensory incomplete; Frankel C, motor function useless, sensory incomplete; Frankel D, motor function useful, sensory incomplete; Frankel E, motor function normal, sensory normal. Bradford and McBride[3] have further divided the Frankel D classification as follows: D1, preserved motor function at lowest functional grade (3+–5+) with or without bowel and bladder paralysis with normal or reduced voluntary motor function; D2, preserved motor function at midfunctional grade (4+–5+) and normal voluntary bowel or bladder function; D3, preserved motor function at high functional grade (4+–5+) and normal voluntary bowel or bladder function.

Damage to specific sections of the spinal cord present as cord syndromes and are categorized by specific physical findings. These syndromes can also present as a combination of two or more syndromes rather than the pure variety as described.

The anterior cord syndrome, which involves the anterior two thirds of the cord, is manifest as loss of all motor function and sensation below the injured level. Only the posterior columns are spared, which provide crude sensation only. This syndrome has a poor prognosis for recovery (Fig. 3–2).

The central cord syndrome is usually seen in older persons who sustain a hyperextension injury to their neck. The spinal cord is injured by a pincer mechanism formed by osteophytes anteriorly and hypertrophied ligamentum flavum posteriorly that compress the spinal cord in the middle. This injury preferentially involves the central portion of the cord more than the peripheral. The anatomic arrangements of the neural tracts providing function to the upper extremity being mostly medial, followed by thoracic, lower extremity, and sacral in a more lateral distribution, these patients will present with more involvement of the hand than of the lower extremity. The majority will have bowel and bladder control and will be able to ambulate, although often with a spastic gait. Most of these patients do not regain fine motor use of their upper extremities (Fig. 3–3).

The Brown-Séquard syndrome results from hemisection of the cord. It is manifest by loss of ipsilateral motor function and contralateral pain, inability to distinguish temperature, and loss of light touch sensation. These patients will regain control of their bowel and bladder function and most will be able to ambulate (Fig. 3–4).

The posterior cord syndrome is rare and involves loss of posterior column function, which provides proprioception and position sense. These persons maintain the ability to ambulate, but rely on visual input for their spatial orientation.

Root injuries can be isolated in the cervical, lumbar, or sacral spine or may be combined with other cord injury. Nerve root injuries have a more favorable prognosis than cord injuries. In the cervical spine the complex of a complete cord injury with varying levels of root injury is frequently seen. Those patients with complete high cervical injuries have a 30% chance of recovery of one nerve root level, those with midcervical injuries have a 60% chance, and almost all patients with low cervical injuries will have recovery of one root level and sometimes two.

SENSORY EVALUATION

Evaluation of the sensory level in each patient should be carefully tested using an alcohol wipe to distinguish temperature and a sterile needle to evaluate pain and light touch. These are functions of the spinothalamic tract whose fibers lie in the anterolateral portion of the spinal cord. Posterior column function of the spinal cord can be tested using a tuning fork to detect vibration or the position of the limb in space. The muscles are innervated by the neural tissues in the corticospinal tracts which are positioned in the anterolateral aspect of the spinal cord (Fig. 3–5). The sensory and motor examination must be performed in a sequential and systematic manner.

Evaluation of sensation begins with the cervical region and proceeds distally with evaluation of specific dermatomal regions (Fig. 3–6; Table 3–1). Unrestricted access to the patient is mandatory. C1 and C2 roots provide sensation from the occipital region to the nape of the neck. C3 and C4 provide sensation in a cape distribution from the neck and shoulders posteriorly to the anterior chest just inferior to the clavicles. C5 innervates the deltoid region of the shoulder and anterolateral aspect of the upper arm. C6 innervates the radial aspect of the forearm, thumb, and index finger. C7 provides sensation to the long finger and a small strip of skin on the dorsal aspect of the hand. C8 innervates the ulnar aspect of the hand, including the fourth and fifth digits and the ulnar aspect of the forearm. T1 provides sensation to the medial aspect of the arm, axilla, and pectoral region of the chest.

The thoracic region and abdomen receive sensory innervation from the thoracic nerve roots with significant sensory overlap in this area due to the dual in-

STANDARD NEUROLOGICAL CLASSIFICATION OF SPINAL CORD INJURY

Figure 3–1 — A, The American Spinal Injury Association (ASIA) neurologic classification of spinal cord injury form is composed of several sections. The initial portion grades five muscle groups in the upper and five muscle groups in the lower extremities on a score of 1 to 5. A composite motor score is then obtained. The next section grades light touch and pinprick. The final section on the first page specifies the level of injury.

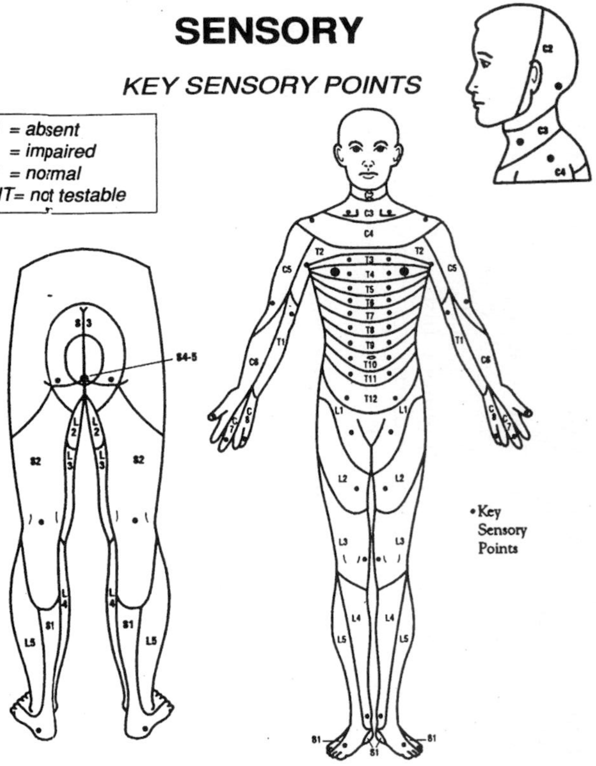

Functional Independence Measure (FIM)

L E V E L S	7 Complete Independence (Timely, Safely) 6 Modified Independence (Device)	No Helper
	Modified Dependence 5 Supervision 4 Minimal Assist (Subject = 75%+) 3 Moderate Assist (Subject = 50%+) **Complete Dependence** 2 Maximal Assist (Subject = 25%+) 1 Total Assist (Subject = 0%+)	Helper

	ADMIT	DISCH
Self-Care		
A. Eating		
B. Grooming		
C. Bathing		
D. Dressing-Upper Body		
E. Dressing-Lower Body		
F. Toileting		
Sphincter Control		
G. Bladder Management		
H. Bowel Management		
Mobility		
Transfer:		
I. Bed, Chair, Wheelchair		
J. Toilet		
K. Tub, Shower		
Locomotion		
L. Walk/Wheelchair	W C	W C
M. Stairs		
Communication		
N. Comprehension	A V V N	A V V N
O. Expression		
Social Cognition		
P. Social Interaction		
Q. Problem Solving		
R. Memory		
Total FIM		

NOTE: Leave no blanks; enter 1 if patient not testable due to risk.

COPY FREELY - DO NOT CHANGE
RESEARCH FOUNDATION OF THE STATE UNIVERSITY OF NEW YORK

B

ASIA IMPAIRMENT SCALE

☐ **A = Complete:** No motor or sensory function is preserved in the sacral segments S4-S5.

☐ **B = Incomplete:** Sensory but not motor function is preserved below the neurological level and extends through the sacral segments S4-S5.

☐ **C = Incomplete:** Motor function is preserved below the neurological level, and the majority of key muscles below the neurological level have a muscle grade less than 3.

☐ **D = Incomplete:** Motor function is preserved below the neurological level, and the majority of key muscles below the neurological level have a muscle grade greater than or equal to 3.

☐ **E = Normal:** Motor and sensory function is normal.

CLINICAL SYNDROMES

☐ Central Cord
☐ Brown-Séquard
☐ Anterior Cord
☐ Conus Medullaris
☐ Cauda Equina

Figure 3–1 *Continued* ═ *B,* Functional independence is compared at admission and discharge. Finally, an impairment scale is specified from A to E and a clinical spinal syndrome is identified, if present. (From the American Spinal Injury Association and Research Foundation of the State University of New York, 1992.)

POSTERIOR

Fasciculus gracilis

Fasciculus cuneatus

Lateral corticospinal tract

Lateral spinothalamic tract

ANTERIOR

Anterior corticospinal tract

Anterior spinothalamic tract

Figure 3–2 = Involvement of the anterior two thirds of the spinal cord leads to loss of motor and sensory function below the lesion. Only deep sensation is present, with this being mediated through the posterior column. (Modified from Keenen TL, Benson DR: Initial evaluation of the spine-injured patient. *In* Browner BD, Jupiter JB, Levine AM, et al (eds): Skeletal Trauma: Fractures, Dislocations, Ligamentous Injuries, vol 1. Philadelphia, WB Saunders, 1992, p 588.)

Figure 3–3 = The central portion of the spinal cord is involved, with sacral sparing due to the arrangements of the fibers in the corticospinal and spinothalamic tracts. In the corticospinal and spinothalamic tracts, the fibers innervating the upper extremity are more medial, with the fibers innervating the distal extremity being located more lateral in each tract. (Modified from Keenen TL, Benson DR: Initial evaluation of the spine-injured patient. *In* Browner BD, Jupiter JB, Levine AM, et al (eds): Skeletal Trauma: Fractures, Dislocations, Ligamentous Injuries, vol 1. Philadelphia, WB Saunders, 1992, p 588.)

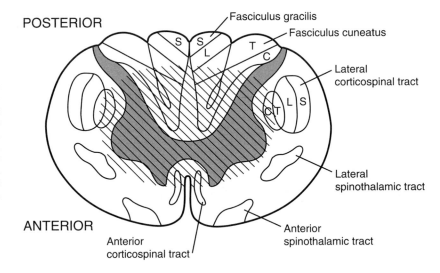

POSTERIOR

Fasciculus gracilis

Fasciculus cuneatus

Lateral corticospinal tract

Lateral spinothalamic tract

ANTERIOR

Anterior corticospinal tract

Anterior spinothalamic tract

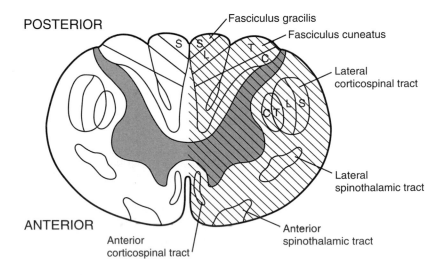

POSTERIOR

Fasciculus gracilis

Fasciculus cuneatus

Lateral corticospinal tract

Lateral spinothalamic tract

ANTERIOR

Anterior corticospinal tract

Anterior spinothalamic tract

Figure 3–4 = Hemisection of the spinal cord leads to loss of motor function on the same side of the lesion, and loss of pain and the ability to distinguish temperature and light touch on the opposite side. (From Keenen TL, Benson DR: Initial evaluation of the spine-injured patient. *In* Browner BD, Jupiter JB, Levine AM, et al (eds): Skeletal Trauma: Fractures, Dislocations, Ligamentous Injuries, vol 1. Philadelphia, WB Saunders, 1992, p 588.)

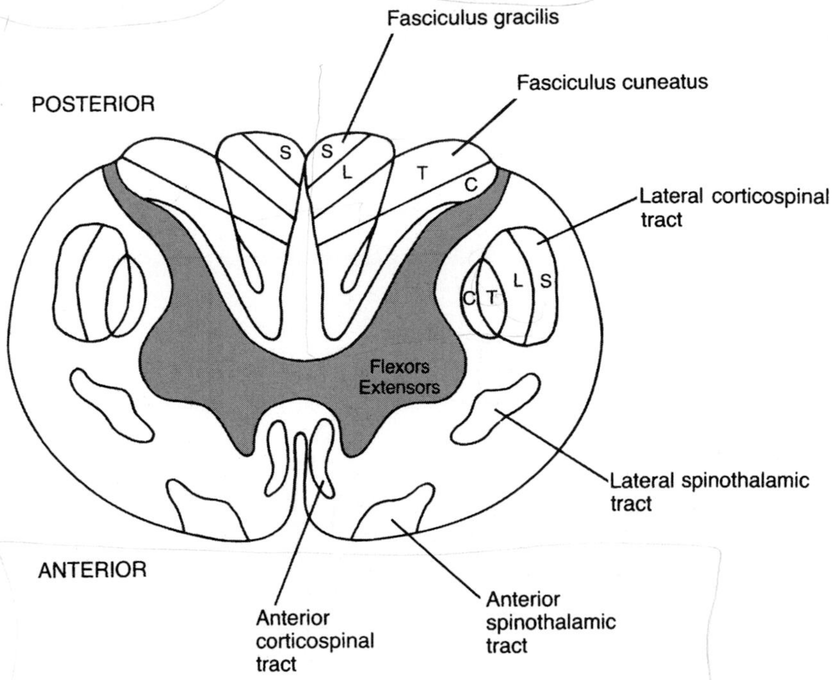

Figure 3–5 = Cross section of the spinal cord noting orientation of the fibers in the spinothalamic and corticospinal tracts. (From Keenen TL, Benson DR: Initial evaluation of the spine-injured patient. *In* Browner BD, Jupiter JB, Levine AM, et al (eds): Skeletal Trauma: Fractures, Dislocations, Ligamentous Injuries, vol 1. Philadelphia, WB Saunders, 1992, p 588.)

nervation of the skin. Anatomically, the skin in this area receives input from the fibers of three different spinal nerve levels. Localizing sensory levels in this region are the nipple line, which represents a T5 level, and the umbilicus, representing the T10 level. The inguinal region receives input from the lower thoracic and upper lumbar region.

The lower extremity and perineum are innervated by the roots making up the lumbosacral plexus (Fig. 3–7). L1 and L2 innervate the skin just below the inguinal ligament and the inner thigh while L3 and L4 provide sensation to the anterior, anterolateral, and knee areas. L5 provides sensation to the lateral aspect of the calf and the dorsomedial skin of the foot and ankle. S1 innervates the posterior calf, and the lateral and plantar aspect of the foot.

The perineum is innervated by sacral nerves S2

through S5 and becomes important as a prognostic indicator of functional recovery in those patients with a spinal cord injury.[8, 9]

MOTOR EVALUATION

Following a thorough evaluation of sensory function, muscles are evaluated and carefully recorded regarding functional strength (Table 3–2; Fig. 3–8). C1 and C2 innervate the musculature of the suboccipital triangle. C3 and C4, in conjunction with the intercostal nerves, provide respiratory function via the diaphragm. Patients with low cervical and thoracic spinal cord injuries often present with paradoxical respiration. The cord injury renders the intercostal and abdominal musculature nonfunctional. With inspiration the diaphragm contracts, which displaces the abdominal contents inferiorly resulting in abdominal distention rather than the flattening of the abdomen and expansion of the chest which takes place normally with inspiration in neurologically intact patients. Should the C3 and C4 roots be nonfunctional, the diaphragm will be paralyzed and severe respiratory compromise may result. C5-innervated muscles include the deltoid, the internal and external shoulder rotators, and the biceps. Muscles innervated by C6 include the biceps, brachioradialis, and wrist extensors (extensor carpi radialis longus, extensor carpi radialis brevis). C7 function evaluates the triceps, wrist flexors (flexor carpi radialis, flexor carpi ulnaris), and finger extensors (extensor digitorum communis). Finger flexors (flexor digitorum superficialis, flexor digitorum profundus) and hand intrinsics are innervated by the C8 root with interossei function being provided by the T1 root.

Thoracic roots innervate the intercostal muscles and

Table 3–1 = **MAJOR SENSORY LEVELS**

LEVEL	REGION
C4	Clavicle
C5	Deltoid region
C6	Radial forearm and thumb
C7	Middle finger
C8	Fifth finger
T1	Medial, proximal arm
T5	Nipples
T7	Costal margins
T10	Umbilicus
T12	Inguinal ligament
L3	Anterior thigh
L4	Medial aspect of knee
L5	Lateral calf, dorsum of foot, big toe
S1	Lateral foot, fifth toe
S2	Posterior thighs
S3–4	Buttocks, perianal region

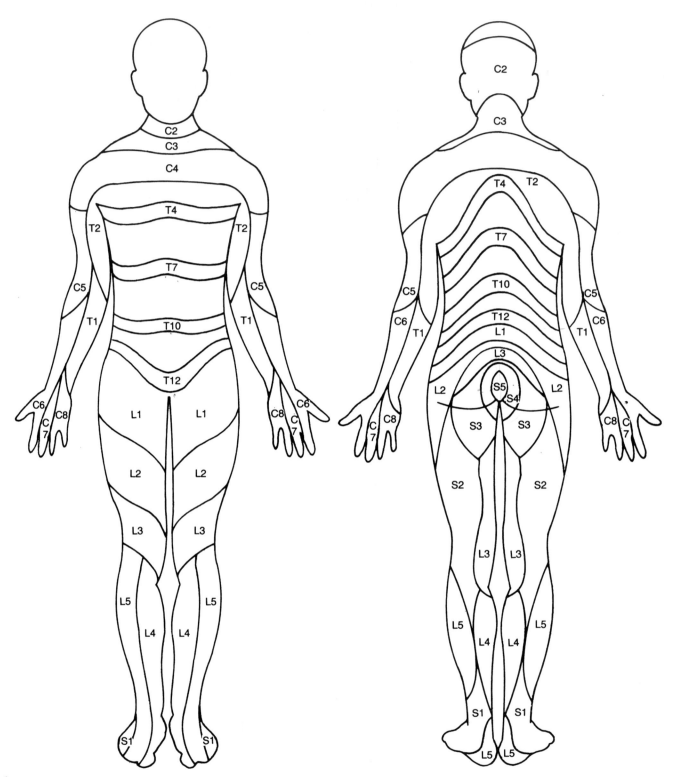

Figure 3–6 = Dermatomes. (From Keenen TL, Benson DR: Initial evaluation of the spine-injured patient. *In* Browner BD, Jupiter JB, Levine AM, et al (eds): Skeletal Trauma: Fractures, Dislocations, Ligamentous Injuries, vol 1. Philadelphia, WB Saunders, 1992, p 595.)

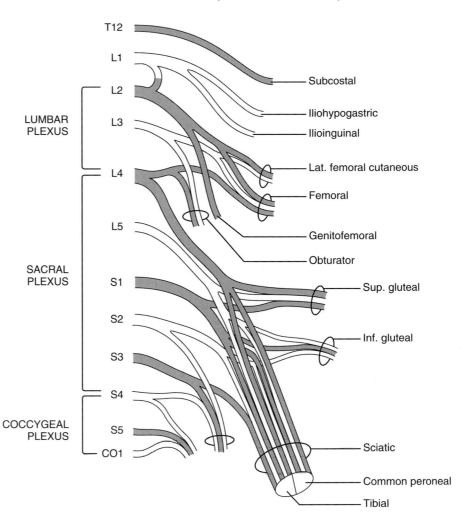

T12

L1

L2 — Subcostal

LUMBAR
PLEXUS

L3 — Iliohypogastric

— Ilioinguinal

L4 — Lat. femoral cutaneous

— Femoral

L5 — Genitofemoral

SACRAL
PLEXUS

— Obturator

S1 — Sup. gluteal

S2

S3 — Inf. gluteal

S4

COCCYGEAL
PLEXUS

S5 — Sciatic

CO1 — Common peroneal

— Tibial

Figure 3–7 = The lumbosacral plexus. (Modified from Gardner E, Gray DJ, O'Rahilly R (eds): Anatomy. Philadelphia, WB Saunders, 1975, p 426.)

the abdominal and paraspinal muscles. Upper abdominal contraction without lower abdominal contraction results in the upward migration of the umbilicus known as Beevor's sign and is indicative of paralysis below T10. L1, L2, and L3 functions are tested by evaluating the hip flexors and adductors. L4 function includes the quadriceps femoris and anterior tibialis. L5 innervates the hip abductors, the hamstring group, and the extensor hallucis longus. S1 function includes hip extensors, the lateral hamstring group, and the gastrocnemius-soleus complex.

Sacral roots 2–5 innervate the sphincter muscles of the perineum.

REFLEX EVALUATION

Following thorough muscle evaluation, the reflex function is tested (Table 3–3; Fig. 3–9). The biceps reflex evaluates C5 function, the brachioradialis evaluates C6 function, and C7 function is evaluated by the triceps reflex.

Table 3–2 = **MAJOR MOTOR LEVELS**

LEVEL	MUSCLE GROUP	ACTION	DEEP TENDON REFLEX
C5	Deltoid, internal and external shoulder rotators	Abduction of shoulder, external rotation of arm	Biceps jerk (C5–6)
C6	Biceps, brachialis, wrist extensors	Flexion of elbow	Brachioradialis jerk (C5–6)
C7	Triceps, wrist flexors	Extension of elbow, wrist	Triceps jerk
C8	Intrinsic hand muscles	Abduction, adduction of fingers	
L2–3	Iliopsoas	Hip flexion	
L4	Quadriceps	Extension of knee	Knee jerk
L5	Tibialis anterior and posterior, extensor hallucis longus	Dorsiflexion of foot and big toe	
S1	Gastrocnemius	Plantar flexion of foot	Ankle jerk
S4–5	Anal sphincter	Voluntary contraction of anal sphincter	

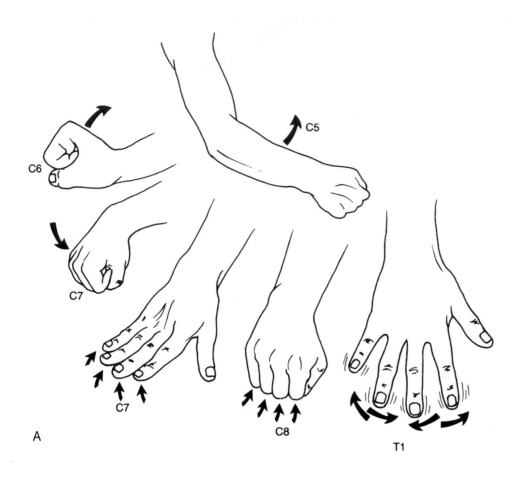

A

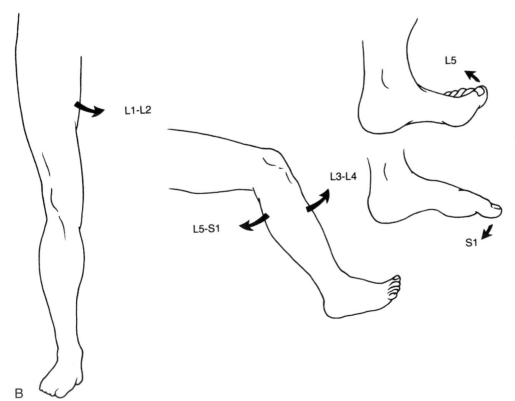

B

Figure 3–8 = *A,* An examination of the upper extremities must include, at a minimum, the muscle groups that are designated by their respective nerve root innervation. These are C5, elbow flexion; C6, wrist extension; C7, finger extension; C8, finger flexion; and T1, finger abduction. The strength (0 to 5) should be listed on the time-oriented flow sheet. *B,* An examination of the lower extremities needs to include at least these muscle groups designated by their respective nerve root innervation: L1–2, hip abductors; L3–4, knee extension; L5–S1, knee flexion; L5, great toe extension; and S1, great toe flexion. (From Keenen TL, Benson DR: Initial evaluation of the spine-injured patient. *In* Browner BD, Jupiter JB, Levine AM, et al (eds): Skeletal Trauma: Fractures, Dislocations, Ligamentous Injuries, vol 1. Philadelphia, WB Saunders, 1992, p 594.)

Table 3–3 = **SEGMENTAL REFLEXES**

REFLEX	LEVEL
Biceps	C6
Triceps	C7
Upper abdominal*	T7–10
Lower abdominal*	T10–12
Cremasteric*	L1
Knee jerk	L4
Posterior tibial jerk	L5
Ankle jerk	S1
Bulbocavernosus†	S2–4
Anocutaneous‡	S4–5

* Cutaneous reflexes: decreased in upper motor neuron lesion.
† Contraction of bulbocavernosus muscle after stimulation of the glans penis.
‡ Contraction of anal sphincter after stroking perineal skin.

Important reflex functions in the lower extremity include the L4 quadriceps reflex or knee jerk and the Achilles reflex, which evaluates S1 function. These deep tendon reflexes are mediated through the anterior horn cells. The cerebral cortex provides an inhibitory function to prevent excessive reaction with stimulation.

The abdominal and cremasteric reflexes are upper motor neuron tests requiring superficial stimulation of the skin and mediated through the central nervous system.

The superficial abdominal reflex is elicited by stroking the skin in each quadrant of the abdomen and noting whether the umbilicus is drawn toward the stimulated area. Innervation of the abdominal musculature is segmental, with the upper musculature innervated by T7–10 and the lower muscles by T10–L1. Asymmetrical loss of this reflex may indicate a localized lower motor neuron lesion.

In men, the superficial cremasteric reflex is elicited by stroking the skin of the inner thigh. If the reflex is intact the scrotum will be drawn upward by the cremasteric muscle. Absence of the reflex is indicative of an upper motor lesion while unilateral absence suggests a lower motor lesion. Anatomically, this reflex involves T12–L2.

Loss of superficial reflexes combined with an exaggerated response of the deep tendon reflexes due to loss of cerebral inhibition is indicative of an upper motor neuron lesion.

Pathologic reflexes are significant because their presence indicates an upper motor neuron lesion. Babinski's test is elicited by stroking the skin on the lateral plantar surface with a sharp object such as a key or the handle of the reflex hammer. A positive response is indicated by extension of the great toe with flexion and splaying of the remaining toes. The Oppenheim reflex is tested in a similar manner. The fingernail or hammer handle is drawn along the tibial crest, a positive test eliciting the same response as Babinski's.

The presence or absence of sacral sparing is extremely important when evaluating spinal trauma patients. It provides an indicator for prognosis of functional recovery in persons sustaining a spinal cord injury.

Sphincter function is tested by inserting a gloved finger into the rectum and noting the resting tone. The patient is then asked to voluntarily contract the sphincter. Sensation to light touch and pinprick are also evaluated at this time. Stimulating the skin around the anus will elicit the superficial anal reflex and contraction of the anal sphincter. This reflex involves S2–4 function (Fig. 3–10).

During the rectal examination in males, the position of the prostate should be noted. An abnormal position is indicative of a possible urethral tear and warrants further evaluation. Special care must be observed during Foley catheter insertion in these patients.

Persons presenting with a neurologic deficit must be evaluated for spinal shock. Spinal shock is often present within 24 hours of injury and is due to edema from the initial trauma to surrounding neural tissues. These patients will exhibit loss of motor, sensory, and reflex function. At this point, determination of whether the neurologic deficit is complete or partial cannot be made.

The bulbocavernosus reflex becomes important in

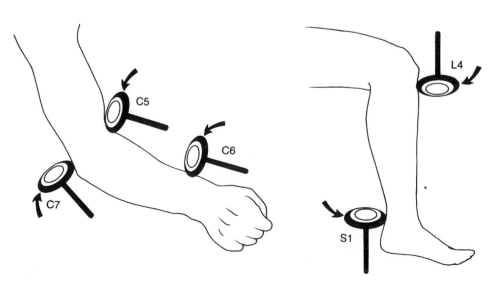

Figure 3–9 = Stretch reflexes and nerve roots of origin. (From Keenen TL, Benson DR: Initial evaluation of the spine-injured patient. *In* Browner BD, Jupiter JB, Levine AM, et al (eds): Skeletal Trauma: Fractures, Dislocations, Ligamentous Injuries, vol 1. Philadelphia, WB Saunders, 1992, p 596.)

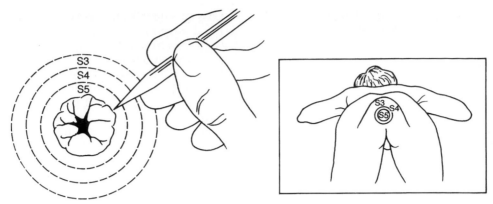

Figure 3–10 = The anal reflex, indicative of S2–4 function, can be elicited by stimulating the perianal skin. (From Keenen TL, Benson DR: Initial evaluation of the spine-injured patient. *In* Browner BD, Jupiter JB, Levine AM, et al (eds): Skeletal Trauma: Fractures, Dislocations, Ligamentous Injuries, vol 1. Philadelphia, WB Saunders, 1992, p 591.)

evaluation of the spinal injury patient because its presence signifies resolution of spinal shock and allows the determination of a complete or incomplete neurologic deficit. This reflex is elicited by stimulation of the penis or clitoris by digital pressure or traction on the Foley catheter while a gloved finger in the rectum notes a resulting contraction of the anal sphincter. A positive response indicates resolution of spinal shock with return of the reflex arc (Fig. 3–11).

In summary, spinal trauma patients must be visually inspected for external evidence that may indicate severe internal injury. Bony palpation must then be per-

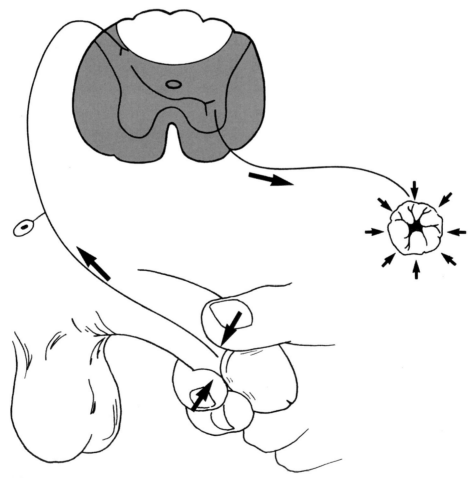

Figure 3–11 = The bulbocavernosus reflex returns following resolution of spinal shock. Once this reflex returns, the determination of whether a neurologic lesion is complete or incomplete can be made. (From Keenen TL, Benson DR: Initial evaluation of the spine-injured patient. *In* Browner BD, Jupiter JB, Levine AM, et al (eds): Skeletal Trauma: Fractures, Dislocations, Ligamentous Injuries, vol 1. Philadelphia, WB Saunders, 1992, p 588.)

formed noting associated soft tissue defects and mal-alignment. Careful attention to detail in motor and sensory evaluation must be undertaken and carefully documented to provide accurate neurologic status.

REFERENCES

1. Bohlman H: Acute fractures and dislocations of the cervical spine: An analysis of 300 hospitalized patients and review of the literature. J Bone Joint Surg Am 61:1119, 1979.
2. Bohlman H: Complications and treatment of fractures and dislocations of the cervical spine. *In* Epps CH (ed): Complications in Orthopaedic Surgery, ed 2. Philadelphia, JB Lippincott, 1985, pp 897–918.
3. Bradford DS, McBride GG: Surgical management of thoracolumbar spine fractures with incomplete neurologic deficits. Clin Orthop 218:201–216, 1987.
4. Davis D, Bohlman H, Walker AE, et al: The pathological findings in fatal craniospinal injuries. J Neurosurg 34:603, 1971.
5. Frankel HL, Hancock GH, Melzak J, et al: Postural reduction in closed injuries of the spine. Paraplegia 7:179–192, 1969.
6. Gertzbein S, Count-Brown C: Flexion-distraction injuries of the lumbar spine. Clin Orthop 227:52–50, 1988.
7. McGuire RA, Neville S, Green BA, et al: Spinal instability and the log rolling maneuver. J Trauma 27:525–531, 1987.
8. Stauffer ES: Neurologic recovery following injuries to the cervical spinal cord and nerve roots. Spine 9:532–534, 1984.
9. Stauffer ES: Spinal cord injury syndromes. Semin Spine Surg 3:87–91, 1991.
10. Vaccaro AR, An HS, Sun S, Balderston RA, et al: Noncontiguous injuries of the spine. J Spinal Disord 5:320–329, 1992.

Radiologic Evaluation of the Spine-Injured Patient

Jeremy W.R. Young ‖ *Joel K. Curé*

Examination of the spinal column in injured patients in the acute setting may be difficult due to combative or uncooperative behavior, secondary to head trauma or intoxication. Plain films are the primary method of evaluation and will detect abnormalities of alignment, as well as the majority of fractures (Fig. 4–1). Additional methods of examination include conventional tomography, computed tomography (CT),[7, 11, 16, 26, 33, 39, 44, 45] and magnetic resonance imaging (MRI).[21, 28, 29, 40] CT is able to clearly identify subtle fractures and small osseous fragments not seen on plain radiographs and has better spatial and contrast resolution than plain films or conventional tomography. The improved contrast resolution allows superior depiction of the soft tissues. CT examinations involve less radiation exposure than conventional tomography and, with the new generation of spiral scanners, take considerably less time.

With state-of-the-art CT scanners, high-quality two-dimensional (2-D) and three-dimensional (3-D) reconstructions may be produced in virtually any plane (Fig. 4–2). Although these images provide excellent 3-D representation, their role in the evaluation of spinal injuries in the acute setting has yet to be fully assessed. The required post-processing is time-consuming and operator dependent. Three-dimensional reconstruction algorithms smooth the edges of the rectangular voxels to produce visually appealing images and thereby tend to obscure subtle fracture lines. Patient motion during the acquisition of CT studies may yield artifactual step-offs or lucent lines in reconstructed images, mimicking fractures. For these reasons, the individual CT slices must still be carefully evaluated.

The development of "spiral" or "helical" CT scanning has provided an improved capability for CT. Traditionally, CT was used only in cases with equivocal plain film findings, and in specific cases, to identify small bone fragments, evaluate the spinal canal, and display the articular pillars more clearly. This under-utilization was largely due to the difficulties in repositioning the patient on the CT scanner, the time taken for the study, and the cost. With spiral scanning, several new options have arisen. The speed of a modern spiral scan, often less than 1 minute, ensures that CT is not only a useful secondary method of evaluation but may indeed become the primary method. Inherent advantages of CT over plain radiography include its independence from technical problems associated with patient positioning and film exposure, its improved potential in visualizing the lower cervical spine in patients with large shoulders, its ability to reconstruct in different planes, and overall, its ability to provide comprehensive and rapid "one-step" examination of the spine. Rapid scanning also increases patient throughput, thereby potentially allowing reduced cost. There are, therefore, many reasons to consider replacing plain radiography with spiral CT scanning.

Understanding that CT, and especially spiral CT, is not universally available, tomography in the lateral projection is still useful for detecting subtle abnormalities of the cervical spine. It is especially effective in delineating the posterior elements, and in cases in which a fracture may lie in the axial plane, particularly when there is little or no displacement (Fig. 4–3). It must be remembered that subtle undisplaced axially oriented fractures can be missed by conventional CT, at least in theory. This is particularly the case when the articular pillars are involved, although this problem has been largely eliminated by the use of thin sections and 2-D reconstructions. CT-myelography with water-soluble contrast has been usually reserved for patients with acute neurologic deficit, or incomplete or progressive neurologic abnormalities. This technique may be extremely helpful in determining the exact location and extent of cord compression or injury, although MRI is proving to be a good alternative in such cases (Fig. 4–4).

MAGNETIC RESONANCE IMAGING OF THE SPINE

Although plain films are useful in the initial diagnosis of spinal injury, they are severely limited in their ability to detect soft tissue injury, both of the surrounding ligaments and of the spinal cord. CT is also limited in this area, although high-quality CT may provide evidence of luniated disc, hematoma and cord displacement compression, or edema, especially if used in conjunction with myelography. It is in this area, however, that MRI has a unique role. The role of MRI in acute spinal injury has yet to be fully evaluated, but results indicate that it has a significant role in detecting

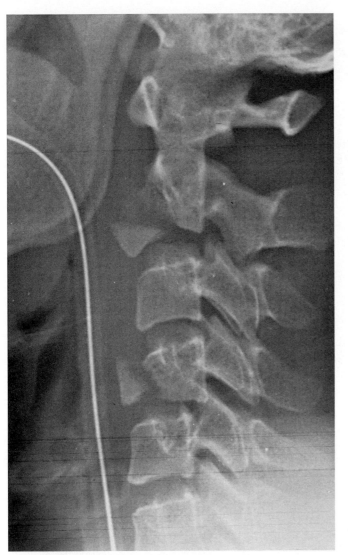

Figure 4–1 = Hyperflexion injury. Plain lateral radiograph of the cervical spine demonstrates hyperflexion teardrop fractures at C2 and C4. There is obvious widening of the intervertebral disc space at C2–3, and posterior displacement at C4 relative to C5, indicative of ligamentous injury. In addition, there is clear widening of the interfacet joint at C4–5, again suggesting complete ligamentous disruption. Marked instability can be inferred at both injury levels.

traumatic disc herniation, hematomas, and cord edema. Advantages of MRI include its ability to visualize all of the soft tissues and the substance of the spinal cord, where subtle injuries may be appreciated[21, 28, 29, 40] (Figs. 4–5 through 4–8). Indeed, the detection of edema or blood within the cord substance yields important prognostic information. Also, newer techniques employing 3-D Fourier magnetic resonance (MR) acquisitions with ultrashort echo times yield images which are significantly more sensitive in detecting osseous abnormalities than conventional MR techniques. MRI allows direct visualization of the anterior and posterior longitudinal ligaments, and provides indirect evidence of ligamentous disruption by depicting prevertebral or dorsal interspinous edema (Fig. 4–9), intradiscal signal abnormalities, and disc widening. High-resolution MRI techniques permit detailed depiction of facet align-

ment. Disadvantages of MRI include its high cost, longer study time, and the relative inaccessibility of the patient within the bore of the magnet. In addition, monitoring and support devices containing ferromagnetic components are not suitable for use in a strong magnetic field. Fortunately, the industry has responded with MR-compatible ventilators and fixation devices, as well as newer techniques, such as echo-planar imaging, which will significantly shorten the time of the study.

RADIOGRAPHIC EVALUATION OF THE SPINE

For convenience, this section is divided into two parts: (1) evaluation of the cervical spine and (2) evaluation of the thoracic and lumbar spine. In practice, the evaluation of the spine is similar in all regions, and so the principles involved are covered in greater depth in the section dealing with the cervical spine.

Spinal Stability

The determination of spinal stability is an important factor in the evaluation of the injured spine. An unstable injury is one in which the spinal canal is unable to maintain its normal relationships under normal physiologic conditions. Radiologic imaging may be helpful in differentiating between stable and unstable spines and thus prevent progression of neural injury. Cervical instability has been described in terms of displacement as a combination of 3.5 mm of horizontal displacement of a vertebra on a lateral radiograph, and greater than 11 degrees of kyphosis, reflecting the posterior[9, 10, 12, 14, 15, 43] ligamentous disruption that must occur to allow this motion. Signs of instability include widening of the intervertebral disc space and splaying of the spinous process. Splaying of the spinous process per se indicates posterior ligamentous disruption, but in mild cases does not necessarily imply disruption of the anterior or posterior longitudinal ligaments. Obvious dislocations and fracture dislocations are invariably inherently unstable.

As in the cervical spine, stability is an important factor in the evaluation of the lumbar and thoracic spine. Clearly, bidirectional displacement of a vertebral body implies ligamentous disruption and hence instability. Problems arise, however, in deciding upon stability in cases of severe compression fractures and burst fractures. In the thoracic and lumbar spine, it has been generally agreed that wedge compression fractures with loss of anterior height of less than 50% are stable.[2, 3, 5, 13, 17, 32] However, the presence of these fractures at more than one level may make the spine mechanically unstable. In addition, crush fractures extending to the posterior aspect of the vertebral body (middle element) may be inherently stable by virtue of intact ligaments but may be unstable practically and may demonstrate displacement of minor fragments into the spinal canal.[5, 13, 17, 32] The three-element concept is thus theoretically useful inasmuch as the integrity of the middle column

Text continued on page 35

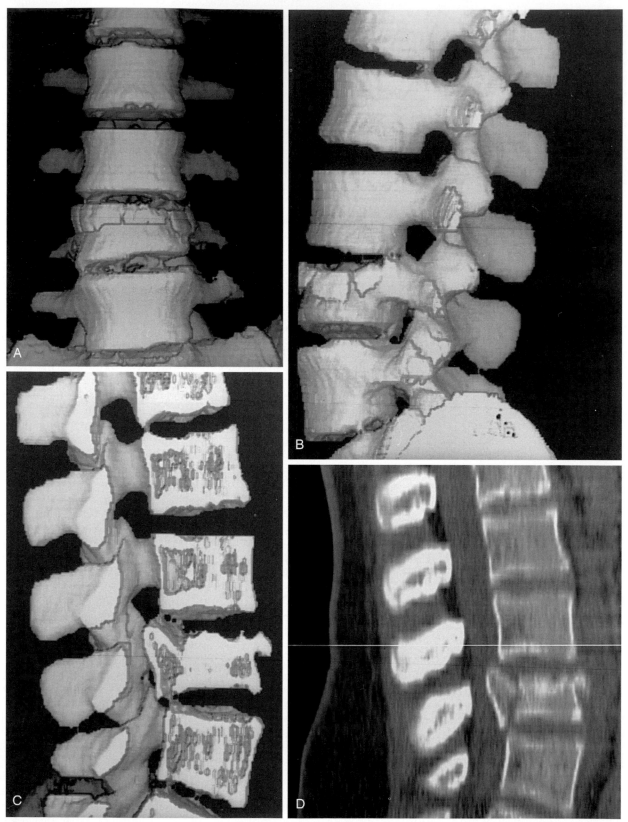

Figure 4–2 = Three-dimensional CT rendering of a compression fracture of L4 in *(A)* frontal and *(B)* lateral projections. *C,* Sagittal cutaway image gives a graphic representation of encroachment of the posterior fragment on the spinal canal. *D,* Two-dimensional (2-D) sagittally reformatted image provides similar information.

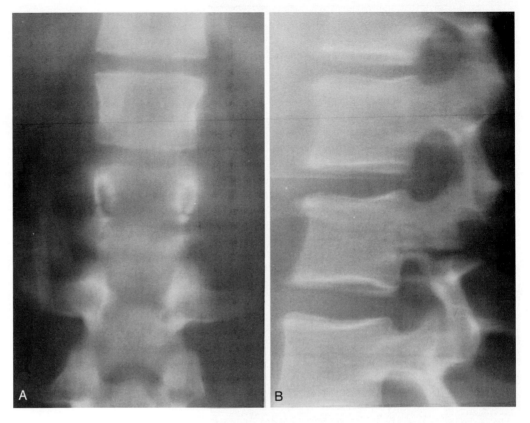

Figure 4–3 = Anteroposterior (A) and lateral (B) tomography of a Chance fracture of L2, indicating the horizontal fractures extending from the posterior vertebral body through the pedicles. Incidentally noted is a mild depressed fracture of the anterosuperior aspect of L2.

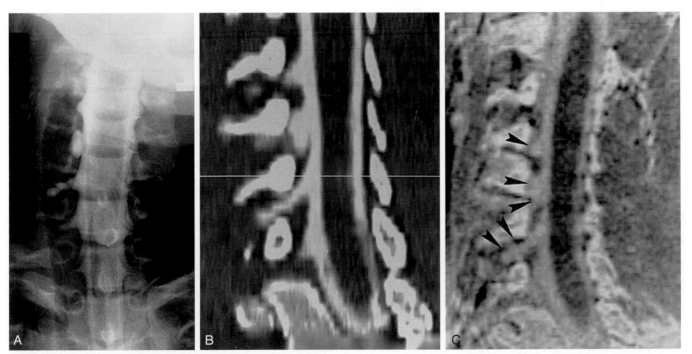

Figure 4–4 = A, Cervical myelogram demonstrates abnormal contrast collections at the nerve root sheath of C5–7 on the right. There has been avulsion of the nerve root at all three levels. B, CT myelogram with 2-D coronal reconstruction demonstrates similar abnormality of the nerve root sheaths. C, MR demonstrates abnormal collection of cerebrospinal fluid in the nerve root sheaths on the right (*arrowheads*), similar to that seen in A and B.

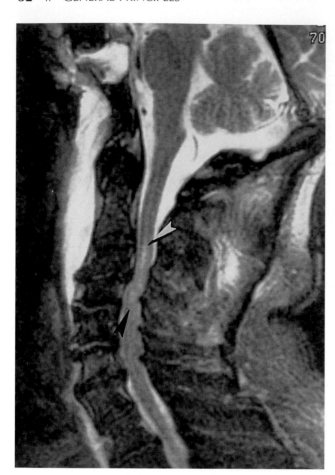

Figure 4–5 = Central cord syndrome. This patient presented with a central cord syndrome after a hyperextension injury. T2-weighted sagittal MRI demonstrates multilevel spondylosis with narrowing of disc and prominent marginal osteophytes, most notably at C3–4. There is edema in the prevertebral soft tissues, often seen in hyperextension injuries due to disruption of the anterior longitudinal ligament. There is also edema within the cord *(arrowheads)* extending above and below the C3–4 disc level where the cord was maximally compressed.

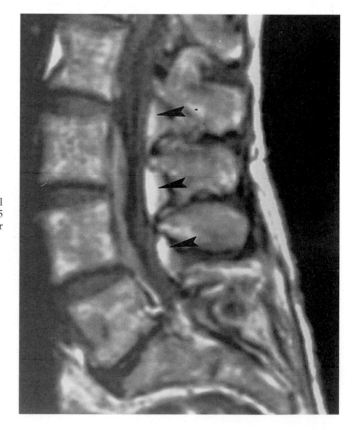

Figure 4–6 = Spinal subdural hematoma. This T1-weighted sagittal MRI demonstrates subdural blood to the lumbar thecal sac at the L3–5 levels *(arrowheads)*. The patient had recently undergone multiple lumbar puncture attempts.

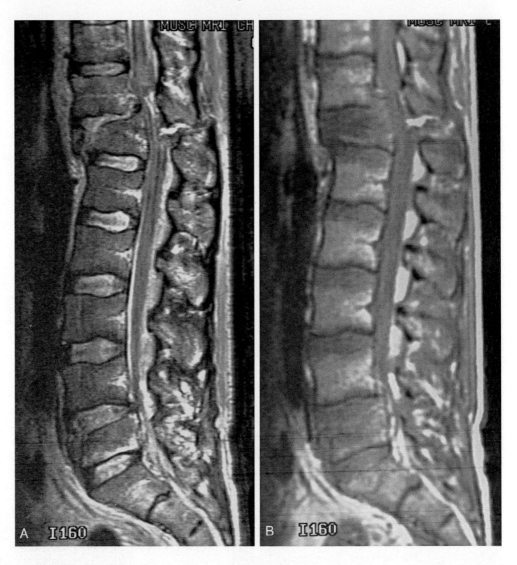

Figure 4–7 = Thoracic fracture subluxation. This patient suffered a fall from a height and sustained a T12 compression fracture associated with subluxation of T11 on T12. There is also a compression fracture at L5. *A,* This T2-weighted sagittal image demonstrates compression fractures of T12 and L5. Note anterior subluxation of T11 with respect to T12. There is heterogeneous signal within the conus medullaris due to contusion. Also note focal increased signal intensity within the interspinous ligament at T11–12 due to ligamentous injury relative to the hyperflexion mechanism. *B,* This T1-weighted image demonstrates abnormal marrow signal at the T12 and L5 compression sites. These changes may be a relatively sensitive indicator of vertebral injury, when plain films or CT is equivocal.

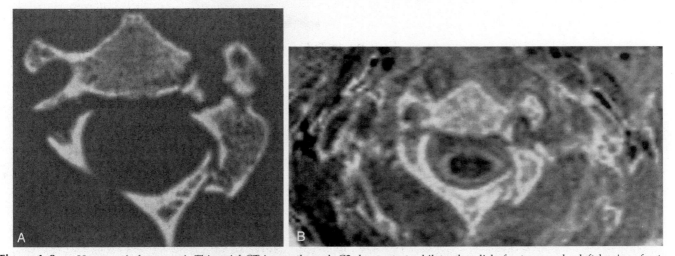

Figure 4–8 = Hangman's fracture. *A,* This axial CT image through C2 demonstrates bilateral pedicle fractures and a left laminar fracture. The fracture passes into the left transverse foramen, placing the patient at risk of a vertebral artery injury. *B,* Axial image from a 3-D gradient echo study of the cervical spine demonstrates findings comparable to the CT study. However, the MRI study also visualizes the spinal cord and subarachnoid space and does not require subarachnoid instillation of myelographic contrast material.

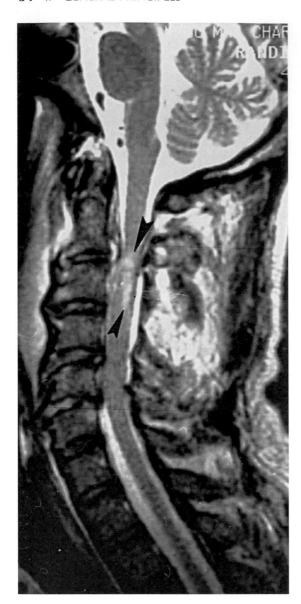

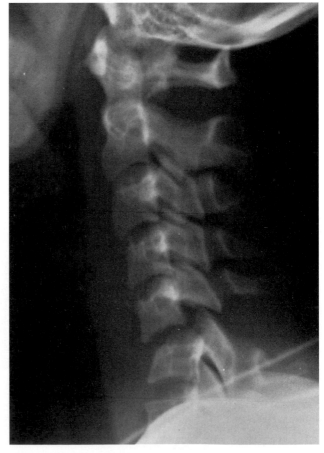

Figure 4–9 = Hangman's fracture with spinal cord edema. This T2-weighted sagittal image demonstrates edema within the cord at the C2 and C3 levels *(arrowheads)*. There is a small disc herniation at the C2–3 level producing spinal canal compromise. Prevertebral edema consistent with a hyperextension mechanism is again noted.

Figure 4–10 = Hyperflexion injury at C5–6. There is obvious splaying of the interspinous distance with subluxation of the interfacet joints at C5–6, approaching perched facets. A localized kyphosis with anterior displacement of C5 is identified indicating ligamentous disruption of all of the posterior ligamentous groups, and either ligamentous disruption or ligamentous stripping of the anterior longitudinal ligament.

in the absence of displacement would indicate stability. However, involvement of the middle element cannot be judged confidently by plain films, even in such cases as wedge compression fractures, and can only be diagnosed accurately by CT, which is therefore indicated in all compression injuries.

CERVICAL SPINE

Despite an unresolved debate regarding the usefulness of routine, protocol-driven cervical spine radiographs in trauma cases, they continue to be obtained. However, ordering more than a single cross-table lateral radiograph as a protocol should be discouraged. The detection rate of fractures in an alert, oriented patient, without pain or neurologic signs, is negligible. On the other hand, the patient with a neurologic deficit requires extensive workup, and unconscious, disoriented, or neurologically impaired patients require careful evaluation. Plain film evaluation will define the majority of bony abnormalities, including fracture of the vertebra, and even damage to posterior elements. Ligamentous damage can also be implied from the radiographs (Fig. 4–10). The supine cross-table lateral view is the single most important radiographic examination and should be made as soon as the patient is stabilized. All seven cervical vertebral bodies should be included on the radiographs[22, 34] (Fig. 4–11). Evaluation of this film alone by an expert in the field will allow diagnosis of abnormality in the vast majority of cases.[4] A normal cervical spine will demonstrate a gentle lordosis, without disruption of the anterior spinal line. Lack of lordosis, however, should not be taken as an infallible sign of abnormality. Although this may be due to muscular spasm and indicate spinal injury, age, prior trauma, radiographic positioning, flexion of the spine, and the wearing of a hard collar (commonly seen today) can all cause alteration in the natural lordosis. The normal cervical lordosis may be lost in up to 20% of normal asymptomatic patients radiographed in the neutral position.[24] In addition, if the "West Point" or military position is adopted, this figure rises to 70%.[42] Assessment of the lateral radiograph of the cervical spine is made by observing the anatomic structures that are visible, and the relationship they bear to one another. Subtle malalignment of the vertebral bodies, articular pillars, or posterior structures may be the only radiographic sign of abnormality. Measurement of prevertebral soft tissues in the upper spine is generally regarded as an important part of the examination of the cervical spine (Fig. 4–12). However, there are many variables that may affect the presence or value of soft tissue swelling, including radiographic technique, time lapse between injury and examination, and position and nature of the injury. There is also a large variation in the reported measurements of what constitutes normal or abnormal. It has been shown that only at measurements above 7 mm is there a statistical likelihood of underlying injury, with the statistical probability of injury rising significantly at measurements of over 10 mm.[41] This sign is therefore of limited diagnostic value. Other signs, such as displacement of the prevertebral fat stripe, and laryngeal or tracheal air

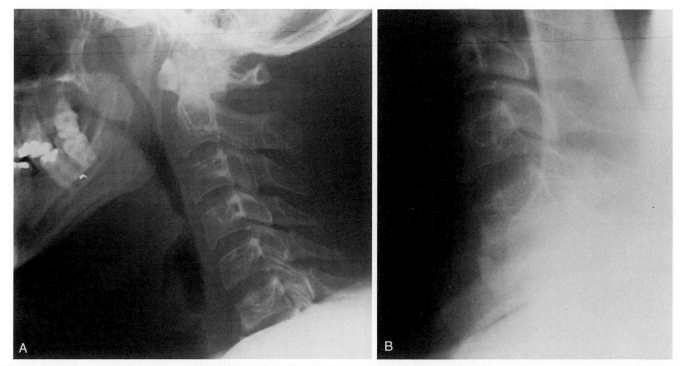

Figure 4–11 = *A,* Only six cervical vertebrae are adequately visualized on this study. There is only the vague impression of a small bone fragment lying anterior and inferior to the anterior vertebral line of C6. There is also the impression of slight compression of C6. *B,* Overpenetrated swimmer's view demonstrates a crush fracture of the body of C7.

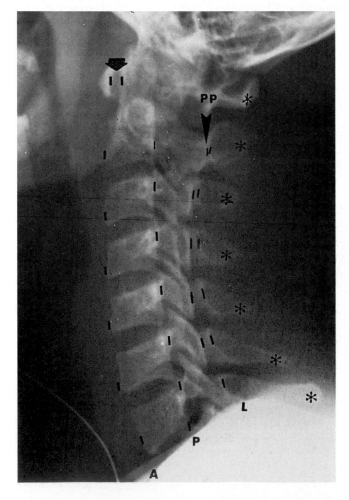

Figure 4–12 = *A,* Marked prominence of the retropharyngeal soft tissues is identified. There is abnormal positioning of the anterior arch of C1, which is displaced anteriorly from the odontoid. A fracture through the ring of C1 is also implied *(arrowhead). B,* Anteroposterior open-mouth odontoid view demonstrates marked lateral displacement of the lateral masses of C1, particularly on the left.

Figure 4–13 = Normal cervical spine demonstrating a normal C1; normal odontoid interspace *(thick arrow);* normal alignment along the anterior vertebral margins *(line A);* normal alignment along the posterior vertebral margins *(line P);* normal spinolaminar line *(line L);* normal relationship of the dorsal spinous processes *(asterisks);* and normal laminar facet interspace *(arrowhead PP).*

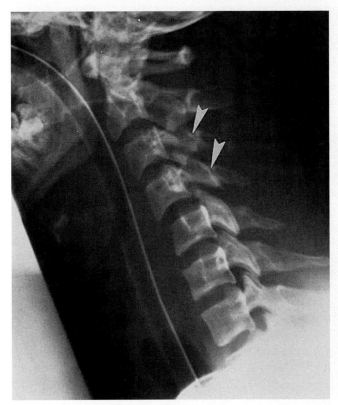

Figure 4–14 = Unilateral disrupted facet. There is mild anterior displacement of C4 relative to C5 with abrupt narrowing of the laminar facet interspace above C5 *(arrowheads)*. The anteriorly displaced articular facet of C4 can be identified overlying the posterior aspect of the C4 vertebral body.

shadows, are also only of occasional value. Traditional teaching stresses visualization of four imaginary lines[22, 34] (Fig. 4–13). These are the anterior and posterior spinal lines, joining the anterior and posterior aspects of the vertebral bodies along the line of the longitudinal ligaments; the spinolaminar line, joining the anterior margins of the junction of the lamina and spinous processes; and the spinous process line, joining the tips of the spinous processes. In addition, a fifth line should be drawn along the posterior margins of the articular pillars. This line defines the posterior aspect of the articular pillars and allows assessment of the laminar space between the posterior pillar and spinolaminar line. Abrupt variation in this space has been shown to be an accurate method of determining rotational abnormality of a vertebral column, or fracture of the articular pillar[47] (Fig. 4–14).

In flexion, the middle and upper segments move forward over the next inferior segment with concurrent sliding of the inferior articular facet over the superior facet of the level below, up to approximately 30% of the length of the articular surface.[36] A special problem arises in children up to the age of 8 years. Approximately 25% will demonstrate a "pseudosubluxation" at the C2–3 level, attributed to laxity of the ligaments.[8] This can be confirmed by examining the spinolaminar line, which will maintain a normal relationship in cases of pseudosubluxation. In addition, in approximately

20% of patients in this age group, over half of the anterior arch of the atlas lies above the tip of the dens. This should not be misinterpreted as atlantoaxial dislocation. Furthermore, the space between the posterior surface of the anterior arch of C1 and the anterior surface of the dens may widen in flexion up to 6 mm in children, although it remains constant in adults.

Kyphosis, or a localized flexion angulation, usually occurs as a result of narrowing of the vertebral bodies anteriorly in both compression fractures and burst fractures (Fig. 4–15). This finding is more common in both burst fractures of the cervical spine and in the thoracic or lumbar spine (Fig. 4–16). Widening of the interspinous distance or interfacet joints is also a sign of a posterior distractive force, commonly associated with a flexion injury pattern (Fig. 4–17). Asymmetry of the disc space is also a useful sign, suggesting ligamentous damage to the longitudinal ligament at the site of widening.

If additional plain radiographic examination is war-

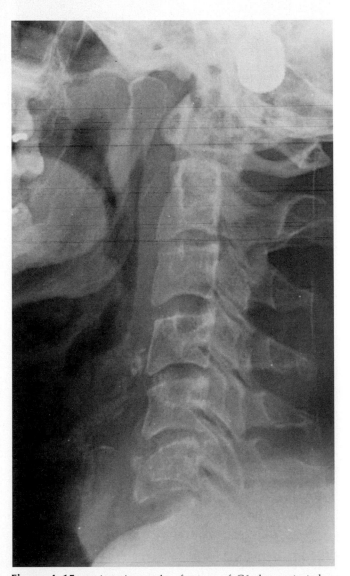

Figure 4–15 = Anterior wedge fracture of C6 demonstrated on lateral radiograph.

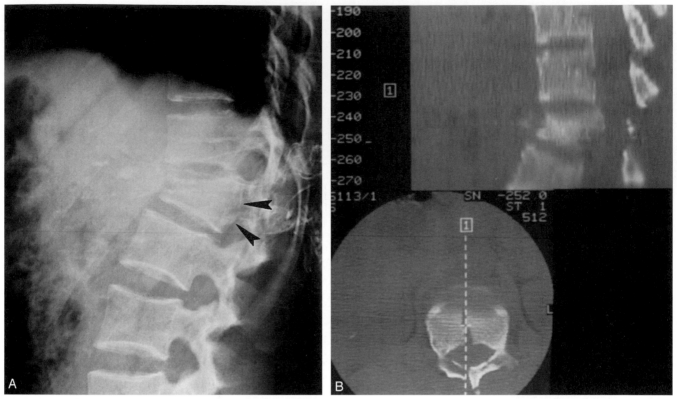

Figure 4–16 = *A,* Burst fracture of L1 seen on a lateral radiograph. There is the impression of posterior bowing of the posterior vertebral body line *(arrowheads). B,* CT image with sagittal reformatting demonstrates the fracture through the body and lamina of L1, with obvious posterior bowing of the dorsal fragment of the vertebral body.

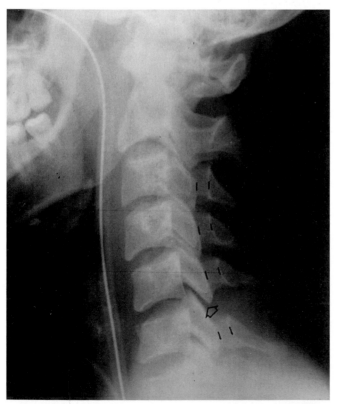

Figure 4–17 = Hyperflexion injury seen on a lateral radiograph. There is a small chip fracture of the superior aspect of C6 anteriorly, with widening of the interspinous distance at C5–6, and of the interfacet joint at this level *(arrow).*

ranted, anteroposterior (AP), and open-mouth AP odontoid views can be obtained (see Fig. 4–12). The incidence of injury to C7 in cervical injuries has been reported to be as high as 30%, although in our experience this figure is too high. Nevertheless, if C7 is not fully visualized, additional radiographic projections should be used. Swimmer's views or caudad pulling of the shoulders may be helpful, but tomography or CT may be needed to visualize this region fully. Oblique views are useful for defining the neural foramina, and may clarify a fracture of the articular pillars. However, in practice we find these views of limited value, as they are usually apparent on the lateral view. "Pillar views" of the cervical spine are also advocated by some authors, although we do not routinely obtain them.[10] If an abnormality is not seen by routine AP and lateral plain film evaluation in a clinical setting, suggesting a fracture or dislocation, more definitive additional studies are mandatory in any case. These include flexion-extension lateral radiographs, multidirectional tomography, or preferably CT. These provide additional information as to normality or abnormality, and are indicated in the symptomatic patient, whether the oblique or pillar views demonstrate abnormality or not. Oblique or pillar views merely add time, expense, and irradiation, without providing the definitive answer so easily obtained with CT.

In the alert, unsedated, and nonintoxicated patient, upright lateral cervical spine films may demonstrate malalignment that is not evident on supine lateral

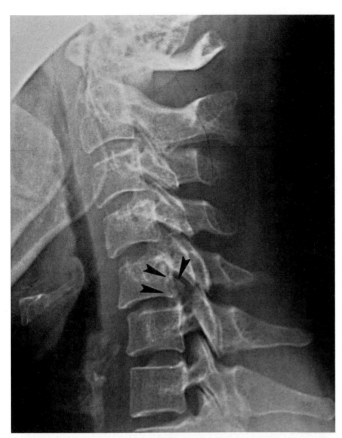

Figure 4–18 = Hyperflexion injury with facet fracture. There is mild kyphotic deformity at C5–6, with disc space narrowing, and mild anterior displacement of C5 relative to C6. In addition, there is an abrupt change in the orientation of the articular pillars at C5, suggesting a localized rotational deformity. The anterosuperior aspect of one of the articular pillars of C6 is also visualized displaced anteriorly, indicating a fracture through the articular pillar *(arrowheads)*.

films. Supervised flexion-extension views may be performed in these patients, preferably with the patient limiting the degree of motion in response to any elicited symptoms.

Hyperflexion Injury Patterns

In hyperflexion injuries, a predictable progression of changes is seen, depending on the severity of ligamentous injury and the ligaments involved. In mild hyperflexion sprain, there is early "fanning" of the dorsal spines, which may be an isolated finding, although there may be associated widening of the interfacet joint (see Fig. 4–17). This indicates interspinous and capsular ligament involvement.[25, 36] Widening of the posterior intervertebral space suggests posterior longitudinal ligament rupture and distal disruption in addition (see Fig. 4–10). Flexion-extension views may also be helpful in determining ligamentous damage in the neurologically intact patient. If subluxation of the vertebra is seen, this indicates rupture or stripping of the anterior longitudinal ligament, although it must be remembered that vertebral subluxation may also be due to articular pillar injury or facet subluxation or dislocation (Fig.

4–18). There may be a localized kyphosis at the level of injury. Although Harris and Mirvis[22] believe that these are stable injuries that may proceed to "delayed instability" in up to 20% of cases, Scher[36] believes that they are unstable, with the degree of displacement on initial radiograph an unreliable indicator of cord injury because of possible spontaneous reduction before examination. When one appreciates the ligamentous damage that must occur in these injuries, the natural reduction applied by positioning a support collar at the site of injury, and the associated edema and spasm in the acute setting, the latter argument seems more likely.

With complete disruption of the disc and posterior ligamentous groups, the "flexed" vertebra is free to ride forward, with the inferior articular facets either coming to rest on top of the superior facets of the vertebra below (perched facets; Fig. 4–19), or leapfrogging over them as in bilateral locked facets (Fig. 4–20). Although most common in the lower cervical spine, this can occur as high as C2 as well as in the thoracic and lumbar regions. The affected vertebra is dislocated by greater than 50% with respect to its inferior neighbor. Neurologic deficit is common, unless fractures through the posterior arch occur, thus decompressing the cord.

A simple wedge fracture occurs as a result of com-

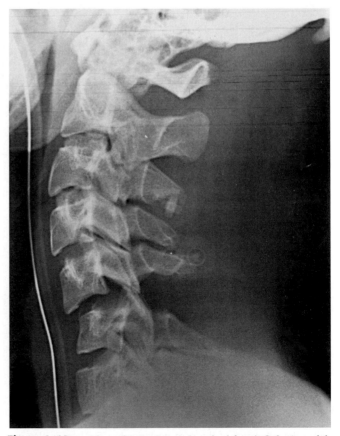

Figure 4–19 = Hyperflexion injury (perched facet). Splaying of the spinous processes at C5–6 is seen with localized kyphotic deformity and anterior displacement of C5 relative to C6. The inferior aspects of the articular pillars of C5 are perched on the superior pillars of C6.

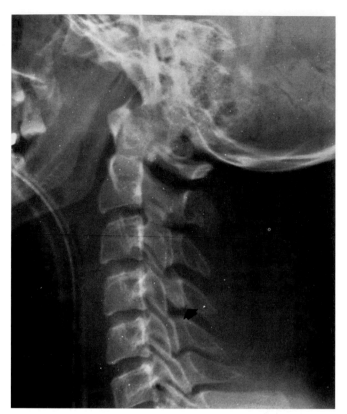

Figure 4–24 ═ Abrupt narrowing of the laminar facet interspace at C4 *(arrow)* is due in this case to posterior displacement of the entire articular pillar. This indicates fracture at the pedicle and the lamina.

this can be mimicked by a fracture dislocation of an articular pillar[46] (Fig. 4–24). Fanning of the spinous process and anterior subluxation of the dislocated vertebra of up to 7 mm with respect to the vertebra below may be seen. These signs, however, are extremely variable in their presentation. The diagnosis may be confirmed by oblique views, tomography, or CT, the last two techniques being useful in determining associated fractures of the articular pillars. Fractures of the articular pillars are commonly associated, and although they may be appreciated on plain radiography, are better seen with CT or tomography (Fig. 4–25).

Hyperextension Injury Patterns

Hyperextension injuries in contrast to flexion injuries involve ligamentous damage which is predominantly anterior. By definition, the anterior longitudinal ligament is disrupted, and there is variable posterior displacement of the vertebra above the level of injury[6, 37] (Fig. 4–26). It must be remembered, however, that stabilization of the head and neck by the emergency team may reduce this dislocation, giving rise to a virtually normal-appearing spine on the lateral radiograph. However, there is usually a mild asymmetry of the intervertebral disc space, with widening anteriorly.[10, 12] The posterior longitudinal ligament is either stripped from the subjacent vertebra or disrupted, and the inter-

vertebral disc is either ruptured or separated from the vertebra and plate. The cord is pinched between the dislocated vertebral body and the buckled ligamentum flavum and lamina, with neurologic damage ranging from transient paresthesia to complete quadriplegia, depending on the severity of the injury. In these injuries, there is generally marked prevertebral soft tissue swelling secondary to disruption of the anterior longitudinal ligament. Fracture of the posterior arch of the atlas may occur as a result of compression between the occiput and spinous process of C2. At the level of injury there may be crush fractures of the articular pillars and lamina that may be subjected to compressive forces (Fig. 4–27). With fractures through the posterior elements, and disruption of the anterior longitudinal ligament, there may be significant instability, giving rise to a misleading anterior displacement at the time of initial examination (see Fig. 4–27). This is similar to the appearances seen in the "low hangman's fracture" (see later).

Hyperextension of the upper cervical spine, often resulting from deceleration injuries with the head striking the windshield or surrounds, results in a form of posterior rotation of the skull. The occiput is driven downward onto the upper cervical spine, giving rise to the hangman's fracture.[30] The superficial resemblance to the victims of hanging furnishes a poor analogy, because the forces are completely at variance, one injury being caused by massive hyperextension and the other by axial distraction and rotation. In a hangman's fracture the result of the injury is a bilateral fracture through the pars interarticularis of C2, which may extend obliquely into the body of C2 (Fig. 4–28). There is variable forward displacement of the cervicocranium with respect to the spine below C2, due to the rotational force on the skull; this delivers an inferiorly and anteriorly directed vector onto the cervical spine. Cord damage is variable owing to the wide canal diameter at this level. Prevertebral soft tissue swelling may occur, but is often absent. The fracture is usually easily diagnosed on lateral radiographs, but CT provides useful additional information as to the presence and nature of the injury to the body of C2 (see Fig. 4–28).

An interesting variation of the hangman's fracture may be seen at lower levels of the spine, and again is due to excessive hyperextension. There is a posterior rotational force of the superior spine in the sagittal plane, giving rise to an apparently paradoxical injury force delivered to the vertebra in an inferior anterior direction. This causes oblique fractures of the articular pillars, or posterior arch, and an anteriorly directed force onto the superior vertebra, exacerbating anterior ligamentous disruption and giving rise to anterior displacement of the vertebra, superior to the site of injury (Fig. 4–29).

True whiplash injuries are of considerable interest, as the mechanism involves both hyperflexion and hyperextension. A combination of hyperflexion and hyperextension injuries is therefore seen (Fig. 4–30). Although not covered in detail in the literature, this is not a rare occurrence, and should always be ruled out in major auto accident injuries.

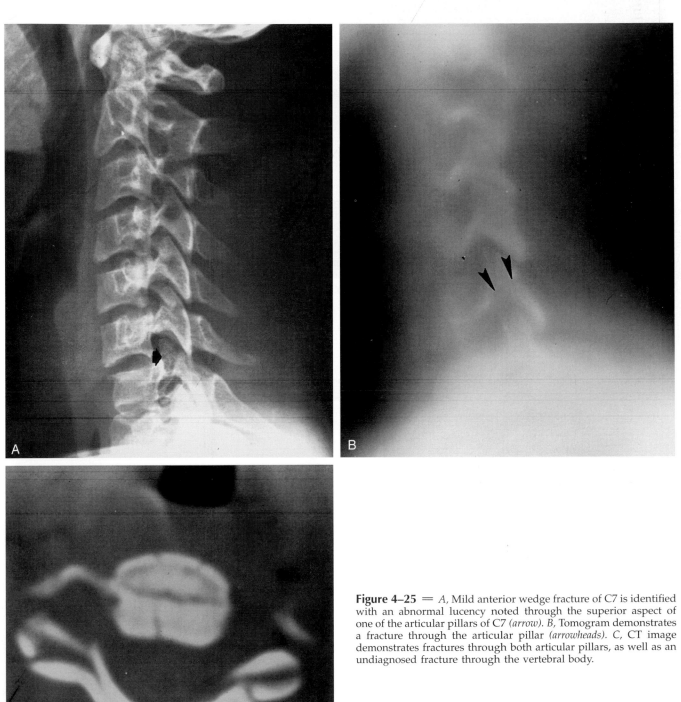

Figure 4–25 = *A*, Mild anterior wedge fracture of C7 is identified with an abnormal lucency noted through the superior aspect of one of the articular pillars of C7 *(arrow)*. *B*, Tomogram demonstrates a fracture through the articular pillar *(arrowheads)*. *C*, CT image demonstrates fractures through both articular pillars, as well as an undiagnosed fracture through the vertebral body.

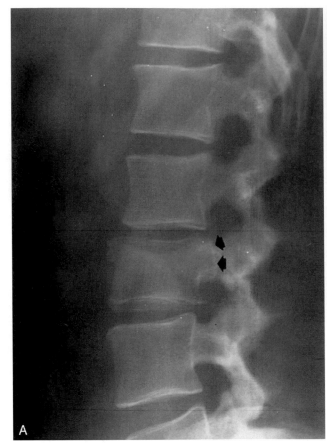

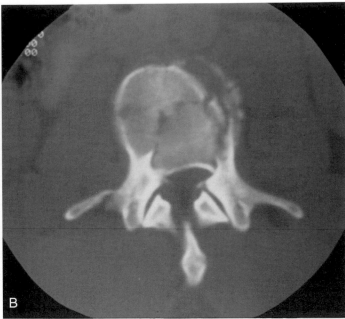

Figure 4–32 = A, Compression fracture of L3 with the suspicion of posterior displacement of the posterior aspect of the vertebral body *(arrows)*. B, CT scan better demonstrates the extent of the fracture of the vertebral body, and near complete occlusion of the spinal canal by the retropulsed fragment.

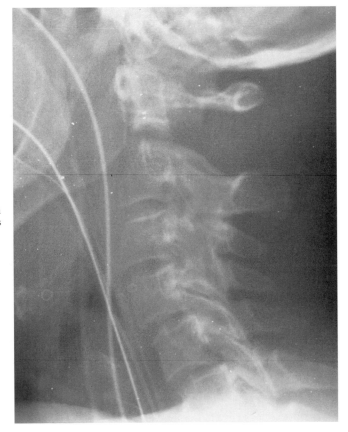

Figure 4–33 = Low odontoid fracture (type II). Lateral radiograph demonstrates obvious fracture through the base of the odontoid process with mild displacement.

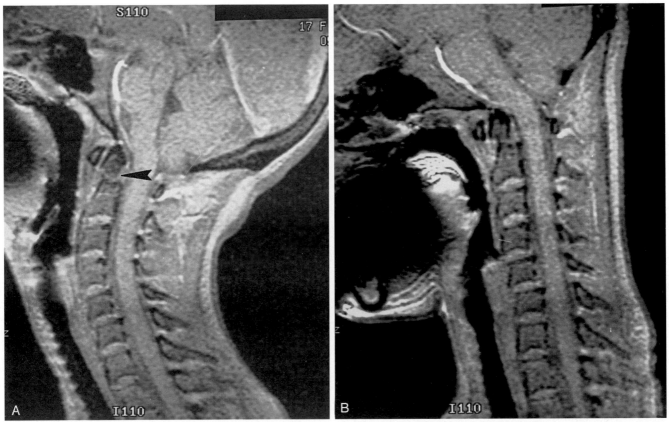

Figure 4–34 = Type II fracture of the odontoid: flexion and extension MRI. *A,* Rapid gradient echo midline sagittal image of the cervical spine demonstrates a fracture through the base of the odontoid, which is anteriorly displaced *(arrowhead). B,* In flexion, the odontoid does not move significantly with respect to the body of C2. There is no evidence of significant impingement on the cervicomedullary junction. Each of these images requires only a few seconds to obtain.

cord. Flexion-extension MRI can also be performed (Fig. 4–34). Nonunited high dens fractures are inherently unstable and, indeed, are postulated as one of the likely causes of os odontoideum[18] (Fig. 4–35). It has also been suggested that os odontoideum is the result of nonunion of a superior ossification center of the dens. However acquired, the radiographic appearance is diagnostic, with a characteristic smooth convex border on the tip of the odontoid stump. Instability may be demonstrated with flexion-extension views (Fig. 4–35).

Low dens fractures are not true odontoid fractures, but involve the body of C2 to a greater or lesser degree. As such, they usually involve cancellous bone, and good bone healing usually occurs. Again, this is an inherently unstable injury. A helpful radiographic sign of low dens injuries is interruption of the axis ring (Fig. 4–36), composed of the cortex of the junction of the pedicle and antrum anteriorly and the cortex of the junction of the odontoid and body superiorly. Harris and co-workers[23] in their series found this sign to be positive in all patients with a low fracture, although in our experience, this is not always the case. Smoker and Dolan[38] suggested that widening of the AP diameter of C2 relative to C3 (the "fat" C2 sign) constitutes another radiographic feature of low C2 fractures. However, in such cases the fracture is almost always evident. In some patients with persistent upper cervical spine pain and nondisplaced odontoid or C2 body fractures, care-

fully supervised flexion-extension lateral views may demonstrate the injury.

Rotatory Subluxation of C1–2

Rotatory subluxation of C1–2 occurs when there is axial rotation of C1 with respect to C2, involving the interfacet joint either unilaterally or bilaterally. It may be suspected on the frontal view (open-mouth odontoid projection) by asymmetry of visualized facet joints, usually in conjunction with asymmetry of the distance between the odontoid and lateral masses of C2 (Fig. 4–37). It must be remembered that the latter sign can also be seen as a normal appearance if the head is mildly rotated, or there is mild lateral flexion. Therefore, both signs should be sought concurrently, and the diagnosis made in the appropriate clinical setting. Tomography is often diagnostic (see Fig. 4–37) and is preferred to CT, where the diagnosis can be missed if the subtle alteration in the axis of C1 and C2 is not appreciated, and 2-D or 3-D reformatting is not performed. Kowalski et al.[27] have suggested that locked rotatory subluxation of C1 on C2 can be established by thin-section axial CT scanning with the patient's head turned first to one side and then to the other. In patients with "locked subluxation," the rotation between C1 and C2 is fixed and will not be altered by changes in head position, as opposed to transient torticollis.

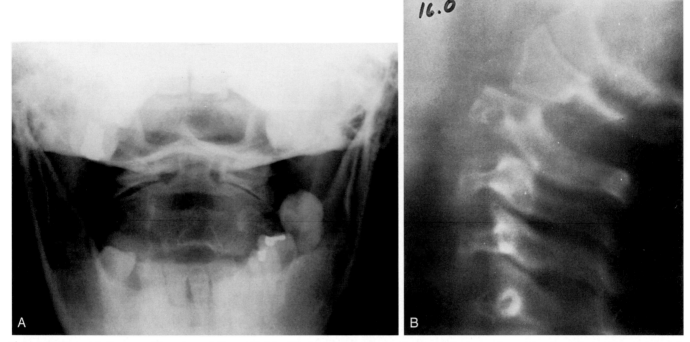

Figure 4–37 = *A,* Rotary subluxation of C1 on C2, identified on the open-mouth odontoid view, where there is obvious asymmetry of the C1–2 joint space bilaterally. *B,* Lateral tomogram demonstrates posterior displacement of the articular facet of C1 relative to C2.

FRACTURES OF THE THORACOLUMBAR SPINE

Injuries to the thoracic and lumbar portions of the spine are similar in many ways, and are discussed together. Plain film examination is the initial method of investigating the thoracolumbar spine. Ideally, AP and lateral views should be obtained, but in traumatized unstable patients or in patients with neurologic deficit, a cross-table lateral view alone should be obtained initially so as to prevent further injury by moving the patient into a lateral position. The lateral radiograph of the lumbar spine is centered at L2–3 and should include the lower thoracic spine. Because of the divergence of the x-ray beam, an additional radiograph centered over the lumbosacral region may be necessary to better define this area. It is often difficult to obtain satisfactory views of the upper two or three thoracic vertebrae on the lateral radiograph because of the superimposed shoulders. To counter this, some authors advocate use of the swimmer's view[34] and others suggest that oblique views of this area may be helpful in defining the anatomic structures.[2, 12] In the patient with neurologic deficit, however, it may be judicious to move directly to CT particularly if a fast CT scanner is available. The AP view of the thoracic spine as a whole may also be poor because of the overlying cardiac and mediastinal shadows. Overpenetrated views may be helpful for better evaluation of the upper thoracic spine.[24] Also, the posterior elements in the thoracic spine are not as easy to evaluate in the AP projection as they are in the lumbar spine because of the more vertical orientation of the articular facets. Extra views

are not routinely obtained in our institution and the examination of this region is tailored to the clinical picture and the appearance of the available AP and lateral radiographs.

The diagnosis of injury to the posterior elements of the spine is an important part of the examination and may be appreciated on the frontal projection by disruption of the pedicles (Fig. 4–38) or neural arch, widening of the interpedicular distance, or by appreciation of a break in the continuity of the bony structures (Fig. 4–39). A "vacant" appearance of a vertebral body may be seen and is due to a posterior ligamentous disruption, allowing superior displacement of a vertebra on its subjacent neighbor, which is no longer overlain by these structures. This last finding is most evident in cases of facet dislocation. Appreciation of the posterior element injury on the frontal view is important, as it may indicate spinal instability. Furthermore, the posterior elements may be difficult to see on a lateral view because of overlying ribs and soft tissues, or a diagnostic lateral view may not be available.[31] Although plain films may indicate the injury (see Fig. 4–32), CT is much more effective in determining the site and extent of injury (see Figs. 4–32*B,* 4–40*B* and *C*) and, as in the cervical spine, CT-myelography or MRI (Figs. 4–41 and 4–42) is useful in defining damage to the cord.

In addition to the examination of the bony structures, signs of soft tissue injury should be sought. These include paravertebral soft tissue prominence (Fig. 4–43), loss of the psoas shadow (Fig. 4–44), and examination of the visible hepatic, splenic, or renal shadows.

Compression fractures, with or without associated hyperflexion, are the commonest injuries to the thora-

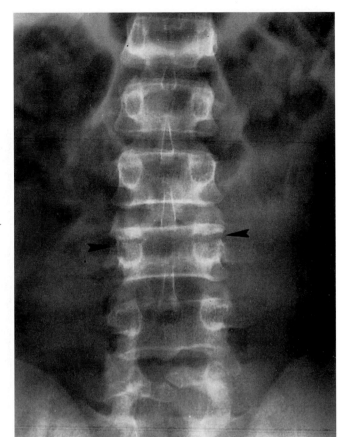

Figure 4–38 = Horizontal fracture through the pedicle of L3 *(arrowheads)* indicative of a lap belt injury.

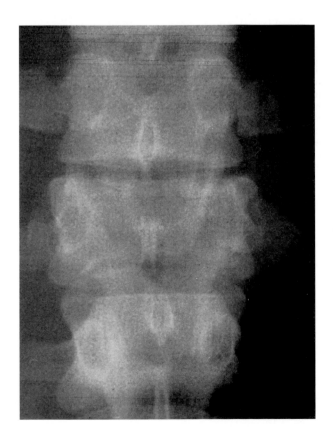

Figure 4–39 = Compression fracture of T12 with "widening" of the vertebral body, and separation of the pedicles as compared to L1.

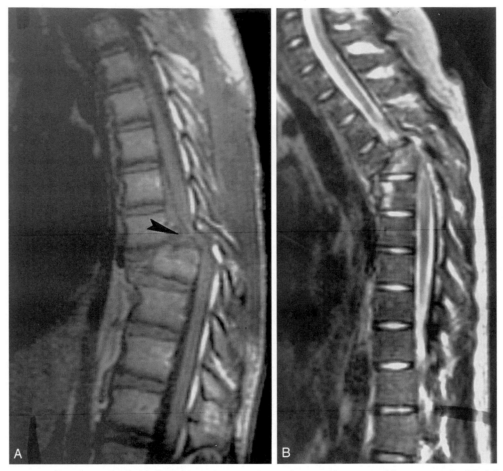

Figure 4–42 = Thoracic fracture-dislocation. *A,* T1-weighted image demonstrates a fracture subluxation at the T8–9 level with significant compromise of the spinal canal and spinal cord compression. The abnormal signal between the posterior surface of T8 and the thecal sac represents an epidural hematoma *(arrowhead). B,* T4–5 fracture subluxation in a different patient demonstrates abnormal signal within the fractured T5 vertebral body and within the compressed spinal cord. The spinal cord was essentially transected in this patient. The abnormal signal intensity within the spinal cord probably represents a combination of edema and hemorrhage.

columbar spine. The fracture pattern depends upon the magnitude of the force.

In simple hyperflexion (stage I), as described by Ferguson and Allen,[17] there is buckling of the anterior vertebral body only. The fulcrum of rotation is at the midportion of the vertebra, and there is, therefore, by simple mechanics, a compressive force anteriorly and a distractive force posteriorly. As a result, there is no posterior ligament damage and the spine is stable. In stage II injuries, there is greater posterior distractive force, leading to posterior ligament disruption, and a greater incidence of neurologic damage (Fig. 4–45). In stage III injuries, there is greater than 50% loss of vertebral height, and the posterior aspect of the vertebral body is involved, often with retropulsion of the posterior fragments. This picture therefore closely resembles the burst fracture, and carries the same implications for repair, necessitating a distractive force.

Although plain radiographs will show anterior wedging, they are not adequate in visualizing the posterior elements. CT is obligatory to assess the bony integrity of the middle and posterior elements, and MRI may prove to be the most effective modality for examining the spinal cord and even the posterior ligaments.

Seat Belt Fractures

A special type of hyperflexion injury occurs as the result of the wearing of seat belts in deceleration accidents. The belt acts as a fulcrum for massive flexion, usually at the L1 or L2 level. This results in a distraction force on the spine, and is further exacerbated by the continued forward motion of the upper torso, which is transferred into an axial distraction by the bending of the lower spine. The result is a distraction force on the posterior spine and an anterior shearing force caused by the continued forward motion of the superior spinal segments, with the inferior portion of the victim's body being held secure by the seat belt. Rarely, there may be anterior wedging of the vertebral body, resulting from the initial hyperflexion component of the injury, although this is usually very mild. In general, the anterior column is regarded as being uninvolved.

The "seat belt syndrome" is a term coined by Garrett and Braunstein[19] to describe an association of injuries found in massive deceleration injuries to passengers wearing seat belts. In addition to the seat belt fracture of the spine, injuries to the spinal cord or cauda equina, ruptures of the spleen, pancreas, and second or third

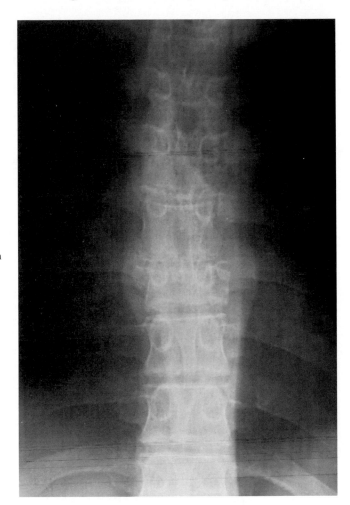

Figure 4–43 = Widening of the paraspinal soft tissues surrounding a fracture of T8 identified on anteroposterior radiograph.

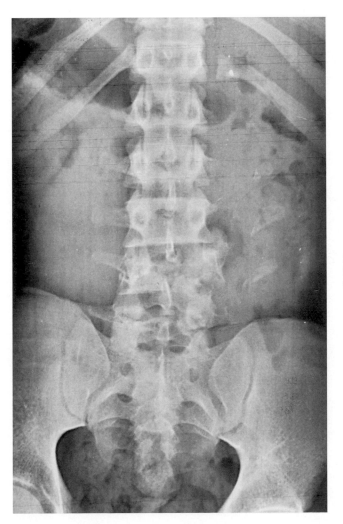

Figure 4–44 = Fracture of L4 and of the lateral processes of L2–4 on the left. There is obliteration of the psoas shadow on the left, indicative of hematoma.

part of the duodenum, tears of the small bowel, rupture of the musculature of the abdominal wall, and abrasions of the abdominal wall at the site of the seat belt may be seen. In addition, rupture of the gravid uterus and circumferential laceration of the serosa of the sigmoid colon have been reported. Thus when a seat belt fracture is seen, a careful search for abdominal visceral injury should be made. CT scanning is particularly useful in the evaluation of associated injuries, but MRI is probably the most effective modality to define the spinal cord injury (see Fig. 4–45).

Hyperflexion Injuries

Upper and midthoracic fractures are less common and are usually seen in severe osteoporosis or as a result of massive trauma. They are associated with a higher incidence of neurologic symptoms than are fractures of the thoracolumbar spine. Many injuries result from hyperflexion. There may be associated anterior dislocation of the vertebra above the level of compression, and fracture may occur at multiple levels. It may be especially difficult to determine involvement of the posterior cortex and posterior elements on plain lateral radiographs, due to factors such as overlying ribs. As in the cervical spine, CT, or if not available, at least tomography, is mandatory for evaluation of the

extent of injury, and MRI may have a role to play in evaluating the nature and extent of cord injury.

As in the cervical spine, dislocations are commonly associated with cord damage. This may be evaluated by CT-myelography, but MRI is proving an effective alternative (see Fig. 4–45).

In adults, fractures of the thoracolumbar junction account for up to 60% of thoracic and lumbar fractures. This is probably due to the transitional nature of this region, with alteration of alignment of the apophyseal joints; alteration from a rigid thoracic spine, protected by ribs and intercostal muscles, to a more mobile lumbar spine; and alteration of spinal curvature. Fractures are generally the result of compression and flexion forces, with the injury pattern following that of the thoracic spine. The integrity or disruption of the dorsal cortex of the vertebral body is of considerable importance, and cannot be judged accurately by plain radiographs. CT, or at least tomography, is required for full evaluation (see Fig. 4–40).

It must be remembered that crush fractures of the vertebra are associated with calcaneal fractures, and patients with these injuries should always be subjected to examination of the spine, as spinal fractures may be masked initially.

Hyperextension injuries of the thoracic and lumbar spine are also seen, but less commonly than in the

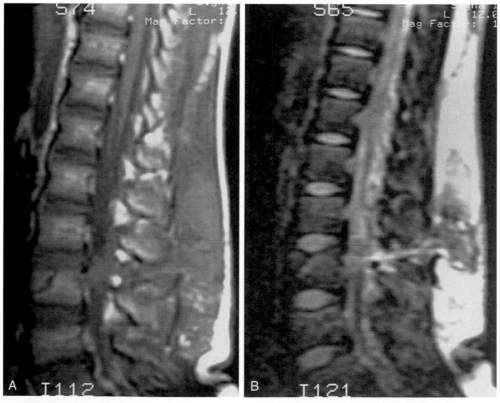

Figure 4–45 = Lap seat belt injury with avulsion of the cauda equina. *A,* T1-weighted sagittal image demonstrates horizontal fracture through the posterior elements of L3, and an anterior compression fracture. The nerve roots of the cauda equina cannot be identified. Abnormal signal intensity within the spinal canal at the L3 level represents clot. *B,* T2-weighted sagittal image demonstrates heterogeneous signal intensity within the thecal sac due to hemorrhage. A horizontally oriented band of bright signal intensity extends through the dorsal elements at the L3 level and there is heterogeneous signal posterior to the spinous processes here as well. At surgery, nerve roots were encountered protruding through the dorsal elements at the L3 level.

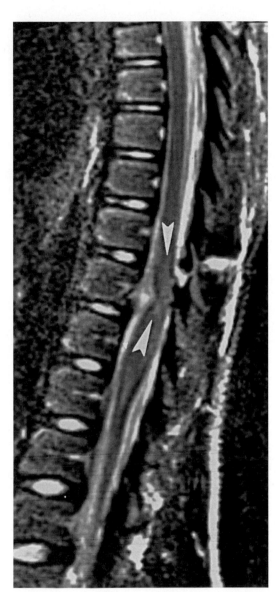

Figure 4–46 ═ Stab wound with cord laceration. This child tried to intervene in a fight between her father and uncle and was accidentally stabbed. This T2-weighted sagittal image demonstrates the trajectory of the knife blade through the dorsal elements and spinal cord *(arrowheads)*. There is abnormal signal intensity within the cord at, above, and below the level of the cord laceration.

cervical spine. Although extremely rare, excessive hyperextension can give rise to a type of low hangman's fracture with oblique fractures through the vertebra, and paradoxical anterior displacement of the spine superior to the site of injury.

Cord damage may also occur as the result of penetrating injuries, and can best be evaluated by CT-myelography or MRI (Fig. 4–46), particularly as there may be little or no overt bony injury.

REFERENCES

1. Anderson LD, D'Alonzo RT: Fractures of the odontoid process of the axis. J Bone Joint Surg Am 56:1663–1672, 1974.
2. Angtuaco EJC, Binet EF: Radiology of thoracic and lumbar fractures. Clin Orthop 189:43–57, 1984.
3. Atlas SW, Regenbogen V, Rogers LF, et al: The radiographic characterization of burst fractures of the spine. AJR 147:575–582, 1986.
4. Berquist TH: Diagnostic Imaging of the Acutely Injured Patient. Baltimore, Urban & Schwarzenberg, 1985, pp 39–68.
5. Brant-Zawadski M, Jeffrey RB, Minagi H, et al: High resolution CT of thoracolumbar fractures. AJR 138:699–704, 1982.
6. Burke DC: Hyperextension injuries of the spine. J Bone Joint Surg Br 53:3–11, 1971.
7. Cacayorin ED, Kieffer SA: Applications and limitations of computed tomography of the spine. Radiol Clin North Am 20:185–206, 1982.
8. Cattell HS, Filtzer DL: Pseudosubluxation and other normal variations of the cervical spine in children. J Bone Joint Surg Am 47:1295, 1965.
9. Chiroff RT, Sachs BL: Discontinuity of the spinous process on standard roentgenographs as an aid in the diagnosis of unstable fractures of the spine. J Trauma 16:313–318, 1976.
10. Cintron E, Gilula LA, Murphy WA, et al: The widened disk space: A sign of cervical hyperextension injury. Radiology 141:639–644, 1981.
11. Daffner RH: Imaging of Vertebral Trauma. Rockville, Md, Aspen, 1988.
12. Daffner RH, Deeb ZL, Rothfus WE: "Fingerprints" of vertebral trauma—A unifying concept based on mechanisms. Skeletal Radiol 15:518–525, 1986.
13. Denis F: The three column spine and its significance in classification of acute thoracolumbar spinal injuries. Spine 8:817–831, 1983.
14. Edeiken-Monroe B, Wagner LK, Harris JH Jr: Hyperextension dislocation of the cervical spine. AJNR 7:335–341, 1986.
15. Evans DK: Anterior cervical subluxation. J Bone Joint Surg Br 58:318–325, 1976.
16. Federle MP, Brant-Zawadski MN (eds): Computed Tomography in the Evaluation of Trauma. Baltimore, Williams & Wilkins, 1983.
17. Ferguson RL, Allen BL: A mechanistic classification of thoracolumbar spine fractures. Clin Orthop 189:77–88, 1984.
18. Fielding JW, Griffin PP: Os odontoideum: An acquired lesion. J Bone Joint Surg Am 56:187–196, 1974.
19. Garrett JW, Braunstein PW: Seat belt syndrome. J Trauma 2:220–227, 1962.
20. Gehweiler JA, Osborne RL, Becker RF: The Radiology of Vertebral Trauma. Philadelphia, WB Saunders, 1980.
21. Goldberg AL, Rothfus WE, Deeb ZZ, et al: Impact of magnetic resonance on the diagnostic evaluation of acute cervicothoracic spinal trauma. Skeletal Radiol 17:89–97, 1988.
22. Harris JH, Mirvis SE (eds): Hyperflexion Injuries, ed 3. Baltimore, Williams & Wilkins, 1995, pp 245–289.
23. Harris JH Jr, Burke JT, Ray RD, et al: Low (type III) odontoid fracture: A new radiologic sign. Radiology 153:353–356, 1984.
24. Harris JH Jr, Harris WM: The Radiology of Emergency Medicine. Baltimore, Williams & Wilkins, 1975.
25. Holdsworth FW: Fractures, dislocations, and fracture dislocations of the spine. J Bone Joint Surg Am 52:1534–1551, 1970.
26. Keene JS, Goletz TH, Lilleas F, et al: Diagnosis of vertebral fracture: A comparison of conventional radiography. J Bone Joint Surg Am 64:586–594, 1982.
27. Kowalski HM, Cohen WA, Cooper P, et al: Pitfalls in the CT diagnosis of atlantoaxial rotatory subluxation. AJR 149:595–600, 1987.
28. Kulkarni MY, McArdle CB, Kopanicky D, et al: Acute spinal cord injury: MR imaging at 1.5T. Radiology 164:837–843, 1987.
29. Mirvis SE, Geisler FH, Jelinek JJ, et al: Acute cervical spine trauma: Evaluation with 1.5T MR imaging. Radiology 166:807–816, 1988.
30. Mirvis SE, Young JWR, Lim C, et al: Hangman's fracture: Radiologic assessment in 27 cases. Radiology 163:713–717, 1986.
31. Nicoll EA: Fractures of the dorso-lumbar spine. J Bone Joint Surg Br 31:376–394, 1949.
32. Rennie W, Mitchell N: Flexion distraction fractures of the thoracolumbar spine. J Bone Joint Surg Am 55:386–394, 1973.
33. Roab IW, Drayer BP: Spinal computed tomography: Limitations and applications. AJR 133:267, 1979.
34. Rogers LR: Radiology of Skeletal Trauma. New York, Churchill Livingstone, 1982.

35. Scher AT: Unilateral lateral facet in cervical spine injuries. AJR 129:45–48, 1977.
36. Scher AT: Anterior cervical subluxation: An unstable position. AJR 133:275–283, 1979.
37. Scher AT: Diversity of radiologic features in hyperextension injury of the cervical spine. S Afr Med J 58:27–36, 1980.
38. Smoker WRK, Dolan KD: The "fat" C2: A sign of fracture. AJNR 8:33–38, 1987.
39. Steppe R, Bellemans M, Boven F, et al: The value of computed tomography scanning in elusive fractures of the cervical spine. Skeletal Radiol 6:175–178, 1981.
40. Tarr RW, Drolshagen LF, Kerner TC, et al: MR imaging of recent spinal trauma. J Comput Assist Tomogr 11:412–419, 1987.
41. Templeton PA, Young JWR, Mirvis SE, et al: The value of retropharyngeal soft tissue measurement in trauma of the adult cervical spine. Skeletal Radiol 16:98–104, 1987.
42. Weir DC: Roentgenographic signs of cervical injury. Clin Orthop 109:9–17, 1975.
43. White AA, Johnson RM, Panjab MD, et al: Biomedical analysis of clinical stability in the cervical spine. Clin Orthop 109:85–93, 1975.
44. Wojcik WG, Edeiken-Monroe BS, Harris JH Jr: Three-dimensional computed tomography in acute cervical spine trauma: A preliminary report. Skeletal Radiol 16:261–269, 1987.
45. Wojcik WG, Harris JH Jr: Three dimensional CT scanning in the evaluation of acute spinal trauma. Radiology 157:236, 1985.
46. Young JWR, Mirvis SE: Cervical spine trauma. *In* Mirvis SE, Young JWR (eds): Imaging in Trauma and Critical Care. Baltimore, Williams & Wilkins, 1992, pp 291–379.
47. Young JWR, Resnik CS, DeCandido P, et al: The laminar space in the diagnosis of rotational flexion injuries of the cervical spine. AJR 152:103–107, 1989.

CHAPTER 5

Vascular Anatomy of the Spine

Glenn Amundson ‖ *Steven R. Garfin* ‖ *Wesley W. Parke*

THE ARTERIAL ANATOMY

Thoracolumbar Anatomy

The descending aorta lies over the left half of the anterior surface of the vertebral bodies from T2–L4. The segmental arteries arise in pairs, millimeters apart, near the posterior midline of the aorta (Fig. 5–1). These are the intercostal and lumbar arteries of the thoracic and lumbar regions, respectively. These vessels have a horizontal course from their origin from T6–L1, ascend to levels T3–5, and descend to the lower lumbar levels. The segmentals are closely applied to the anterolateral aspect of the midportion of the vertebral bodies, coursing toward the intervertebral foramina (Fig. 5–2).

On the vertebral body, two sets of branches are apparent (see Fig. 5–1). Anterior central branches enter vascular foramina subjacent to the segmental artery and penetrate radially to the midportion of the vertebral body. Ascending and descending branches form dense networks on the anterolateral aspects of the vertebral body and anterior longitudinal ligament. These vessels terminate by penetrating the vertebrae adjacent to each end plate.

Prior to entering the intervertebral foramen the segmental artery divides into three main sets of branches: anterior, intermediate, and posterior[3] (see Fig. 5–1). The anterior branch supplies the body wall, intercostal spaces, and lumbar region.

The intermediate (spinal canal) branches are derived from the posterior branch as it passes lateral to the intervertebral foramen. This branch may enter the fora-

men as a single vessel or it may arise from the dorsal segmental branch as a number of independent rami.[29] This represents the origin of the blood supply of the vertebral canal and neuromeningeal structures and is a site of great vascular vulnerability. The intermediate branches have three components. The anterior spinal branch divides immediately on entering the foramen, one limb ascending over the lateral one third of the disc, the other descending to course near the superior border of the inferior vertebral body's pedicle, anastomosing with the ascending limb of the lower segment. Transverse anastomoses between the two axes run over the middle of the vertebral body forming a network of collaterals in quadrangular fashion around the vertebrae. This arterial network penetrates posterior foramina as posterior central arteries, completing the blood supply to the vertebral body (Fig. 5–3).

The second intermediate branch supplies the vessels to the neuromeningeal structures of the thoracolumbar cord and cauda equina, best described by Parke and co-workers[27] most recently (Fig. 5–4). The neural branch accompanies the spinal nerve in the intervertebral foramen to supply the plexus of the dorsal root ganglion. This plexus is the origin of the dorsal and ventral distal radicular arteries which supply the distal two thirds of their respective roots (see Figs. 5–4 and 5–5). The dorsal ganglion plexus is also the source of the ventral and dorsal medullary arteries, when present. The medullary arteries course along the internal aspects of their respective roots, but give no branches to them in their midcourse. The ventral and dorsal medullary arteries anastomose and thereby supply the anterior spinal ar-

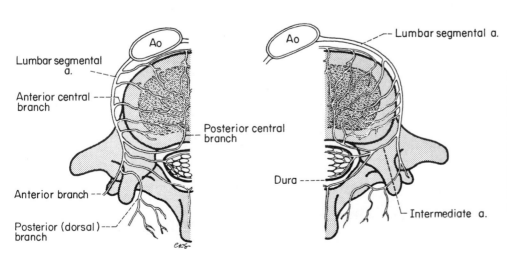

Figure 5–1 = Cross section through a typical lumbar vertebra at the level of the cauda equina, depicting the arterial supply at this level. The paired segmental vessels leaving the aorta (Ao) near the center of the body anterolaterally to the left of the midline are shown. The drawing on the left includes the anterior and posterior branches of the segmental artery. The right includes more details of the intermediate artery branch.

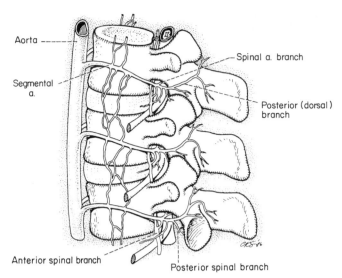

Figure 5–2 ═ Lateral depiction of three typical lumbar vertebrae with their arterial supply. The view is from the left side of the vertebral body. The segmental arteries course along the midline of the body in the concavity. A thin lateral arcade connects these segmental vessels. The segmental vessels enter the neuroforamen along the course of the spinal nerve as it exits the canal through the foramen.

tery and paired posterolateral spinal arteries, respectively. The anterior spinal artery (ASA) is supplied by fewer, but larger, medullary arteries than the posterolateral vessels. The medullary feeder vessels follow the obliquity of the spinal nerve roots to reach the cord. The posterolateral spinal arteries form a more plexiform and often-interrupted network on the dorsolateral

surface of the cord, receiving more numerous, but smaller, nutritive contributions from various segmental levels.

The ASA supplies most of the internal substance of the cord and almost all the gray matter (see Figs. 5–5 and 5–6A and B). In the midthoracic and thoracolumbar regions of the cord, this major blood source is often supplied by only a single feeder artery.[5, 20, 27] Both the anterior and posterior spinal arteries, through a highly anastomotic plexus (vasa corona), supply the circumferential medullary white matter. From the plexus of the vasa corona, the emerging ventral root fibers receive true proximal ventral radicular arteries that supply the proximal one third of each ventral root. The posterior spinal arteries, coursing just ventral to the merging rootlets, supply true proximal dorsal radicular arteries to the upper one third of the dorsal root. The proximal and distal radicular arteries anastomose in step-down fashion, creating an area where the directional flows abut and therefore approach a near-zero flow rate at the anastomoses or distally according to variations in the collateral demand. Though originally thought to be an area of relative hypovascularity, this anastomotic section, near the midportion of each dorsal and ventral root, is not hypovascular, but just demonstrates low directional flow[27] (see Fig. 5–4).

The third and final branch of the intermediate arterial branches is the posterior spinal (prelaminar) branch, which courses on and supplies the anterior surface of the lamina and ligamentum flavum (see Fig. 5–1). A laminar branch penetrates the posterior arch at its junction with the pedicle and bifurcates into a shorter ascending and a longer descending limb. Both

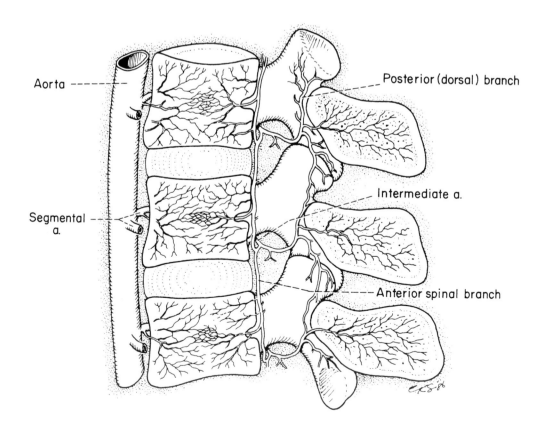

Figure 5–3 ═ Depiction of a sagittal cross section through the midportion of the vertebral bodies shown in Figure 5–2. Vessels within the cancellous body are graphically shown as they enter anteriorly and posteriorly. An anastomosis of the anterior, posterior, and central radiating vessels occurs at the level of the neuroforamen.

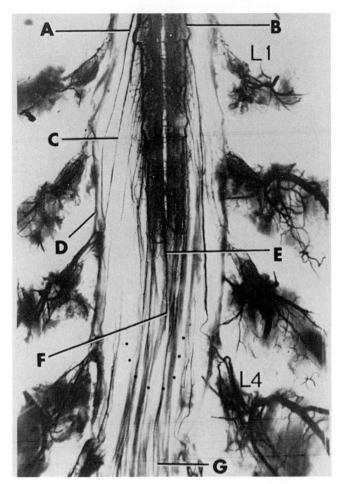

Figure 5–4 = This photograph shows the proximal source of blood supply from the anterior spinal artery and the distal source coming from the distal radicular arteries. The originally named area of "relative hypovascularity" has proved to be an unfortunate name as the vascular bed is rather uniform in length. The term was originally meant to indicate that there was some point near the middle of the root where the blood in the distal and proximal longitudinal radicular arteries met in an anastomotic channel, and the directional flow in the longitudinal segments at this level was near zero; but there is no true hypovascularity. This point may shift proximally or distally according to variations in the collateral demand. This photograph is a transillumination of the dorsal aspect of the fetal lumbosacral spinal cord under low magnification, showing the termination of the conus opposite the third lumbar ganglion. Below this point, the content of the vertebral canal consists only of the lumbosacral roots. The last dorsal medullary artery is seen following the right fourth lumbar nerve root, and all other vessels inferior to this are true radicular arteries. The area of "hypovascularity" (decreased directional flow) occurs between the radicular vessels and the proximal descending vessels, which is marked by the dotted U-shaped area distal to the conus. *A,* Small dorsal medullary artery of the third lumbar level. *B,* Right dorsolateral spinal artery. *C,* Ventral medullary artery from the third lumbar level. *D,* Strip of lateral dura left to preserve relationships. *E,* Anterior spinal artery terminating in the filum terminale *(F)*. *G,* Distal radicular vessels in the lower part of the cauda equina. These vessels ascend toward the proximal descending vessels. (From Parke WW, Gammell K, Rothman RH: Arterial vascularization of the cauda equina. J Bone Joint Surg Am 63:53, 1981.)

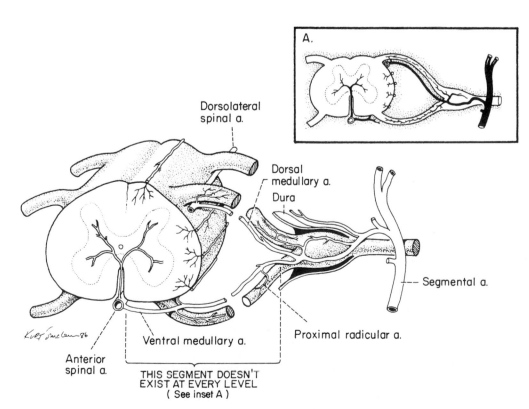

Figure 5–5 = The arterial blood supply to the spinal cord and nerve roots is depicted, but only those arteries supplying the spinal cord are labeled here. Similar arcades and communications occur along the spinal nerves and dorsal root ganglia. The anterior spinal artery is the major blood supply to the gray matter of the spinal cord. *Inset A* demonstrates vessels coursing along the anterior and posterior rami.

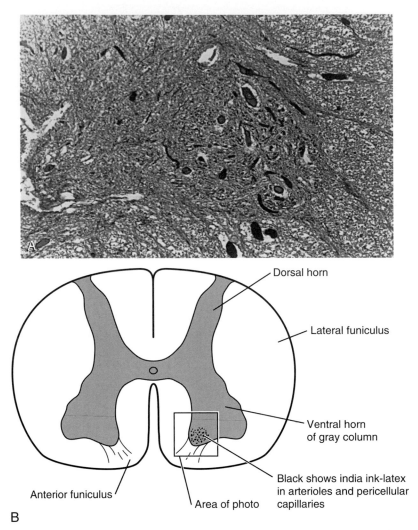

B

Figure 5–6 = *A,* This photomicrograph (×30) was taken from a cross section of the lumbosacral region of a human spinal cord that had an arterial injection with an India ink–latex mixture. It shows a group of motor nuclei localized in the medial tip of the ventral horn spinal gray matter and illustrates well a significant capillary concentration. The amount of capillaries increases in association with increased neuron cell bodies (see text). The dark-black ovals are areas where India ink–latex became affixed in the arterials and pericellular capillaries. *B,* Artist's depiction of cross section of the lumbosacral region of the human spinal cord. The squared area in the anterior gray matter is the section that the photomicrograph in *A* was taken from.

course in the center of the cancellous bone to their respective inferior and superior apophyseal joints. A central branch penetrates the base of the spinous process and runs toward its tip. Small branches supply the epidural fat and posterior dura.

The final division of the segmental artery is the posterior (dorsal) branch (see Fig. 5–1). It courses over the pars interarticularis and supplies the lamina, spinous process, apophyseal joint, and finally the sacrospinalis muscles.

The divisions and distribution of the posterior branch are well described by Macnab and Dall.[23] A knowledge of its course is important in anticipation and minimization of blood loss during posterior procedures, particularly intertransverse fusions.

The first division of the posterior branch is the interarticular artery, which passes along the lateral aspect of the pars interarticularis, curving medially over its posterior surface. It continues into the fibrofatty tissues immediately overlying the interlaminar space terminat-

ing in the sacrospinalis muscle. Two superior articular arteries are the next branches, passing posteriorly adjacent to the superolateral aspect of the facet joints. A larger communicating artery courses over the medial portion of the transverse process connecting the superior articular arteries to a single inferior articular artery. The inferior articular artery travels along the inferolateral aspect of the facet joint and pierces the intermediate layer of the fascia, and serves to anastomose with the adjacent level.

Other sources of potential hemorrhage include the intertransverse artery, which is a large branch of the lumbar artery originating at the level of the intervertebral foramen. It passes laterally along the anterior surface of the middle layer of the lumbar fascia midway between the transverse processes. The anterior transverse artery is another significant branch of the lumbar artery coursing adjacent to the anterior surface of the transverse process. Coagulation of these posterior vessels and avoidance of dissection anterior to the plane of the transverse processes minimize blood loss during intertransverse fusions and other posterior procedures.

There has been debate as to the vascular competence to the thoracic cord; the earliest anatomic studies suggested that there was a vascular fragility of the blood supply to the thoracic cord. Dommisse[5] and Dommisse and Grobler[6] showed that every nerve root enjoys an abundant arterial supply, which it receives in the form of small arteries, arterioles, precapillaries, and capillary vessels. However, these studies found an inconsistent and incomplete blood supply to the cord due to the absence of medullary feeder vessels accompanying the nerve roots at each segmental level. Similarly, Feeney and Watterson[7] observed that there exists a very close relationship between the metabolic requirements of the nervous tissue and the final distribution of the intraneural vessels in the adult. Apparently, the nervous system has a blood supply which is just adequate for its "needs." Regarding this limited blood supply, descriptions of the blood supply to the lumbosacral portion of the spinal cord refer to the existence of a single main artery known as the arteria medullaris magna (formerly the arteria radicularis magna) or artery of Adamkiewicz. It arises from an intercostal or lumbar artery (slightly more often from the left side), generally at the level of T8–L2, though occasionally from the fourth lumbar or first sacral artery. It was long believed that ligation of the artery of Adamkiewicz would lead to acute postoperative ischemia and paraplegia. Consequently, there were concerns that the thoracic spinal cord was highly prone to injury from vascular insults because of its marginal vascular supply from too few vessels supplying long areas.

Later studies of the anastomotic network of the spinal arteries led to an assessment of the risk of medullary ischemia, which was believed to be lower than initially thought.[19, 22] These studies were believed to demonstrate arteries of the cauda equina with anastomoses between branches in the region of the intervertebral foramina constituting a blood supply system supplementary to the anterior and posterior spinal arteries. Crock and Yoshizawa[4] believed that in anatomic studies prior to their own, the smallest-caliber arteries were not consistently injected and thus only larger vessels were identified. Louis's studies,[22] in agreement, demonstrated the presence of branches of the intermediate artery of varying caliber accompanying each spinal nerve to the spinal cord. Further demonstrating the adequacy of the blood supply to the thoracic cord and diminishing the importance of the artery of Adamkiewicz are reports that, following complete embolization of it to obliterate intramedullary arteriovenous aneurysms, no compromise of spinal cord function occurred. This is supportive of the work of Fried and others[8] showing that experimental ligation of the artery of Adamkiewicz in monkeys did not greatly impair spinal cord blood flow. These observations and other studies have led some investigators to refute the notion that an extremely tenuous vascular supply to the spinal cord in general, and the thoracic cord in particular, exists.[22]

Perhaps the most essential concept concerning the knowledge of the vascular supply to the spinal cord is the awareness of the ranges of individual variability. The work on the rhesus monkey by Fried and colleagues[8] and the numerous successful surgical cases in which the artery of Adamkiewicz had been inadvertently interrupted without producing a disastrous spinal cord ischemia certainly give the impression that an adequate collateral vascularity may protect the cord in most persons when a single major artery is compromised. However, in procedures involving the interruption of blood flow in numerous consecutive segmental branches of the aorta, such as aortic cross-clamping for abdominal vascular surgery, the maintenance of adequate spinal cord blood flow, particularly in the thoracic area, appears to be more dependent on the regional competence of the ASA than on the number of collateral sources to the cord. Spinal cord injury following cross-clamping without adjunct vascular support has been reported to vary between 15% and 25% depending on the series of cases reviewed.[26, 35] Proximal-to-distal aortic pressures have been measured in cross-clamped aortic segments. Hypertension develops proximal to the first clamp, and hypotension develops in the segments distal to the second clamp. Distal aortic hypotension allows blood to drain away from the spinal cord rather than supplying it longitudinally. The work of Molina and others[26] on dogs indicates that the shunt capacity should provide more than 60% of the baseline descending aortic flow and have a diameter greater than half that of the descending aorta to be effective.

Of particular significance was a study by Svensson and co-workers[33] on the blood flow in the baboon spinal cord and its implications in aortic cross-clamping. This animal was chosen because its spinal vascularity is similar to the human in that its ASA is a continuous vessel without the occasional interruptions noted in some quadrupeds. Nevertheless, the authors' work indicated that in the baboon, as in man, the caliber of the ASA is often critically narrowed where the thoracic ASA joins the lumbar segment of this vessel at their common junction with the artery of Adamkiewicz. The functional implication here is that the shunting of the cross-clamped aorta may help maintain an adequate flow in the lumbosacral sections of the cord, but it is of little help to the supply of the lower sections of the thoracic cord because of the marked discrepancy that usually exists between the ASA diameters above and below the junction of the artery of Adamkiewicz. In accordance with the hemodynamic principles of Poiseuille's equation, the resistance to blood flow upward from the junction of the artery of Adamkiewicz was over 50 times greater than the flow resistance downward into the lumbosacral ASA in the baboon. As a series of direct measurements showed that this discrepancy in the ASA diameters was even greater in the human, Svensson and his associates conclude that even the lowest segments of the thoracic cord are dependent on a blood flow from the superior end of the thoracic ASA in spite of the shunting.

The investigations of Parke and colleagues,[27] as pre-

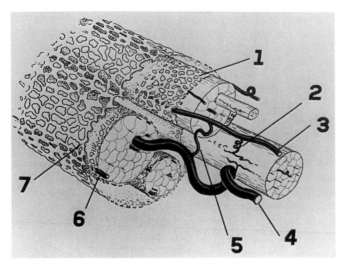

Figure 5–7 = An artist's depiction of the essential elements and relationships of the intrinsic spinal nerve root vasculature. *1,* The fascicular pia arachnoid. *2,* Intra- and interfascicular arteries have compensating coils to allow for intrafascicular motion before supplying precapillary arterials. *3,* A major longitudinal radicular artery. *4,* Spiraling radicular vein. *5,* Relatively large arterial venous anastomosis. *6,* Collateral radicular artery. These often accompany the longitudinal radicular artery *(3). 7,* Radicular pia-arachnoid. Note that the fascicular pia-arachnoid is relatively thicker and less open-meshed than the radicular pia-arachnoid. (From Parke WW, Watanabe R: Lumbosacral nerve roots. Spine 10:508–515, 1985.)

viously described, identify a consistent, adequate vascular pattern supplying the nerve root at each segmental level (see Figs. 5–4 and 5–7). Additionally, it identifies an area of relative hypovascularity near the midportion of each root. These areas of root hypovascularity provide an anatomic rationale for the neuroischemic manifestations accompanying degenerative lumbar spine disease. The authors did not believe that the collateral vascular supply provided by the nerve root could adequately support an area of ischemic cord caused by loss of a medullary feeder vessel. Supporting the work of Dommisse,[5] their studies found a paucity and variability of medullary feeder vessels. They explain the presence of the large longitudinal spinal arteries of the conus as being due to their supplying the proximal radicular arteries of the cauda equina rather than the reverse, as formerly supposed. Finally, Parke and associates[27] think that there is no vascularly "safe" area of the cord.

The previously described arterial distribution to the thoracolumbar spine is present only for those vertebrae adjacent to the aorta. The cervical and sacral spines and transitional cervicothoracic and craniocervical regions have other sources and patterns of arterial supply.

CERVICAL SPINE

The vertebral arteries represent the major blood supply to the cervical spine and cord (Figs. 5–8 and 5–9). The paired vertebral arteries arise bilaterally as the first and largest branches of the subclavian arteries at the level of T1. The arteries enter the foramen transversaria

of C6 ascending to and passing posterior to the lateral masses of the atlas. The vertebral arteries then pass over the arch of the atlas, through the posterior atlanto-occipital membrane, continue cephalad through the foramen magnum, and anastomose forming the basilar artery. The vertebral arteries represent a lateral longitudinal fusion of the original segmental vessels, which provide an arterial supply to the subaxial cervical vertebrae similar to the pattern of that provided by the segmentals in the thoracolumbar spine.

At each segmental level the vertebral arteries supply a ventrally coursing transverse anterior central branch which passes beneath and supplies the longus colli muscle and then courses along the upper ventral edge of its respective intervertebral disc. Longitudinal branches connect adjacent levels forming a well-developed rectangular mesh of vessels that supply the anterior vertebral body at each level.

The vertebral arteries also supply a posterior central branch that enters the intervertebral foramen to supply the posterior vertebral body at each level. Other vessels enter the intervertebral foramina and supply the inner

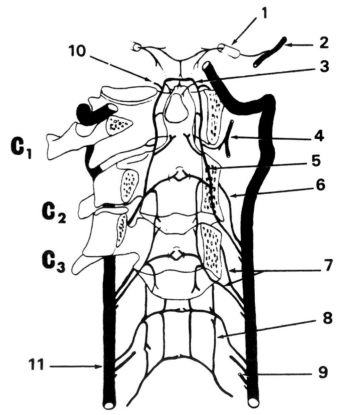

Figure 5–8 = An artist's depiction of the arterial supply to the upper cervical vertebrae and the odontoid process. *1,* Hypoglossal canal passing meningeal artery. *2,* Occipital artery. *3,* Apical arcade of odontoid process. *4,* Ascending pharyngeal artery giving collateral branch beneath anterior arch of atlas. *5,* Posterior ascending artery. *6,* Anterior ascending artery. *7,* Precentral and postcentral arteries to typical cervical vertebral body. *8,* Anterior spinal plexus. *9,* Medullary branch of vertebral artery. Radicular, prelaminar, and meningeal branches are also found at each level. *10,* Collateral to ascending pharyngeal artery passing rostral to the anterior arch of the atlas. *11,* Left vertebral artery. (From Parke WW: The vascular relations of the upper cervical vertebrae. Orthop Clin North Am 9:879–889, 1978.)

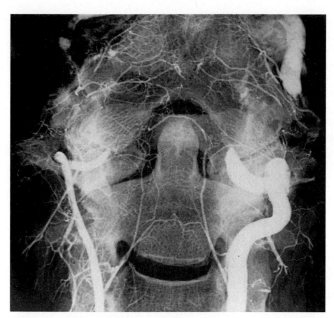

Figure 5–9 = Latex-barium arterially injected radiograph of the upper cervical vertebrae. The vessels should be compared with those shown in Figure 5–8. (From Parke WW: The vascular relations of the upper cervical vertebrae. Orthop Clin North Am 9:879, 1978.)

(anterior) portion of the lamina (prelaminar branches). Other *variable* branches supply the cord as medullary feeder arteries. The final branch of the vertebral artery at each subaxial level passes dorsally to supply the outer surface of the lamina and the posterior muscles of the neck (postlaminar branches).[32]

Lateral Spinal Arteries of the Cervical Cord

The highest three to four segments of the cervical spinal cord receive blood from a unique pair of vessels, the lateral spinal arteries. Although ontogenetically these appear to be the most rostral expressions of the dorsolateral spinal arteries, they have a more extensive distribution and are without equivalents in other levels of the cord. They usually arise from the intradural parts of the vertebral arteries near the origins of the posterior inferior cerebellar arteries (PICAs), or they may arise from the proximal sections of the PICAs themselves. Their typical course carries them anterior to the posterior roots of the cervical spinal nerves C1–4, dorsal to the denticulate ligaments and parallel to the spinal components of the 11th cranial nerve. Their general distribution is to the dorsolateral and ventrolateral cord regions caudal to the olives.

Although these vessels were observed in the late 19th century,[14] they were usually regarded as variants, and their functional significance was not appreciated. Lasjaunias and associates[18] have compiled an extensive report on the variations and selective angiography of these important vessels.

OCCIPITOATLANTOAXIAL REGION

Owing to its complex developmental history and functional demands, the occipitoatlantoaxial articula-

tion demonstrates the most atypical vascular pattern of all vertebrae (Figs. 5–10, 5–11A–C, and 5–12). The odontoid process represents the first cervical vertebral body isolated by synovial cavities. Direct branches to the odontoid are rare, probably because of its isolation by these development synovial cavities, because of the motion (rotation) of the atlas, and because of the transient cartilaginous plate (C1–2 vestigial disc), which is present early and prevents ingrowth from the axis.[28]

Schiff and Parke[31] demonstrated that the odontoid process is supplied primarily by pairs of ascending anterior and posterior central branches that originate from the vertebral artery at the level of the C2–3 foramen (see Figs. 5–8, 5–9, and 5–11A–C). The posterior ascending arteries are the larger members of these two sets of vessels.

The posterior ascending artery courses cephalad on the dorsal surface of the axis and crosses the posterior surface of the transverse ligament 1.5 mm lateral to the neck of the odontoid process (see Fig. 5–11A–C). It continues dorsal to the alar ligament and sends an anterior anastomotic branch over this ligament to collateralize with the anterior ascending artery (see Figs. 5–8, 5–9, and 5–11A–C). The posterior ascending artery terminates medially as it courses toward its contralateral counterpart, forming an apical arcade over the odontoid process.

The anterior ascending artery originates from the vertebral artery at the same level as the posterior ascending artery. It passes anterior to the body of the axis (C2) (see Fig. 5–11A–C). Central perforating branches supply the body of the axis. The cephalad continuation of the anterior ascending artery delivers the vessel to the anterior arch of the atlas. Terminal branches perforate the anterolateral aspect of the "waist" of the odontoid process and the median synovial atlantoaxial joint capsule (see Figs. 5–8, 5–9, and 5–11A–C).

The atlantoaxial and craniovertebral articulations are

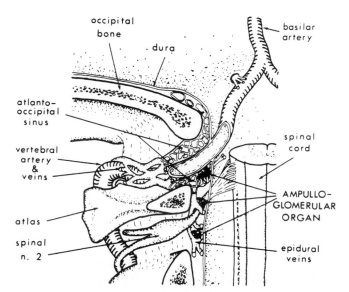

Figure 5–10 = Lateral drawing through the upper cervico-occipital spinal canal. (From Parke WW: The vascular relations of the upper cervical vertebrae. Orthop Clin North Am 9:879, 1978.)

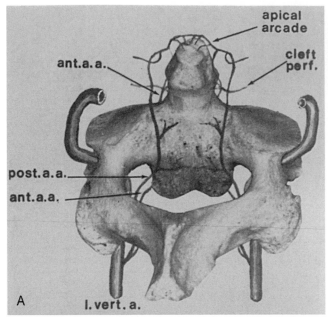

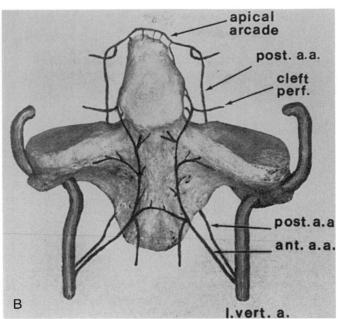

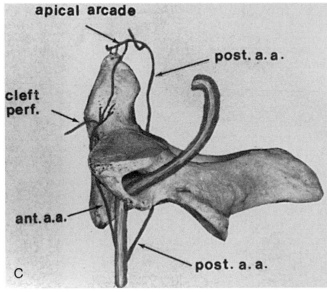

Figure 5–11 = Fixed section of C2 with arterial supply shown. *A*, Posterior view looking into the spinal canal over the posterior spinous process of C2. *B*, Anterior view looking at the anterior aspect of C2 and the odontoid process. The ring of C1 has been removed. *C*, Lateral view of C2 with a significant arterial blood supply. post.a.a., posterior ascending artery; ant.a.a., anterior ascending artery; l.vert.a., left vertebral artery; cleft perf., a perforating artery that enters through the cleft between the odontoid neural centrum. (From Parke WW: The vascular relations of the upper cervical vertebra. Orthop Clin North Am 9:879, 1978.)

therefore supplied to some degree by fine branches from the anterior and posterior ascending arteries. Branches of the vertebral and occipital arteries supply the majority of the blood supply to the atlanto-occipital articulations.

The ascending pharyngeal artery sends a branch along the inner aspect of the carotid sheath that becomes recurrent at the base of the skull. It descends deep to the prevertebral fascia supplying the prevertebral cervical muscles. Branches pass both superior and inferior to the arch of the atlas to anastomose with the apical arcade, ascending arteries, and anterior spinal plexus.

The meningeal branch of the occipital artery enters the skull through the hypoglossal canal and provides a spray of small vessels descending from the foramen magnum to anastomose with the apical arcade. They also supply the periforaminal dura, tectorial membrane, and alar and apical ligaments.

CERVICOTHORACIC REGION (C6–T2)

The cervicothoracic region is a transitional region of the lower two cervical and upper two thoracic vertebrae. The costocervical and thyrocervical trunks of the subclavian artery provide auxiliary blood supply to this region. The pattern of supply is often variable and bilaterally dissimilar.

SACRUM

The sacral spine, like the cervical spine, does not have the typical segmental supply provided by the aorta in the thoracolumbar region. The sacral blood supply is provided by paired lateral sacral and singular middle sacral arteries. The lateral sacral arteries are derived from the superior gluteal arteries or, less frequently, from the hypogastric arteries. They course on the anterolateral surface of the sacrum just lateral to the anterior sacral foramina sending sequential branches dorsally through each foramen. The arterial supply provided by this foraminal artery is similar to that provided by the segmentals in the thoracic and lumbar spine.

The first branch of the foraminal artery follows the anterior surface of each vertebral body segment providing penetrating anterior central branches. They also anastomose with the middle sacral artery and the anterior central branch from the opposite side.

As the main foraminal branch arrives at the level of the intervertebral foramen, it provides branches to the sacral spinal canal and cauda equina. On the floor of the canal the typical longitudinal arcade pattern persists with posterior central arteries providing penetrating branches to the dorsal portion of the vertebral body. Radicular branches accompany the nerve roots of the cauda equina, and intermittent medullary feeder vessels are supplied.

The foraminal branch exits the posterior sacral foramen supplying the postlaminar branches which course to the fused posterior elements and low back muscles.

The middle sacral artery originates from the aorta near its bifurcation between L2 and L5. It is of inconsistent length and course, but does anastomose with and supply anterior central branches to the vertebral bodies and anterior longitudinal ligament. It travels near the midline, anterior to the sacrum and coccyx. In some cases the middle sacral artery gives rise to the fifth lumbar artery.

CERVICAL SPINAL CORD BLOOD SUPPLY

The spinal cord has two major sources of blood supply: the anterior and posterior spinal arteries. Each vertebral artery, prior to coalescing to form the basilar artery, supplies a descending branch that combines with its contralateral counterpart to form the ASA. It descends in the ventral median fissure of the spinal cord, supplying its anterior portion.

Dorsally the paired posterior spinal arteries descend from their respective vertebral artery source lying on the posterolateral cord and forming transverse plexiform channels. The anterior and posterior spinal arteries also receive medullary feeder vessels from the vertebral artery. These vessels are inconstant in distribution, but are larger and exist more commonly in the cervical spine than in any other area.

INTRINSIC VASCULARITY OF THE SPINAL CORD

The tissues of the spinal cord are supplied by two systems of vessels that enter its substance. The first is a centripetal arrangement of arteries that supplies the superficial tracts of the ventral and lateral funiculi, all of the dorsal funiculus, and the extremities of the dorsal horns. They are radially penetrating branches of the vasa corona and the dorsolateral spinal arteries which serve but little more than one fourth of the cord. The greater part of the cord and almost all of its gray matter is supplied by a second centrifugal system of vessels derived from the sulcal (or central) arteries. These arteries are a repetitive series of branches derived from the dorsal aspect of the ASA that penetrate the depths of the anterior median fissure. In the midsagittal plane they form a close palisade of vessels that occurs with a frequency of 3 to 8 arteries per centimeter in the cervical region, 2 to 6 in the thoracic cord, and are densest in the lumbar region where they number 5 to 12 per centimeter of the ASA (see Fig. 5–6A and B). Not surprisingly, the average diameters of the sulcal arteries are greater in the cervical (0.21 mm) and lumbosacral region (0.23 mm) than in the thoracic cord (0.14 mm).[11] As these vessels approach the anterior commissure, the majority turn either to the right or to the left and supply only their corresponding side of the cord. This unilateral proclivity reflects their origins

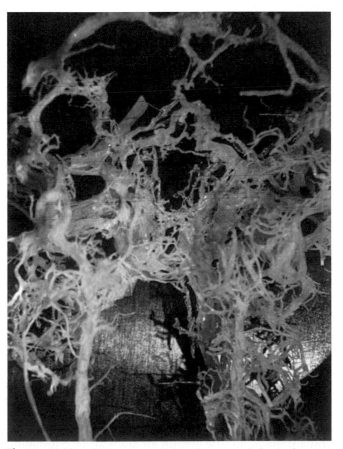

Figure 5–12 = This photograph, of a corroded vinyl acetate injection of the upper cervical region in a term fetus, shows the ubiquity of the epidural arteries and veins, particularly in the upper cervical areas. The plastic medium was injected into the arterial system but partially filled the tortuous venous channels of the suboccipital sinuses by passing through arterial venous arcades. The large artery on the lower left is the vertebral artery giving way proximally to the posterior ascending artery. (From Parke WW: The vascular relations of the upper cervical vertebrae. Orthop Clin North Am 9:879, 1978.)

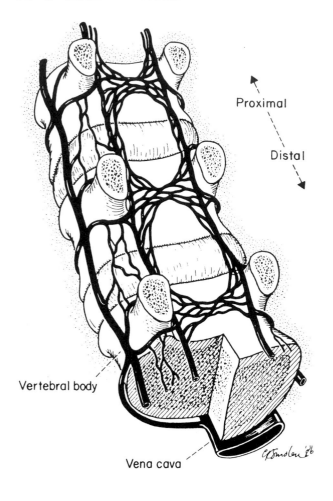

Proximal

Distal

Vertebral body

Vena cava

Figure 5–14 = The venous system is shown from the posterior view with the lamina and pedicles removed. This forms a steplike arcade over the posterior vertebral bodies anterior to the dura. Centrally, over the disc, there is a paucity of veins, though they anastomose in an arcade-like fashion over the posterior aspect of the bodies. The arterial system is similar, though less complex, at this level.

and eventually emptying into a segmental vein (see Fig. 5–16).

The cervical region differs in that the internal venous plexus gives rise to the origin of the vertebral veins, a plexiform sheath of vessels that surrounds each vertebral artery, from its point of dural penetration to C7, where it reaches Pirogoff's venous angle. Near their origin, the vertebral veins anastomose with the intraspinal plexus, intracranial sinuses, and the condylar, mastoid, occipital, and posterior jugular veins. The plexiform vertebral veins constitute the longitudinal axis of the external cervical venous plexus, which is

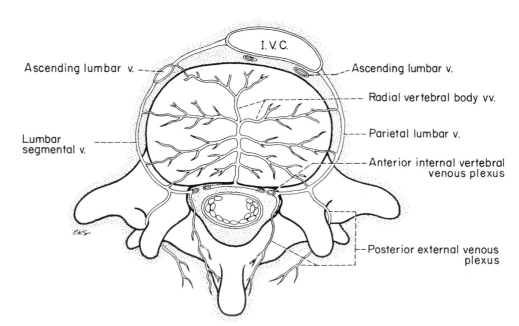

I.V.C.

Ascending lumbar v.

Ascending lumbar v.

Radial vertebral body vv.

Parietal lumbar v.

Lumbar segmental v.

Anterior internal vertebral venous plexus

Posterior external venous plexus

Figure 5–15 = Cross section through a lumbar vertebral body demonstrating the venous system. This is at the level of the cauda equina. The radially directed vertebral veins allow blood to flow (exit from the body and neural elements) in all directions. I.V.C., inferior vena cava.

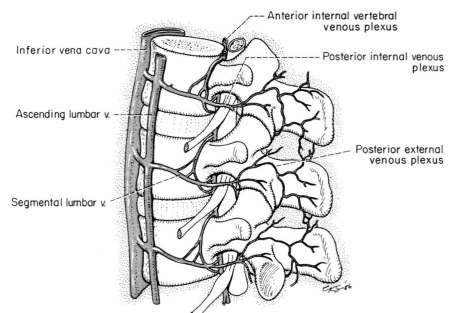

Inferior vena cava

Ascending lumbar v.

Segmental lumbar v.

Anterior internal vertebral venous plexus

Posterior internal venous plexus

Posterior external venous plexus

Figure 5–16 = This illustration demonstrates the venous system lateral to the vertebral column looking from the right side. The veins surround the spinal nerves at the level of the neuroforamen. Communication to the vena cava is through the ascending lumbar veins and segmental veins.

connected to the internal system by a complicated pattern of venous channels completely ensheathing each nerve root as it courses through the intervertebral foramen.

The final connection between the internal and external system is accomplished by transverse veins that course from the basivertebral system obliquely through the cancellous bone of the vertebral body to the anterior external plexus (see Figs. 5–13 and 5–15).

The external vertebral venous plexus consists of a small anterior and larger posterior set of veins (see Figs. 5–13, 5–15, and 5–16). The external system is arranged in the same distribution as the anterior central and posterior laminar arterial supply. The small anterior external plexus receives the venous drainage of the vertebral body via tributaries that perforate the anterior and lateral sides of the vertebral body. The venous pattern within the centrum of the vertebral body consists of the basivertebral system of veins which are oriented horizontally, accompanying the radiate arteries (see Fig. 5–15). The vertical veins of the vertebral body are large and flow toward each end plate. The central veins of the vertebral bodies converge anteriorly and posteriorly, draining into the external vertebral plexus and anterior internal vertebral plexus, respectively. Subjacent to the vertebral end plate, large-caliber tributaries of the vertical veins of the centrum turn abruptly to run horizontally forming a horizontal subarticular collecting venous system. A final terminal vascular network exists as a capillary bed in the cartilaginous plate overlying the perforated cortical vertebral end plate. This serves to drain blood and metabolic products from the vertebral end plate and cartilage into the subarticular collecting vein system.[3]

The posterior vertebral arches are drained by a central vein of the spinous process and by veins of the laminae. These channels subsequently drain toward the pedicles and intervertebral foramen to anastomose with the internal and external vertebral venous plexus.

The larger posterior external venous system drains the region supplied by the posterior branch of the segmental artery (see Figs. 5–15 and 5–16). The system is bilaterally symmetrical, lying in the costovertebral grooves with cross-anastomoses between the spinous processes. The posterior external plexus is most extensive in the posterior nuchal region, eventually draining into the deep cervical and jugular veins. In the thoracic and lumbar spine the external vertebral venous plexus receives a venous return that has followed the arterial supply from the periphery to drain into the intercostal and lumbar veins. These veins accompany the segmental arteries coursing over the midportion of the vertebral bodies. The venous return differs from the arterial supply in its mode of confluence with the great veins. Blood drains into the ascending lumbar and azygos system of veins in the lumbar and thoracic regions, respectively. There are three azygos vessels in the region of the thoracic spine: the azygos (right side), hemiazygos (left T3–6), and accessory hemiazygos (left T7–12). These eventually drain into the superior vena cava, completing the venous drainage of the thoracic and lumbar spine.

INTRINSIC VENOUS DRAINAGE OF THE SPINAL CORD

Compared to the arterial anatomy, the structural and functional aspects of the venous drainage of the spinal cord have been relatively neglected. Unlike in other organ systems where the equivalent orders of veins and arteries tend to course in a common vascular bundle, the veins of the CNS are generally less numerous than the arteries and are larger than their corresponding efferent vessels; the larger branches may not show

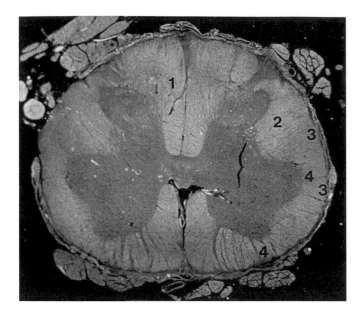

Figure 6–2 = This photograph depicts a transverse section through the lumbar spinal cord. Note the increased proportion of gray matter in the caudal lumbar cord compared with more rostral sections of the spinal cord. The posterior funiculus of the lumbar cord is solely composed of the fasciculus gracilis *(1),* for the fasciculus cuneatus commences rostral to T6. The lateral corticospinal *(2)* tract makes up a large proportion of the lateral funiculus. However, contributions from the spinocerebellar *(3)* and spinothalamic *(4)* tracts can be seen along the periphery of the white matter. The dorsal and ventral nerve roots enter and exit the gray matter via the dorsal and ventral horns.

and contains the anterior, intermediate, and posterior horns depending on the level examined. Cross-communications occur through a thin commissure. The white matter is composed of three funiculi (Latin dim. of *funis,* cord) or columns: the posterior, lateral, and anterior columns,[69] which house the various ascending and descending nerve tracts of the spinal cord (Figs. 6–1 through 6–5).

In general, the fiber tracts of the human spinal cord follow a basic neuroanatomic tenet referred to as the Bell-Magendie law. This law affirms that primary afferent nerve fibers are contained within the dorsal roots, while motor efferent fibers are contained primarily within the ventral roots. Studies in cats and observation in humans, however, have found that this may not be entirely true, with evidence that some finely

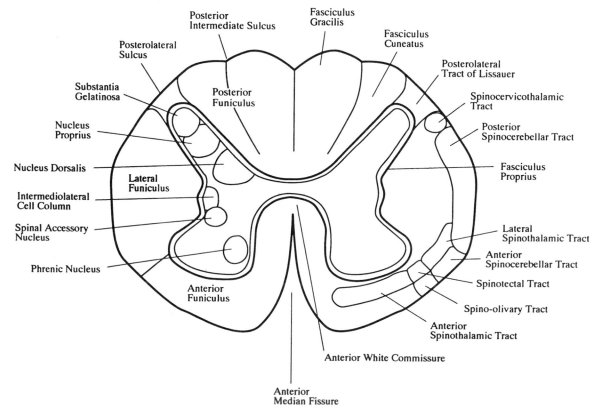

Figure 6–3 = The transverse section of the spinal cord showing the various ascending tracts of the three funiculi (anterior, lateral, and posterior) of the spinal white matter. The various subdivisions of the anterior, intermediate, and posterior horns of the spinal gray matter are also shown.

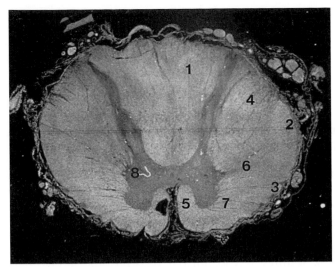

Figure 6–4 = A transverse section through the thoracic spinal cord. Since the fasciculus cuneatus commences rostral to T6, the posterior funiculus is solely composed of the fasciculus gracilis *(1)*. The lateral funiculus consists of the posterior *(2)* and anterior *(3)* spinocerebellar tracts, the lateral *(4)* and anterior *(5)* corticospinal tracts, and the lateral *(6)* and anterior *(7)* spinothalamic tracts. The intermediolateral cell column *(8)*, composed of preganglionic sympathetic nerve cell bodies, is easily seen in sections through the thoracic cord.

myelinated or unmyelinated afferent fibers traverse within the ventral root fibers.[39]

Humans' earliest venture into the understanding of the anatomy and function of the spinal cord can be dated back to 4000 BC when Egyptian physicians accurately noted the correlation between loss of motor function and spinal cord injury. Galen, in the 2nd century AD, was one of the first to experimentally produce in animals specific loss of motor function by transecting spinal cords. In the mid-19th century, anatomic localization of spinal cord function was realized when Brown-Séquard correlated motor losses with specific cord lesions.[57, 73] These investigators were the true pioneers in the understanding of the anatomy and function of the human spinal cord, and laid the groundwork for future research into the pathophysiology of spinal cord dysfunction related to traumatic and nontraumatic causes.

SPINAL GRAY MATTER

The gray matter of the human spinal cord appears as the letter H embedded within the white matter tracts on transverse histologic sectioning (see Fig. 6–3). The gray matter is composed primarily of nerve cell bodies and their processes, connective tissue, and interspersed vascular components. Three distinct regions are identified within the gray matter, referred to as the posterior, intermediate, and anterior horns. Further subdivision is predicated on morphologic correlation with specific cord function, with the posterior horn divided into four groups, or columns, and the anterior horn divided into three.[69] A less clinically useful, and more antiquated, classification system involves dividing the gray matter into laminations referred to as the lamina of Rexed,[76] which are discussed later.

Posterior Gray Matter

The posterior horn is composed primarily of interneurons and tract cells whose processes collect to

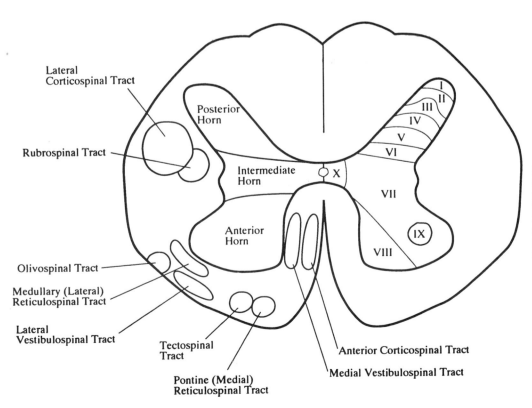

Figure 6–5 = The transverse section of the spinal cord, illustrating the various descending tracts of the spinal white matter. The lamina of Rexed is illustrated contralateral to the three horns (posterior, intermediate, and anterior) of the spinal gray matter.

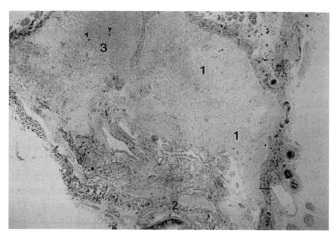

Figure 6–10 = A histologic transverse section obtained through the level of cord injury (cervicothoracic) demonstrating an architecture distorted by compression with subsequent atrophic loss of cord matter. Demyelination and cystic degeneration are evidenced by lack of staining and the spongiform appearance of most of the section (1). Additionally, focal areas of reactive gliosis are revealed as darker areas, secondary to an increased number of activated astrocytes, particularly in the peripheral portions of the cord (2). Foci of old hemorrhage are punctate, demarcated by small clusters of macrophages laden with phagocytosed hemosiderin (3).

their discussion of specific cord lesions and their histopathologic manifestations over time, reported a 53-year-old woman who developed a T9 paraplegia after thrombosis of her anterior spinal artery following a lumbar sympathectomy for severe high blood pressure. Histologic evaluation at necropsy 10 months later revealed significant degeneration of the ascending tracts in the anterior and lateral funiculi, beginning with their origin in the gray matter, with associated degeneration of some descending tracts (see Fig. 6–11). Tract degeneration manifests itself as generalized pallor on histologic review (Figs. 6–8 and 6–9).

A debated topic in mammalian spinal cord injury is the potential for regeneration after injury.[19] It is known that lower vertebrates such as fish and amphibians show remarkable plasticity for central nervous system regeneration. Unfortunately, little potential for neural recovery has been realized after complete cord injuries

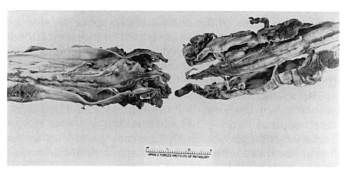

Figure 6–11 = A pathologic specimen of a transected spinal cord with its dural sheath opened and reflected revealing the late appearance or final phase of spinal cord injury. Normal remnants of spinal cord tissue may be seen above and below the level of cord transection.

in humans.[57] Studies by Saunders and colleagues,[78] using a fetal rat model, demonstrated their remarkable potential for rapid and extensive axonal regrowth after injury unlike their adult counterparts, testifying to the differences in the immature and mature mammalian central nervous systems. Numerous investigators have shown in animal models that in an ideal environment, axonal sprouting may occur with growth of these processes into, or onto, an appropriate substrate, that is, similar to that seen with the peripheral nervous system through transplanted Schwann cell tubes or fetal nerve transplant tissue.* A physical barrier to axonal regrowth is thought to be the wallerian zone where remnants of myelin debris, neuroglial profileration, and other obstructive inhibitory substances are thought to block further growth of these nervous structures.[9, 87] Studies have demonstrated significant decreased growth activity in the regenerating central nervous system in the transition between the zone of injury and the wallerian zone.[20] Also, the lack of appropriate trophic and stimulatory substrates, most notably receptive astrocytes, makes regeneration more improbable.[10, 90] Investigators have shown that the astrocyte, once thought to be an inhibitor to axonal growth, actually releases factors that stimulate axon formation while at the same time being stimulated by the presence of axons themselves.[5, 24, 33, 57] Interestingly, purified populations of astrocyte cell lines have supported axonal growth in vitro, while in vivo the presence of scar tissue inclusive of these cells has prevented growth, thereby suggesting the presence of additional factors responsible for neuronal growth inhibition.[57]

In vitro studies have shown the ability of axonal processes to grow within the gray matter of the central nervous and peripheral nervous systems, but to be markedly retarded in the white matter of the central nervous system. Possibly the presence of nondigested myelin remnants and remaining oligodendrocytes within the wallerian zone are the inhibitory factors which must be neutralized prior to successful axonal growth.[90] Work in vivo, noting the potential for regeneration of the corticospinal tracts, demonstrates that with neutralization of two minor proteins within the central nervous system myelin, and a portion of the oligodendrocyte membrane, regrowth is possible.[57, 63, 81]

It is clear that the histopathologic changes which occur after closed spinal cord injury are dependent on many factors, most notably the severity of force impact, the duration of continued spinal cord compression, and the body's physiologic capacity to respond to this injury with its intrinsic biomolecular repair mechanisms. By noting these changes and delving into the biomolecular and physiologic processes of spinal cord injury, we may be better able to alter the natural history of functional neural return after significant cord injury. Promising basic and clinical research exploring the role of various agents of inflammation[12, 66]; tissue eicosanoids, that is, thromboxane and leukotrienes[25, 44]; free radical formation[4, 17, 25, 26, 35, 64, 67]; endogenous opiate production[30, 31, 43, 60, 61, 93]; excitatory amino acids[32, 66, 83];

*References 16, 18, 22, 23, 34, 57, 74, 75, 82, and 90.

gangliosides[37, 59]; and steroid function[14, 92, 93] have once again illustrated the potential for prevention of further neural damage after injury and the possibility of axon regeneration with improvement in neural function.[3, 11, 38, 40, 42, 52, 53, 72]

REFERENCES

1. Allen AR: Surgery of experimental lesion of spinal cord equivalent to crush injury of fracture dislocation of spinal column. A preliminary report. JAMA 57:878–880, 1911.
2. Allen AR: Remarks on the histopathological changes in the spinal cord due to impact. An experimental study. J Nerv Ment Dis 41:141–147, 1914.
3. Alvin MS, White RJ, Acosta-Rua G, et al: Study of functional recovery produced by delayed localized cooling after spinal cord injury in primates. J Neurosurg 29:113–120, 1968.
4. Anderson DK, Means ED: Lipid peroxidation in the spinal cord: FeCl(2) induction and protection with antioxidants. Neurochem Pathol 1:249–264, 1983.
5. Assouline JG, Bosch P, Lim R, et al: Rat astrocytes and Schwann cells in culture synthesize nerve growth factor–like neurite-promoting factors. Dev Brain Res 31:103–118, 1987.
6. Balentine JD: Pathology of experimental spinal cord trauma: 1. The necrotic lesion as a function of vascular injury. Lab Invest 39:236–253, 1978.
7. Balentine JD: Hypotheses in spinal cord trauma research. CNS Status Rep 31:445–461, 1985.
8. Balentine JD: Impact injuries of the spine and spinal cord. *In* Leestma JE (ed): Neuropathology. New York, Raven Press, 1988, pp 254–275.
9. Bernstein JJ, Getz R, Jefferson M, et al: Astrocytes secrete basal lamina after hemisection of rat spinal cord. Brain Res 327:135–141, 1985.
10. Bjorklund A, Stenevu U: Regeneration of monoaminergic and cholineric neurons in the mammalian central nervous system. Physiol Rev 59:62–100, 1979.
11. Black P, Markowitz RS: Experimental spinal cord injury in monkeys: Comparison of steroids and local hypothermia. Surg Forum 22:409–411, 1971.
12. Blight AR: Delayed demyelination and macrophage invasion: A candidate for secondary cell damage in spinal cord injury. CNS Trauma 2:299–315, 1985.
13. Blight AR: Macrophages and inflammatory damage in spinal cord injury. J Neurotrauma 9(suppl 1):S83–91, 1992.
14. Bracken MB, Collins WF, Freeman DF, et al: Efficacy of methylprednisolone in acute spinal cord injury. JAMA 251:45–52, 1984.
15. Bresnahan JC, King JS, Martin GF, et al: A neuroanatomical analysis of spinal cord injury in the rhesus monkey. J Neurol Sci 28:521–542, 1976.
16. Campbell JB, Bassett CA, Husby J, et al: Regeneration of adult mammalian spinal cord. Science 126:929–930, 1957.
17. Chan PK, Fishman RA: Brain edema: Induction in cortical slices by polyunsaturated fatty acids. Science 201:358–360, 1978.
18. Clemente CD, Windle WF: Regeneration of severed nerve fibers in the spinal cord of the adult cat. J Comp Neurol 101:691–731, 1954.
19. Collins GH, West NR: Prospects for axonal regrowth in spinal cord injury. Brain Res Bull 22:89–92, 1989.
20. Collins GH, West NR, Parmely JD: The histopathology of freezing injury to the rat spinal cord. A light and electron microscope study. 2. Repair and regeneration. J Neuropathol Exp Neurol 45:742–757, 1986.
21. Curati WL, Kingsley DP, Kendall BE, et al: MRI in chronic spinal cord trauma. Neuroradiology 35:30–35, 1992.
22. Das GD: Neuronal transplantation in mammalian brain: Some conceptual and technical considerations. *In* Wallace RB, Das GD (eds): Neural Tissue Transplantation Research. New York, Springer-Verlag, 1983, pp 1–4.
23. David S, Aguayo AJ: Axonal elongation into peripheral nervous system "bridges" after central nervous system injury in adult rats. Science 214:931–933, 1981.
24. David S, Miller RH, Patel R, et al: Effects of neonatal transection

25. Demediuk P, Faden AI: Traumatic spinal cord injury in rats causes increases in tissue thromboxane but not peptidoleukotrines. J Neurosci Res 20:115–121, 1988.
26. Demopoulos HB, Flamm ES, Pietronegro DD, et al: The free radical pathology and microcirculation in the major central nervous system disorders. Acta Physiol Scand Suppl 492:91–119, 1980.
27. Dohrmann GJ, Wagner FC Jr, Bucy FC: The microvasculature in transitory traumatic paraplegia. An electron microscope study in the monkey. J Neurosurg 35:263–271, 1971.
28. Dohrmann GJ, Wagner FC Jr, Bucy FC: Transitory traumatic paraplegia: Electron microscopy of early alterations in myelinated nerve fibers. J Neurosurg 36:406–415, 1972.
29. Ducker TB: Experimental injury of the spinal cord. *In* Vinken PJ, Bruyn GW (eds): Handbook of Clinical Neurology, vol 25. Amsterdam, Elsevier North-Holland, 1976, pp 9–26.
30. Faden AI: Opioid and nonopioid action mechanisms may contribute to dynorphin's pathophysiological actions in spinal cord injury. Ann Neurol 27:67–74, 1990.
31. Faden AI, Jacobs TP, Mougey E, et al: Endorphins in experimental spinal injury. Ann Neurol 10:326–332, 1981.
32. Faden AI, Simon RP: A potential role for excitotoxins in the pathophysiology of spinal cord injury. Ann Neurol 23:623–626, 1988.
33. Fallon JR: Neurite guidance by non-neuronal cells in culture: Preferential outgrowth of peripheral neurites on glial as compared to non-glial surfaces. J Neurosci 5:3169–3177, 1985.
34. Feringa ER, Shuer LM, Vahlsing HL, et al: Regeneration of corticospinal axons in the rat. Ann Neurol 2:315–321, 1977.
35. Fong KL, McCay PB, Poyer JL, et al: Evidence that peroxidation of lysosomal membranes is initiated by hydroxyl free radicals produced during flavin enzyme activity. J Biol Chem 248:7792–7797, 1973.
36. Geisler FH: GM-1 ganglioside and motor recovery following human spinal cord injury. J Emerg Med 11:45–55, 1993.
37. Geisler FH, Dorsey FC, Coleman WP: Recovery of motor function after spinal cord injury—a randomized, placebo controlled trial with GM-1 ganglioside. N Engl J Med 324:1829–1838, 1991 [erratum appears in N Engl J Med 325:659–660, 1991; letters in N Engl J Med 326:493–494, 1992].
38. Gerber AM, Olson WL, Harris JH: Effect of phenytoin on functional recovery after experimental spinal cord injury in dogs. Neurosurgery 7:472–476, 1980.
39. Gilman S, Newman SW: Manter and Gatz's Essentials of Clinical Neuroanatomy and Neurophysiology, ed 8. Philadelphia, FA Davis, 1992, pp 54–97.
40. Giulian D, Robertson C: Inhibition of mononuclear phagocytes reduces ischemic injury in the spinal cord. Ann Neurol 27:33–42, 1990.
41. Griffiths IR, McCulloch MC: Nerve fibers in spinal cord impact injuries. Part 1. Changes in the myelin sheath during the initial five weeks. J Neurol Sci 58:335–349, 1983.
42. Harvey JE, Srebnix HH: Locomotor activity and axon regeneration following spinal cord compression in rats treated with L-thyroxine. J Neuropathol Exp Neurol 236:661–668, 1967.
43. Holaday JW, Faden AI: Naloxone acts on central opiate receptors to reverse hypotension, hypothermia, and hypoventilation in spinal shock. Brain Res 189:295–299, 1980.
44. Hsu CY, Halushka PV, Hogan EL, et al: Alteration of thromboxane and prostacyclin levels in experimental spinal cord injury. Neurology 35:1003–1009, 1985.
45. Hughes JT: Pathology of the Spinal Cord. Philadelphia, JB Lippincott, 1966, pp 59–69.
46. Hughes JT: Disease of the spine and spinal cord. *In* Adams JH, Corsellis JA, Duchen LW (eds): Greenfield's Neuropathology. London, Edwards Arnold, 1984.
47. Hughes JT: Neuropathology of the spinal cord. Neurol Clin 9:551–571, 1991.
48. Iwasaki Y, Iizuka H, Yamamoto T, et al: Alleviation of axonal damage in acute spinal cord injury by a protease inhibitor: Automated morphometric analysis of drug effects. Brain Res 347:124–126, 1985.

on glial cell development in the rat optic nerve: Evidence that the oligodendrocyte–type 2 astrocyte cell lineage depends on axons for its survival. J Neurocytol 13:961–974, 1984.

49. Jellinger K: Traumatic vascular disease of the spinal cord. *In* Vinken PJ, Bruyn GW (eds): Handbook of Clinical Neurology, vol 12. Amsterdam, North Holland Elsevier, 1972, pp 556–630.

50. Jellinger K: Neuropathology of cord injuries. *In* Vinken PJ, Bruyn GW (eds): Handbook of Clinical Neurology, vol 25. Amsterdam, North Holland, 1976, pp 43–123.

51. Jellinger K: Pathology of spinal cord trauma. *In* Errico TJ, Bauer D, Waugh T (eds): Spinal Trauma. Philadelphia, JB Lippincott, 1991, pp 455–495.

52. Joyner JJ, Freeman LW: Urea and spinal cord trauma, Neurology 13:69–72, 1963.

53. Kajihara J, Kawanaga H, de la Torre JC, et al: Dimethyl sulfoxide in the treatment of experimental acute spinal cord injury. Surg Neurol 1:16–22, 1973.

54. Kakulas BA, Bedrock GM: Pathology of injuries of the vertebral column with emphasis on the macroscopic aspect. *In* Vinken PJ, Bruyn GW (eds): Handbook of Clinical Neurology, vol 25. Amsterdam, North Holland, 1976, pp 27–42.

55. Kawata K, Morimito T, Ohashi T, et al: Experimental study of acute spinal cord injury: A histopathological study. No Shinkei Geka 21:45–51, 1993.

56. Kholin AV, Makarov AIU, Amelina OA, et al: Magnetic resonance tomography in spinal cord trauma. Zh Vopr Neirokhir Im N N Burdenko 6:32–37, 1992.

57. Kliot M, Lustgarten JH: Strategies to promote regeneration and recovery in the injured spinal cord. Neurosurg Clin North Am 1:751–759, 1990.

58. Lampert PW, Cressman M: Axonal regeneration in the dorsal columns of the spinal cord of rats. Lab Invest 13:825–834, 1964.

59. Ledeen RW: Ganglioside structures and distribution: Are they localized at the nerve ending? J Supramol Struct 8:1–17, 1978.

60. Long JB, Kinney RC, Malcolm DS, et al: Intrathecal dynorphin A (1-13) and dynorphin A (3-13) reduce rat spinal cord blood flow by non-opioid mechanisms. Brain Res 436:374–379, 1987.

61. Long JB, Martinez-Arizala A, Petras JM, et al: Endogenous opioids in spinal cord injury: A critical evaluation. CNS Trauma 4:295–315, 1986.

62. Marburg O: Die traumatischen Erkrankungen des Gehirns und Rückenmarks. *In* Bumke O, Foerster O (eds): Handbuch der Neurologie, vol. 11. Berlin, Springer-Verlag, 1936, pp 1–177.

63. Martinez-Arizala A, Green BA, Bunge RP: Experimental spinal cord injury: Pathophysiology and treatment. *In* Rothman RH, Simeone FA (eds): The Spine. Philadelphia, WB Saunders, 1992, pp 1247–1276.

64. McCord JM: Oxygen-derived radicals: A link between reperfusion injury and inflammation. Fed Proc 46:2402–2406, 1987.

65. McVeigh JF: Experimental cord crushes with special references to the mechanical factors involved and subsequent changes in the areas affected. Arch Surg 7:573–600, 1923.

66. Means ED, Anderson DK: Neuronophagia by leukocytes in experimental spinal cord injury. J Neuropathol Exp Neurol 42:707–719, 1983.

67. Misra HP, Fridovich I: The role of superoxide anion in the autooxidation of epinephrine and a simple assay for superoxide dismutase. J Biol Chem 247:3170–3175, 1972.

68. Nathan PW, Smith MC, Cook AW: Sensory effects in man of lesions of the posterior columns and of some other afferent pathways. Brain 109:1003–1041, 1986.

69. Nolte J: Spinal Cord. *In* Nolte J (ed): The Human Brain. St. Louis, Mosby–Year Book, 1988, pp 114–145.

70. Olliver GP: Über das Rückenmark und seine Krankheiten. Leipzig, L Voss, 1824.

71. Panter SS, Yum SW, Faden AI: Alteration in extracellular amino acids after traumatic spinal cord injury. Ann Neurol 27:96–99, 1990.

72. Politis MJ, Zanakis MF: The short term effects of delayed application of electric fields in the damaged rodent spinal cold. Neurosurgery 25:71–75, 1989.

73. Puchala E, Windle WF: The possibility of structrual and functional restitution after spinal cord injury. A review. Exp Neurol 55:1–42, 1977.

74. Reier PJ, Bregnian BS, Wujek JR: Intraspinal transplantation of embryonic spinal cord tissue in neuronal and adult rats. J Comp Neurol 247:275–296, 1986.

75. Reier PJ, Eng LF, Jakeman L: Reactive astrocyte and axonal outgrowth in the injured CNS: Is gliosis really an impediment to regeneration? *In* Seil FJ (ed): Neural Regeneration and Transplantation. New York, Alan R Liss, 1989, pp 183–209.

76. Rexed B: The cytoarchitectonic organization of the spinal cord in the cat. J Comp Neurol 96:415–495, 1952.

77. Rothman SM, Olney JW: Glutamate and pathophysiology of hypoxic-ischemic brain damage. Ann Neurol 19:105–111, 1986.

78. Saunders NR, Balkwill P, Knott G, et al: Growth of axons through a lesion in the intact CNS of fetal rat maintained in long term culture. Proc R Soc Lond B Biol Sci 250:171–180, 1992.

79. Schmaus H: Commotio spinalis. *In* Lubarsch O, Ostertag R (eds): Ergenbnisse der allemeinen Pathologie und pathologischen Anatomie des Menschen und der Tiere. Wiesbaden, JF Bergman, 1890, pp 674–713.

80. Schmaus H: Beiträge zur pathologischen Anatomie der Rückenmarkerschutterung. Virchows Arch 122:470–495, 1890.

81. Schnell L, Schwab ME: Axonal regeneration in the rat spinal cord produced by an antibody against myelin-associated neurite growth inhibitors. Nature 343:269–273, 1990.

82. Schreyer DJ, Jones EJ: Growth of corticospinal axons on prosthetic substrates introduced into the spinal cord of neonatal rats. Dev Brain Res 35:291–299, 1987.

83. Simon RP, Griffiths T, Evans MC, et al: Calcium overload in selectively vulnerable neurons of the hippocampus during and after ischemia: An electron microscopy study in the rat. Cereb Blood Flow Metab 4:350–361, 1984.

84. Snell RS: Clinical Neuroanatomy for Medical Students, ed 3. Boston, Little, Brown, 1992.

85. Spiller WC: A critical summary of recent literature on concussion of the spinal cord with some original observations. Am J Med Sci 118:190–198, 1899.

86. Tator CH: Review of experimental spinal cord injury with emphasis on the local and systemic circulatory effects. Neurochirurgie 37:291–302, 1991.

87. Vick RS, Neuberger TJ, DeVries GH: Role of adult oligodendrocytes in remyelination after neural injury. J Neurotrauma 9(suppl 1):S93–103, 1992.

88. Wagner FC, Dohrmann GJ, Bucy PC: Histopathology of transitory traumatic paraplegia in the monkey. J Neurosurg 35:272–276, 1971.

89. Wallace MC, Tator CH, Frazee P: Relationship between posttraumatic ischemia and hemorrhage in the injured rat spinal cord as shown by colloidal carbon angiography. Neurosurgery 18:433–439, 1986.

90. West NR, Collins GH: Relationship of wallerian degeneration to regrowing axons. J Neuropathol Exp Neurol 50:693–703, 1991.

91. Wolman L: The disturbances of circulation in traumatic paraplegia in acute and late stages. Paraplegia 2:231–236, 1965.

92. Young W, Flamm ES: Effect of high-dose corticosteroid therapy on blood flow, evoked potentials, and extracellular calcium in experimental spinal injury. J Neurosurg 57:667–673, 1982.

93. Young W, Flamm ES, Demopoulos HB, et al: Effect of naloxone on post-traumatic ischemia in experimental spinal contusion. J Neurosurg 55:209–219, 1981.

CHAPTER 7

Experimental Spinal Cord Injury

Alberto Martinez-Arizala ‖ *Barth A. Green*

Although advancements in the surgical techniques for spinal stabilization and the clinical care of the patient in specialized spinal cord injury (SCI) units have effectively reduced the morbidity and mortality associated with spinal injuries, our capability to prevent the loss, or to promote the restoration, of neural function following spinal trauma remains limited. Since the early 1970s, skillfully planned laboratory research has provided knowledge that has dramatically improved our understanding of the pathophysiology of SCI. This has fostered recent developments of specific pharmacologic therapies that have proven to be effective in the treatment of acute SCI. Specifically, the beneficial effect of methylprednisolone noted in animal models of SCI resulted in its successful use in the Second National Acute Spinal Cord Injury Study.[36] This landmark study was the first documented successful pharmacologic treatment of human SCI. We can expect that further advances in our understanding of factors influencing successful nerve regeneration and central nervous system (CNS) transplantation will offer therapeutic alternatives for acute, subacute, and chronic SCI.

SPINAL CORD INJURY MODELS

Limitations in the current neurophysiologic methods and neuroimaging techniques make assessment of the pathophysiology of acute human SCI difficult. Therefore, our understanding of SCI will continue to rely on the use of experimental animal models. Animal models of SCI attempt to mimic human SCI as closely as possible. This in itself is quite complex because human injuries are multifactorial. The following are examples of the variables involved in human SCI: (1) age, (2) sex (most human injuries occur in males), (3) level of injury, (4) open vs. closed injuries, (5) completeness of injury, (6) force of impact and type of force (e.g., flexion, extension, compression, distraction, rotation),[51, 257] (6) rate of compression of the spinal cord tissue, (7) presence of associated bony and ligamentous damage producing vertebral column disruption and instability, (8) duration of compression, (9) occurrence of other associated injuries, and (10) presence of pre-existing conditions (e.g., vascular disease, hypertension, spinal stenosis). In addition, animal models of SCI usually require certain conditions that produce deviation from the human condition (e.g., utilizing a posterior approach via laminectomy to create the injury and use of anesthesia).

The majority of human SCIs are closed. They rarely involve direct severance of cord tissue; they more commonly derive from contusive forces that do not interrupt the continuity of the cord but lead to internal tissue loss.[148] Contusive types of injuries, in which hemorrhage and tissue necrosis evolve into a fluid-filled cyst, are mimicked by several animal models. Figure 7–1 shows such a lesion produced by the Allen, or weight-drop, technique.

Although early models of experimental SCI provided information about the neurologic and histopathologic changes associated with experimental spinal cord lesions, the first model that allowed quantification of the severity of SCI was introduced by A.R. Allen in 1911. Allen produced SCI in dogs by dropping a known weight through a tube that was placed on the exposed thoracic cord.[1] This model thus become known as the Allen or "weight-drop" model of SCI. In this model, the severity of the spinal injury can be graded by varying either the weight or the height of the drop, and the magnitude of the injuries are expressed as the gram-centimeters product. This method allows investigators to produce fairly reproducible graded injuries and has been modified to successfully produce contusive spinal cord lesions in various species.[32, 33, 40, 72, 105, 263, 271] Despite its wide acceptance, the weight-drop technique has several disadvantages: (1) the energy of the impact is not adequately represented by the gram-centimeter product; a 40-g mass dropped 10 cm transfers more that 100 times more energy to the cord than a 5-g mass dropped 80 cm, although both are "400 g-cm injuries"[68]; (2) compression of the cord occurs from the posterior aspect, which differs from the more common anterior or circumferential compression seen in human injuries; and (3) the weight-drop technique has been noted by some investigators to produce variable results.[152, 169] Despite this, the weight-drop mimics some of the biomechanics of the human SCI and has been effectively utilized by investigators who have carefully controlled experimental variables.[101, 110, 203, 204, 209, 271]

Besides the weight drop, a variety of other models have also been developed to produce SCI in animals. A highly sophisticated device, consisting of a feedback-controlled electromechanical impactor, has been reported to produce highly reproducible and graded le-

cium overload was first suggested as a mechanism of cellular injury in liver cells by McLean and colleagues[191] in 1965, and the phenomenon of the "calcium paradox" as a mechanism of cell death in the heart was described by Zimmerman and colleagues.[283, 284] He demonstrated that perfusion of isolated rat hearts with a calcium-free medium produced electromechanical dissociation without significant morphologic changes. However, the introduction of calcium into the medium produced substantial intracellular calcium influx, cellular contracture, and cell death.

The initial observation of the potential involvement of calcium in SCI was made by Balentine and Spector in 1977; they described the occurrence of selective intra-axonal calcification in SCI in rats.[17, 19] Calcium accumulation was noted to occur as early as 30 minutes after trauma and became more profuse in the late necrotic phases of the injury.[17, 19] Similar findings were also reported in injured spinal cords of monkeys, cats, and humans.[20] Additional observations support the detrimental role of calcium in spinal cord injury: (1) a rapid decrease in the extracellular calcium concentration occurs in the injured cord,[252, 280, 281] (2) the total calcium concentration in the injured spinal cord segment is significantly elevated after injury,[128] and (3) dripping calcium chloride onto the exposed spinal cord produces morphologic alterations and behavioral deficits similar to those seen following spinal cord trauma.[21, 22] In addition, post-traumatic spinal cord ischemia is likely to potentiate the role of calcium in SCI because calcium has also been implicated as a mediator of cellular death in CNS hypoxic-ischemic injury.[62, 242] Although the mechanisms for calcium accumulation in the injured spinal cord are not well defined, the following hypotheses have been advanced: (1) leakage through either the voltage-dependent calcium channels or the excitatory amino acid, N-methyl-D-aspartate (NMDA) receptor channel, (2) failure of Ca^{2+}-ATPase–mediated calcium extrusion, and (3) release of calcium from intracellular organelles (i.e., endoplasmic reticulum and mitochondria), which normally bind cytosolic calcium.[49]

Excess intracellular calcium produces deleterious effects on cellular function because increases in free cytosolic calcium disrupt the normal regulation of the function of calcium-dependent proteases and nucleases and adversely affect mitochondrial energy production.[173] Activation of calcium-dependent proteases can lead to the degradation of neurofilament and myelin proteins.[24, 25] In addition, activation of the calcium-dependent phospholipase enzymes, phospholipase C and A_2, results in the breakdown of cellular membranes and the production of arachidonate by phospholipase A_2.[219] The metabolism of arachidonate yields thromboxanes, leukotrienes, and free radicals, which promote tissue injury via their effects on the vasculature and the inflammatory response.

Endogenous Opiates

While studying spinal shock in 1980, Holaday and Faden observed that the opioid antagonist naloxone reversed the hypotension produced by cervical spinal cord transection.[140] Based on this observation, it was hypothesized that if naloxone would raise arterial pressure following SCI, spinal cord blood flow would improve and the extent of the injury would be reduced. Indeed, several investigations found naloxone to be beneficial in the treatment of experimental SCI,[80, 278] and although it improved post-traumatic SCBF, this effect was independent of its effect on systemic blood pressure.[278] These findings suggested the possibility of the involvement of endogenous opiates in SCI. In support of this, large elevations in plasma of the endogenous opiate β-endorphin have been found to occur following SCI.[81]

The exact nature of opiate involvement in SCI is unclear, because when naloxone is given in the high doses used to treat SCI, it is active at the three principal types of opiate receptors, the mu, delta, and kappa receptors.[180, 211] In lower doses, naloxone is typically more selective for the opiate mu receptor. The results from studies from Faden (1990) have implicated the endogenous opioid dynorphin A (1–17), the ligand for the kappa opioid receptor, as the opioid most likely to be involved in SCI for the following reasons: (1) dynorphin immunoreactivity selectively increased following SCI and the increase correlated with the severity of injury,[90] (2) significant time-dependent increases in kappa opioid receptor occur with spinal trauma,[171] (3) opiate antagonists more selective for the kappa receptor have been increasingly effective in the treatment of experimental spinal cord injury and ischemia,[27, 88, 91] and (4) dynorphin is the only endogenous opioid that produces hindlimb paralysis in the rat following its intrathecal injection into lumbar subarachnoid space.[84, 182, 217] It is clear, however, that dynorphin-induced hindlimb paralysis is in part a nonopiate effect, as it is not reversible by either naloxone or other more specific kappa antagonists.[183, 250] Furthermore, unlike the paralysis produced by spinal trauma, dynorphin-induced paralysis is not affected by pretreatment with thyrotropin-releasing hormone (TRH).[187] The intrathecal injection of dynorphin in paralytic doses in the rat is associated with marked decrease in SCBF, and this may in part explain its paralytic actions.[181]

Free Radicals

Free radicals are molecules that possess an unusual reactivity due to the presence of unpaired electrons in their outer orbits. A peculiar aspect of this reactivity is their ability to propagate via chain reactions.[57] Phospholipid and cholesterol components of biologic membranes are very susceptible to damage by free radical reactions,[59] and the involvement of fatty acids in oxygen free radical chain reactions is known as *lipid peroxidation*. Normal cellular metabolic pathways for oxygen reduction generate the following oxygen free radicals: superoxide anion (O_2^-), hydroxyl radical $OH^\cdot$, and hydrogen peroxide (H_2O_2). Normally, cells control the harmful effects of free radical production with a number of naturally occurring antioxidant compounds such as superoxide dismutases, catalases, glutathione peroxidase, ascorbic acid, α-tocopherol, steroids, cysteine, and selenium. Superoxide dismutases scavenge the superoxide anion by catalyzing its conversion into hydrogen peroxide and oxygen, whereas catalases reduce hydrogen peroxide to water.

Lipid peroxidation can result in the fragmentation of cellular membranes in pathologic states such as CNS ischemia, in which excess free radicals are generated.[59, 268, 277] In addition, these processes have also been implicated in brain and spinal cord trauma.[59, 168] Several observations support the role of free radical lipid peroxidation in SCI because of the observation of the following after spinal trauma: (1) increase in peroxidized polyunsaturated fatty acid breakdown products,[172, 196] (2) decrease in cholesterol accompanied by the appearance of cholesterol oxidation products,[8] (3) activation of guanylate cyclase and increase in cyclic guanosine monophosphate (cGMP),[124, 172] (4) decrease in levels of tissue antioxidants, such as α-tocopherol, and ascorbic acid,[214, 235] and (5) inhibition of the phospholipid-dependent membrane-bound Na$^+$-K$^+$-ATPase.[50] In addition, antioxidants have been shown to be effective in the treatment of experimental SCI.[8, 10, 123]

Among the possible potential sources of oxygen radicals in SCI is the depletion of adenosine triphosphate (ATP) and production of adenosine monophosphate (AMP) which is degraded to hypoxanthine.[160] During ischemia, xanthine dehydrogenase converts to its oxidase form, and in the presence of hypoxanthine catalyzes the formation of O$_2$.[189] Two other potential sources of oxygen free radicals are coenzyme Q (a component of the electron transport chain), and the metabolism of arachidonate in the cyclooxygenase pathway, which generates superoxide radicals. This effect is probably enhanced by the calcium-mediated activation of phospholipase A$_2$ that occurs following injury. In addition, the respiratory burst of invading neutrophils, the auto-oxidation of catecholamines, and the release of hemoglobin from the hemorrhage that accompanies SCI are also potential sources of oxygen free radicals.[190, 197] Hemoglobin can also stimulate lipid peroxidation and provide a source of iron to catalyze oxygen radical and lipid peroxidation reactions.[7, 15, 233] Besides injury to cellular membranes, free radicals can contribute to tissue injury by disrupting lysosomal membranes,[104] promoting tissue edema,[47, 48] and inhibiting mitochondrial function.[59]

Excitatory Amino Acids

The concept of excitatory amino acid–mediated cell death, or excitotoxicity, was introduced in 1969 when Olney[206] described the neurotoxic effects of systemically administered glutamate on the endocrine hypothalamus. This concept now embraces the deleterious actions of the excitatory amino acid transmitters, glutamate and aspartate, at their receptors. Specific evidence now implicates excitotoxicity in the pathophysiology of CNS hypoxic-ischemic injury[230] as well as in brain and spinal trauma.[92, 94, 130, 212, 272, 273]

Of the three well-characterized excitatory amino acid receptors, the majority of data suggest that the N-methyl-D-aspartate (NMDA) receptor complex is predominantly involved in excitotoxicity in spinal trauma.[229, 242, 243] However, it must be emphasized that glutamate also acts as an agonist at the kainate and the quisqualate receptors, and recent evidence suggests that non-NMDA receptors are also involved in SCI.[272, 273] The following observations support the role of excitatory amino acid toxicity in SCI: (1) excitatory amino acid concentrations increase following spinal trauma[210]; (2) spinal ischemia is associated with SCI, and excitotoxicity has been shown to occur in models of CNS ischemia; and (3) administration of excitatory amino acid receptor antagonists as a form of treatment in experimental SCI and ischemia is effective in improving neurologic outcome.[93, 167, 188]

Other

Studies in the histologic evolution of SCI have shown that an infiltration by polymorphonuclear leukocytes occurs early.[194] In fact, polymorphonuclear leukocytes are deleterious because they can actively engage in neuronophagia acutely after spinal injury,[194] and their respiratory burst serves as a source of free radicals.[190] The macrophage, which heavily infiltrates the lesions after the acute period, may also play a role in the demyelination that occurs in SCI. The eicosanoids thromboxane and leukotrienes may also play a role in SCI. Levels of thromboxane, which stimulates platelet aggregation and vasoconstriction, are elevated in SCI.[58, 145] Leukotrienes are potent mediators of inflammation and have been reported to either increase or remain unchanged after SCI.[58, 198]

THERAPY OF ACUTE EXPERIMENTAL SPINAL CORD INJURY

Unfortunately, studies in the therapy of experimental SCI have occasionally yielded conflicting results, and this raises difficulties when trying to transfer specific therapies from the laboratory to the clinical arena. In large part these conflicts are due to the different injury models, animal species, anesthetics, and methods utilized to measure neurologic outcome by the various investigators. The anatomic and physiologic bases for the recovery function following SCI are unclear because most studies do not include detailed morphologic analysis. Our understanding of the anatomic requirements for the preservation of locomotive capacity in animals suggests that as little as 10% of the white matter permits locomotion.[32, 78, 261] Following SCI in cats, a preferential loss of the axons, which are large and are located toward the center of the lesion, occurs.[32] Moreover, conduction across the lesion for the surviving axons is absent or abnormal,[33] which suggests that demyelination plays an important role in SCI.

The first measures employed in the treatment of experimental SCI were surgical, not pharmacologic. Allen described the beneficial effects of myelotomies as early as 1911.[1, 2] The application of hypothermia was based on the observation that it decreased cerebral metabolic demand and reduced brain volume,[195, 227] and it became popular in the treatment of experimental SCI in the 1960s.[3, 30, 116, 144] The technique of hypothermia fell out of favor because it is technically difficult to implement in humans.[30, 116, 144]

Steroids

Steroids were one of the earlier pharmacologic agents utilized in the treatment of both experimental and human SCI based on their anti-inflammatory actions and their effectiveness in treating cerebral edema.[102, 133] Reviews of studies that assessed some form of functional outcome, such as the neurologic status of the animal, have shown the beneficial effects of steroids in the treatment of experimental SCI.[30, 38, 45, 56, 71, 77, 117, 129, 193, 274, 278] Some studies have reported negative or no effects.[77, 86, 135, 231] Conflicting results are secondary to the following factors: (1) the use of different injury models, (2) the use of different measures of outcome, and (3) the use of different treatment protocols. For example, investigators used different steroids (methylprednisolone vs. dexamethasone), doses, routes of administration (intravenous vs. intrathecal), or combinations with surgical therapeutic modalities (myelotomy or dural decompression).[71, 231]

The particular actions of the different steroids have become important since it has been shown that methylprednisolone is a stronger inhibitor of lipid peroxidation.[38] The fact that a specific dose is also required to obtain the desired effect was also shown in studies in which high doses of methylprednisolone (30 mg/kg) improved neurologic recovery following SCI. This led to its incorporation in the second human SCI cooperative study[36, 37, 281] (Young and co-workers, 1982; Braughler and colleagues, 1982).

The beneficial actions of steroids in SCI include the following: (1) prevention of the loss of potassium from the injured cord tissue and facilitation of the recovery of the extracellular level of calcium ions[176, 281]; (2) amelioration of post-traumatic spinal cord ischemia[6, 125, 281]; (3) enhancement of the post-injury activity of neuronal Na^+-K^+-ATPase[37]; (4) enhancement of the excitability of the CNS, including the motor neuron[37, 122, 270]; and (5) inhibition of lipid peroxidation,[37, 121] which is perhaps the most significant beneficial action of steroids in SCI.

A new class of steroid compounds, the 21-aminosteroids, which are potent inhibitors of lipid peroxidation and are devoid of glucocorticoid activity, have been developed.[39, 147] These compounds have already shown efficacy in the treatment of experimental brain ischemia and brain and spinal trauma.[9, 127] In fact the prototype of these compounds, tirilazad mesylate, has already been incorporated into the third National Acute Spinal Cord Injury Study clinical trial.

Opiate Antagonists

Based on the initial observations of the effect of naloxone on spinal shock, Faden and colleagues[91] showed it was beneficial in the treatment of experimental spinal cord injury (see section on secondary mechanisms). Various investigators also confirmed the positive effects of naloxone in SCI[80, 81, 83, 103, 278]; however, as in the case of steroids, conflicting results have been obtained.[31, 120, 267] The differences in methodologies, therapeutic regimens, and SCI models must be taken into consideration when interpreting these conflicting results.

The actions of naloxone are not necessarily at opiate receptors, because naloxone has also been demonstrated to have the following effects: (1) reversal of post-traumatic calcium and ascorbic acid derangements,[215, 252] (2) inhibition of neutrophil superoxide release and iron-catalyzed lyposomal lipid peroxidation,[170, 240] and (3) inhibition of proteolysis and stabilization of lysosomal membranes.[53] Because recent evidence has implicated the endogenous opioid dynorphin A in SCI, more selective kappa opiate receptor (the receptor for dynorphin A) antagonists have been developed and proved to be efficacious in the treatment of experimental SCI.[27, 91, 93] Results from the second National Acute Spinal Cord Injury Study did not show naloxone to be beneficial in human injury[36]; however, antagonists more selective for the kappa receptor may be efficacious.

Like naloxone, TRH was beneficial in models of circulatory shock and spinal injury,[82, 141] and various studies have shown TRH to be effective in the treatment of experimental SCI.[85] Because TRH has a short half-life, more stable analogues have been developed and successfully utilized in the treatment of experimental SCI.[27, 89, 95, 218] As in other drug studies, there have been negative results in the treatment of SCI with TRH.[142, 143] Although it was initially hypothesized that TRH acted as a physiologic opiate antagonist,[141] the actual mechanisms by which TRH improves neurologic function in SCI are unknown. It has been documented to potentiate spinal reflexes and to have trophic effects on cholinergic spinal neurons.[109, 237]

Excitatory Amino Acid Antagonists

Excitotoxicity, specifically the actions of glutamate and aspartate at the NMDA receptor complex, have been implicated in the pathophysiology of SCI. Two types of NMDA receptor antagonists have been used in the therapy of experimental SCI: competitive antagonists that act at glutamate's binding site and noncompetitive antagonists that act at a site located in the NMDA receptor ion channel.[158] Theoretically, noncompetitive antagonists offer the advantage of functioning in an agonist-dependent fashion (i.e., the receptor must be activated for the antagonist to bind). This is favorable for the treatment of pathologic conditions such as CNS trauma and ischemia, in which excessive receptor activation is thought to occur.[269] A variety of competitive and noncompetitive NMDA receptor antagonists have been tested and shown to be protective in models of spinal cord trauma and ischemia.[92, 167, 188, 273] In addition, one study has reported beneficial effects in SCI treated with non-NMDA receptor antagonists.[273]

Calcium Channel Antagonists

As discussed in previous sections, the intracellular accumulation of calcium plays an important role in the mediation of neural injury, and calcium channel blockers have been successfully used in certain models of brain ischemia.[247, 248] The actions of calcium channel blocking drugs cannot be ascribed to the prevention of calcium movement into the neuron because calcium may enter cells via other receptor channels (such as the NMDA receptor) or by nonspecific leakage through the damaged cell membrane. Moreover, calcium that is normally bound to intracellular organelles may be released into the cytosol after injury. The actions of calcium channel blockers on the vascular smooth muscle can also produce a vasodilatory improvement in perfusion and thereby improve neurologic outcome.[259] These effects, however, raise concerns over their application in the treatment of SCI, because mean arterial pressure could be lowered to the point of being detrimental to the perfusion of the injured cord (which cannot autoregulate). The significance of this issue is greater in cervical and high thoracic cord lesions, in which neurogenic hypotension is likely to occur. Although nimodipine has been reported to increase blood flow and restore neurophysiologic function in the traumatized spinal cord,[99, 228] it has not improved neurologic function in models of spinal cord trauma or ischemia.[87, 106, 142, 143]

GM₁-Ganglioside

GM₁-ganglioside, a major component of the neuronal membranes in the CNS, was found to be beneficial in models of CNS ischemia,[12, 155, 254] in clinical stroke trials and, on a more limited basis, in models of SCI.[35, 114] Based on these observations, it was utilized in a human SCI study that contained a small number of subjects with positive results.[111] An interesting aspect was that it appeared to be of benefit when administered up to 72 hours postinjury. This study had several limitations and its results have been questioned. In addition, a clinical trial of GM₁-ganglioside in stroke in a limited number of patients did not find it to be of value.[139] Nevertheless, a major study of the effects of GM₁-ganglioside in human SCI has been undertaken and will hopefully resolve this issue. The actions of GM₁-ganglioside in SCI are not known, and the following theories have been proposed: (1) it increases neurite outgrowth in vitro,[61, 149] (2) it can reduce retrograde and anterograde fiber degeneration,[232, 246] (3) it can induce regeneration and sprouting in neurons,[232] and (4) it reduces amino acid–induced neurotoxicity.[202]

Other Therapies

Based on the monoamine theory of spinal cord injury,[207, 208] catecholamine blockade has been tried in SCI with compounds such as α-methyltyrosine, phenoxybenzamine, or clonidine. Results from these experiments have been inconsistent.[135, 144, 200, 208] A number of other pharmacologic therapies have been used in the treatment of acute experimental SCI and they have provided either limited data or conflicting results: urea,[150] levothyroxine,[131, 258] dimethyl sulfoxide,[56, 151] enzymes,[119] phenytoin,[113] leupeptin,[146] and electrical fields.[216]

SUMMARY

Only since 1990 has an effective clinical therapy for human SCI been available. Nonetheless, the institution of methylprednisolone therapy marked the first application of a pharmacologic agent, the treatment regimen of which was developed from sound laboratory research. A number of promising compounds aimed at specific deleterious processes in SCI are presently on the horizon. The recent development of the 21-aminosteroid tirilazad and its applications to human injury is an excellent example.

REFERENCES

1. Allen AR: Surgery of experimental lesion of spinal cord equivalent to crush injury of fracture dislocation of spinal column. JAMA 57:878–880, 1911.
2. Allen AR: Remarks on the histopathological changes in the spinal cord due to impact: An experimental study. J Nerv Ment Dis 41:141–147, 1914.
3. Alvin MS, White RJ, Acosta-Rua Gaston, et al: Study of functional recovery produced by delayed localized cooling after spinal cord injury in primates. J Neurosurg 29:113–120, 1968.
4. Alvin MS, Bunegin L: Catecholamine synthesis rates in traumatized spinal cord. Anat Rec 178:296–297, 1974.
5. Anderson DK, Means ED, Waters TR, et al: Spinal cord energy metabolism following compression trauma to the feline spinal cord. J Neurosurg 53:375–380, 1980.
6. Anderson DK, Means ED, Waters TR, et al: Microvascular perfusion and metabolism in injured spinal cord after methylprednisolone treatment. J Neurosurg 56:106–113, 1982.
7. Anderson DK, Means ED: Lipid peroxidation in the spinal cord: FeCl₂ induction and protection with antioxidants. Neurochem Pathol 1:249–264, 1983.
8. Anderson DK, Saunders RD, Demediuk P, et al: Lipid hydrolysis and peroxidation in injured spinal cord: Partial protection with methylprednisolone or vitamin E and selenium. CNS Trauma 2:257-267, 1985.
9. Anderson DK, Braughler JM, Hall ED, et al: Effects of treatment with U-74006F on neurological outcome following experimental spinal cord injury. J Neurosurg 69:562–567, 1988.
10. Anderson DK, Hall ED, Braughler JM, et al: Effect of delayed administration of U74006F (tirilazad mesylate) on recovery of locomotor function after experimental spinal cord injury. J Neurotrauma 8:187–192, 1991.
11. Anderson TE: A controlled pneumatic technique for experimental spinal cord contusion. J Neurosci Methods 6:327–333, 1982.
12. Argentino C, Sachetti ML, Toni D, et al: GM₁ ganglioside therapy in acute ischemic stroke: Italian acute stroke study– Hemodilution + Drug. Stroke 20:1143–1149, 1989.
13. Assenmacher DR, Ducker TB: Experimental traumatic paraplegia: The vascular and pathological changes seen in irreversible and reversible spinal-cord lesions. J Bone Joint Surg Am 53:671–680, 1971.
14. Auckland K, Bower BF, Berliner RW: Measurement of local blood flow with hydrogen gas. Circ Res 14:164–187, 1964.
15. Aust SD, Morehouse LA, Thomas CE: Role of metals in oxygen radical reactions. J Free Rad Biol Med 1:3–25, 1985.
16. Baker PF: The regulation of intracellular calcium. Symp Soc Exp Biol 30:67–88, 1976.
17. Balentine JD, Spector M: Calcifications of axons in experimental spinal cord trauma. Ann Neurol 2:520–523, 1977.

effects of dynorphin and dynorphin related peptides after their intrathecal injection in rats. Neuropeptides 3:233–240, 1983.

218. Puniak MA, Freeman GM, Agresta CA, et al: Comparison of a serotonin antagonist, opioid antagonist, and TRH analog for the acute treatment of experimental spinal trauma. J Neurotrauma 8:193–203, 1991.

219. Rasmussen H: The calcium messenger system (first of two parts). N Engl J Med 314:1094–1101, 1986.

220. Rawe SE, Roth RH, Boadle-Biber M, et al: Norepinephrine levels in spinal cord trauma: I. Biochemical study of hemorrhagic necrosis. J Neurosurg 46:350–357, 1977.

221. Rawe SE, Roth RH, Collins WF: Norepinephrine levels in experimental spinal cord trauma: II. Histopathological study of hemorrhagic necrosis. J Neurosurg 46:350–357, 1977.

222. Rawe SE, Lee WA, Perot PL: Spinal cord glucose utilization after experimental spinal cord injury. Neurosurgery 9:40–47, 1981.

223. Reivich M, Jehle J, Sokoloff L, et al: Measurement of regional cerebral blood flow with antipyrine-^{14}C in awake cats. J Appl Physiol 27:296–300, 1969.

224. Rivlin AS, Tator CH: Effect of duration of acute spinal cord compression in a new acute cord injury model in the rat. Surg Neurol 9:39–43, 1978.

225. Rivlin AS, Tator CH: Regional spinal cord blood flow in rats after severe cord trauma. J Neurosurg 49:844–853, 1978.

226. Rosenthal M, Lamanna J, Yamada S, et al: Oxidative metabolism, extracellular potassium, and sustained potential shifts in cat spinal cord in situ. Brain Res 162:113–127, 1979.

227. Rosomoff HL, Gilbert R: Brain volume and cerebrospinal fluid pressure during hypothermia. Am J Physiol 183:19–22, 1955.

228. Ross IB, Tator CH: Further studies of nimodipine in experimental spinal cord injury in the rat. J Neurotrauma 8:229–238, 1991.

229. Rothman SM, Olney JW: Excitotoxicity and the NMDA receptor. Trends Neurol Sci 10:299–302, 1987.

230. Rothman SM, Olney JW: Glutamate and the pathophysiology of hypoxic-ischemic brain damage. Ann Neurol 19:105–111, 1988.

231. Rucker NC, Lumb WV, Scott RJ: Combined pharmacologic and surgical treatments for acute spinal cord trauma. Am J Vet Res 42:1138–1142, 1981.

232. Sabel BA, Del Mastro R, Dunbar GL, et al: Reduction of anterograde degeneration in brain damaged rats by GM$_1$-gangliosides. Neurosci Lett 77:360–366, 1987.

233. Sadrzadeh SM, Graf E, Panter SS, et al: Hemoglobin, a biological Fenton reagent. J Biol Chem 259:14354–14356, 1984.

234. Sandler AN, Tator CH: Review of the effect of spinal cord trauma on the vessels and blood flow in the spinal cord. J Neurosurg 45:638–646, 1976.

235. Saunders RD, Dugan LL, Demediuk P, et al: Effects of methylprednisolone and the combination of alpha tocopherol and selenium on arachidonic acid metabolism and lipid peroxidation in traumatized spinal cord tissue. J Neurochem 49:24–31, 1987.

236. Schanne FAX, Kane AB, Young EE, et al: Calcium dependence of toxic cell death: A final common pathway. Science 206:700–702, 1979.

237. Schmidt-Achert KM, Askansas V, Engel WK: Thyrotropin-releasing hormone enhances choline acetyl transferase and creatine kinase in cultured spinal ventral horn neurons. J Neurochem 43:586–589, 1984.

238. Senter HJ, Venes JL: Altered blood flow and secondary injury in experimental spinal cord trauma. J Neurosurg 49:569–578, 1978.

239. Senter HJ, Venes JL: Loss of autoregulation and posttraumatic ischemia following experimental spinal cord trauma. J Neurosurg 50:198–206, 1979.

240. Simpkins CO, Alailima ST, Tate EA: Inhibition by naloxone of neutrophil superoxide release: A potentially useful anti-inflammatory effect. Circ Shock 20:181–191, 1986.

241. Singer JM, Russel GV, Coe JE: Changes in evoked potentials after experimental cervical spinal cord injury in the monkey. Exp Neurol 29:449–461, 1970.

242. Simon RP, Griffiths T, Evans MC, et al: Calcium overload in selectively vulnerable neurons of the hippocampus during and after ischemia: An electron microscopy study in the rat. J Cereb Blood Flow Metab 4:350–361, 1984.

243. Simon RP, Swan JH, Griffith T, et al: Blockade of N-methyl-D-aspartate receptors may protect against ischemic damage in the brain. Science 226:850–852, 1984.

244. Smith DR, Smith HJ, Rajjoub RK: Measurement of spinal cord blood flow by the microsphere technique. Neurosurgery 2:27–30, 1978.

245. Smith AJK, McCreery DB, Bloedel JR, et al: Hyperemia, CO$_2$ responsiveness, and autoregulation in the white matter following experimental spinal cord injury. J Neurosurg 48:239–251, 1978.

246. Sofroniew MV, Pearson RCA, Cuello AC, et al: Parenterally administered GM$_1$ ganglioside prevents retrograde degeneration of the rat basal forebrain. Brain Research 398:393–396, 1986 .

247. Steen PA, Newberg LA, Milde JH, et al: Nimodipine cerebral blood flow and neurologic recovery after complete global ischemia in the dog. J Cereb Blood Flow Metab 3:38–43, 1982.

248. Steen PA, Gisvold SE, Milde JH, et al: Nimodipine improves outcome when given after complete cerebral ischemia in primates. Anesthesiology 62:406–414, 1985.

249. Stern MD: In vivo evaluation of microcirculation by coherent light scattering. Nature 254:56–58, 1975.

250. Stevens CW, Yaksh TL: Dynorphin A and related peptides administered intrathecally in the rat: A search for putative kappa opiate receptor activity. J Pharmacol Exp Ther 238:833–838, 1986.

251. Stokes BT, Garwood M: Traumatically induced alterations in the oxygen fields in the canine spinal cod. Exp Neurol 75:665–677, 1982.

252. Stokes BT, Fox P, Hollinden G: Extracellular metabolites: Their measurement and role in the acute phase of spinal cord injury. In Dacey RG Jr, Winn HR, Rimmel RW, et al (eds): Trauma of the Central Nervous System. New York, Raven Press, 1985, pp 309–323.

253. Studer RK, Welch DM, Siegel BA: Transient alteration of the blood-brain barrier: Effect of hypertonic solutions administered via carotid artery injection. Exp Neurol 44:266–273, 1974.

254. Tanaka K, Dora E, Urbanics R, et al: Effect of the ganglioside GM$_1$, on cerebral metabolism, microcirculation, recovery kinetics of EcoG and histology, during the recovery period following focal ischemia in cats. Stroke 17:1170–1178, 1986.

255. Tarlov IM, Klinger H, Vitale S: Spinal cord compression studies: I. Experimental techniques to produce acute and gradual compression in dogs. Arch Neurol Psychiatry 70:813–819, 1953.

256. Tator CH: Acute spinal cord injury in primates produced by an inflatable extradural cuff. Can J Surg 16:222–231, 1972.

257. Tator CH: Spine-spinal cord relationships in spinal cord trauma. Clin Neurosurg 30:479–494, 1983.

258. Tator CH, van der Jagt RH: The effect of exogenous thyroid hormones on functional recovery of the rat after acute spinal cord compression injury. J Neurosurg 53:381–384, 1980.

259. Van Neuten JM, Wauquier A, De Clerk F, et al: Vascular reactivity of selective calcium-entry blockers. In Lenzi S, Descovich GC (eds): Atherosclerosis and Cardiovascular Disease. Boston, MTP Press, 1984, pp 93–105.

260. Vyklicky L, Sykova E: The effects of increased extracellular potassium in the isolated spinal cord on the flexor reflex of the frog. Neurosci Lett 19:203–207, 1975.

261. Windle WF, Smart JO, Beers JJ: Residual function after subtotal spinal cord transection in adult cats. Neurology 8:518–521, 1958.

262. Wagner FC, Dohrmann GJ, Bucy PC: Histopathology of transitory traumatic paraplegia in the monkey. J Neurosurg 35:272–276, 1971.

263. Wagner FC Jr, VanGilder JC, Dohrmann GJ: Pathological changes from acute to chronic in experimental spinal cord trauma. J Neurosurg 48:92–98, 1978.

264. Wagner FC Jr, Stewart WB: Effect of trauma dose on spinal cord edema. J Neurosurg 54:802–806, 1978.

265. Walker JG, Yates RR, O'Neill JJ, et al: Canine spinal cord energy state after experimental trauma. J Neurochem 29:929–932, 1977.

266. Walker JG, Yates RR, Yashon D: Regional canine spinal cord energy state after experimental trauma. J Neurochem 33:397–401, 1979.

267. Wallace MC, Tator CH: Failure of blood transfusion or naloxone to improve clinical recovery after experimental spinal cord injury. Neurosurgery 19:489–494, 1986.

268. Watson BD, Busto R, Goldberg W, et al: Lipid peroxidation in vivo induced by reversible global ischemia in rat brain. J Neurochem 42:268–274, 1984.

269. Wong EH, Knight AR, Woodruff GN:[³H]MK-801 labels a site on the N-methyl-D-aspartate receptor channel complex in rat membrane. J Neurochem 50:274–281, 1988.
270. Woodbury DM, Vernadakis A: Effects of steroids on the central nervous system. Methods Horm Res 5:1–56, 1966.
271. Wrathall JR, Pettegrew RK, Harvey F: Spinal cord contusion in the rat: Production of graded, reproducible, injury groups. Exp Neurol 88:108–122, 1985.
272. Wrathall JR, Teng YD, Choiniere D, et al: Evidence that local non-NMDA receptors contribute to functional deficits in contusive spinal cord injury. Brain Res 586:140–143, 1992.
273. Wrathall JR, Bouzoukis J, Choiniere D: Effect of kynurenate on functional deficits resulting from traumatic spinal cord injury. Eur J Pharmacol 218:273–281, 1992.
274. Xu J, Qu ZX, Hogan EL, et al: Protective effect of methylprednisolone on vascular injury in rat spinal cord injury. J Neurotrauma 9:245–253, 1992.
275. Yammada S, Sanders D, Maeda G: Oxidative metabolism during and following spinal cord ischemia. Neurol Res 3:1–16, 1981.
276. Yashon D, Bingham G Jr, Faddoul E, et al: Edema of the spinal cord following experimental impact trauma. J Neurosurg 38:693–697, 1973.
277. Yoshida S, Abe K, Busto R, et al: Influence of transient ischemia on lipid soluble antioxidants, free fatty acids and energy metabolites in the rat brain. Brain Res 245:307–316, 1982.
278. Young W, Flamm ES, Demopoulos HB, et al: Effect of naloxone on posttraumatic ischemia in experimental spinal contusion. J Neurosurg 55:209–219, 1981.
279. Young W, Koreh I, Yen V, et al: Effect of sympathectomy on extracellular potassium activity and blood flow in experimental spinal cord contusion. Brain Res 253:115–125, 1982.
280. Young W, Yen V, Blight AR: Extracellular calcium activity in experimental spinal cord contusion. Brain Res 253:115–125, 1982.
281. Young W, Flamm ES: Effect of high dose corticosteroid therapy on blood flow, evoked potentials, and extracellular calcium in experimental spinal injury. J Neurosurg 57:667–673, 1982.
282. Young W: Blood flow, metabolic and neurophysiological mechanisms in spinal cord injury. In Becker PB, Povlishock JT (eds): Central Nervous System Trauma Report. National Institute of Neurological and Communicative Disorders and Stroke, Bethesda, Md, 1985, pp 463–473.
283. Zimmerman ANE: Paradoxical influence of calcium ions on the permeability of the cell membranes of the isolated rat heart. Nature 211:646–647, 1966.
284. Zimmerman ANE, Daems W, Hülsmann WC, et al: Morphological changes of heart muscle caused by successive perfusion with calcium-free and calcium-containing solutions (calcium paradox). Cardiovasc Res 1:201–209, 1967.
285. Zivin JA, Doppman JL, Reid JL, et al: Biochemical and histochemical studies of biogenic amines in spinal cord trauma. Neurology 26:99–107, 1976.
286. Zivin JA, Degirolami V: Spinal cord infarction: A highly reproducible stroke model. Stroke 11:200–204, 1980.

CHAPTER 8

Biomechanics of Spinal Cord and Nerve Root Injury

Björn L. Rydevik ‖ *Richard Skalak†* ‖ *Michael K. Kwan*
Kjell Olmarker

ANATOMY OF THE SPINAL CORD AND NERVE ROOTS

The spinal cord is the extension of the central nervous system caudal to the cranium. The spinal cord is located within the vertebral column and is, therefore, relatively well protected from external trauma by the enclosing bony structures. When the axons that run within the spinal cord longitudinally are about to exit the spine to the periphery, they first leave the spinal cord as small bundles called rootlets. These rootlets join segmentally and form the somewhat larger nerve roots. The nerve roots in turn are transformed to spinal nerves which continue as peripheral nerves beyond the spinal column (Fig. 8–1). The nerve roots at these locations are supplied with protective connective tissue layers which are continuations from the surrounding meninges.[95] Unlike peripheral nerves, the intraspinal structures, such as the spinal cord and the nerve roots, have a paucity of surrounding protective connective tissue layers.[32, 33, 56] Hence, the nerve roots might be well protected from external trauma, but they are extremely vulnerable when exposed to direct trauma due to intraspinal conditions such as disc herniation and tumors, or when the surrounding vertebral protection fails, as in spine trauma.[75, 94, 99]

Impulses from the central nervous system are propagated down through the spinal cord, and linked to the motor cell bodies, located in the ventral horn of the spinal cord (see Fig. 8–1). The axons of the motor cells leave the spinal cord through nerve roots from the ventral side of the spinal cord, called ventral or motor roots. Conversely, impulses to the central nervous system from the periphery enter the spinal cord in the dorsolateral corner, through the dorsal, or sensory, nerve roots. The nerve cell bodies of the sensory axons, located in the respective dorsal root ganglion at each spinal level, constitute an enlargement of the sensory roots in, or close to, the intervertebral foramina. From these cell bodies there are two axons, one directing impulses toward the spinal cord, within the sensory root, called the preganglionic axon, and one running toward the periphery, called the postganglionic axon.

The microscopic anatomy of the spinal cord is similar to that of the brain, with axons surrounded by glia cells. However, in the nerve roots there is a transitional zone some millimeters after the roots leave the spinal cord where the axons become surrounded by Schwann cells.[10, 32, 89] In this respect, the microanatomy of the compartment within the nerve roots in which the axons are located, called the endoneurium, closely resembles that of the peripheral nerves.

The surface of the spinal cord is covered by the pia mater, which in turn is surrounded by cerebrospinal fluid (see Fig. 8–1). The cerebrospinal fluid and the nerve tissue are enclosed by the dura and the arachnoid. Between these two layers is a strong diffusion barrier called the neurothelium.[7, 15, 102]

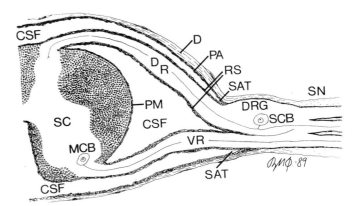

Figure 8–1 = Cross section of a segment of the spinal cord *(SC)*, a ventral *(VR)* and a dorsal *(DR)* spinal nerve root. The cell bodies *(MCB)* of the motor axons, which run in the ventral nerve root, are located in the anterior horn of the gray matter of the spinal cord. The cell bodies *(SCB)* of the sensory axons, which run in the dorsal nerve root, are located in the dorsal root ganglion *(DRG)*. The ventral and dorsal nerve roots blend just caudal to the dorsal root ganglion, and form the spinal nerve *(SN)*. The spinal cord is covered with the pia mater *(PM)*. This sheath continues out on the spinal nerve roots as the root sheath *(RS)*. The root sheath reflects to the pia-arachnoid *(PA)* at the subarachnoid triangle *(SAT)*. Together with the dura *(D)*, the pia-arachnoid forms the spinal dura. The spinal cord and nerve roots are floating freely in the cerebrospinal fluid *(CSF)* in the subarachnoid space. (From Olmarker K: Thesis, Gothenburg, Sweden, 1990.)

Supported by grants from the Swedish Medical Research Council (8685, 9758), the Asker's Research Foundation, and Gothenburg University, Gothenburg, Sweden.
†Professor Skalak died on Aug 17, 1997.

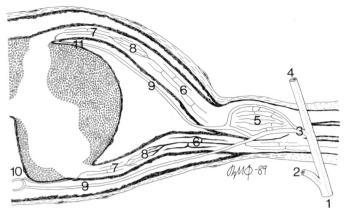

Figure 8–2 = Schematic drawing of the vascular supply to the spinal cord and nerve roots. When the intermediate branch of the segmental artery *(1)* enters the spinal canal it divides into an anterior spinal canal branch *(2)*, a nervous system branch *(3)*, and a posterior spinal canal branch *(4)*. The nervous system branch joins the nerve root and forms a ganglionic plexus *(5)* and caudal nerve root arteries running craniad *(6)*. From the vasa corona of the spinal cord cranial nerve root arteries *(7)* run caudad. The caudal and cranial nerve root arteries anastomose within the cranial half of the nerve root *(8)*. From the nervous system branch there are also medullary feeder arteries *(9)*. These vessels run craniad through the subarachnoid space, without any connections to the nerve root arteries, to the vasa corona of the spinal cord. *10*, Anterior spinal artery. *11*, One of the two dorsolateral spinal arteries. (From Olmarker K: Thesis, Gothenburg, Sweden, 1990.)

The nerve roots have an organization of surrounding tissues similar to the spinal cord. However, the distal parts of the nerve roots are enclosed by an extension of the spinal dura mater which becomes narrow and thereby tightly encloses the nerve roots just prior to leaving the spinal canal. Also, the pia mater that covers the spinal cord transforms to the pia-arachnoid, or root sheath. This provides a weak diffusion barrier which is 5 to 15 cellular layers thick.[38, 42, 83] The barrier properties are located in the innermost cell layers. These cells, together with the neurothelium from the spinal dura, constitute the perineurium of the peripheral nerves, a strong diffusion barrier which encloses every peripheral nerve fascicle.[51, 75, 86]

The spinal cord and nerve roots have a special vascular arrangement.[18, 47, 48, 70, 71] From the abdominal aorta there are segmental vessels which approach the spinal canal (Fig. 8–2). Besides branches which supply the vertebral column, there is a specific branch from each segmental vessel that enters the intervertebral foramen. This branch first gives off vessels to the nerve roots and dorsal root ganglion and then continues, with no branches, to the spinal cord.[70] There are four of these medullary feeder branches at each vertebral level at the early embryologic stages, but in adult life only three may be of importance. The most commonly known of these vessels supplies the spinal cord in the lower thoracic spine and is usually referred to as the artery of Adamkiewicz.[2, 3]

The spinal cord is surrounded by a network of vessels called the vasa corona. This network is supplied by the medullary feeder vessels. The vasa corona send off vessels that follow the nerve roots. These intrinsic nerve root vessels anastomose with similar vessels coming from the distal parts of the nerve roots.[71] It has been suggested that the anastomosing site is particularly vulnerable due to a relative paucity of vessels. However, the presence of this "watershed" area has been debated.[103]

BIOMECHANICAL PROPERTIES OF THE SPINAL CORD AND DURA

The spinal cord, like many soft tissue structures, has specific biomechanical properties which are important for its functional integrity. In flexion of the spinal column, the spinal cord tends to stretch and its cross-sectional area is reduced. Local compression and bending can also occur, or increase, when the cord passes over an osteophytic spur in this mode.[99] In extension of the spinal column, the spinal cord can be compressed while the cross-sectional area of the cord increases, as occurs with an incompressible material. Under normal conditions, these motions of the spinal column would not lead to detrimental stresses or strains in the spinal cord. In pathologic situations, however, as occurs, for example, with thickening of the ligamentum flavum, disc herniation, osteophyte formation, and spinal stenosis, the same functional movements may result in abnormal stresses and strains in the spinal cord and cause neurologic disturbances. In order to analyze such pathologic conditions and changes of the spinal cord, it is important to understand its normal biomechanical properties. For example, a simplified model studying the stress patterns in the spinal cord, caused by direct compression applied transversely, showed a distribution of shear stress with maximum value centrally and not in the periphery.[73] These results correspond well with neurologic dysfunction seen from trauma, where central areas of the spinal cord are injured more often than peripheral areas.

Studies of the biomechanical properties of the spinal cord began with the pioneer work of Breig.[12, 13] He studied the biomechanics of the spinal cord and column in a series of experiments, using fresh cadavers appropriately prepared to show the movement and deformation of the spinal cord. The cord exhibits a nonlinear stress-strain behavior characteristic of most soft tissues.[16] When suspended freely from the upper end in the air, the spinal cord by its own weight has been shown to elongate by more than 10%. The cord is very extensible initially when placed under tension, even with forces less than 0.01 N. Such flexibility is due to the accordion-like folding and unfolding of the cord. The folds are more distinct on its posterior surface, where maximal decrease in length occurs, than on its anterior surface. However, when the spinal cord is stretched further it stiffens and becomes resistant to tension and deformation. Measurements have shown that the spinal cord can support 20 to 30 N in tension before mechanical breakage occurs. Because of the incompressibility of the cord, the length changes are accompanied by changes in the cross-sectional area of the cord, as indicated earlier. This corresponding cross-

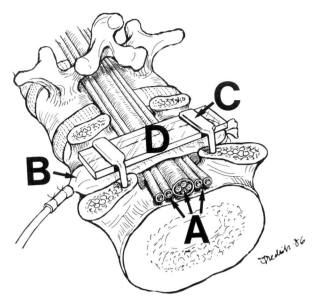

Figure 8–5 = Schematic drawing of an experimental model of nerve compression in the pig. The cauda equina *(A)* is compressed by an inflatable balloon *(B)* that is fixed to the spine by two L-shaped pins *(C)* and a Plexiglas plate *(D)*. (From Olmarker K, Rydevik B, Holm S: Edema formation in spinal nerve roots induced by experimental graded compression. An experimental study on the pig cauda equina with special reference to differences in effects between rapid and slow onset of compression. Spine 14:569–573, 1989.)

induces some venular congestion even at low pressure levels, that is, 5 to 10 mm Hg.[62, 67] Capillary stasis occurs at a slightly higher pressure level, but the blood flow in the endoneurial capillaries is intimately linked to the flow in the connected venules (Fig. 8–6). Arteriolar stasis is induced at a pressure close to the mean systemic arterial blood pressure. During decompression it is evident that full recovery of the blood flow is not achieved until the pressure is lowered to 5 mm Hg or less.[62] Under normal conditions part of the nutritional supply to the intrathecal nerve roots is provided by diffusion from the cerebrospinal fluid.[76] However, Olmarker and associates,[65] in a study which addressed the nutritional contribution provided by both the blood vessels and the cerebrospinal fluid, found no indications that the cerebrospinal nutritional pathway might compensate for a compression-induced reduction in blood flow. On the contrary, a significant overall nutritional reduction was seen with 10 mm Hg compression.

Decompression of nerve tissue can allow improved blood flow to the endoneurial blood vessels. However, owing to ischemic and mechanical injury to the endothelial cells, which leads to increased permeability of the endoneurial vessels, the recirculation phase might also include formation of endoneurial edema.[66, 75] An increase in vascular permeability may result in leakage of fluid from the vessels into the endoneurial space, with subsequent formation of an intraneural edema (Fig. 8–7). Such edema may increase the endoneurial tissue fluid pressure and thus reduce the intrafascicular blood flow like a "miniature compartment syndrome."[53, 57, 79] Edema may also be transformed into an intraneural fibrotic scar which is more likely to interfere over the long term with the nutrition and function of the nerve tissue. Using the compression model shown in Figure 8–5, the formation of intraneural edema following acute compression injury was studied by Olmarker and associates.[66] They found that edema is induced at 50 mm Hg applied for 2 minutes, which is a surprisingly low pressure level. The edema was mainly localized to the edges of the compression zones, which is in agreement with similar studies on peripheral nerves performed by Rydevik and Lundborg.[75] There was much more edema formation in nerve roots exposed to compression with a rapid outset (i.e., 0.05 to 0.1 second) than in nerve roots compressed at a slower onset rate (20 seconds). This effect was believed to be due to the viscoelastic behavior of the nerve tissue during the compression-induced displacement of nerve tissue at compression onset.

A similar increase in the effects of a rapid-onset compression compared to slow onset was also noted for nerve conduction. The effects on muscle action potential amplitude, recorded on tail muscle electromyography (EMG) following stimulation of the cauda

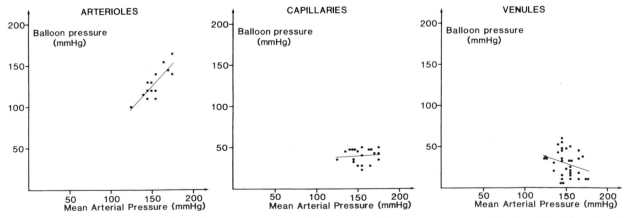

Figure 8–6 = Diagrams showing correlation between mean arterial pressure and the pressure required to stop blood flow in arterioles, capillaries, and venules. (From Olmarker K, Rydevik B, Holm S, et al: Effects of experimental graded compression on blood flow in spinal nerve roots. A vital microscopic study on the porcine cauda equina. J Orthop Res 7:817–823, 1989.)

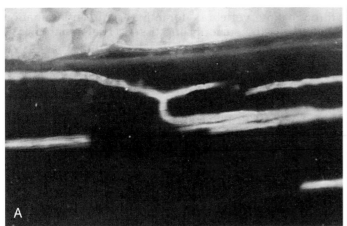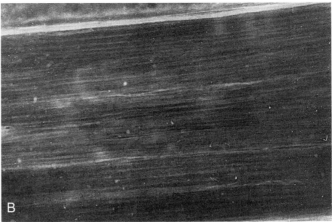

Figure 8–7 = Fluorescence microscopy of spinal nerve roots following intravenous injection of albumin labeled with Evans blue. *A,* Control nerve root. The Evans blue–albumin complex (here white) is confined to the vascular lumina. *B,* Nerve root subjected to mechanical compression. The Evans blue–albumin complex has penetrated the vessel walls owing to increased vascular permeability resulting from the mechanical injury. This indicates the presence of edema in the nerve root tissue.

equina cranial to the maintained compression levels zone, were more pronounced for rapid onset than slow onset at 50, 100, and 200 mm Hg compression for 2 hours[61] (see Fig. 8–8). The importance of the compression onset rate was further emphasized by data which showed that 600 mm Hg compression for only 2 seconds, that is, compression onset only and no continued compression, which might mimic a spine trauma situation, induced a progressive decrement of nerve conduction.[63] No similar effect was noted at 200 mm Hg compression, which indicates that 600 mm Hg probably induced mechanical effects sufficient to create a progressive post-traumatic impairment of nerve function. Since there were no immediate functional changes observed, which would indicate severe mechanical injury, for example, axonal breakage, it was postulated that the functional deterioration was due to vascular injury with gradual formation of intraneural edema.[63]

In a series of studies by Olmarker, Rydevik, and their associates it was demonstrated that the nerve roots are particularly susceptible to double level compression, that is, compression at two locations.[17, 55, 64, 88] Compression at two levels, as compared to only one level, induces more pronounced effects on nerve conduction and blood flow. This is probably due not only to the fact that the nerve roots are compressed at one additional location but also that there is a reduction of blood flow in the segment between the compression sites similar to the reduction in the directly compressed nerve segments.

MODELING OF NERVE COMPRESSION INJURIES

The distribution of stress and strain in the component tissues of the spinal cord and nerve root during compression, or with other mechanical injury, has not been extensively described by purely mathematical modeling. This is due in part to the fact that the struc-

tures involved are complex and their individual properties are not known in detail. Nevertheless, some concepts and conclusions aimed at understanding the nature of mechanical injuries can be drawn from simple idealized models.

Several different theoretical types of mechanical stress systems can be defined that may have relevance to nerve injuries, as illustrated in Figures 8–9, 8–10, and 8–11. In Figure 8–9*A,* axial tension is indicated, which tends to stretch the spinal cord or nerve root, as discussed earlier. In Figure 8–9*B,* the possible shortening of a nerve due to axial compression is indicated. This is an unlikely mechanism of spinal cord or nerve root damage. No test results are available, but one can assume that the spinal cord is very easily compressed axially and will likely buckle laterally if the length of the segment is long.

Figure 8–9*C* illustrates a shearing action by forces, F_s, acting transversely to the axis of the spinal cord. This type of stress may occur in the spinal cord in trauma which translates or rotates adjacent vertebrae with respect to each other.

Figure 8–9*D* shows the stress distribution that occurs when a bending moment or couple, *M,* is applied to a straight beam or other structure like a nerve. The beam is bent and this produces tension stress on one side and compression on the other. No basic data are available on the bending stiffness of the spinal cord or nerve roots, but it may be expected that they may be easily bent and that the bending stresses, even in severe trauma, probably play a minor role. Probably the more severe hazards are the stretching (see Fig. 8–9*A*) that may accompany bending, or the shear (see Fig. 8–9*C*) or transverse compression (see Fig. 8–10 and 8–11) which accompanies the forces that may also produce bending.

Transverse compression may be applied in various ways resulting in different patterns of stress and deformation. The two main experimental and clinically important modes are shown in Figures 8–10 and 8–11.

prognostic significance of this subdivision remains unclear (Fig. 9–11). The classification of *burst fractures*, also proposed by Denis,[21] has proved quite useful, both prognostically and in aiding the surgeon's decision about the optimal surgical construct for stabilization of these injuries (Fig. 9–12). Type A fractures involve comminution of both end plates, and they constitute approximately 40% of all burst fractures. They are generally the result of axial compression resulting in comminution of the pedicles and posterior elements. Type B fractures involve the superior end plate and most often result from a combination of flexion and axial compression with retropulsion of the posterior superior corner of the body into the spinal canal. This is the other commonly seen burst fracture pattern, also constituting 40% of burst fractures. In Type C fractures, the comminution occurs at the inferior end plate; this also results from a flexion and compression mechanism and is decidedly uncommon. Type D fractures would be better classified as shear injuries, whereas type E fractures are lateral burst fractures, again a relatively uncommon injury pattern.

Flexion-distraction injuries have been classified by a number of different radiographic methods. The general theme is similar in all systems; that is, differentiation of bony from ligamentous components. Denis' classifi-

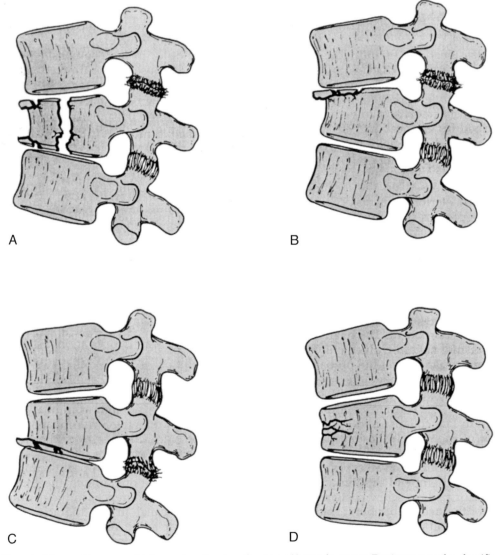

Figure 9–11 = Although it has not been as widely used as the classification of burst fractures, Denis proposed a classification of compression fractures. The critical feature of all four types is that the posterior wall of the vertebral body is intact with the fracture line either involving the end plates or the anterior portion of the body. *A,* These fractures may involve both end plates, with or without a coronal plane fracture. *B,* The most common type involves fractures of the superior end plate alone. *C,* However, isolated fracture of the inferior end plate can occur. *D,* The final pattern is a buckling fracture of the anterior cortex with both end plates intact. This type must be carefully differentiated from a minimally displaced flexion-distraction injury. (From Eismont FJ, Garfin SR, Abitbol J-J: Thoracic and upper lumbar spine injuries. *In* Browner BD, Jupiter JB, Levine AM, et al (eds): Skeletal Trauma: Fractures, Dislocations, Ligamentous Injuries, vol 1. Philadelphia, WB Saunders, 1992, p 746.)

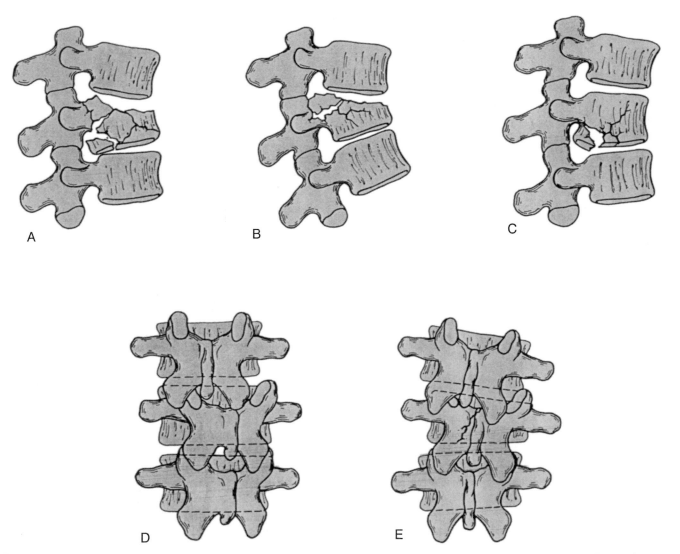

Figure 9–12 = The Denis classification of burst fractures is used to describe the majority of injuries of this type and is helpful in subdividing the injuries according to differing treatment patterns. The common element is disruption of the posterior wall of the vertebral body in all cases. The type A fracture is predominantly an axial loading injury with minimal kyphosis. A comminution of both end plates occurs, and there may also be fractures in the posterior elements. Type B fractures tend to have more kyphosis and sparing of the posterior elements. Comminution of the superior end plate and upper portion of the vertebral body occur, with retropulsion of the posterosuperior portion into the canal. The first two types represent 80% to 90% of all burst fractures. Type C fractures involve the inferior portion of the vertebral body and end plate with retropulsion of the posterior inferior corner of the body into the canal. These are extremely uncommon. The Type D fracture is a combination of a type A fracture with rotation, which is best appreciated on an anteroposterior (AP) radiograph. This type must be carefully differentiated from a shear injury. Type E is a lateral burst fracture that results from a combination of axial loading and lateral bending and is again best appreciated on AP x-ray. (From Eismont FJ, Garfin SR, Abitbol J-J: Thoracic and upper lumbar spine injuries. *In* Browner BD, Jupiter JB, Levine AM, et al (eds): Skeletal Trauma: Fractures, Dislocations, Ligamentous Injuries, vol 1. Philadelphia, WB Saunders, 1992, p 753.)

cation[21] consists of four parts (Fig. 9–13): (1) one level through bone, (2) one level through ligaments, (3) two levels with the middle column injured through bone, and (4) two levels with the middle column injured through ligament. The classification of Gertzbein and Court-Brown[28] allows more precision, specifying individually the injury to the anterior elements, posterior elements, and body (Fig. 9–14). In reality, the route of the fracture line from posterior to anterior determines the late stability of the injury. Thus, injuries that can be considered to involve only bone from posterior to anterior have the best prognosis for stability with pri-

mary healing. Injuries that involve ligaments posteriorly and bone anteriorly have an intermediate probability for stability. The final type of flexion-distraction injury goes through the interspinous ligament, facet capsule, and disc, and mimics the injury seen in the cervical spine. As a result of the severe translation and high probability of neurologic deficit, as well as the absolute need for surgical reduction and stabilization, these injuries should be considered as a separate subtype[40] and noted as a bilateral facet dislocation.

The final major type of injury in the thoracic, thoracolumbar, and lumbar spine is sometimes denoted as

42. Levine AM, Mazel C, Roy-Camille R: Cervical spine fracture separation of the articular mass. Spine 17:447–454, 1992.
43. Lind B, Nordwall A, Sihlbom H: Odontoid fractures treated with halo-vest. Spine 12:173–177, 1987.
44. Lucas JT, Ducker TB: Motor classification of spinal cord injuries with mobility, morbidity and recovery indices. Am Surg 1979, pp 151–158.
45. Maiman DJ, Larson SJ: Management of odontoid fractures. Neurosurgery 11:471–476, 1982.
46. McAfee PC, Yuan HA, Fredrickson BE, et al: The value of computed tomography in thoracolumbar fractures. J Bone Joint Surg Am 65:461–466, 1983.
47. McAfee PC, Yuan HA, Lasda NA: The unstable burst fracture. Spine 7:365, 1982.
48. McCormack T, Karaikovic E, Gaines RW: The load sharing classification of spine fractures. Spine 19:1741–1744, 1994.
49. McEvoy R, Bradford DS: The management of burst fracture of the thoracic and lumbar spine. Spine 10:631–637, 1985.
50. Miller MD, Gehweiler JA, Martinez S, et al: Significant new observations on cervical spine trauma. AJR 130:659–663, 1978.
51. Nicoll EA: Fractures of the dorsolumbar spine. J Bone Joint Surg Br 31:376–394, 1949.
52. Powers B, Miller MD, Kramer RS, et al: Traumatic anterior atlanto-occipital dislocation. Neurosurgery 4:1:12–17, 1979.
53. Rogers WA: Treatment of fracture-dislocation of the cervical spine. J Bone Joint Surg Am 24:245, 1942.
54. Roy-Camille R, Mazel C, Saillant G: Fractures et luxations du rachis dorsal et lombaire de l'adulte, vol A: In Encyclopedie Medico-Chirurgicale 15829. Paris, Masson, 1985, pp 1–12.
55. Roy-Camille R, Saillant G, Gagna G, et al: Transverse fracture of the upper sacrum: Suicidal jumper's fracture. Spine 10:838–845, 1985.
56. Ryan MD, Taylor TKF: Odontoid fractures: A rational approach to treatment. J Bone Joint Surg Br 64:416–421, 1982.
57. Sabiston CP, Wing PC: Sacral fractures: Classification and neurologic implications. J Trauma 26:1113–1115, 1986.
58. Schmidek HH, Smith DA, Kristiansen TK: Sacral fractures. Neurosurgery 15:735–746, 1984.
59. Schneider RC, Kahn EA: Chronic neurological sequelae of acute trauma to the spine and spinal cord: I. The significance of the acute flexion or "teardrop" fracture-dislocation of the cervical spine. J Bone Joint Surg Am 38:985, 1956.
60. Smith WS, Kaufer H: Patterns and mechanisms of lumbar injuries associated with lap seat belts. J Bone Joint Surg Am 51:239–254, 1969.
61. Southwick WO: Current concepts review: Management of fractures of the dens (odontoid process). J Bone Joint Surg Am 62:482–486, 1980.
62. Taylor AR, Blackwood W: Paraplegia in hyperextension cervical injuries with normal radiographic appearance. J Bone Joint Surg Br 30:245, 1948.
63. Taylor AR: Mechanism of injury to the spinal cord in the neck without damage to the vertebral column. J Bone Joint Surg Br 33:543, 1951.
64. Trafton PG, Boyd CA: Computed tomography of thoracic and lumbar spine injuries. J Trauma 24:506, 1984.
65. Traynelis VC, Marano GD, Dunker T, et al: Traumatic atlanto-occipital dislocation: Case report. J Neurosurg 65:863–870, 1988.
66. Triantafyllou SJ, Gertzbein SD: Flexion distraction injuries of the thoracolumbar spine: A review. Orthopedics 15:357–364, 1992.
67. Watson-Jones R: Fractures and Joint Injuries, ed 3. Edinburgh, E & S Livingstone, 1943.
68. Whitesides TE: Traumatic kyphosis of the thoracolumbar spine. Clin Orthop 128:77–92, 1977.
69. White AA, Panjabi MM: The clinical biomechanics of the occipitoatlantoaxial complex. Orthop Clin North Am 9:867–878, 1978.
70. White AA III, Panjabi MM: Clinical Biomechanics of the Spine. Philadelphia, JB Lippincott, 1978.
71. Whitley JE, Forsyth HF: The classification of cervical spine injuries. Am J Roentgenogr Radiat Ther Nucl Med 83:633–44, 1960.

Surgical Approaches to the Cervical Spine

Scott H. Kitchel

Surgical treatment of cervical spine disease requires an understanding of cervical anatomy, the disease process, and a comprehensive review of the imaging studies. Once the decision to undertake surgical treatment has been made, the importance of positioning and the appropriate surgical approach cannot be overemphasized. In this chapter, the current knowledge regarding surgical approaches to the cervical spine is presented. Many lesions of the cervical spine may be approached from more than one route. This chapter does not deal with indications for each approach, but rather summarizes the anatomy and technique for anterior, lateral, and posterior approaches to the cervical spine. The decision as to which approach is used must be individualized, depending on the surgical lesion as well as the expertise and experience of the operating surgeon. Whichever approach is chosen, the positioning and technique will have a major effect on the overall success of the surgical procedure.

POSTERIOR APPROACHES

History

Posterior approaches to the cervical spine were developed before other approaches.[14] Most authors believe this is because of the immediate accessibility of the posterior cervical structures.[23] Despite the apparent simplicity of the exposure, adequate positioning and technique are critical. Posterior approaches allow excellent exposure of the posterior elements of the cervical spine, including the spinous processes, laminae, and facet joints. The posterior spinal cord is also readily exposed as well as the posterolateral corner of the cervical discs.[4]

Positioning for posterior cervical approaches requires placing the patient in the prone position once the patient has been adequately anesthetized. This may be a formality in the patient with a lateral cervical disc herniation or of critical importance in a patient with unstable cervical fractures. I prefer that all patients to be positioned prone have placement of Gardner-Wells tongs or a Gardner head holder. This allows maintenance of accurate alignment of the cervical spine during turning.[14] A Stryker frame may still be utilized in patients with extreme instability or in whom combined anterior and posterior approaches are to be made in one surgical setting. However, because of the cumbersome nature of this device it is not routinely recommended.

Once adequate anesthesia has been ensured, the tongs are applied. The patient is then logrolled into the prone position using an attachment to the operating table appropriate to the tongs. Under routine conditions, four assistants are required to safely turn the patient, with the surgeon being responsible for stabilizing the head and neck. As soon as the patient is positioned, it is critical that pressure on the face and eyes be checked. The eyes must be kept free of any direct pressure from the frame, as prolonged pressure may result in intraocular damage or blindness.[23] Once the face and eyes have been checked, traction may be applied as needed.

The thorax is supported by chest rolls, which allow slight flexion of the hips. The knees are padded and also flexed. Equal pressure must be assured and no direct contact with metal table parts is allowed. The table is then put into a reversed Trendelenburg position to raise the cervical spine to the surgeon's level. The neck is positioned in adequate flexion for exposure and to eliminate the skin folds. The amount of flexion is individualized to the pathologic findings. For improved radiographic visualization of the lower cervical spine, the shoulders may be taped in a depressed position or Boger straps may be placed on the wrists. In either case, the surgeon must bear in mind that excessive traction may cause stretching of the brachial plexus.

Many surgeons continue to perform posterior cervical approaches with the patient in the sitting position. This is particularly popular for posterior cervical foraminotomy and discectomy. However, there have been a number of occurrences of air embolism related to this positioning.[19] As this may represent a fatal complication, I prefer the prone position for posterior cervical approaches.

Once adequate positioning (Fig. 10–1) has been assured and reconfirmed, the posterior cervical surface is prepared in a sterile fashion. Localization of the appropriate level is done through a combination of palpating anatomic landmarks and radiography. The occipital protuberance and prominent posterior spinous process of C2 are easily palpated. Similarly, the

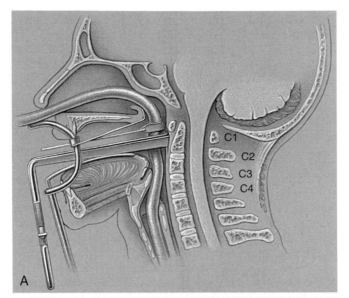

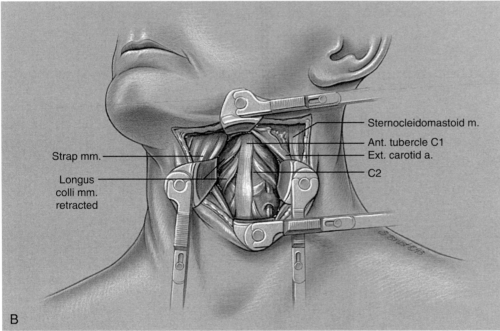

Figure 10–7 = *A* and *B*, Transoral retractors in position. (Drawing by Susan E. Brust, M.S., Tualatin, Ore.)

OTHER ANTERIOR AND ANTEROLATERAL APPROACHES

The Smith-Robinson anterior approach affords excellent visualization of the middle and lower cervical spine. However, it must be modified or other approaches may be needed for the upper cervical spine and the cervicothoracic junction. The remainder of this chapter deals with those other approaches by anatomic location.

Transoral Approach

History

Over the years many different anterior approaches to the craniocervical junction have been described. In 1962, Fang and Ong[8] described the transoral direct approach to the cervical spine. This has been the standard with which all other approaches to this region must be compared. In 1987, Archer and colleagues[1] described their transmaxillary approach. However, this approach allows no exposure below the foramen magnum. Derome presented his transbasal approach in 1988.[7] Most observers believe it is too extensive for the craniocervical junction. Gockard described an extended maxillotomy approach in 1991.[9]

After reviewing all of the approaches, I believe that only the widely used transoral approach has withstood the test of time. This technique will be described in detail as will the lateral retropharyngeal approach to the upper cervical spine. The reader is directed to the references for descriptions of the other techniques.

Positioning

Positioning for transoral surgery requires immobilization of the head as well as adequate access to the mouth. Most surgeons prefer either the supine or lateral position. As compared to the sitting position, this decreases the drainage down via the esophagus into the stomach. Although the lateral position allows the surgeon to sit, I prefer the supine position because of the easier orientation to the anatomic structures.

The head may be immobilized with Gardner-Wells tongs or in a Gardner headrest. Once anesthesia has been induced and the positioning is adequate, the mouth is cleaned out with oral chlorhexidine solution and a transoral retractor is placed (Fig. 10–7A and B). Great care must be taken not to impinge on the tongue and the lower teeth. The mouth is opened as far as possible and the soft palate is retracted with the curved palatal retractor. Another palatal retractor is used to retract the nasogastric and nasotracheal tubes into the tonsillar fauces.

Surgical Approach

The key anatomic landmark for palpation is the tubercle of the ring on C1.[8] Once this has been identified the area is injected with epinephrine in a concentration of 1:200,000. This injection will create a plane between the pharynx and prevertebral tissues. A midline longitudinal incision is then made from the tubercle to the base of C2. In the midline, one should not encounter any bleeding.[5] The tissue can then be elevated in the plane between bone and the cervical mucosa laterally in each direction. An additional palatal retractor is now placed.

The insertion of the longus colli and the anterior longitudinal ligament into the tubercle of C1 is divided (Fig. 10–8) with electrocautery. Electrocautery is additionally used to dissect free the C1 arch and C2 anterior body. The surgeon may then proceed with the indicated procedure.

Once the procedure is completed, the wound is copiously irrigated with antibiotic solution. The muscle and fascial layers are closed with one layer. The pharyngeal mucosa is then closed with absorbable sutures in a separate layer.

If further exposure is required, the mandibular-tongue-pharynx–splitting approach as described by Stauffer[22] may be utilized. A vertical incision is made from the center of the lower lip to the prominence of the chin, which is circumscribed, and the incision is then continued to the back of the chin. The mucous membrane is split and the mandible predrilled and cut in a step-cut fashion to facilitate reapproximation. The tongue is split longitudinally through its central raphe (Fig. 10–9). The halves of the mandible and tongue are retracted laterally on each side. The vertebral prominences are palpated in the midline and the mucosa is split in the middle, creating laterally based flaps. This allows anterior exposure from the clivus to C6.[22] Preoperative tracheostomy is required.

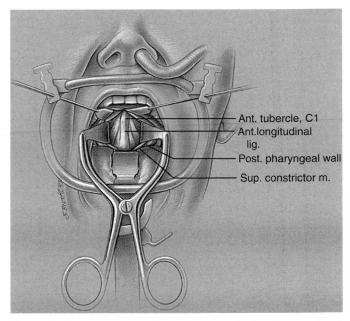

Figure 10–8 = Location of the anterior longitudinal ligament and longus colli muscles in the transoral approach. (Drawing by Susan E. Brust, M.S., Tualatin, Ore.)

Anterior Retropharyngeal Approach to the Upper Cervical Spine

History

Because of the high risk of infection in transoral surgery, the anteromedial retropharyngeal approach to the upper cervical spine is preferred.[8] This approach really represents an extension and evolution of the Smith-Robinson anteromedial approach to the midcervical spine.[13–20] In 1973, Riley described the extensile retropharyngeal approach utilizing division of the stylohyoid and digastric tendons and dislocation of the ipsilateral temporomandibular joint.[15] Southwick and Robinson[21] further modified this by using a transverse submandibular skin incision.

Positioning

Positioning considerations for this procedure are identical to those outlined in the discussion of anterior approaches.

Surgical Approach

A modified transverse submandibular incision is used[13] (Fig. 10–10). This is made on the patient's right side if the surgeon is right-handed, allowing easier exposure.[13] This incision and the subsequent exposure are a logical cephalad extension of the traditional anterior Smith-Robinson incision. The dissection is carried sharply through the platysma muscle and flaps are mobilized in the subplatysmal plane of the superficial fascia.

The marginal mandibular branch of the facial nerve is found with a nerve stimulator and protected. By ligating the retromandibular vein and keeping the dis-

Intraoperative Evaluation: Somatosensory Evoked Potentials and Motor Evoked Potentials

Cor J. Kalkman || *John C. Drummond*

The aim of intraoperative physiologic monitoring of the spinal cord is to prevent neurologic injury by early detection of spinal cord dysfunction and institution of corrective measures before irreversible damage has occurred. There are data to confirm that intraoperative somatosensory evoked potential (SSEP) monitoring can reduce the incidence of neurologic deficit. Meyer and co-workers[68] reviewed 295 patients who were surgically treated for acute spinal injuries in the thoracic and lumbar regions and observed a 6.9% incidence of new neurologic deficits in 145 patients who were unmonitored or had only a wake-up test. In contrast, 6 of 150 (4%) patients who had intraoperative SSEP monitoring showed intraoperative deterioration of their SSEPs that prompted intervention. Only one patient (0.7%) in this group revealed a new neurologic deficit postoperatively. More recently, a large survey showed that experienced sensory evoked potential (SEP) spinal cord monitoring teams had less than one half as many neurologic deficits per 100 cases compared with teams with relatively little monitoring experience. Definite neurologic deficits, despite stable SEPs (false-negative monitoring), occurred during surgery in only 0.063% of patients in these centers.[77]

This chapter reviews the current status of SSEP monitoring during spinal surgery and introduces the clinical application of intraoperative motor evoked potential monitoring (MEP). The emphasis is on the acquisition and interpretation of SSEP and MEP waveforms, as well as factors that can influence the recording of responses adequate for reliable interpretation.

SOMATOSENSORY EVOKED POTENTIALS (SSEPs)

SSEPs are the electrical responses of the nervous system to stimulation of a peripheral nerve. They depend on an intact conducting pathway between the site of stimulation and the site of recording. The premise underlying the use of spinal cord function monitoring with SSEPs is that changes in latency and amplitude indicative of spinal cord dysfunction will occur early, while spinal cord injury is still in a reversible stage. It is most likely that the greatest risk to the spinal cord during spinal surgery results from stretching or compression of neural and vascular structures which ultimately leads to spinal cord ischemia or mechanical damage. The most widely used system for intraoperative monitoring of spinal cord function during spinal surgery entails the recording of cortical responses after electrical stimulation of the posterior tibial or peroneal nerve. It was popularized by Nash and colleagues in 1977,[72] and has been in clinical use for more than 15 years. In some centers SSEP monitoring has superseded the wake-up test, although many groups prefer to err on the safe side and still perform a wake-up test after high-risk maneuvers. SSEPs are most commonly recorded from the scalp (cortical and subcortical SSEP), but can also be obtained from needles placed in the interspinous ligaments or from electrodes placed in the epidural space. Since cortical SSEP recording is noninvasive and can be employed throughout the entire perioperative period, in the United States it has been more widely applied than other techniques. However, since the cortical SSEP traverses more synapses, it is more sensitive to depression by anesthetic agents, and accordingly the anesthetic constraints are more rigid. A large number of reports have been published to date summarizing clinical experience with SSEP monitoring.*

Technical Aspects of Acquisition of SSEPs

Evoked potentials from the nervous system are invariably of much less amplitude than the combined

---

*References 1, 7, 10, 19, 23, 24, 35, 68, 69, 72, 84, 98, and 109.

noise of other biologic signals, including the electrocardiogram (ECG), the electroencephalogram (EEG), the electromyogram (EMG), and random noise generated by electrical equipment in the operating room. With the exception of the motor evoked response recorded from muscle, signal averaging techniques are usually necessary to extract evoked responses from the background noise. The principle of signal averaging is that the signal of interest is time-locked to the stimulus, while the background noise is random. The amplified raw signal is digitized and successive trials are averaged. With an increasing number of trials the random background noise will gradually approach zero, while the recurrent event (the SSEP) is preserved. The signal-to-noise ratio, that is, the ratio of the signal amplitude to the background noise, increases in proportion to the square root of the number of trials. Usually several hundred stimuli need to be averaged to extract the evoked potential waveform from the background activity. Several early publications reported disappointing results (up to 28% failure rate) with acquisition of cortical SSEPs in the operating room,[96] while more recently success rates of 96% and higher have become standard.[7, 44, 60, 109] This probably reflects the increased experience of personnel involved in acquiring SSEPs in the operating room, as well as increased awareness of the effects of anesthetic drugs on SSEPs.

Stimulation Sites, Stimulus Intensity, and Stimulus Frequency

The preferred stimulation site for spinal cord monitoring is a peripheral nerve in the leg, usually the posterior tibial nerve at the ankle, and less often, the peroneal nerve. Some groups routinely record median nerve SSEPs as a "control" for anesthetic and other systemic factors that may alter SSEPs. Stimulation electrodes can be either subcutaneous needle electrodes or standard EEG disc electrodes, applied over the peripheral nerve. Subdermal needles have a more constant electrical impedance. This allows consistent stimulus delivery, which is important during long operations. Electrical stimuli used to elicit SSEPs are usually square wave pulses of short duration (100 to 200 μs). Constant-current stimulators are necessary to ensure constant stimulus delivery in the face of changes in electrode impedance occurring over time. Alternating unilateral stimulation is recommended.[4] Simultaneous bilateral stimulation produces SSEPs of larger amplitude and can be employed when small amplitude SSEPs of insufficient reproducibility are produced by unilateral stimulation. With bilateral stimulation, unilateral injury to the spinal cord may remain undetected. As an alternative to peripheral nerve stimulation, direct electrical stimulation of the conus medullaris via an electrode inserted through an epidural catheter has also been employed.[99] This technique results in high-amplitude SSEPs recorded from spinal cord or scalp. It may be preferable during spinal cord monitoring for procedures in which peripheral nerve ischemia is expected, for example, during cross-clamping of the aorta. However, because of the invasive nature of the technique, it has not been employed widely.

SSEP amplitude increases with increasing stimulus intensity. For the posterior tibial nerve the sensory threshold is usually around 1 to 2 mA, while the threshold for a motor response varies between 2 and 4 mA. Tsuji and colleagues[103] found that in awake patients posterior tibial nerve cortical SSEPs (PTN-SSEPs) were maximal at three times sensory threshold, while amplitudes of spinal and subcortical PTN-SSEPs increased with stimulus intensities from sensory threshold to five times sensory threshold. In their study stimulus intensities between 1.2 and 8.0 mA were used, which is much lower than those commonly used intraoperatively. During anesthesia SSEP amplitude increases linearly with increasing stimulus intensity until a plateau is reached at 20 mA.[75] For intraoperative spinal cord monitoring it is advisable to use these higher stimulus intensities as they maximize the chance of obtaining optimal recordings.

The *rate of stimulation* also has an important influence on SSEP amplitude. Nuwer and Dawson[75] compared peroneal nerve cortical SSEP amplitude with stimulus rates ranging from 1.1 to 11.1 Hz. There was a progressive decline in amplitude with increasing stimulus rates. Compared with a stimulus rate of 1.1 Hz, a rate of 5.1 Hz caused 25% amplitude attenuation, while there was 80% attenuation with a stimulus rate of 11.1 Hz. The authors recommended 5.1 Hz as the optimum "tradeoff" between amplitude and speed of acquisition. In most centers a stimulus rate between 3.1 and 5.1 Hz is employed during spinal cord SEP monitoring.

Recording Electrodes and Recording Sites

Standard silver–silver chloride or gold-plated electrodes filled with electrode jelly are used to record the signals from the different recording sites. Electrode impedance should be kept at a minimum (less than 2 kΩ) to prevent artifacts. Alternatively, stainless steel or platinum subdermal needles can be used for recording. However, they have a higher electrode impedance than well-applied surface electrodes and may be more susceptible to artifacts. Recording electrodes may be positioned along the ascending sensory pathway on the skin, in the popliteal fossa, or overlying the vertebral column, the neck, and the scalp. For intraoperative spinal cord monitoring, SSEPs from cortex and subcortex (both recordable from scalp electrodes) are the most frequently recorded, because they are noninvasive and can be recorded preoperatively, intraoperatively, and postoperatively. During spinal surgery SSEPs can also be recorded invasively from needle electrodes placed in the interspinous ligaments or from special electrodes placed in the epidural space. Epidural recording electrodes[13] must be positioned under direct vision by the surgeon, or inserted percutaneously before the operation via a Tuohy needle. Recordings can also be made from electrodes positioned below the level of potential spinal cord injury, for example, lumbar spinal cord or tibial nerve in the popliteal fossa, to verify appropriate stimulus delivery.

Figure 12–1 shows two superimposed cortical posterior tibial nerve SSEPs recorded during spinal surgery

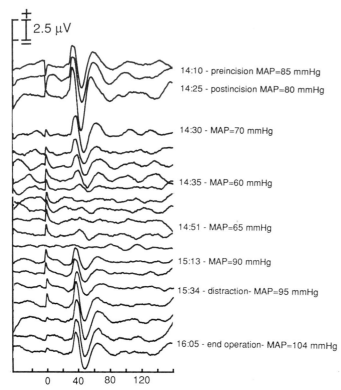

Figure 12–6 = Loss of posterior tibial nerve SSEPs in a 14-year-old female patient during institution of controlled hypotension after positioning in a Cotrel-Dubousset frame with 15 kg of traction. MAP, mean arterial pressure.

becomes additive and may shift the balance between oxygen supply and demand toward ischemia. This has been confirmed both experimentally[14, 30] and clinically.[31, 32, 102] Figure 12–6 shows loss of posterior tibial nerve SSEPs in a 14-year-old girl during institution of controlled hypotension after positioning in a Cotrel-Dubousset frame with 15 kg of traction.

Criteria for Abnormality: When to Intervene

When significant impairment of spinal cord function occurs intraoperatively, the most common pattern is a rapid increase in latency paralleled by a decrease in amplitude, and eventually total loss of the SSEP waveform (see Figs. 12–6 and 12–7). On empirical grounds it has been advocated that an increase in latency of the first cortical peak P1, occurring around 35 to 45 ms post stimulus by more than 3 ms or by 10% of baseline value, should be an indication for intervention.[15, 76] Likewise, a decrease in the cortical P1N1 peak-to-peak amplitude of more than 50% should be a reason for intervention. However, no prospective studies have been performed to assess the validity of these criteria. The use of SSEPs for the prevention of neurologic complications is based on the assumption that significant changes in latency and amplitude will occur while spinal cord ischemia is still in a reversible stage. Immediate action, for example, diminishing distraction, removal of instrumentation, and increasing mean arterial

blood pressure, may then restore blood supply to the cord, restore conduction, and prevent paraplegia. New SSEP waveforms are continuously compared with baseline values that typically were recorded after induction of anesthesia and positioning of the patient, but before surgical intervention. Forbes and co-workers[24] reported their clinical experience with 1168 cases of spinal cord monitoring using SSEPs recorded in the epidural space. They observed no postoperative neurologic changes when SSEP amplitude remained above 50% of control or was only transiently decreased below 50%, whereas mild to severe neurologic complications were observed when persistent loss of amplitude greater than 50% occurred.

SSEP Variability

It is extremely important to record SSEPs at regular intervals during the entire surgical procedure.[4] This allows the assessment of trends in latency and amplitude and gives an indication of spontaneous variability. Whether significant changes from control have occurred should be determined with respect to several recent waveforms rather than a single control waveform recorded earlier. Monitoring should be continu-

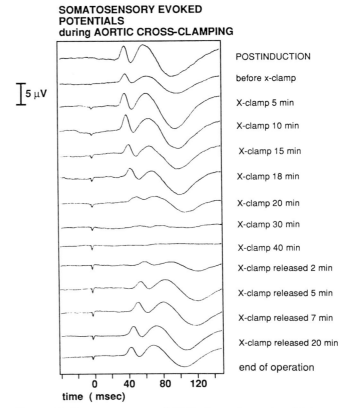

SOMATOSENSORY EVOKED POTENTIALS during AORTIC CROSS-CLAMPING

POSTINDUCTION
before x-clamp
X-clamp 5 min
X-clamp 10 min
X-clamp 15 min
X-clamp 18 min
X-clamp 20 min
X-clamp 30 min
X-clamp 40 min
X-clamp released 2 min
X-clamp released 5 min
X-clamp released 7 min
X-clamp released 20 min
end of operation

Figure 12–7 = Limitations of SSEPs: loss of posterior tibial nerve SSEPs during repair of a traumatic aortic rupture in a 19-year-old male patient. Cross-clamp time was 55 minutes; SSEPs were absent for 25 minutes. The patient sustained paraplegia, despite return of a near-normal SSEP after release of the cross-clamp. (From Kalkman CJ: Intraoperative spinal cord function monitoring with somatosensory evoked potentials: Influence of anesthetic and physiologic factors. Doctoral thesis, University of Amsterdam, 1990.)

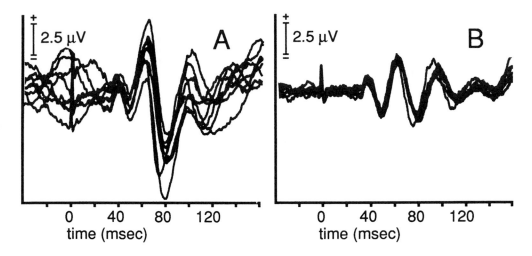

Figure 12–8 = Effect of digital 30-Hz high-pass filtering on variability of posterior tibial nerve SSEPs. *A,* Eight superimposed waveforms recorded over 30 minutes. *B,* The same waveforms after digital filtering. Anesthesia: N_2O and continuous infusion of alfentanil. (From Kalkman CJ, ten Brink SA, Been HD, et al: Variability of somatosensory cortical evoked potentials during spinal surgery: Effects of anesthetic technique and high-pass digital filtering. Spine 16:924–929, 1991.)

ous during those stages of surgery that have been shown to be associated with the highest risk of SSEP abnormalities, for example, distraction or the passage of sublaminar wires.[80, 106] Although absolute changes in amplitude and latency are the most important parameters of intraoperative SSEP monitoring, the *variability* between successive recordings will determine the magnitude of changes from control that can be detected with confidence. Reliable spinal cord function monitoring can only be achieved when the spontaneous "within-patient" variability does not exceed the criteria for intervention. Spontaneous amplitude variability of cortical PTN-SSEPs has been reported to be as high as 40% to 50% in some circumstances.[60, 109] Within-patient amplitude variability is highly correlated with absolute amplitude: the lower the absolute amplitude, the higher the variability. It is therefore important to try to maintain amplitudes of the primary cortical peaks above 1 μV. Variability can be reduced by eliminating from the SSEP waveform those frequencies that do not contain relevant information.[38] For instance, the variability of cortical PTN-SSEPs could be decreased to 20% by digital filtering or modification of the anesthetic technique[44] (Fig. 12–8).

Modification of the anesthetic technique early in the course of an operation may occasionally improve SSEP amplitudes. Substitution of a continuous infusion of propofol for nitrous oxide has been shown to result in a more than twofold increase in P1N1 amplitude of PTN-SSEP[45] (Fig. 12–9). In one instance in which posterior decompression and placement of Cotrel-Dubousset instrumentation was planned, no reproducible SSEPs could be recorded during midazolam-alfentanil anesthesia, and substitution of midazolam by etomidate increased SSEP amplitudes to a level sufficient for intraoperative monitoring.[93] The latter agent should be used with due consideration of its inhibiting effect on cortisol synthesis.[17]

A successful and widely applied anesthetic technique for SSEP monitoring consists of the following: benzodiazepine premedication; barbiturate induction; bolus plus continuous infusion of fentanyl, sufentanil or alfentanil; and nitrous oxide 50% to 66% with or without low concentrations (less than 0.5 minimal alve-

olar concentration), of volatile agents. Muscle relaxation can be given as necessary. The latter will decrease residual EMG noise in SSEP waveforms. In patients with spinal cord injury and pre-existing spinal cord dysfunction it may be advisable to use etomidate or propofol as the induction agent and avoid volatile anesthetics.

Improving Quality of Intraoperative SSEPs

Increasing the Signal Amplitude

As stated previously, the key to successful acquisition and accurate interpretation of evoked potentials in

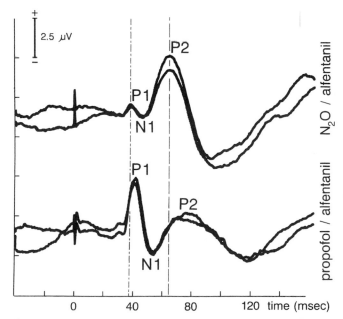

Figure 12–9 = Increased P1N1 amplitude of posterior tibial nerve SSEPs recorded from one patient during N_2O-alfentanil anesthesia and 15 minutes after substitution of N_2O by a continuous infusion of propofol. (From Kalkman CJ, Traast H, Zuurmond WW, et al: Differential effects of propofol and nitrous oxide on posterior tibial nerve somatosensory cortical evoked potentials during alfentanil anesthesia. Br J Anaesth 66:483–489, 1991.)

the operating room is to maximize the signal-to-noise ratio from the outset. Unfortunately, pre-existing neurologic abnormalities and recent injury to the spinal cord may have decreased signal amplitude to abnormally low values. In addition, commonly used anesthetic techniques invariably decrease amplitudes. However, the latter influence can be minimized by selection of anesthetic drugs that only minimally influence SSEPs, and by maintaining constant plasma levels of these anesthetics by means of continuous infusion techniques. Table 12–1 presents the effects of commonly used anesthetic drugs on SSEPs.

There are large differences in the amplitude of SSEPs among individual patients. Obviously it is important to ensure adequate stimulus delivery by applying a supramaximal stimulus. Patients with spinal cord injury or pre-existing neurologic abnormalities usually have low-amplitude evoked potentials that may show "fatigue" of the response at higher stimulus frequencies. In these patients it may be necessary to employ slower stimulation rates, for example, 1.1 to 2.1 Hz, to obtain responses of adequate amplitude. Stimulation at a rate of 5.1 Hz was observed to have a markedly detrimental influence on amplitude in a population of patients with incomplete spinal cord injuries.[89] Figure 12–10 shows decreasing posterior tibial nerve SSEP amplitude with increasing stimulus frequencies.

Decreasing the Noise

Attempts at improving the quality of intraoperative SSEPs or MEPs can also be aimed at decreasing the noise level (Table 12–2). The electrode-skin interface is extremely important. Maintaining impedance of recording electrodes below 2 kΩ and preventing imbalance between the active and reference electrodes can make the difference between high fidelity and extremely noisy recordings. Use of preamplifiers with a very high input impedance will alleviate some of the problems due to electrode imbalance and poor contact. It is best to avoid stimulus repetition rates that are a

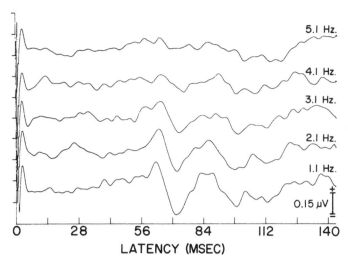

Figure 12–10 = The effect of stimulus frequency on posterior tibial nerve cortical SSEPs in a patient with spinal cord dysfunction. Note the low absolute amplitude of P1N1 and significant decrease in amplitude at stimulus rates in excess of 3.1 Hz. (From Schubert A, Drummond JC, Garfin SR: The influence of stimulus presentation rate on the cortical amplitude and latency of intraoperative somatosensory-evoked potential recordings in patients with varying degrees of spinal cord injury. Spine 12:969–973, 1987.)

multiple of the alternating current line frequency (United States, 60 Hz; Europe, 50 Hz). Line frequency interference should be eliminated by identifying the equipment responsible for it, and removing or repositioning it. The 60 Hz "notch" filter should not be used to eliminate 60 Hz interference from cortical SSEP waveforms, since it may result in resonance or "ringing," which can simulate an evoked response, even when the waveform is flat.[74, 110] The use of diathermy during acquisition of an evoked response will always reduce the signal-to-noise ratio. Even when all sweeps containing high-voltage artifacts are automatically rejected by the computer, amplifier saturation and low-amplitude degradation of the EEG signal will result in suboptimal SSEP waveforms. The solution is either to refrain from diathermy during evoked potential acquisition, or to interrupt acquisition during the use of diathermy either manually or automatically until the amplifiers have recovered. This may take up to several seconds after diathermy is stopped. The latest generation of extremely small, battery-powered biologic amplifiers uses optical transmission of the recorded signals via a fiberoptic link. These devices can be placed in close proximity to the patient, which dramatically decreases the sensitivity to electrical interference.[39]

Limitations of SSEP Monitoring

It is important to realize that a normal SSEP throughout the operation does not guarantee normal motor function. SSEPs only measure condition in ascending sensory tracts, predominantly the dorsal columns and, to a lesser extent, dorsolateral pathways. From the outset there has been a theoretical objection to the use of intraoperative SSEP monitoring for the prevention of motor deficits. Selective injury to the anterior parts

Table 12–1 = **EFFECTS OF ANESTHETIC DRUGS ON SOMATOSENSORY EVOKED POTENTIALS (SSEPs) IN ORDER OF DECREASING EFFECT OF AMPLITUDE OF PRIMARY CORTICAL SSEP PEAKS**

DRUG	AMPLITUDE	LATENCY
Halothane/ enflurane/ isoflurane[82, 107]	↓ ↓ ↓ (Dose dependent)	↑ ↑
Nitrous oxide[92]	↓ ↓	=
Thiopental[21, 66]	↓	↑
Midazolam[91]	↓	↑
Fentanyl/sufentanil/ alfentanil/ morphine[47, 81]	↓ =	= ↑
Propofol[45]	=	↑
Muscle relaxants	=	=
Etomidate[50]	↑	↑ ↑

↑, Moderate increase; ↑ ↑, marked increase; ↓, moderate decrease; ↓ ↓, marked decrease; =, no change.

Table 12–2 = **IMPROVING THE QUALITY OF INTRAOPERATIVE SOMATOSENSORY EVOKED POTENTIALS (SSEPs)**

PROBLEM	POSSIBLE CAUSES	SOLUTION
Excessive noise	Recording electrode impedances high or mismatched	Check recording electrode impedance and balance
	EMG artifact	Administer relaxant
	Frequent diathermy	Automated or manual interruption of SSEP acquisition during diathermy
Low-amplitude SSEP	Normal variation	Adjust anesthetic technique
	Inadequate stimulus delivery	Check stimulation electrode location and contact
		Increase stimulus intensity or duration or both
	Antecedent spinal cord dysfunction	Decrease stimulus frequency
		Modify anesthetic technique, e.g., eliminate volatile agent; substitute etomidate or propofol
	Anesthetic depression	Decrease concentration of volatile anesthetic
		Change anesthetic technique
Large variability	Low-amplitude SSEP	See text
	Residual random low-frequency components	Increase low-frequency filter setting, e.g., from 1 to 30 Hz

of the spinal cord can go undetected, resulting in a false-negative result. Given the well-known distinct differences in blood supply to the anterior and dorsal parts of the spinal cord, it is remarkable that SSEPs have proved to be extremely sensitive in detecting spinal cord dysfunction in experimental spinal cord injury[8, 14, 18, 20, 30, 73, 87] and during spinal surgery.[19] This supports the notion that the majority of insults to the spinal cord during spinal surgery result in global injury to the cord rather than selective ischemia of the anterior horns. However, apparently normal SSEPs have been recorded in the presence of a spinal artery syndrome[118] and a number of false-negative results of SSEP monitoring have been reported.[6, 52] During thoracic aortic surgery reappearance of a near-normal SSEP after release of the cross-clamp has been observed despite the presence of postoperative paraplegia[40, 97] (see Fig. 12–7).

MOTOR EVOKED POTENTIALS (MEPs)

Since a major threat of spinal surgery is damage to the motor pathways, several groups have developed techniques that allow direct monitoring of pyramidal tracts concurrent with SSEP recording. There are two potential avenues for monitoring conduction in motor pathways. The motor tracts can be stimulated transcranially using electrical[67] or magnetic stimulators,[5] with recordings made either from spinal cord, peripheral nerve, or muscle. The other approach utilizes electrical stimulation of the spinal cord proximal to the operative field with recording either from peripheral nerve or muscle. At present these techniques of intraoperative MEP monitoring are still in development stages, and there have been no formal comparisons of the various methods in humans.

Spinal Cord Stimulation

Initial attempts at recording MEPs have employed epidural electrodes for rostral spinal cord stimulation with recordings made from the caudal spinal cord.[53, 57]

This technique is highly invasive and it is usually applicable only during a limited period of operation. Moreover, it may not be specific for the motor tracts because of antidromic conduction in nonpyramidal (sensory) tracts.[62, 95]

"Neurogenic" MEPs

Owen and others[78, 79] have described a system of motor tract monitoring that utilizes rostral spinal cord stimulation via needle electrodes inserted into the lamina of the cervical vertebrae and recording of action potentials from the sciatic nerve. They term these responses "neurogenic motor evoked potentials" (NMEPs). In this system, as with compound muscle action potential (CMAP) recording, the signal has traversed one synapse between the descending motor tracts and alpha motor neuron. The technique requires averaging of about 200 responses. Unlike CMAPs, NMEPs can be recorded in the presence of complete neuromuscular blockade. In fact, Schwentker and co-workers[90] recently demonstrated that it is necessary to maintain a deep level of neuromuscular blockade, because the NMEP waveform may be obscured by the superimposed CMAP when the level of blockade decreases. NMEPs were more sensitive and specific to the effects of experimental spinal cord compression, ischemia, and distraction than SSEPs.[79] Owen and colleagues were able to elicit NMEPs in 90% of 111 patients undergoing spine surgery and concluded that NMEPs are a valuable complement to SSEP monitoring (Fig. 12–11). However, a recent report suggested that high thoracic spinal cord stimulation may produce antidromic sensory pathway conduction. Su and associates[95] observed that the dorsal root and sciatic nerve responses were abolished after dorsal column transection in dogs, while there was only minimal alteration of the spinal cord evoked potential recorded from L2. Another study showed that dorsal rhizotomy abolished the ipsilateral peroneal nerve action potential to high thoracic spinal cord stimulation, indicating antidromic conduction via afferent fibers.[33] Groups that routinely use the NMEP technique are now aware that this

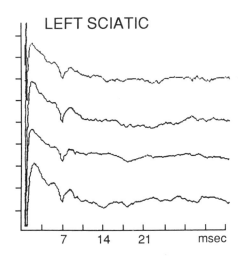

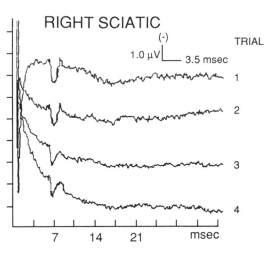

LEFT SCIATIC / RIGHT SCIATIC figure with msec scales 7 14 21

Figure 12–11 = Neurogenic motor evoked potentials recorded from the left and right sciatic nerves after electrical stimulation of the spinal cord elicited in a patient undergoing surgery for spinal deformity. (From Owen JH, Laschinger J, Bridwell K, et al: Sensitivity and specificity of somatosensory and neurogenic-motor evoked potentials in animals and humans. Spine 13:1111–1118, 1988.)

method monitors a combination of motor and retrograde sensory conduction.

Motor Evoked Potentials to Transcranial Stimulation (tc-MEPs)

The development of stimulators that are capable of stimulating the motor cortex transcranially, using either electrical current (tc^e-MEP) or a transient magnetic field(tc^{mag}-MEP), has given a large impetus to the investigation of noninvasive techniques for evaluating the motor pathways intraoperatively. The depolarization of cortical motor neurons or their axons produces a descending volley in the corticospinal tracts that can be recorded from the spinal cord, peripheral nerve, and muscle (CMAP). Techniques for intraoperative tc-MEP monitoring are currently being evaluated in several centers in the United States and Europe.[16, 22, 42, 113, 114]

Electrical Transcranial Stimulation

It has proved difficult to stimulate the motor cortex transcranially using conventional constant-current stimulators. The resistance of the skull is very high; current applied to the scalp is dispersed by volume conduction, and the majority of available (somatosensory) stimulators have insufficient output to achieve stimulation. However, Levy and others[58] developed a system for the recording of intraoperative MEPs with a conventional constant-current stimulator. It involved electrical stimulation of the cortex via electrodes placed on the vertex and hard palate. Several hundred stimuli were required to record a reproducible response from the spinal cord. A special stimulator is now commercially available that uses high-voltage capacitor discharges (Digitimer D180, Digitimer Ltd, Welwyn Garden City, UK) to stimulate the motor cortex via standard EEG electrodes applied to the scalp. With this stimulator, a large CMAP (several millivolts) can be recorded from hand or leg muscles after a single transcranial stimulus. This stimulator has been used clinically for intraoperative tc^e-MEP monitoring, using both epidural recording techniques,[11, 49, 114] and recording of CMAPs in the unparalyzed or partly paralyzed patient.*

Magnetic Stimulation

An alternative technique for stimulating neural structures is the use of a strong transient magnetic field. This approach was pioneered by Bickford and Fremming[9] and adapted by Barker and Jalinous[5] for transcranial stimulation of the motor cortex. A strong transient current (peak current, 6000 A; duration, 100 μs) in the coil of the magnetic stimulator produces a transient magnetic field (1.5 to 2.0 T) that reaches the motor cortex unattenuated by the skull. This rapidly changing magnetic field induces a current in underlying brain tissue. With the coil positioned appropriately over the scalp, this current is capable of depolarizing neurons in the motor cortex. Transcranial magnetic stimulation has clear advantages for diagnostic purposes in awake patients, since, in contrast to transcranial electrical stimulation, it is not painful. However, this difference is irrelevant in the anesthetized patient, and it is not yet clear whether either of these two modes of transcranial stimulation is superior with respect to eliciting tc-MEPs during intraoperative monitoring or with respect to possible complications.

The first report describing initial experiences with tc^{mag}-MEP monitoring during scoliosis surgery found that tc^{mag}-MEPs were recordable in 9 of 11 patients intraoperatively during nitrous oxide–opioid anesthesia, but the large-amplitude variability both among and within patients was perceived to be a significant limitation.[22] Using etomidate anesthesia in patients undergoing surgical removal of spinal tumors, Herdmann and co-workers[34] were able to record tc^{mag}-MEPs in 10 of 13 patients, 12 of whom were initially neurologically impaired. Subtle changes in position and angulation of the stimulating coil have a large influence on tc^{mag}-MEP amplitude.[25] The development of a skull-mounted coil holder, for example, a "helmet," may obviate this problem.[51] However, factors other than coil location, for instance, depth of anesthesia, may contribute to the

---

*References 16, 42, 46, 100, 108, 112, 113, 116, and 117.

amplitude variability that has been observed. Additional studies will be necessary to define the variables that contribute to amplitude variability and determine which method of transcranial stimulation produces the most consistent intraoperative tc-MEPs.

Where to Stimulate and What to Record?

At present it is unclear whether transcranial or spinal cord stimulation has different sensitivities with respect to early detection of impending damage to motor pathways. There is evidence to suggest that recordings made from nerve or muscle, that is, *after* the signal has traversed the alpha-motor neuron, may be more sensitive to injury. Levy and associates[55] observed in cats that potentials recorded from peripheral nerve and muscle were more sensitive to injury than potentials recorded from the spinal cord. Based on their experience with this technique in patients they[54] concluded that spinal cord potentials can change so little in amplitude and latency with injury conditions that their reliability for intraoperative monitoring may be limited. Similar results were observed in studies by Machida and colleagues.[61, 63] They reported that in dogs, CMAPs were immediately abolished after cross-clamping of the aorta above the artery of Adamkiewicz, while spinal MEPs remained unchanged. In another study in which cats were subjected to maneuvers similar to those used in scoliosis surgery, Machida and others[63] reported that CMAPs recorded from the soleus muscle were a much better predictor of spinal cord injury than the signal recorded from the caudal spinal cord. In patients undergoing Cotrel-Dubousset instrumentation, Machida and colleagues stimulated the rostral spinal cord via an epidural electrode and recorded spinal MEPs from the distal spinal cord and CMAPs from the soleus muscle.[63] In 3 of the 30 patients the derotation maneuver decreased the amplitude of CMAPs, but not of spinal MEPs. A possible explanation for this discrepancy may be that the signal recorded from the spinal cord is at least in part conducted by pathways other than the corticospinal tracts.[111]

Nonetheless, some investigators have reported satisfactory experiences with epidurally recorded responses. Kitagawa and co-workers[49] recorded tc-MEPs during upper cervical spine surgery from electrodes in the dorsal epidural space in 20 patients. One patient, who was paraplegic postoperatively, showed irreversible loss of the MEP after tightening of sublaminar wires at C3–5. However, others have had less consistent success with epidural recording. Zentner and others[114] reported a 65% success rate with epidurally recorded tc-MEPs, while recording from cauda equina allowed recording of MEPs in 85%. In the latter study a permanent reduction in amplitudes of more than 50% of the baseline or loss of potentials correlated with postoperative deterioration of the motor status in three patients. A more extensive experience will be required to determine the true potential in humans for the false-negative responses observed in animals by Levy and

colleagues and Machida and co-workers while recording responses of spinal origin.

The attractiveness of CMAP recording is that the muscle acts as a biologic amplifier of the small action potential traveling in the nerve. A CMAP in response to transcranial stimulation may have an amplitude of several millivolts, and accordingly can be acquired without signal averaging. In contrast, the epidural and peripheral nerve signals are relatively small (1 to 10 μV) and up to 200 transcranial or spinal cord stimuli have to be administered for the acquisition of one epidural or peripheral nerve MEP waveform. For these reasons we currently favor CMAP recording rather than recording from spinal cord or peripheral nerve.

Effects of Anesthetics on Motor Evoked Potentials

The effects of anesthetics on MEPs have recently been studied extensively. It appears that responses elicited by both tc^e-MEP and tc^e-MEP (TCS) are extremely sensitive to amplitude depression by anesthetic drugs, although the anatomic locus of this depression has not been defined. Inhalation of nitrous oxide 60% results in CMAP amplitude depression to 10% of baseline.[28, 112, 115] During nitrous oxide–narcotic anesthesia tc^e-MEPs can be recorded readily, although the amplitude is only 10% to 20% of awake baseline values. Tc^e-MEPs have also been recorded during spinal surgery under propofol anesthesia, which reduced amplitudes to 7% of baseline.[37] Addition of even very low concentrations of isoflurane (< 0.5%) during opioid–nitrous oxide anesthesia abolishes the tc^e-MEP[16, 42] (Fig. 12–12). MEPs also appear to be sensitive to benzodiazepines and some other intravenous anesthetics. Midazolam and the intravenous anesthetic agent propofol produce severe amplitude depression of tc-MEPs, while amplitudes are well preserved after etomidate and ketamine.[26, 27, 43, 86] In monkeys, an induction dose of midazolam also increased the stimulation threshold, resulting in a smaller scalp area where magnetic stimulation produces contralateral movement.[29] The amplitude of neurogenic MEPs to spinal cord stimulation in swine was unaffected after ketamine or opioids, but significantly decreased after propofol.[83] tc^e-MEPs recorded from the epidural space appear to be relatively resistant to depression by halothane or propofol.[59]

Muscle Relaxants. When CMAPs are recorded, either no muscle relaxants should be administered, or administration of the relaxant should be titrated to maintain a steady state of incomplete neuromuscular blockade that will allow recording of CMAPs from the muscle of interest.[16, 94] In the latter instance a CMAP response to supramaximal stimulation of the relevant peripheral nerve should be employed to verify the level of depression of neuromuscular transmission at the recording muscle (e.g., peroneal nerve stimulation when MEPs are recorded from the tibialis anterior muscle). When MEPs are recorded from the spinal cord there are no restrictions on the use of muscle relaxants. In fact, complete paralysis may facilitate recording by

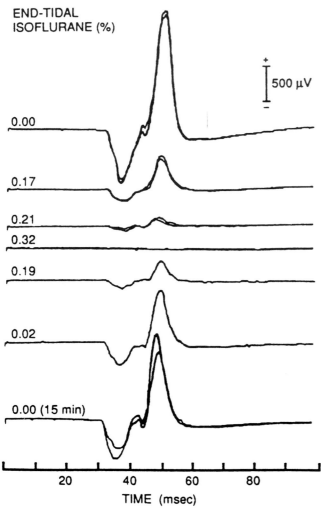

END-TIDAL ISOFLURANE (%)

500 µV

0.00

0.17

0.21

0.32

0.19

0.02

0.00 (15 min)

20　40　60　80

TIME (msec)

Figure 12–12 = Motor evoked responses to transcranial electrical stimulation in one patient during N_2O sufentanil anesthesia before, during, and after administration of isoflurane, 0.3% end-tidal volume. Duplicate waveforms are superimposed to show reproducibility, except during recovery (isoflurane concentrations 0.19% and 0.02%) when only one waveform was recorded. (From Kalkman CJ, Drummond JC, Ribberink AA: Low concentrations of isoflurane abolish motor evoked responses to transcranial electrical stimulation during nitrous oxide/opioid anesthesia in humans. Anesth Analg 73:410–415, 1991.)

eliminating artifact from contraction of paraspinal muscles.

In conclusion, at present the most feasible anesthetic technique for monitoring tc-MEPs or neurogenic MEPs appears to be a continuous infusion of an opioid, for example, fentanyl or sufentanil, supplemented with nitrous oxide. We use etomidate for induction of anesthesia, since it lacks the major depressive effects of tc-MEPs. The use of etomidate as part of a total intravenous anesthetic technique is limited by its depressant effect on cortisol synthesis. However, in patients who receive methylprednisolone for spinal cord protection[12] we are willing to supplement the standard opioid–nitrous oxide regimen with etomidate by infusion. Alternatively, ketamine can be given as an anesthetic supplement.

Improved Amplitude and Reproducibility of MEPs Using Multipulse Stimulation

Recently several groups have concentrated on overcoming anesthetic-induced depression of conduction in the motoneuronal system by employing facilitation techniques. Myogenic responses to transcranial electric or magnetic stimulation increase in amplitude when two or more stimuli are applied in rapid succession. This mechanism is known as "temporal summation." The optimal stimulus interval appears to be between 2 and 5 ms[46] (Fig. 12–13). Similarly, myogenic responses to spinal cord stimulation increase in size, and the stimulus intensity needed to elicit a response decreases when paired stimuli are administered.[101] We have incorporated a double-pulse stimulus paradigm in our routine myogenic MEP monitoring protocol, and since that time the success rate of achieving recordable responses of sufficient amplitude for reliable intraoperative monitoring in neurologically intact patients has been better than 95%. Manufacturers of both electrical and magnetic transcranial stimulators now make devices that have multipulse capabilities. The user can

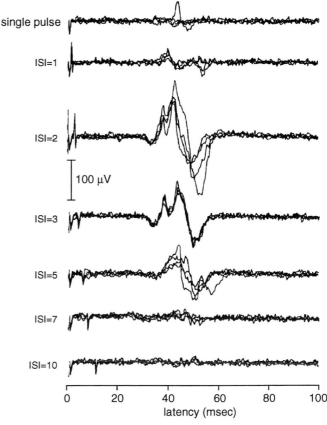

single pulse

ISI=1

ISI=2

100 µV

ISI=3

ISI=5

ISI=7

ISI=10

0　20　40　60　80　100

latency (msec)

Figure 12–13 = Influence of interstimulus interval on amplitude of myogenic motor evoked responses with paired transcranial electrical stimuli. Maximal amplitude augmentation occurred with interstimulus intervals between 2 and 5 ms. (From Kalkman CJ, Ubags LH, Been HD, et al: Improved amplitude of myogenic motor evoked responses after paired transcranial electrical stimulation during sufentanil/nitrous oxide anesthesia. Anesthesiology 83:270–276, 1995.)

select a number of pulses from 1 to 10 (electrical) or 1 to 4 (magnetic), and specify the interstimulus interval.

Safety of Transcranial Stimulation

Electrical and magnetic TCS have been used extensively in clinical neurophysiology for more than 8 years. There is no convincing evidence that the use of TCS in the circumstances of clinical monitoring results in neural damage or produces seizures. Damage to neural structures as a result of prolonged and intense electrical stimulation appears to be proportional to the total net charge delivered.[56] The safety record of low-frequency TCS (<0.3 Hz) is encouraging, especially with respect to the risk of provoking seizures.[3, 48, 56] Pending a more extensive experience with TCS, we prefer the recording of CMAPs for intraoperative MEP monitoring. Because this technique does not require averaging, it greatly reduces the total number of transcranial stimuli delivered to the patient and consequently the net charge delivered to the brain.

Limitations of MEPs

Although the clinical application of MEPs for intraoperative monitoring will probably reduce the incidence of undetected serious damage to the motor pathways, each of the available techniques has its limitations. Interpretation of tc-MEPs, especially when recorded from nerve or muscle, is limited by great variability in the transfer characteristics of the motor system, since it is subject to synaptic amplification and appears to be influenced by the excitatory state of the motor neuron pool. We have observed that light anesthesia may be associated with a sudden increase in the tc^e-MEP amplitude to values above 200% of control. This may represent the influence of facilitative mechanisms similar to those observed during voluntary contraction of the muscle.[2] Therefore, in order to reduce variability, it is probably appropriate to average three to five single responses, even when single stimuli produce MEPs of sufficient amplitude.

CONCLUDING REMARKS

Over the last decade SSEP monitoring during spinal surgery has grown from an experimental procedure to an accepted clinical technique for the prevention of postoperative neurologic deficits.[70, 71, 77] Both the validity and the limitations of the technique of SSEP monitoring for the early detection of impending spinal cord damage have become apparent.[52] The latter has prompted the search for techniques that can be employed clinically to monitor the motor tracts directly. Recently, promising results have been obtained with MEPs recorded from sciatic nerve or muscle after TCS or epidural spinal cord stimulation. It is our opinion that these evolving motor evoked response recording methods should serve as a complement, rather than an alternative, to SSEP recording. It is important that both

ascending and descending pathways in the spinal cord be monitored concurrently.

Future evoked potential equipment for intraoperative use may have various levels of automation that could govern the process of SSEP and MEP acquisition, interpretation, and automatic generation of alarms.[36, 38, 105] Such systems may alleviate the tedious task of repetitive SSEP or MEP acquisition during long surgical procedures. However, it is highly unlikely that they will ever replace the dedicated evoked potential consultant, who will remain essential for "troubleshooting" the plethora of technical, physiologic, surgical, and anesthetic factors that can alter intraoperative evoked potentials. Extensive communication between surgeon, anesthesiologist, and electrophysiologist both before and during the case regarding anesthetic management is essential. A spinal cord monitoring team with adequate equipment and sufficient experience for the acquisition and interpretation of intraoperative SSEPs and MEPs remains a major prerequisite for any reliable system of monitoring intraoperative spinal cord function.

REFERENCES

1. Abel M, Mubarak S, Wenger D, et al: Brainstem evoked potentials for scoliosis surgery: A reliable method allowing use of halogenated anesthetic agents. J Pediatr Orthop 10:208–213, 1990.
2. Ackermann H, Scholz E, Koehler W, et al: Influence of posture and voluntary background contraction upon compound muscle action potentials from anterior tibial and soleus muscle following transcranial magnetic stimulation. Electroencephalogr Clin Neurophysiol 81:71–80, 1991.
3. Agnew WF, McCreery DB. Considerations for safety in the use of extracranial stimulation for motor evoked potentials. Neurosurgery 20:143–147, 1987.
4. American Electroencephalographic Society: Guidelines for intraoperative monitoring of sensory evoked potentials. J Clin Neurophysiol 4:397–416, 1987.
5. Barker AT, Jalinous R: Nonivasive magnetic stimulation of human motor cortex. Lancet 2:1106–1107, 1985.
6. Ben-David B, Haller G, Taylor P: Anterior spinal fusion complicated by paraplegia. A case report of a false-negative somatosensory-evoked potential. Spine 12:536–539, 1987.
7. Bennett HL, Benson DR: Somatosensory evoked potentials for orthopaedic spine trauma. J Orthop Trauma 3:11–18, 1989.
8. Bennett MH: Effects of compression and ischemia on spinal cord evoked potentials. Exp Neurol 80:508–519, 1983.
9. Bickford RG, Fremming BD: Neural stimulation by pulsed magnetic fields in animals and man. In Digest of the Sixth International Conference on Electronics and Biological Engineering Tokyo, 1965; paper 7-6.
10. Bieber E, Tolo V, Uematsu S: Spinal cord monitoring during posterior spinal instrumentation and fusion. Clin Orthop 229:121–124, 1988.
11. Boyd SG, Rothwell JC, Cowan JM, et al: A method of monitoring function in corticospinal pathways during scoliosis surgery with a note on motor conduction velocities. J Neurol Neurosurg Psychiatry 49:251–257, 1986.
12. Bracken MB, Shepard MJ, Collins WF, et al: A randomized, controlled trial of methylprednisolone or naloxone in the treatment of acute spinal-cord injury. Results of the Second National Acute Spinal Cord Injury Study [see comments]. N Engl J Med 322:1405–14011, 1990.
13. Britt RH, Ryan TP: Use of a flexible epidural stimulating electrode for intraoperative monitoring of spinal somatosensory evoked potentials. Spine 11:348–351, 1986.
14. Brodkey JS, Richards DE, Blasingame JP, et al: Reversible spinal

cervicothoracic orthoses (SOMI and a four-poster orthosis) using flexion-extension radiographs and a goniometric technique. Their study provided the first level-by-level assessment of motion segments in the spine. In addition, they studied pressures on the chin and occiput after application of orthosis with forced motion. They concluded that the pressures were an extremely important determinant of the limitation of motions in the use of these devices. Additionally, they noted a poor correlation between goniometric measurements and total bony motion observed radiographically.

The Philadelphia collar may be the most popular cervical orthosis on the market. Its shape and contour allow it to make limited contact with the superoanterior and posterior thorax. When applied, the collar produces minimal flexion of the neck.[53] In general, this collar restricts flexion and extension 71%, lateral bending 34%, and axial rotation 56%.[40, 41] Immobilization is inadequate for rigid control of the upper cervical spine. The Philadelphia collar is well tolerated by patients and is used frequently in both prehospital and hospital settings. Unfortunately, its use in comatose patients

may result in occipital scalp ulcerations due to elevated occipital skin pressures when worn by a person in the supine position.[72]

The SOMI brace has been found to restrict cervical flexion-extension motion by approximately 72%, lateral bending by 34%, and axial rotation by 66%. This brace is especially useful in immobilizing flexion instability patterns between C1 and C5, but is much less useful in limiting cervical extension.

In a well-designed study, Johnson and associates[40, 41] evaluated various means of cervical immobilization (Fig. 13–15). They compared a soft collar, a Philadelphia collar, a four-poster cervical orthosis, a four-poster cervicothoracic orthosis, a Yale brace, and halo brace affixed to a vest in 44 volunteers. Each subject was used as his or her own control. Radiographic assessment was used to evaluate cervical motion, except for rotation. Statistical analysis was provided by the authors, as was a level-by-level assessment. Evaluation of the device included only seven subjects, all of whom had partial cervical fusions. In their report, detailed recommendations for the use of cervical orthoses at each level of the cervical spine were given. Of interest

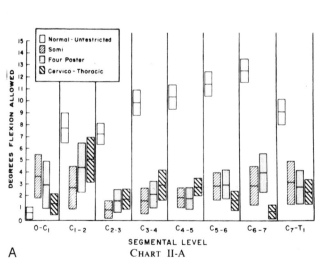

A — CHART II-A

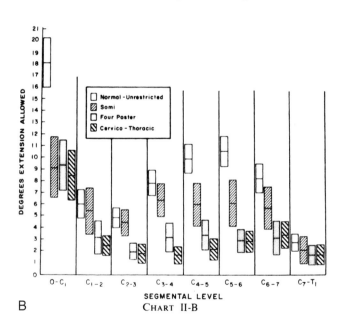

B — CHART II-B

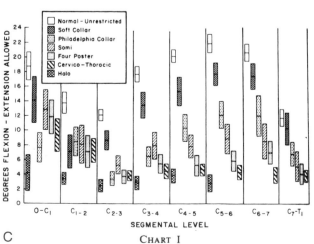

C — CHART I

Figure 13–15 = Graphs of normal cervical spine motion compared to motion observed in a variety of orthoses applied to normal volunteers. Degrees of flexion *(A)* and extension *(B)* allowed in SOMI, four-poster, and cervicothoracic orthoses compared to the normal unrestricted cervical spine. *C,* Degrees of flexion-extension allowed at each cervical motion segment level in a variety of orthotics compared to the normal unrestricted cervical spine. (From Johnson RM, Hart DL, Simmons EF, et al: Cervical orthoses: A study comparing their effectiveness in restricting cervical motion in normal subjects. J Bone Joint Surg Am 59:332–339, 1977.)

was the finding that the motion between the occiput and C1 increased from the normal motion of the unrestricted spine for all braces. This paradoxical, or "snake," motion has been noted by others in various parts of the spine.[19, 38, 57, 89] It was also noted that the length of the orthosis and the rigidity of the connections improved rotational as well as flexion-extension control, but lateral bending and total flexion-extension motions were not affected by these factors. In their conclusions they stated that the halo brace provided the best overall control of the cervical spine and should be used for truly unstable injuries. They also observed little difference (less than 2 degrees) in the immobilization of the C2–3 level between the halo brace, four-poster device, and the Yale brace. The Yale brace in general limits flexion and extension by 87%, lateral bending by 61%, and axial rotation by 75%.[41] Owing to its comfort, this brace has a high rate of patient compliance when compared to other cervicothoracic orthoses.

Devices that immobilize the cervical spine in the acute trauma setting have also been studied.[18, 73] Ninety-two volunteers were studied by Cline and co-authors,[18] utilizing the Hare extrication collar, the Philadelphia collar, and their own system for immobilization, which consisted of a short board with a forehead and a chin strap.[18] In their study, it was concluded that a board and straps (consisting of Kerlix rolls) provided the best acute immobilization. The authors did not provide a statistical analysis or a level-by-level analysis of motion. Podolsky and colleagues[73] used goniometry to assess the immobilization provided by the Hare device, the Philadelphia collar, the soft collar, and their own technique of using a board, two sandbags, and forehead tape. In this study, the authors felt that a Philadelphia collar provided the best immobilization in the flexion-extension mode. Recently, newer innovations in cervical orthosis design have contributed to improved patient comfort and, therefore, compliance as well as to decreased morbidity as a result of lessened brace-skin contact pressures.

The Malibu cervical orthosis is designed with thoracic (anterior and posterior) extensions slightly longer than those of the Philadelphia collar, therefore providing greater stability in the flexion-extension plane.[53] The Stifneck collar is a one-piece cervical orthosis used in prehospital clinical settings. This orthosis limits flexion-extension by approximately 70%, lateral bending by 50%, and axial rotation by 57%.[6, 36] Unfortunately, brace-skin contact pressures with this orthosis were found to be greater than the minimal capillary skin pressures at both the occipital and mandibular contact sites in the erect and supine positions.[72] The Miami J collar is a two-piece cervical orthosis that has been found to limit flexion-extension by 73%, lateral bending by 51%, and axial rotation by 65%.[6] This orthosis was found to statistically limit the degree of cervical motion, especially in the flexion-extension plane, greater than the Philadelphia, Stifneck, and Aspen collars. Patient compliance with the Miami J collar is similar to that of the Philadelphia collar and appears to be more suitable for use in patients with altered sensorium, because collar-skin contact pressures are

well below maximal capillary skin pressures.[72] The Aspen or Newport collar is a two-piece orthosis with an anterior thoracic extension that limits flexion-extension by approximately 62%, lateral bending by 31%, and axial rotation by 38%.[6] This collar is found to be extremely comfortable by patients owing to brace-skin contact pressures that are well below capillary closing pressures. The NecLoc collar is a two-piece cervical orthosis that is well liked by paramedics due to its acceptable restriction of cervical motion and its ease of application. This collar has been found to limit flexion-extension by 80%, lateral bending by 60%, and axial rotation by 73%.

The majority of cervical orthoses, excluding the hard or soft collars, are useful in the prehospital phase of cervical immobilization due to their ease of application, storage, and effectiveness. These include the NecLoc, the Philadelphia, Miami J, Stifneck, and Aspen collars. Of these, the NecLoc collar has proved somewhat superior to the others in its ability to limit cervical range of motion and is therefore favored for use by many prehospital caregivers.

The Miami J, NecLoc, Stifneck, and Philadelphia collars are popular orthoses utilized in the postoperative period. The Miami J collar, though, because of its low brace-skin contact pressures, is useful in patients with an altered sensorium.

The Minerva cervical brace is a cervicothoracic orthosis that has been found to limit flexion-extension by approximately 79%, lateral bending by 51%, and axial rotation by 88%.[76] This brace poorly immobilizes the occipital-C1 junction, but it limits motion at the C1 and C2 level to a greater degree than do other cervicothoracic braces. Table 13–2 is a summary of the percent motion restriction for various cervical and cervicothoracic orthoses.

The halo cervical immobilizer provides the most rigid stabilization of the cervical spine. Various studies have been performed evaluating restriction of motion in the cervical spine with a halo brace applied. Unfortunately, some caution must be made in assessing these investigations because the patients had concurrent cervical spine pathology, which perhaps also led to limitation in motion. In light of this, Whitehall and associates noted a 14% incidence of loss of cervical alignment in a retrospective review of 101 patients with halo braces.[91] The reported range of motion allowed by an appropriately applied halo vest ranges from 4% to 70% of normal. The greatest absolute range of cervical motion reported within a halo is approximately 7.2 degrees at the C4–5 level, and the greatest percent of normal range of motion is 42% at the C2–3 level, with the least being 20% at the C7–T1 level.[5, 48, 56] Thirty-three percent of normal cervical motion may occur within a halo when going from the upright to supine position.[48] Although results of some of the reports conflict, most agree that the halo provides the least amount of restriction above the C2 level and is best in restricting motion at or below C4–5. A careful review of the literature failed to identify the level in the thoracic spine at which the device ceases to be beneficial.

The halo brace was initially designed to provide

Table 13–2 = **PERCENTAGE OF MOTION RESTRICTED FOR VARIOUS COLLARS**

ORTHOSIS	% OF MOTION RESTRICTED				
	Combined Flexion-Extension	Flexion	Extension	1-Directional Lateral Bending	1-Directional Axial Rotation
Soft	26	23	20	8	17
Hard	27	28	27	33	34
Philadelphia	71	74	59	34	56
NecLoc	80	86	78	60	73
Stifneck	70	73	63	50	57
Aspen	62	59	64	31	38
Miami J	73	85	75	51	65
Malibu	NA	NA	NA	NA	NA
Two-poster*	90	NA	NA	90	90
SOMI	72	93	42	34	66
Four-poster	79	89	82	54	73
Yale	87	NA	NA	61	75
Minerva	79	78	78	51	88

*Results determined through cineradiography.
NA, not available; SOMI, sterno-occipitomandibular immobilizer.

distraction across the cervical spine. However, measurements of both distraction and compression have been demonstrated across the cervical spine. Average distraction force varies according to body position and activity.[48, 86] The average distraction force has been shown to vary according to position by nearly 20 lb when attached to a vest and by more than 30 lb when a cast supports the superstructure.[48] Additionally, significant changes in the forces across the cervical spine occur as a result of gravity when the head and body change position; when the vest is distorted from changes in body shape; with direct pressure from the abdomen, arms, or shoulders; or from contact with external surfaces. Bending from a seated position and reaching sideways while lying down also significantly alters the forces across the spine. Mediolateral forces have been determined to be small in comparison with the larger anteroposterior forces.[86]

Table 13–3 lists our modification of the recommendations made by the aforementioned studies, based on literature review and personal experience.[40, 41, 59] It must be pointed out that all of the devices that have been studied appear to lose effectiveness at the ends of the motion segments.

Halo

The halo skeletal fixator provides the most rigid type of immobilization for the cervical spine. It was first introduced by Perry and Nickel in 1959.[69] Its effectiveness in immobilization has been well established.* Following its introduction, few changes were made in the design or recommended method of application for many years.[39, 66, 67, 69, 94] Despite its being a very effective device, problem areas, especially pin loosening and infection, became apparent.[9, 14, 29, 30, 70, 79, 91] Studies emphasizing complications and analyzing biomechanical aspects of the device have generated scientific guidelines for its design and application.[10, 13–15, 28, 31–33, 75, 85]

Historical Development

During World War II, Frank Bloom, M.D., developed a device similar to the halo brace used today. His system consisted of an incomplete ring that opened posteriorly, which was fixed by pins to the skull. It was used on pilots who had inwardly displaced facial fractures and multiple skin burns. It was utilized to stabilize and apply traction to these fractures by the use of pins placed into the facial bones, with outward traction being applied through the ring. The pin design utilized in this device was very similar to those that are used today.

The device that Bloom designed was the inspiration for the development of halo skeletal fixation by Vernon Nickel, M.D., and first reported by Perry and Nickel in 1959.[69] The halo cervicothoracic orthosis originally consisted of a complete ring that was attached to a

Table 13–3 = **RECOMMENDED ORTHOSES FOR IMMOBILIZATION OF THE CERVICAL SPINE**

	TOTAL FLEXION-EXTENSION	FLEXION	EXTENSION
Occipital–C1	Halo	Halo	Halo
C1–2	Halo	Halo	Halo
	CTO	SOMI	CTO
C2–3	Halo	Halo	Halo
	CTO		CTO
C3–7	Halo	Halo	Halo
	CTO	CTO	CTO
	CO	CO	CO
C7–T2	Halo	CTO	CTO
	CTO		

CTO, cervicothoracic orthosis; SOMI, sterno-occipitomandibular immobilizer; CO, cervical orthosis.
From Lavernia CJ, Botte MJ, Garfin SR: Spinal orthoses for traumatic and degenerative disease. *In* Rothman RH, Simone FA (eds): The Spine, ed 3. Philadelphia, WB Saunders, 1992.

*References 1, 21, 34, 45, 48–50, 55, 58, 66, 70, 74, 79, 83, 90, and 94.

body cast. It utilized skeletal pins that were placed through holes with a complete ring anchoring the skull to the ring. It was first used to immobilize the cervical spine in poliomyelitis patients with paralytic cervical muscles.[66, 67, 69] The halo was subsequently used in the cervical spine of both adults and children for stabilization in trauma, infection, tumors, inflammatory and degenerative diseases, congenital malformations, and surgical fusions.*

The original ring was manufactured out of metal and was available in multiple sizes. Several holes were available for pin insertion. The ring was curved upward in the posterior aspect to afford a greater surgical exposure to the upper cervical spine with the ring in place. This ring was attached to a plaster body jacket by two upright anterior posts.[69]

Changes in materials and design have led to the availability of multiple halo fixators from a variety of manufacturers. Composite materials have allowed the fabrication of radiolucent rings, adjustable rings, convertible tong-to-ring designs, and open rings or crowns (tiaras) that encircle only a portion of the head. The latter designs are open in the back and avoid the need to pass the head through the ring, allowing easier application and thereby improving safety. In some of the incomplete rings, the posterior ends are angled inferiorly to ensure posterior pin placement below the equator of the skull.

Recent advances in plastic technology have allowed the development of lightweight, durable, yet adjustable and quickly applied vests, which have replaced plaster body casts.[38, 69] Cross-straps, as well as shoulder and trunk supports, stabilize the structure and decrease the shear stress between the anterior and posterior portions. A low-profile design for the uprights and connecting rods provides a manageable and "tolerable" frame. Specialized coating of the rods helps avoid seizing of the metal during tightening. In addition, connecting bolts on the vest are able to be tightened with wrenches that ratchet or give way at a set amount of torque (e.g., 28 ft-lb). These wrenches can potentially minimize overtightening, prevent bolt stripping, and save time. Currently utilized plastic vests and connecting-rod systems allow cervical spine adjustment in multiple planes. Knurled adjustment knobs, two-point flexion-extension supports with ratchets, and lightweight metals, allow "fine" adjustments that are useful in the alignment of fractures after application.

Despite the advantages provided by these prefabricated vests, they do not always fit adequately, especially if availability is limited by inventory restrictions. Occasionally, form-fitting plaster body casts or custom-manufactured thoracolumbosacral orthoses (TLSOs) should be considered when a proper vest size is not available. This is especially true for extremely thin or obese patients. Triggs and associates[84] evaluated the significance of vest length on cervical spine stability between a commercially available halo vest and a well-molded fiberglass body cast in a cadaver model. They found little difference in cervical angulation between a vest length down to the level of the iliac crest vs. down to the sternal xiphoid. The authors concluded that cervical immobilization may be optimally restricted in a well-fitted commercially available halo vest extending to the level of the xiphoid.[84] Wang and co-workers[87] also found that a vest length down to the level of the nipples was effective in cervical instability patterns above the C5 level.

Very few changes have been made in the design of the halo pin since it was originally described. It has been shown that altering this design can improve the mechanical quality of the pin-bone interface.[32] Bullet-type pins with broader shoulders may provide more rigidity at the pin-bone tip; these are under investigation and are not commercially available.

Break-away torque wrench handles for the pins, designed for one time use, have been introduced. These wrenches are designed to break off at a specific torque (e.g., 8 in-lb, 0.90 N-m) and can potentially save time. They are smaller than the standard torque wrenches and allow tightening despite limited access to the posterior aspect of the skull (e.g., when the patient is placed on a Rotobed). Although preliminary results demonstrate that they are accurate, rechecking the pin torque with a calibrated torque screwdriver is prudent. Some desirable features for a halo apparatus are listed in Table 13–4.[15]

Pin Insertion

The preferred sites for halo pin insertion have been evaluated in cadaver skull and in radiographic studies combined with clinical reviews of complications.[14, 28, 30, 33]

Table 13–4 = DESIRABLE FEATURES OF THE HALO SKELETAL FIXATOR

Ring and pins
  Maximum number of threaded holes structurally possible (to ease pin-site selection)
  Occipital area open (to ease ring placement)
  Radiolucent
  MRI compatible (nonferrous, nonmagnetic)
  Pins placed with break-away wrenches set at 8 in-lb
  Easy connections to upright posts
  Holes allow pin placement at 90 degrees to skull
  Pins have "shoulders"
Upright posts
  Low profile with length above ring kept to minimum
  Do not interfere with lateral roentgenograms (radiolucent or strategically placed)
  Multiplane adjustment of head and neck
  Fine tuning not essential
Vest
  Lightweight, conforming, yet rigid enough to provide support
  Compatible sizes with additional pediatric and extra-large sizes available
  Bridges or cross-straps connecting anterior and posterior components to prevent shear motion
  Radiolucent buckles and attachments
  Easy to apply, particularly in an unstable or anesthetized patient
  Provision for emergency access to the anterior chest

From Botte MJ, Garfin SR, Byrne TP, et al: The halo skeletal fixator: Principles of application and maintenance. Clin Orthop Rel Res 239:12–18, 1989.

---

*References 1, 21, 23, 34, 45, 48, 49, 50, 60, 61, 66, 70, 74, 75, 79, 83, 90, and 94.

Optimal positioning for anterior pins have been elucidated on the basis of anatomic structures at risk as well as on skull thickness. The preferred location is in the anterolateral aspect of the skull, approximately 1 cm superior to the orbital rim (eyebrow), cephalad to the lateral two-thirds of the orbit, and below the greater circumference of the skull. This is a safe zone for pin placement (Fig. 13–16). Placement of these pins below the level of the greatest skull diameter helps prevent cephalad migration.[15, 28, 30, 33] This position avoids violating the frontal sinuses and injuring the supraorbital and supratrochlear nerves medially and the zygomaticotemporal nerve laterally.

The temporalis muscle and fossa lie in the lateral aspect of the safe zone. Avoidance of this muscle and fossa is desirable for two reasons: (1) penetration of the temporalis muscle by the pin may result in painful mandibular motion (particularly with mastication) as well as localized pain, and (2) the bone in this area is thin, often being a single shell without a cancellous component, which makes skull penetration or loosening more likely than in a more anterior position (Fig. 13–17).

The supraorbital and supratrochlear nerves lie along the medial aspect of the safe zone adjacent to the front sinus. Placement of the pins lateral to the medial one-third of the orbit should avoid injury to these nerves and decreases the chance of penetration into the frontal sinus[15, 28, 30, 33] (see Fig. 13–16).

Posterior pin placement appears to be less critical, because vulnerable neuromuscular structures are lacking, the skull is thick, and bony contours are more uniform. In our experience, penetration in the posterolateral aspect of the skull appears optimal at the 4- and 8-o'clock positions[15, 28, 30, 33] (see Fig. 13–16).

The angle of insertion of the pin influences the fixa-

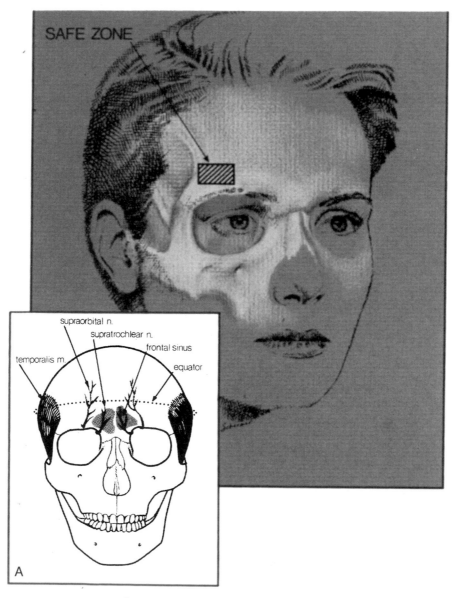

Figure 13–16 = *See legend on opposite page*

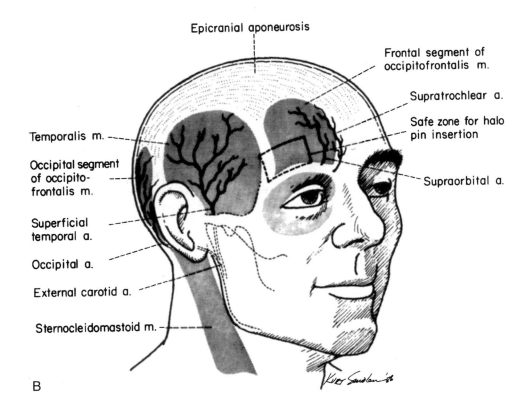

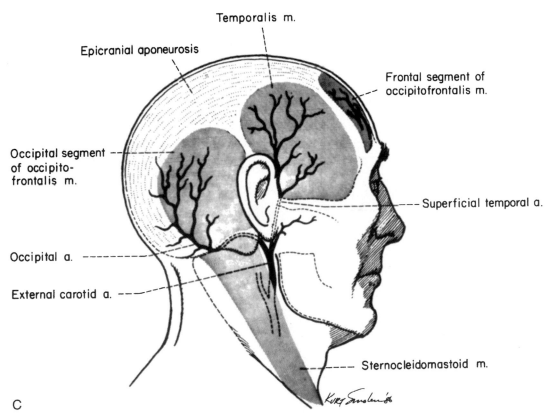

Figure 13–16 = *A–C,* Drawings depicting the "safe zone" for placement of halo fixator pins. The anterior pins are placed anterolaterally, approximately 1 cm above the orbital rim, below the equator of the skull, and cephalad to the lateral two thirds of the orbit. The safe zone avoids the temporalis muscle and fossa laterally and avoids the supraorbital and supratrochlear nerves and the frontal sinus medially. (*A* from Garfin SR, Botte MJ, Nickel VL, et al: Complications in the use of the halo fixation device. J Bone Joint Surg Am 68:320–325, 1986; *B* from Ballock RT, Botte MJ, Garfin SR: Complications of halo immobilization. *In* Garfin SR (ed): Complications of Spine Surgery. Baltimore, Williams & Wilkins, 1989.)

CHILD   ADULT

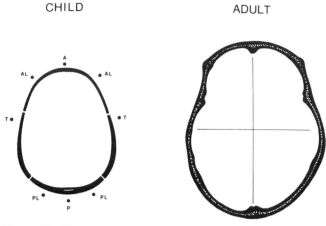

Figure 13–17 = Drawings of transverse sections through the skull (as shown by computed tomographic scanning) at the level of halo pin-site insertion in children and adults. A, anterior; AL, anterolateral; T, temporal fossa; PL, posterolateral; P, posterior. (From Garfin SR, Roux R, Botte MJ, et al: Skull osteology as it affects halo pin placement in children. J Pediatr Orthop 6:434–436, 1986.)

tion characteristics.[85] Loading studies of these pins inserted at different angles have demonstrated that perpendicularly inserted pins appear to provide more rigidity of fixation when compared to those placed at 15 or 30 degrees to the skull surface. The broader pin-bone interface afforded by this insertion angle provides increased contact area. Any angulation of the pin allows the shoulder of the pin to intercept the skull's outer cortex before the tip is fully seated.[85] Since the pin angle is fixed, or predetermined by the ring in most halo devices, placement of the ring over a flat portion of the skull is desirable.

The utilization of a skin incision prior to pin placement has been studied. There appears to be no advantage to cutting the skin before inserting the pin into the skull.[14] The complications of pin placement without an incision include loosening, infection, discomfort, and resultant scar: these were not altered by inserting the pin through a small incision. Additionally, we found that the placement of the skin incision causes occasional problems with bleeding, which delays, at least momentarily, the halo application procedure. Routine placement of skin incisions for halo pin placement does not seem warranted.[14]

The correct torque recommended for insertion of the pins was felt to be 5 to 6 in-lb (0.57 to 0.68 N-m).[67, 69, 70] Empirical observations were the basis for these recommendations. Because of clinical problems, such as pin loosening, anatomic studies on cadaver human skulls were performed and demonstrated that pins inserted at up to 10 in-lb (1.13 N-m) barely penetrate the outer table.[13] Additional mechanical testing of the pin-bone interface (cyclic loading and load-to-failure) have revealed that a torque of 8 in-lb (0.9 N-m) improved the mechanical qualities over those achieved with 6 in-lb (0.68 N-m).[32] In addition, clinically, 8 in-lb of insertion torque was shown to be safe and effective in lowering the incidence of loosening and infection when compared with 6 in-lb of torque.[13] From these studies, it appears that 8 in-lb is preferable to the 5 or 6 in-lb of torque originally recommended.

Application Techniques

Three persons is the preferred number for appropriate halo application.[15] Positioning pins and mechanical head-holders are also helpful. The physician in charge, who is holding the head, should be aware of the type of fracture and be comfortably positioned while keeping the unstable cervical spine and the halo in place. This is one of the most important tasks of the procedure, and it should not be relegated to an inexperienced member of the team.

Once appropriate ring and vest sizes are determined, the equipment should be checked carefully.[15] Ring size can be determined by selection of a ring that gives 1 to 2 cm of clearance circumferentially around the head. The suggested list of materials for application is shown in Table 13–5. The determination of vest size is based on chest circumference.

The patient can be lightly sedated if the neurologic and medical status permit, but he or she should be kept sufficiently conscious to make an accurate report of any changes in neurologic status during the maneuver. General anesthesia is not recommended for this procedure.

The patient should be placed on the bed in a supine position with the head positioned slightly beyond the edge. When a crown-type halo ring is employed, the patient's head can remain on the bed. A head-ring support aids in the application.[15]

Once the anterior pin sites are selected in the anterolateral aspect of the skull, the area should be appropriately marked. The skin sites are then prepared with a cleansing solution of choice.

The posterior sites are then selected as described in the prior section. Although these posterior sites are less critical, they should be placed approximately diagonal to the contralateral anterior pins. These sites should be placed inferior to the equator of the skull, yet superior enough to prevent impingement of the upper helix of the ear by the ring. An optimally placed ring should

Table 13–5 = MATERIALS FOR HALO APPLICATION

3-Person minimum recommended
Halo ring or crown (in preselected size)
Sterile halo pins (5, including 1 spare)
Halo torque screwdrivers (2) or "break-away" wrenches (4)
Halo vest (in preselected size)
Halo upright post and connecting rods
Head board
Spanners or ratchet wrenches (3)
Preparation razors (2)
Povidone-iodine solution
Sterile gloves (2 pairs)
Sterile gauze (4 packs of 2, 4 × 4-in size)
Syringes (2, 10 mL)
Needles (4, 25 gauge)
Lidocaine hydrochloride (10 mL of 1% solution)
Crash cart (including manual resuscitator, endotracheal tube)

From Botte MJ, Garfin SR, Byrne TP, et al: The halo skeletal fixator: Principles of application and maintenance. Clin Orthop Rel Res 239:12–18, 1989.

pass a centimeter cephalad to the top of the ear. Hair should be shaved in the posterior portion of the head, around the pin sites, and the skin should also be prepared with a solution of choice.[15]

The ring is then slipped over the head and held in position. The center hole, if present in the anterior portion of the ring, can be an aid to centering the anterior portion of the ring. Once the skin is prepared, infiltration with 1% lidocaine should be performed. Pins are then advanced directly through the skin, utilizing the desired torque screwdriver, and inserted perpendicular to the skull surface. During anterior pin advancement, the eyes of the patient should be closed and the forehead should be relaxed. This technique helps avoid skin or eyebrow tenting. Alternating in a diagonal fashion, the pins are tightened in 2 in-lb intervals until an 8 in-lb (0.9 N-m) torque is reached.[13] If the newer disposable type (break-away) handles are used, the final torque should be checked utilizing a calibrated torque screwdriver.[31] Lock nuts are then applied over the pin ends. Avoidance of overtightening the lock nut is important to prevent the halo pin from backing out.

When applying the vest, the patient's trunk should be elevated to allow placement of the posterior half of the vest.[12] The anterior half is then placed, and the neck and head are positioned and the bolts secured. The ratchet-type wrenches that give way at a set torque can be used to speed the application of the device. All of the application tools should be kept at bedside at all times in case emergency removal of the vest is required, such as for cardiopulmonary resuscitation. We recommend a roentgenogram of the spine after placement of the device.

After initial application, all the pins should be retightened 24 to 48 hours after application. Normally we do not utilize dressings around the pin sites. However, we do recommend that the sites are kept clean with hydrogen peroxide cleansing every other day, or as needed. Table 13–6 details the steps in the application of a halo fixator.

Complications

Significant complications can occur following the application of the halo external fixator[9, 14, 29, 30, 35, 70, 79, 91] (Table 13–7). The most common complications include pin loosening and pin-site infection.

If the pins become loose during the course of treatment, retightening to the 8 in-lb force is indicated if resistance is met within the first two complete rotations of the pin. If, in the process of retightening a loose pin, no resistance is met, placement of a new pin in an adjacent or nearby location should be considered.[15, 29] We recommend the placement of a new pin prior to removing a loose pin in order to maintain rigid ring fixation prior to pin-site change.

Bacterial cultures should be obtained if drainage develops around the pin and appropriate oral antibiotic therapy started; local pin care procedures should be emphasized to the patient. Drainage not responding to treatment, cellulitis, or abscess development suggests

Table 13–6 ═ PROCEDURE SUMMARY FOR APPLICATION OF THE HALO SKELETAL FIXATOR

1. Determine ring or crown size (hold ring or crown over head, visualize proper fit)
2. Determine vest size (from chest circumference measurement)
3. Identify pin-site locations (while holding ring in place)
4. Shave hair at posterior pin sites
5. Prepare pin sites with povidone-iodine solution
6. Anesthetize skin at pin sites with 1% lidocaine hydrochloride
7. Advance sterile pins to level of skin
8. Have patient close eyes
9. Tighten pins at 2 in-lb increments in diagonal fashion
10. Seat and tighten pins to 8 in-lb torque
11. Apply lock nuts to pins
12. Maintain cervical traction and raise patient trunk to 30 degrees
13. Apply posterior portion of vest
14. Apply anterior portion of vest
15. Connect anterior and posterior portions of vest
16. Apply upright posts and attach ring to vest
17. Recheck fittings, screws, and nuts
18. Tape vest removing tools to vest or keep at bedside
19. Obtain cervical spine roentgenograms

From Botte MJ, Garfin SR, Byrne TP, et al: The halo skeletal fixator: Principles of application and maintenance. Clin Orthop Rel Res 239:12–18, 1989.

the need for pin removal and insertion of a new pin at a different site. Intravenous antibiotics should be started and irrigation, debridement, and drainage performed as necessary.[15, 29, 30]

Bleeding complications have been reported at pin sites in patients taking anticoagulant medication. Anticoagulation occasionally has to be regulated by tapering the dose if this is a problem. Packing of the pin sites has not been shown to be effective as long as anticoagulation medication is continued.[15, 29]

Dysphagia or difficulty in swallowing has been reported to occur if the head and neck are placed in too much extension. Readjustment is often necessary to diminish the extension if this problem develops.[29]

Falls and trauma to the halo can cause dural puncture.[15, 29, 30] Symptoms associated with a dural puncture include headache, malaise, visual disturbances, and, on occasion, other local or systemic symptoms. Fluid leakage around loose or too deeply seated pins should

Table 13–7 ═ COMPLICATIONS ASSOCIATED WITH THE HALO IMMOBILIZATION DEVICE

COMPLICATION	% OF PATIENTS
Pin loosening	36
Pin site infection	20
Severe pin discomfort	18
Pressure sores	11
Severe scars	9
Nerve injury	2
Dysphagia	2
Bleeding at pin sites	1
Dural puncture	1

From Garfin SR, Botte MJ, Nickel VL, et al: Complications in the use of the halo fixation device. J Bone Joint Surg Am 68:320–325, 1986.

suggest this possibility. Plain radiographs and possibly a computed tomographic (CT) scan should be taken to discover or assess the possibility of fractures. If this complication is identified, the patient should be hospitalized and placed with the head in an elevated position, and a regimen of antibiotics should be started.[30]

Sores under the vest or cast can develop if it is not appropriately padded or if the patient is left in one position for long periods of time.[29] Patients with sensory deprivation (e.g., spinal cord injury, diabetes) are particularly at risk for this complication. Surgical stabilization of the cervical spine, if possible, should be considered in patients at high risk for pressure sores to avoid the use of the halo device. This, however, is a relative indication for any surgical procedure.

Loss of reduction has been shown to occur with this device.[48, 66, 91] The most commonly reported injuries associated with loss of reduction are those involving the posterior elements, especially unilateral facet fractures.[91] This is mostly due to the inability of the halo device to control rotation within the spine. In addition, large patients with poor-fitting vests can be at risk for loss of reduction and/or alignment.[91]

The Halo in Pediatric Trauma

The use of the halo brace in children is an effective means of cervical immobilization.[49, 60, 77] General anesthesia is a helpful adjunct in halo application in this age group. In children, recommended pin application torque should be between 2 to 5 in-lb.[49, 60] In pediatric patients younger than 3 years, a multiple-pin low-torque technique has been recommended to allow a greater range of pin placement and distribution of forces to the immature skull. In these patients, the young skull is too thin (weak) to accept high torque forces (see Fig. 13–17).[60] Other than this exception and the size of the orthosis, the hardware required for the pediatric population and techniques of application are similar to those recommended for older patients. Due to the patient's small size and infrequent need, manufacturers may not have complete inventory of parts. Custom-made components might be required.[60] Mubarak and associates have outlined the use of custom halo devices in young patients.[60] The size and shape of the head can be measured by using a flexible wire placed around he perimeter of the head. The halo ring is then fabricated by constructing it 2 cm in diameter larger than the wire impression. A plaster mold of the trunk can be obtained to custom manufacture a bivalve polypropylene vest. Linear measurements should also be done to ensure appropriate length of the suprastructure, which should be made of a lightweight anodized material. The use of 10 to 12 standard pins is recommended (Fig. 13–18). Custom-constructed halo rings in this population should be applied under general anesthesia. The 10 pins should be inserted to two-finger tightness or to a torque of 2 in-lb, avoiding the temporal regions and the frontal sinus.[33] The vest and the superstructure are then carefully applied. CT scans and skull radiographs can be obtained to visualize (and thereby avoid) suture lines or bone fragments

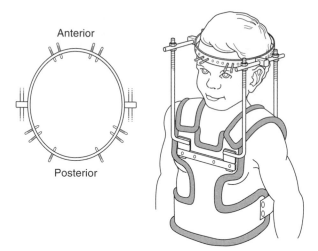

Figure 13–18 = *A*, Drawing of a young child with custom-molded halo vest and specially sized ring in place. *B*, "Crown-of-thorns" appearance of the ring with multiple pins anterolaterally, laterally, and posterior.

occasionally found in congenital malformations.[60] Pin care is identical to that for the adult patient.[60] The development of the skull is a pertinent consideration when planning anticipated halo pin sites.[60] In this group, cranial suture interdigitation can be incomplete, and the fontanels may open anteriorly (patients younger than 18 months) or posteriorly (patients younger than 6 months). Cranial distortion may result in these patients on application of the halo device if too great a force is applied.

THORACOLUMBAR SPINE

Orthotic use in the thoracolumbar spine can be divided into three categories, depending on the functional requirements of the orthosis.[17]

1. Braces may have a dynamic function, in which their purpose is to actively correct an existing deformity or actively prevent its progression. Examples of this may include bracing for idiopathic scoliosis or adolescent kyphosis. Biomechanically, these braces work through end-point surface contact and transverse loading to aid in curve correction.[62]
2. Braces may have a postural functional purpose in relieving discomfort associated with painful movements related to osteoporosis, low back pain, or following surgery in which postural realignment may promote improved function.
3. Braces may also function in a static fashion, providing physiologic support to allow healing following spinal trauma or a surgical fusion. Static brace support may also be useful in preventing progression of certain neuromuscular spinal disorders. Braces in this mode exert their influence through total truncal contact with or without pelvis support.

In summary, thoracolumbar braces collectively function through providing pain relief, correction of deformity, spinal immobilization, and truncal support. Their ability to successfully accomplish these goals is determined in part by the contact pressures they exert on the truncal soft tissues. The mechanical properties of these soft tissues (i.e., their patient-specific stiffness characteristic and the pain threshold or discomfort level of the patient) ultimately determines the degree of patient compliance and, therefore, brace success rate.

THORACIC SPINE

Few devices are available to immobilize the thoracic spine. If limited rigidity is necessary, the Jewett brace is most commonly utilized in the immobilization of this area of the spine (Fig. 13–19). This device includes a proximal rotating sternal and a distal rigid suprapubic symphysis pad. In addition, posterior and lateral components provide three-point fixation. The Jewett brace restricts flexion of the lower thoracic and upper lumbar spine and can be utilized to apply hyperextension forces. The James orthosis, also used for thoracic spine disorders, consists of a posterior aluminum frame with proximal straps that encircle the shoulders and an anterior abdominal pad that attaches to a pelvic band. This brace exerts an anterior force on the upper torso and abdominal region, pivoting on a third point of posterior contact in the midthoracolumbar spine, preventing thoracic flexion. These two orthoses are best utilized for symptomatic relief of compression fractures in which there is little evidence of instability. Unfortunately, Jewett braces do not appear to provide strong

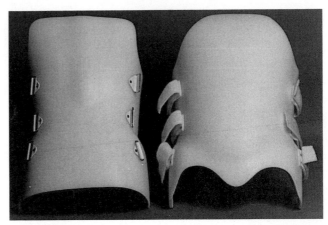

Figure 13–20 = Photograph of a custom-molded rigid thoracolumbosacral orthosis or body jacket: dorsal and frontal views. Note the presence of Velcro straps that hold the anterior and posterior shells in place.

rigidity against flexion forces. These devices are poorly tolerated by the older patient population.

When rigid immobilization is desired in this area of the spine, a custom-molded body jacket made of Kydex (polyvinyl chloride), Plastizote, low-molecular-weight polyethylene, or block leather (Fig. 13–20) is indicated. Thoracolumbar orthoses (including body jackets) provide restriction of motion up to the T8 level proximally and distally to the level of L4. Upper thoracic spine injuries should be treated with cervical extensions to these (TLSO) braces (Fig. 13–21). Below L4 a hip-thigh extension is commonly utilized, as some surgeons believe it assists in decreasing pelvic rotation and motion.

The usefulness of bracing and the appropriate duration of wear has been evaluated by Johnsson and colleagues,[42] who found that patients (N = 11) who were immobilized in a rigid lumbosacral orthosis for approximately 5 months following lumbosacral fusion had a higher success rate than patients (N = 11) immobilized for only 3 months. Johnsson and associates utilized three-dimensional roentgen stereophotogrammetric analysis 1 year postoperatively to evaluate intersegmental motion in the supine and erect positions.

The addition of a thigh cuff has been reported by some authors to improve successful fusion rates following surgery in the lumbosacral spine.[47, 63] Lumbar orthoses paradoxically tend to increase motion at the lumbosacral junction, motivating many treating physicians to apply this additional brace appendage. However, other researchers have cited no additional benefit in arthrodesis outcome and have noted the additional inconvenience in terms of patient discomfort during ambulation and subsequent poor compliance with its use.[80]

In symptomatic treatment of back pain or in osteoporotic compression fractures, corsets acting in postural functional manner may be useful (Figs. 13–22 and 13–23). These braces are composed generally of a cloth cylinder, with or without ancillary straps or posterior metal struts. Although adverse changes in the electromyographic characteristics of abdominal muscles in

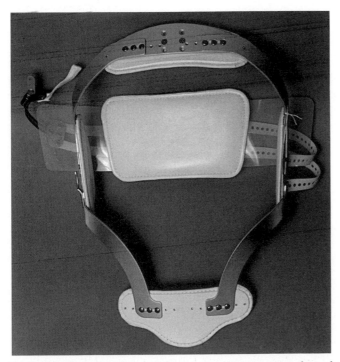

Figure 13–19 = Jewett brace. Frontal view demonstrating the pads that press over the sternum and pubic symphysis. The single posterior strap attempts to apply pressure to extend the spine and prevent kyphosis.

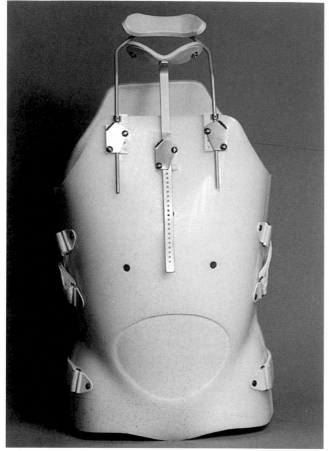

Figure 13–21 = Custom-molded thoracolumbosacral orthosis or body jacket with a cervical extension attached: frontal view.

patients wearing these corsets for more than 6 weeks have been identified in some studies, their use is advocated by some. Structurally, corsets do not stabilize the bony column of the thoracic spine. They do, however, provide some soft tissue support to the trunk and may, in this way, provide symptomatic relief.

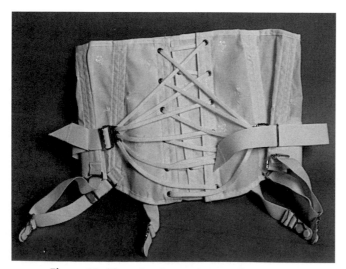

Figure 13–22 = Lumbosacral corset: frontal view.

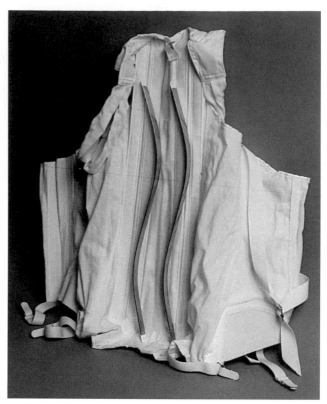

Figure 13–23 = Thoracolumbosacral corset: dorsal view.

Flexible Braces

Sacroiliac, lumbosacral, cervicothoracolumbosacral, and thoracolumbosacral orthoses may be used in rigid or flexible forms. Flexible orthoses are constructed in a shape similar to that of more rigid ones in terms of the overall architecture. Flexible sacroiliac orthoses usually encircle the whole pelvic bony structure, between the iliac crest and the trochanters. In addition, perineal straps are often added to avoid upward displacement of the devices. Lumbosacral orthoses are similar in design, but they may extend to the xiphoid process anteriorly and to the inferior angle of the scapula posteriorly (Fig. 13–24). Flexible thoracolumbosacral orthoses extend even higher with their posterosuperior border at the level of the midscapula, whereas the anterosuperior border remains at the costal margin (Fig. 13–25). These garments are circumferentially adjustable by the use of front and back laces or hooks and, more recently, with straps made of Velcro.

The indications for the use of flexible sacroiliac orthoses include postpartum traumatic separation of the symphysis pubis. The flexible LSO and TLSO are often used for low back pain. These devices, as stated previously, do decrease the myoelectric activity of the paraspinal muscle groups and possibly increase intra-abdominal pressure by exerting a static upward force to the diaphragm, theoretically diminishing the loads on the disc in the low back.[52, 59, 64, 68, 88] These findings, however, are controversial, and some authors have reported increased myoelectric activity in certain paraspinal muscle groups when specific activities are per-

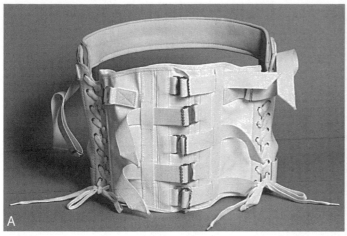
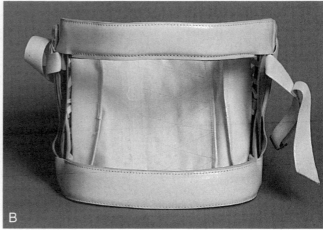

Figure 13–24 = Flexible lumbosacral orthosis. *A,* Frontal view. *B,* Dorsal view.

formed.[52] Although flexible TLSOs and LSOs do provide a certain amount of immobilization, the limitation of motion is minimal and should not be used when rigidity is needed.[52, 57, 88] Low-temperature thermoplastic polymers are used in the fabrication of custom-molded flexible devices in the treatment of back pain. This form-fitting plastic, when placed within a Lycra envelope, can be fastened with Velcro. The use of these thermoplastics has made these orthoses light, better fitting, better tolerated, and more affordable than the older orthoses.[52, 88]

Rigid Thoracolumbar Orthosis

The medical literature has not given thoracolumbar orthoses as much attention as cervical orthoses. Conventional thoracolumbosacral orthoses exert most of their effect in a flexion-extension mode and are less restrictive in the prevention of rotation and lateral bending motions. The Jewett hyperextension brace, a typical thoracolumbosacral orthosis, is shown in Figure 13–19. This device utilizes a three-point truncal force and two anterior supports, one on the pubis and another at the sternum. A posterior support is located across the thoracolumbar junction. Another device, the Knight-Taylor brace, is a classic example of a commonly prescribed thoracolumbosacral orthosis. This device appears similar to a thoracolumbosacral corset; however, it has lateral as well as posterior metal uprights with over-the-shoulder straps that attempt to limit lateral bending and flexion-extension (Fig. 13–26). A cervical extension may also be added to add further control proximal to the T8 vertebral level (Fig. 13–27). The addition of crossed uprights increases the rigidity of these devices. The rotational control, however, is poor.

To obtain adequate rotational control, a thoracolum-

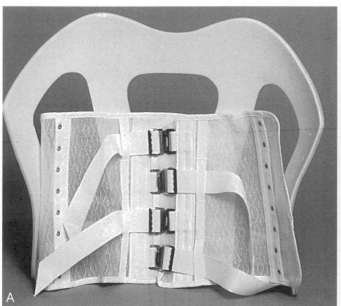
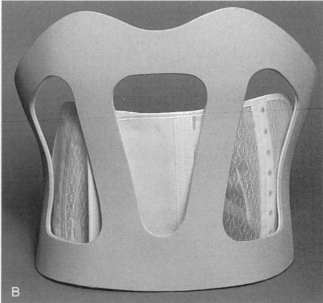

Figure 13–25 = Flexible thoracolumbosacral orthosis. *A,* Frontal view. *B,* Dorsal view.

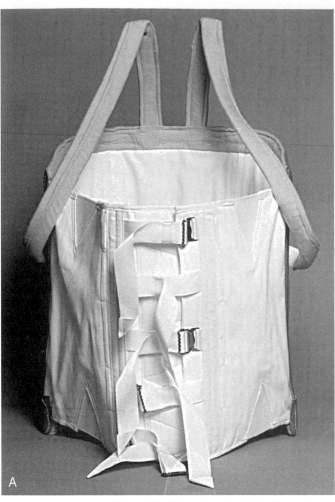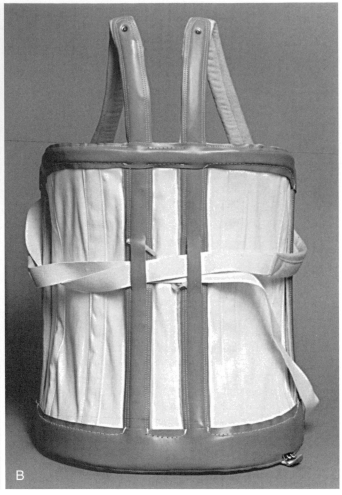

Figure 13–26 ═ Knight-Taylor thoracolumbosacral orthosis. *A,* Frontal view. *B,* Dorsal view.

bosacral orthosis needs to be fully custom molded (Fig. 13–28). High-temperature polyform thoracolumbosacral orthoses are made from a custom plaster shell that has been molded on the patient's body. These devices should not be used to immobilize the thoracic spine above the T8 level.[89] To gain control of this area (above T8), a cervical extension must be added to the polyform jacket.[89] Distally, the immobilization of these orthoses ends at L4.[68, 82, 89]

Rigid lumbosacral orthoses are frequently prescribed for low back pain. However, the use of these devices following the surgical treatment of the lumbosacral region for trauma is also very common. The most common lumbosacral orthosis is similar in shape to the corset-type flexible orthosis with the addition of anterior, posterior, and lateral uprights to achieve restraint of motion in flexion-extension, rotation, and lateral bending. A molded thermoplastic lumbosacral orthosis with adjustable anterior Velcro straps is also popular (Fig. 13–29). These devices provide poorest control in the rotational mode. All of these braces have been shown to decrease activity in the abdominal musculature.

Lantz and Schultz examined various braces (lumbosacral corset, chair-back brace, lumbosacral orthosis,

and molded thoracolumbosacral orthosis) in terms of their effect on gross body motions and myoelectric activity[51] in five volunteers who performed various tasks while wearing the braces. Surface electrodes were utilized to monitor muscle activity. The restriction of function as reflected by myoelectric activity was strictly dependent on the task performed, and no consistent pattern could be observed among the different subjects. Unfortunately, in this study only five subjects were used, and the variability reported can be easily attributed to the sample size. They did find that all braces restricted upper body gross motion (20% of flexion and 45% of rotation, lateral bending, and extension), which may decrease compressive forces across the lumbar spine by lessening muscle tension required for equilibrium. The molded thoracolumbosacral orthosis was most effective in all motions tested except flexion in the standing position, which was most affected by the lumbosacral corset. Unfortunately, no segmental information or statistical analysis was provided by their study.

The effects of these devices on the myoelectric activity of the erector spinal muscles has not been conclusively studied. There is general agreement in the literature, however, that the myoelectric activity in the

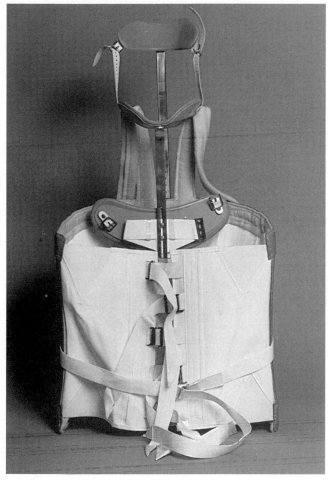

Figure 13–27 = Knight-Taylor brace with cervical extension.

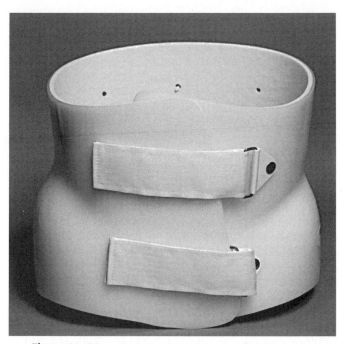

Figure 13–29 = Rigid lumbosacral orthosis: frontal view.

abdominal musculature appears to be decreased with all of the braces.[59, 64, 88]

The lumbar spine has been studied independently.[2, 24, 52, 57, 82, 93] Norton and Brown published a scientific study on the use of braces to restrict motion in the lumbar spine.[68] Four types of lumbosacral orthoses, as well as a thoracolumbosacral orthosis, were evaluated by them. Specific types of orthoses included in the study were the Taylor, Jewett, Goldthwait, Arnold-Abbott, and Williams braces, as well as the group's own design, and a custom-fit plaster brace. The measurements of motion were done by Kirschner wires placed in the spinous processes of the subjects, and angles were measured between the wires. Radiographic measurements were also made. They observed that motion across the lumbosacral junction increased with the use of all of the braces. In addition, they also observed increased motion at the L4–5 level when the subjects

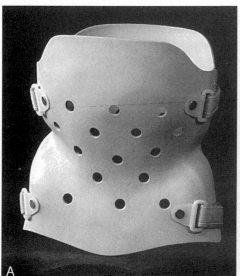
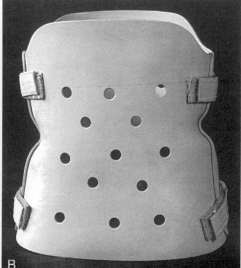
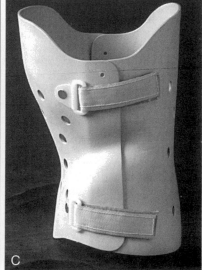

Figure 13–28 = Custom-molded rigid thoracolumbosacral orthosis or body jacket of Kydex (polyvinyl chloride). *A*, Frontal view. *B*, Dorsal view. *C*, Lateral view with Velcro straps holding the anterior and posterior shells in place.

were in a sitting position. Additionally, flexion developed at the L4–5 and L5–S1 interspaces in standing subjects when compared to extension in an unbraced state. These authors also attempted to measure forces between the body and the braces. Pressure points were modified in their experimentally designed brace and succeeded in eliminating some of the flexion in the lower spine that was observed while subjects wore the standard braces. Unfortunately, no motion analysis was done above L4, and the study was limited to flexion-extension; translation and rotation were not assessed. This paradoxical increase in intersegmental lower lumbar motion with bracing (canvas corset with molded plastic posterior support, metal struts, and a molded rigid thoracolumbosacral orthosis) was also reported by Axelsson and colleagues[7] using three-dimensional roentgen stereophotogrammetric analysis. This group studied seven patients following a lumbosacral fusion without instrumentation 1 month after surgical implantation of 0.8-mm tantalum metal spheres. Intervertebral motion in the sagittal and vertical planes increased slightly compared to a nonbraced control when patients went from the supine to erect position. The workers concluded that fixation to the pelvis must be necessary to counteract transmission of proximal forces to more distal levels of the spine.

The rotational motion of the lumbosacral spine was studied by Lumsden and Morris.[57] Steinmann pins were inserted in the posterosuperior iliac spine of volunteer subjects. Numerous measurements of pin rotation and motion seen radiographically were performed. The braces studied by this group included the chairback brace as well as a lumbosacral corset. Their conclusion, similar to that of Norton and Brown, was that conventionally used braces actually increased motion at the lumbosacral level.

Motion restriction in the lumbosacral region achieved with a corset, a brace, and a plaster jacket, with and without the thigh cuff, was reported by Fidler and Plasmans.[24] Lateral radiographs were utilized to study motion by this group. They reported that custom-molded plaster jackets were the most effective of the devices in restricting motion from the L1–3 interspaces; however, to immobilize L4–S1 levels, a thigh cuff needed to be included. Their study, as others, has limitations in that only five volunteers were used, and very limited statistical analysis was provided. Axelsson and colleagues reported their three-dimensional roentgen stereophotogrammetric analysis on nine patients following a lumbosacral fusion without instrumentation, with implantation of tantalum spheres 1 month following surgery, utilizing a thoracolumbosacral orthosis with a unilateral hip spica. No significant effect on sagittal, vertical, or transverse intervertebral motion was noted compared to a nonbraced control. A paradoxical increase in motion was not observed, as it had been in patients previously braced without a thigh cuff.[8]

In summary, the mechanical effectiveness on an orthosis may be measured by its ability to decrease load through direct transfer from the truncal soft tissue structures and, therefore, the spine or by restricting intersegment or gross body motions, thereby decreasing stresses on the spinal column.[51] Studies have confirmed that compressive loads on the spine are favorably dissipated with the use of an orthosis through decreases in intradiscal pressures,[4, 62] but no beneficial effect on truncal myoelectric activity or intrabdominal pressure changes with orthosis use has been proved conclusively. The obvious benefit of brace wear appears to be its effect on gross body movements through patient cooperation, thereby decreasing adverse force moments. Large force moments may result in potentially deleterious motion, predisposing to delayed or unsuccessful fracture or fusion mass healing.

From this review of the literature, the reader can appreciate that no brace available today provides ideal immobilization. Table 13–8 lists our recommendations for immobilization.

COST ANALYSIS

With economic factors affecting the availability and type of medical care, physicians must be aware of the financial impact of a brace prescription. Table 13–9 illustrates the approximate cost of fitting patients with some of the most common spine orthoses in the Philadelphia region in 1996. Some of the newer, untested orthoses are extremely expensive. Physicians should be

Table 13–8 = **RECOMMENDED ORTHOSES FOR IMMOBILIZATION OF THE THORACOLUMBOSACRAL SPINE**

SPINAL SEGMENT	ORTHOSIS
T2–7	Plastic TLSO with attached chin and occiput support
T8–L3	Plastic TLSO
L4–S1	Plastic TLSO with a thigh cuff

TLSO, thoracolumbosacral orthosis.

Table 13–9 = **ESTIMATED AVERAGE COST FOR ORTHOSES IN PHILADELPHIA IN 1996***

ORTHOSIS	COST ($)
Soft collar	18.21
Hard collar	42.57
Philadelphia collar	91.13
Malibu collar	248.22
SOMI	322.79
Dennison 2-poster CTO	248.22
Minerva CTO	1,332.13
Halo with vest	1,702.05
Jewett orthosis	263.49
Molded TLSO	1,158.06
TLSO with cervical extension	1,480.85
TLSO with leg extension	1,506.57

*Data presented for comparative purposes only.
SOMI, sterno-occipitomandibular immobilizer; CTO, cervicothoracic orthosis; TLSO, thoracolumbosacral orthosis.

aware of the advantages as well as the relative cost when selecting one of these orthoses.

CONCLUSION

Our extensive review of the literature, combined with our experience, demonstrates a growing need for better, more rigorous studies of spinal orthotic devices. We think that studies should use radiographic techniques that minimize radiation to evaluate the actual motion of the skeleton in various braces. A larger number of subjects should be studied and a statistical analysis should be provided. The brace fit should be normalized by pressure measurements obtained during maximal effort in bending and other motions. Further studies of the halo brace should also be done on the normal spine and utilized as a baseline for comparison with other devices. The effect of body fat on fit should also be correlated with limitation of motion. Objective fat-quantifying techniques, such as triceps skin-fold thickness, might be used.

REFERENCES

1. Abitbol JJ, Botte MJ, Garfin SR, et al: The treatment of multiple myeloma of the cervical spine with a halo vest. J Spinal Disord 2:263–267, 1989.
2. Allbrook D: Movement of the lumbar spinal column. J Bone Joint Surg Br 39:339–345, 1957.
3. Andriacchi T, Schults A, Belytschoco T, et al: A model for studies of the mechanical interaction between the human spine and ribcage. J Biomech 7:497–507, 1974.
4. American Academy of Orthopaedic Surgeons: Atlas of Orthotics. St Louis, CV Mosby, 1975.
5. American Academy of Orthopaedic Surgeons: Atlas of Orthotics, ed 2. St Louis, CV Mosby, 1985.
6. Akins V, Eismont FJ: Comparison of Four Cervical Collars in their Effectiveness in Restricting Cervical Motion. Tampa, Florida Orthopaedic Society, Oct 20, 1994.
7. Axelsson P, Johnson R, Stromqvist B: Effect of lumbar orthosis on intervertebral mobility: A roentgen stereophotogrammetric analysis. Spine 17:678–681, 1992.
8. Axelsson P, Johnson R, Stromqvist B: Lumbar orthosis with unilateral hip immobilization: Effect on intervertebral mobility determined by roentgen stereophotogrammetric analysis. Spine 18:887–879, 1993.
9. Ballock RT, Botte MJ, Garfin SR: Complications of halo immobilization. In Garfin SR (ed): Complications of Spine Surgery. Baltimore, Williams & Wilkins, 1989, p 376.
10. Ballock RT, Lee TQ, Triggs KJ, et al: The effect of pin location on the rigidity of the halo pin-bone interface. Neurosurgery 26:238–241, 1990.
11. Barnes JW, Harwell AD: Technical note: The use of low heat thermoplastics in vacuumforming. Orthot Prosthet 40:58–63, 1986.
12. Botte MJ, Byrne TP, Abrams RA, et al: Review: The halo skeletal fixator: Current concepts of application and maintenance. Orthopedics 18:463–471, 1995.
13. Botte MJ, Byrne TP, Garfin SR: Application of the halo fixation device using an increased torque pressure. J Bone Joint Surg Am 69:750–752, 1987.
14. Botte MJ, Byrne TP, Garfin SR: Use of skin incisions in the application of halo skeletal fixator pins. Clin Orthop 246:100–101, 1989.
15. Botte MJ, Garfin SR, Byrne TP, et al: The halo skeletal fixator: Principles of application and maintenance. Clin Orthop 239:12–18, 1989.
16. Chase AP, Bader DL, Houghton GR: The biomechanical effectiveness of the Boston brace in the management of adolescent idiopathic scoliosis. Spine 14:636–642, 1989.
17. Chase A, Pearcy M, Balder D: Spinal orthoses. In Bowker P, Wallace W (eds): Biomechanical Basis of Orthotic Management. Boston, Butterworth-Heinemann, 1993, pp 234–251.
18. Cline JR, Scheidel E, Bigsby EF: A comparison of methods of cervical immobilization used in patient extrication and transport. J Trauma 25:649–653, 1985.
19. Colachis SC, Strohm BR: Radiographic studies of cervical spine motion in normal subjects. Arch Phys Med Rehabil 46:253, 1965.
20. Colachis SC, Strohm BR, Ganter EL: Cervical spine motion in normal women: A radiographic study of effect of cervical collars. Arch Phys Med Rehabil 54:161–169, 1973.
21. Cooper PR, Maravilla KR, Sklar FH, et al: Halo immobilization of cervical spine fractures: Indications and results. J Neurosurg 50:603–610, 1979.
22. Edwards JW: Orthopaedic Appliances Atlas. St Louis, American Academy of Orthopaedic Surgeons, 1952.
23. Ewald FC: Fracture of the odontoid process in a 17-month-old infant treated with a halo. J Bone Joint Surg Am 53:1636–1640, 1971.
24. Fidler MW, Plasmans CMT: The effect of four types of support on the segmental mobility of the lumbosacral spine. J Bone Joint Surg Am 65:943–947, 1983.
25. Fisher SV, Bowar JF, Awad EA, et al: Cervical orthoses effect on cervical spine motion: Roentgenographic and goniometric method of study. Arch Phys Med Rehabil 58:109–115, 1977.
26. Fisher SV: Proper fitting of the cervical orthosis. Arch Phys Med Rehabil 59:505–507, 1978.
27. Food and Drug Administration: Medical Device Amendments, 2nd ed. Washington, DC, FDA, 1986.
28. Garfin SR, Botte MJ, Centeno RS, et al: Osteology of the skull as it affects halo pin placement. Spine 10:696–698, 1985.
29. Garfin SR, Botte MJ, Nickel VL, et al: Complications in the use of the halo fixation device. J Bone Joint Surg Am 68:320–325, 1986.
30. Garfin SR, Botte MJ, Triggs KJ, et al: Subdural abscess associated with halo-pin traction. J Bone Joint Surg Am 70:1338–1340, 1988.
31. Garfin SR, Botte MJ, Woo SL, et al: Reliability after repeated use of a torque screwdriver employed for halo pin fixation. J Orthop Res 3:121–123, 1985.
32. Garfin SR, Lee TO, Roux RD, et al: Structural behavior of the halo orthosis pin-bone interface: Biomechanical evaluation of standard and newly designed stainless steel halo fixation pins. Spine 11:977–981, 1986.
33. Garfin SR, Roux R, Botte MJ, et al: Skull osteology as it affects halo pin placement in children. J Pediatr Orthop 6:434–436, 1986.
34. Garret A, Perry J, Nickel VL: Stabilization of the collapsing spine. J Bone Joint Surg Am 43:474–484, 1961.
35. Glaser JA, Whitehall R, Stamp WG, et al: Complications associated with the halo-vest. J Neurosurg 65:762–769, 1986.
36. Graziano AF, Schneider EA, Cline JR, et al: A radiographic comparison of prehospital cervical immobilization methods. Ann Emerg Med 16:1127–1131, 1987.
37. Hannah RE, Cottrill D: The Canadian collar: A new cervical orthosis. Am J Occup Ther 39:171–177, 1985.
38. Hartman JT, Palumbo F, Hill BJ: Cineradiography of the braced normal cervical spine. Clin Orthop 109:97–102, 1975.
39. Houtkin S, Levine DB: The halo yoke: A simplified device for attachment of the halo to a body cast. J Bone Joint Surg Am 54:881–883, 1972.
40. Johnsson RM, Hart DL, Simmons EF, et al: Cervical orthoses: A study comparing their effectiveness in restricting cervical motion in normal subjects. J Bone Joint Surg Am 59:332–329, 1977.
41. Johnsson RM, Owen JR, Hart DL, et al: Cervical orthoses. Clin Orthop 154:34–45, 1981.
42. Johnsson RM, Stromqvist B, Axelsson P, et al: Influence of spinal immobilization on consolidation of posterolateral lumbosacral fusion: A roentgen stereophotogrammetric and radiographic analysis. Spine 17:16–21, 1992.
43. Johnsson RM: The use of orthoses in lumbar spine fusion. Acta Orthop Scand 64:92–93, 1993.
44. Jones MD: Cineradiographic studies of the collar-immobilized cervical spine. J Neurosurg 17:633–637, 1960.
45. Kalamchi A, Yau ACMC, O'Brien JP, et al: Halo-pelvic distraction apparatus: An analysis of 150 consecutive patients. J Bone Joint Surg Am 58:1119–1125, 1976.

46. Kaufman WA, Lunsford TR, Lunsford BR, et al: Comparison of three prefabricated cervical collars. Orthot Prosthet 39:21–28, 1986.

47. Kim SS, Denis F, Lonstein JE, et al: Factors affecting fusion rate in adult spondylolisthesis. Spine 15:979–984, 1990.

48. Koch RA, Nickel VL: The halo vest: An evaluation of motion and forces across the neck. Spine 3:103–107, 1978.

49. Kopits SE, Steingass MH: Experience with the "halo-cast" in small children. Surg Clin North Am 50:935–943, 1970.

50. Kostuik JP: Indications for the use of the halo immobilization. Clin Orthop 154:46–50, 1981.

51. Lantz SA, Schultz AB: Lumbar spine orthosis wearing: I. Restriction of gross body motions. Spine 11:834–837, 1986.

52. Lantz SA, Schultz AB: Lumbar spine orthosis wearing: II. Effect on trunk muscle myoelectric activity. Spine 11:838–842, 1986.

53. Lavenia CJ, Botte MJ, Garfin SR: Spinal orthosis for traumatic and degenerative disease. *In* Rothman RH, Simeone FA (eds): The Spine, ed 3. Philadelphia, WB Saunders, 1992, pp 1197–1224.

54. Levine AM: Spinal orthoses. Am Fam Physician 29:277–280, 1984.

55. Lind B, Nordwall A, Sihlbom H: Odontoid fractures treated with halo-vest. Spine 12:173–177, 1987.

56. Lind B, Sihlbom H, Nordwall A: Forces and motions across the neck in patients treated with the halo vest. Spine 13:162–167, 1988.

57. Lumsden RM II, Morris J: An in vivo study of axial rotation and immobilization at the lumbosacral joint. J Bone Joint Surg Am 50:1591–1602, 1974.

58. Lyddon DW Jr: Experience with the halo and body cast in the ambulatory treatment of cervical spine fractures. Ill J Med 146:458–461, 1974.

59. Morris JM, Lucas DB: Biomechanics of spinal bracing. Ariz Med 2:170–176, 1964.

60. Mubarak SJ, Camp JF, Vuletich W, et al: Halo application in the infant. J Pediatr Orthop 9:612–614, 1989.

61. Muller I, Varmuzkova O, Vlach O, et al: Halo. Another method of treatment and care for cervical spine injuries. Acta Chir Orthop Traumatol Cech 46:161–166, 1979.

62. Nachemson AL, Morris J: In vivo measurements of intradiscal pressure. J Bone Joint Surg Am 46:1072–1092, 1964.

63. Nachemson AL: Orthotic treatment for injuries and diseases of the spinal column. Phys Med Rehabil 1:11–24, 1987.

64. Nachemson A, Schultz A, Anderson GB: Mechanical effectiveness of lumbar spine orthoses. Scand J Rehabil Med 9(suppl):139–149, 1983.

65. Nakamura T, Oh-Hama M, Shingu H: A new orthosis for fixation of the cervical spine: Fronto-occipito-zygomatic orthosis. Orthot Prosthet 38:41–45, 1984.

66. Nickel VL, Perry J, Garrett A, et al: The halo: A spinal skeletal traction fixation device. J Bone Joint Surg Am 50:1400–1409, 1968.

67. Nickel VL, Perry J, Garrett AL, et al: Application of the halo. Orthop Prosthet Appliance J 14:31–35, 1960.

68. Norton PL, Brown T: The immobilizing efficiency of back braces. J Bone Joint Surg Am 39:111–139, 1957.

69. Perry J, Nickel VL: Total cervical spine fusion for neck paralysis. J Bone Joint Surg Am 41:37–60, 1959.

70. Perry J: The halo in spinal abnormalities: Practical factors and avoidance of complications. Orthop Clin North Am 3:69–80, 1972.

71. Pieron AP, Welpy WR: Halo traction. J Bone Joint Surg Br 52:119–123, 1970.

72. Plaisler B, Graham SGA, Schwartz RJ, et al: Prospective evaluation of craniofacial pressure in four different cervical orthoses. J Trauma 37:714–720, 1994.

73. Podolsky S, Baraf LJ, Simon RR, et al: Efficacy of cervical spine immobilization methods. J Trauma 23:461–465, 1983.

74. Prolo DJ, Rennels JB, Jameson RM: The injured cervical spine: Immediate and long-term immobilization with the halo. JAMA 224:591–594, 1973.

75. Sears W, Fazi M: Prediction of stability of cervical spine fracture managed in the halo vest and indications for surgical intervention. J Neurosurg 72:426–432, 1990.

76. Sharpe KP, Rao S, Ziogas A: Evaluation of the effectiveness of the Minerva cervicothoracic orthosis. Spine 20:1475–1479, 1995.

77. Sherk HH, Nicholson JT, Chung SMK: Fractures of the odontoid process in young children. J Bone Joint Surg Am 60:921–924, 1978.

78. Smith GE: The most ancient splints. Br Med J 1:732–734, 1908.

79. Sneddon MH, Giammatei F: Pitfalls in halo application and management. Scientific exhibit at the Annual Meeting of the American Academy of Orthopaedic Surgeons, Anaheim, Calif, March 10–15, 1983.

80. Stauffer RN, Coventry MB: Posterolateral lumbar-spine fusion rate in adult spondylolisthesis. Spine 15:979–984, 1990.

81. Sypert GW: External spinal orthotics. Neurosurgery 20:642–649, 1987.

82. Tanz SS: Motion of the lumbar spine: A roentgenologic study. AJR 69:399, 1953.

83. Thompson H: Halo traction apparatus: A method of external splinting of the cervical spine after surgery. J Bone Joint Surg Br 44:655–661, 1962.

84. Triggs KJ, Ballock T, Byrne T, et al: Length dependence of a halo orthosis on cervical immobilization. J Spinal Disord 6:34–37, 1993.

85. Triggs KJ, Ballock RT, Lee TO, et al: The effect of angled insertion on halo pin fixation. Spine 14:781–783, 1989.

86. Walker PS, Lamser D, Hussey RW, et al: Forces in the halo-vest apparatus. Spine 9:773–777, 1984.

87. Wang GJ, Moskal JT, Albert T, et al: The effect of halo-vest length on stability of the cervical spine. J Bone Joint Surg Am 70:357–360, 1988.

88. Waters RL, Morris JM: Effect of spinal supports on the electrical activity of muscles of the trunk. J Bone Joint Surg Am 52:51–60, 1970.

89. White AA, Panjabi MM: Clinical Biomechanics of the Spine. Philadelphia, JB Lippincott, 1978.

90. White R: Halo traction apparatus. J Bone Joint Surg Br 48:592, 1966.

91. Whitehall R, Richman JA, Glaser JA: Failure of immobilization of the cervical spine by halo vest. J Bone Joint Surg Am 68:326–332, 1986.

92. Willners S: The effect of the Boston thoracic brace on the front and sagittal curves of the spine. Acta Orthop Scand 55:457–460, 1984.

93. Wiltse LL, Kikaldy-Willia WH, McGiver GW: The treatment of spinal stenosis. Clin Orthop 115:83–91, 1976.

94. Zwerling MT, Riggins RS: Use of the halo apparatus in acute injuries of the cervical spine. Surg Gynecol Obstet 138:189–193, 1974.

Cervical Injuries

Craniocervical Trauma

Frank J. Eismont ‖ *Daveed D. Frazier*

Injuries to the craniocervical junction are commonly seen in the coroner's office but are seen only rarely in the emergency room.

In a postmortem study of 112 victims of trauma, Bucholz and Burkhead[11] found that 9 (8%) had atlanto-occipital dislocations. In a similar study of 50 consecutive fatal craniospinal injuries, Davis and co-workers[14] also found that 6 of the victims (12%) had head-on-neck dislocations. Alker and co-workers,[1] in a review of 146 fatalities from traffic accidents, found occipitoatlantal dislocations in 8 victims (5%). In this and in most series, this injury occurs most commonly in pedestrians struck by cars.

In contrast, only 2 of Bohlman's 300 hospitalized patients with cervical fractures or dislocation or both, had occipitocervical dislocations (an 0.67% incidence) and both patients died after a short period of time.[9] Similarly, Clark and others[13] reviewed 236 patients seen at their hospital and found only 2 occipitocervical dislocations (incidence of 0.85%) with both patients dying as a result of the injury.

Occipitocervical instability is also seen as the result of certain diseases of the spine,[18] including ankylosing spondylitis[31] and rheumatoid arthritis,[37, 46] but these patients present with a chronic history of progressive symptoms. This chapter is limited to those patients affected by acute traumatic occipitocervical instability.

There are now many case reports and small series of patients with occipitoatlantal dislocations surviving long enough to be treated.* Many of these patients survive over a long term. With the skills and availability of emergency medical services continually improving, it is probable that a higher percentage of patients with this injury will survive long enough to be seen in our emergency rooms. Although many will not survive because of the intrinsic nature of the injury, it is important that this injury be promptly recognized and properly treated in order to maximize the number of patients surviving with this injury and to minimize their neurologic deficit.

NORMAL ANATOMY

The occipitocervical junction has been thoroughly studied from both the anatomic and radiographic viewpoints.

The bony constraints are limited to the convex occipital condyles articulating with the congruent concave superior lateral masses of the atlas. These joints are flatter and less restrictive in children than in adults and hence children less than 12 years of age have increased joint mobility[5, 12] and are more predisposed to injury at this level. Another bony constraint is the posterior arch of the atlas, which provides a limit to occiput–C1 (C0–1) extension when it abuts against the base of the skull.[60]

There are many ligamentous constraints,[60] but the most formidable are the paired alar ligaments coursing from the superolateral aspect of the odontoid process to the medial aspects of the occipital condyles. The tectorial membrane, which is a superior continuation of the posterior longitudinal ligament, is also very important. Lesser ligamentous restraints include the anterior and posterior atlanto-occipital membrane, the C0–1 articular joint capsules, and the insignificant apical ligament extending from the tip of the odontoid to the basion (Fig. 14–1).

The motion available at the occipitocervical junction is 21 degrees extension, 3 degrees flexion, 7 degrees rotation to each side, and 5 degrees lateral bending to each side.[42, 60]

RADIOGRAPHIC EVALUATION

Many articles have been written concerning the radiographic assessment of the upper cervical spine and the normal ligamentous and osseous constraints.*

The lateral radiograph should show the basion over the posterior aspect of the odontoid process. It is often stated that the distance from the basion to the top of the odontoid process should be 5 mm or less, but this is not always true. Greater distances are frequently seen in the normal population. In the original study of Wholey and others,[62] the average distance in normals was 5 mm, but distances up to 10 mm were observed in infants.

The Powers ratio[43, 44] is also useful for assessing occipitocervical alignment (Fig. 14–2). Lines are drawn from the opisthion to the anterior arch of the atlas (line OA) and from the basion to the posterior arch of the atlas (line BC). The ratio of distances BC/OA should be 1.0 or less. If the ratio exceeds 1.0, there is probably an anterior occipitoatlantal dislocation. Unfortunately,

---

*References 3, 6, 9, 10, 13, 15, 17, 19, 21–23, 36, 38, 40, 41, 48, 57–59, 64.

*References 12, 24, 29, 33, 34, 37, 43, 44, 50, 51, 62–64.

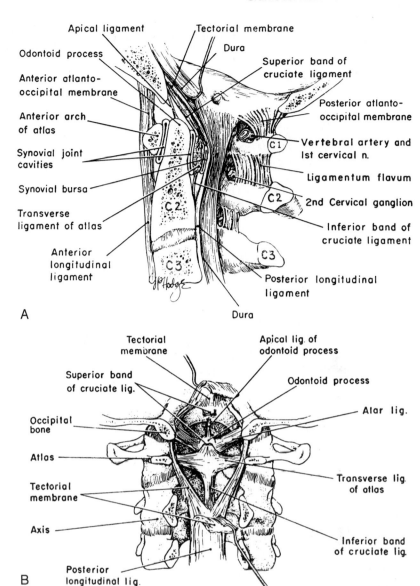

Figure 14–1 = *A*, A midsagittal section through the craniocervical junction. This shows the appropriate relationship of the basion or anterior aspect of the foramen magnum to the ring of C1 and the odontoid process. This nicely illustrates the ligaments at the occipitocervical junction. *B*, A coronal section demonstrating the ligaments at the craniocervical junction. Note especially the alar ligaments and the tectorial membrane. (From Martel W: The occipito-atlanto-axial joints in rheumatoid arthritis and ankylosing spondylitis. AJR 86:223–240, 1961.)

this ratio will not be helpful in diagnosing the much less common occipitoatlantal posterior dislocation or pure distraction injuries.

Although seldom indicated in acute cervical injuries, flexion-extension cervical radiographs should reveal C0–1 translation of 1 mm or less. Translation greater than 1 mm indicates occipitoatlantal instability.[63]

The lateral radiograph should show a smooth gently curved line posteriorly from the opisthion to the inner aspect of the lamina of the atlas, the axis, and the more caudal cervical vertebrae. Any sharp deviation of this line at the C0–1 level could signify an occipitoatlantal dislocation.

A retropharyngeal space exceeding 5 mm measured anterior to C3 is seen with most upper cervical spine injuries and occipitoatlantal injuries are no exception. Many of these patients will have marked retropharyngeal swelling (Figs. 14–3 and 14–4; see also 14–9). In many of the postmortem studies, free air is seen in the retropharyngeal space as a result of concomitant rupture of the posterior pharyngeal wall.

Computed tomographic (CT) scans[24] with sagittal and coronal reconstruction can also be diagnostic as can standard anteroposterior (AP) and lateral tomograms.

Fractures may be seen with occipitoatlantal dislocations and the most typical would be avulsion fractures related to the alar ligaments. This could be from the superolateral portion of the odontoid process as described by Anderson and D'Alonzo's type I odontoid fracture[2] (see Fig. 14–4). They considered it to be an uncommon fracture but of no clinical significance. Most would now agree that this fracture could very well be associated with severe and life-threatening occipitocervical instability, and Scott and colleagues[50] have correctly emphasized the significance of this type I odontoid fracture. The other associated fracture can be an avulsion fracture of the medial aspect of the occipital condyle (see Fig. 14–3). Anderson and Montesano classified this as their type III occipital condyle fracture and recognized its association with head-on-neck dislocations.[3]

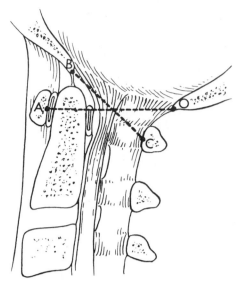

Figure 14–2 = This drawing represents a midsagittal section through the craniocervical junction. B, basion; O, opisthion; A, anterior arch of atlas; C, posterior arch of atlas. The ratio BC/OA should always equal 1 or less. If it is greater than 1 the patient most likely has an anterior occipitocervical subluxation dislocation. (From Powers B, Miller MD, Kramer RS, et al: Traumatic anterior atlanto-occipital dislocation. Neurosurgery 4:12–17, 1979.)

Any widening of the occipitoatlantal joints should also alert the clinician to possible head-on-neck instability (see Figs. 14–3 and 14–4). Kaufman and others[33] have reviewed this joint in children on cross-table lateral skull radiographs and found that a joint space of 4.5 mm or less is normal and that a joint space of 5 mm or more suggests occipitocervical distraction or dislocation injury.

PATHOLOGY OF OCCIPITOCERVICAL SUBLUXATION AND DISLOCATION

The pathologic findings in these head-on-neck dislocations have been accurately described in the literature and are a combination of clinical findings of those who survived this injury and gross pathologic findings of those who did not survive.[1, 11, 14, 52, 56]

Many of the gross anatomy dissections reveal disruption of all occipitocervical ligaments, as would be expected. The injury may be limited to soft tissue or it may involve bone avulsion, as with the alar ligament attachments, or it may involve occipital condyle fractures.

The extent of neural and vascular damage varies from normal to complete disruption. The neural tissue at this level includes the brain stem with its respiratory and cardiovascular centers, the nuclei and tracts of various cranial nerves, and all sensory and motor tracts including the very prominent decussation of the corticospinal tracts (Fig. 14–5). In surviving patients it is common to see respiratory and cardiovascular instability[35] cranial nerve palsies, and various degrees of sensorimotor impairment[17, 19] (see Fig. 14–4). Those patients with incomplete motor paralysis can have very bizarre clinical pictures depending on which part of the pyramidal decussation is involved.[7] This can include weak arms and normal legs, weak legs, and normal arms, and even weakness in one arm and the contralateral leg; hence the term "cruciate" paralysis.[39]

CLASSIFICATION OF OCCIPITOCERVICAL SUBLUXATION AND DISLOCATION

Based on a review of the literature and a personal case, Traynelis and co-workers[57] developed a classification system for occipitocervical subluxation and dislocation (Fig. 14–6). It is graded type I through III. Type I involves anterior displacement of the occiput with respect to the atlas. Type II is a longitudinal distraction injury with separation of the occiput from the atlas. Type III, which is quite rare, involves posterior displacement of the occiput with respect to the atlas.[57] This classification helps to provide some rationale for treatment. In a type II injury, primarily a longitudinal distraction injury in which good alignment is maintained, initial traction might not be indicated because it could lead to a progressive neurologic deficit. However, in type I or type III injuries 5 lb of traction might be indicated to realign the bone structures and decompress the brain stem or spinal cord. Eismont and Bohlman[17] reported a type III dislocation where placement of longitudinal traction led to significant improvement of quadriparesis over several hours.

Figure 14–3 = This 21-year-old woman was involved in a high-speed motor vehicle accident and presented with a mandible fracture, renal contusion, talar neck fracture, bimalleolar ankle fracture, and ipsilateral Lisfranc fracture dislocation. Physical examination revealed that she was alert, had suboccipital tenderness, diffuse mild weakness of the upper and lower extremities, increased deep tendon reflexes, and positive Hoffmann's signs. A, The initial lateral radiograph reveals significant soft tissue swelling at the level of C1–3. B, The patient was placed in Gardner-Wells tong traction because of a suspected cervical spine injury. A follow-up film several hours later reveals markedly increased retropharyngeal soft tissue swelling and in 5 lb of traction there is a mild distraction at the occiput-C1 junction. C, This anteroposterior (AP) tomogram reveals an avulsion fracture of the origin of the alar ligament from the medial aspect of the occipital condyle (*arrow*). D, This lateral tomogram reveals an avulsion fracture of the basion (*arrow*). There is presumably also an injury to the tectorial membrane. E, The patient was taken to surgery for an occiput-to-C2 fusion. At the same time she was placed in a halo vest. At the time of surgery it was thought that there was instability at the C1–2 level in addition to that at the occiput-C1 level. On this follow-up film, taken 3½ years later, the posterior fusion is obviously solid. It should also be noted that the distance at this time between the basion and the tip of the odontoid is markedly reduced compared with her earlier films. On follow-up the patient was neurologically normal with negative Hoffmann's signs and reflexes in a normal range.

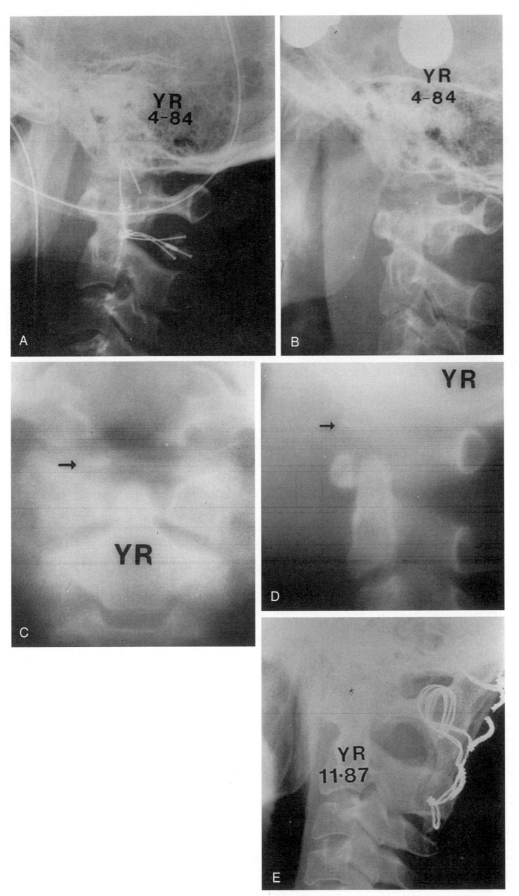

Figure 14–3 = *See legend on opposite page*

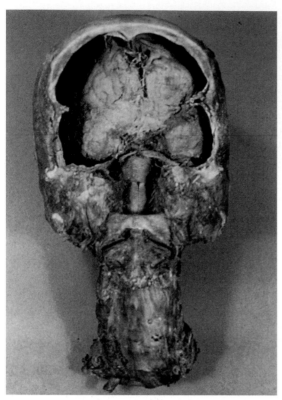

Figure 14–4 = This cadaver dissection shows the relationship of the brain stem to the occipitocervical junction. The decussation of the corticospinal tracts is clearly seen. It should be emphasized that these tracts are extremely superficial and very vulnerable to injury.

TREATMENT OF OCCIPITOATLANTAL DISLOCATIONS AND SUBLUXATIONS

As with all injuries, treatment begins with assessment and immobilization at the injury scene. All patients with major trauma and especially those with a neurologic deficit should be suspected of having an occipitocervical injury. Initial management should consist of maintaining an adequate airway as per the ABCs of trauma and immobilizing the cervical spine in a neutral position. In the emergency room, once this injury is suspected, the ideal treatment is application of a halo vest. If tong traction is applied, no more than 5 lb should be used and a radiograph should be taken immediately because these injuries are very easily overdistracted (see Fig. 14–4). If the patient is a child, care should be taken to use the split-mattress technique described by Herzenberg and associates[30] to maintain normal alignment and avoid forced forward flexion of the head.

If a patient with this injury requires intubation, it is recommended that this be nasotracheal rather than orotracheal. It is also recommended that no axial traction be applied but rather that the head and neck be stabilized in a neutral position to minimize the risk of neurologic injury.[8]

This injury can occasionally be treated with 3 months of halo vest immobilization provided the initial ligamentous and bone injury is relatively limited and sta-

ble. After 3 months of immobilization, flexion and extension radiographs can be done to assess stability, and a delayed occipitocervical fusion can then be performed if it is needed. One case was successfully treated with 3 weeks of traction after reduction with traction, but this is certainly uncommon.[6]

Since this is normally an extremely unstable injury, a posterior occipitocervical fusion is usually indicated[17, 19, 23, 38] (see Figs. 14–3 and 14–4). A fusion from the occiput to the atlas is theoretically adequate treatment, but this is most often not realistic because of other associated injuries to the upper cervical spine and because a fusion just from the occiput to the atlas usually is not biomechanically solid enough to stabilize this severe injury. A fusion from the occiput to the axis is most often necessary. Of the four patients surgically treated by the senior author (F.J.E.),[17, 38] a fusion to a lower level was always necessary because of associated injuries. The timing of surgery should be individualized, and it is normally performed as soon as the patient is medically stable enough to tolerate it.

The technique of posterior occipitocervical fusion depends on the surgeon's preference. Each technique gives predictably good results when performed as outlined by the author. Some authors have recommended posterior wiring with or without a rod and more recently posterior plates and screws have been promoted. We present each of the three techniques.

Operative Setup

These patients are always placed in a halo vest and the spine is reduced prior to surgery. The injuries are unstable and these patients are therefore intubated fiberoptically with a nasotracheal tube. Intubation is done with the patient awake and the patient is kept awake until transfer to the prone position on the surgical table and the patient has been neurologically assessed in this new position. Once positioning is complete a lateral radiograph is taken to ensure adequate alignment of the occipitocervical junction.[53] Intraoperative somatosensory evoked potential monitoring or motor evoked responses are used to assess the physiologic status of the spinal cord during the procedure.

Occipitocervical Wiring Technique

A posterior, midline incision is made from the midocciput to just below the level to be fused. Subperiosteal dissection is used to expose the squamous portion of the occipital bone, the foramen magnum, the posterior ring of C1, and the spinous processes, laminae, and facets of the lower vertebrae to be fused. Care is taken to preserve all ligaments and joint capsules below the level of the fusion.

Wertheim and Bohlman[61] described a triple wiring technique which avoids passage of intracranial wires. Their technique is a modification of a technique originally described by Robinson and Southwick.[47] In the modified procedure a high-speed burr is used to make a trough on either side of the external occipital protuberance. Care is taken to avoid the transverse and

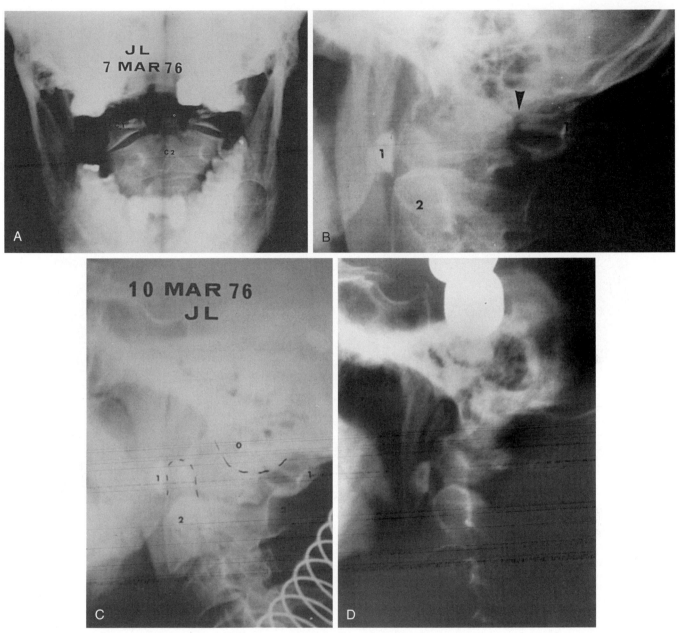

Figure 14–5 = This 68-year-old man was involved in a high-speed motor vehicle accident and was ejected at the time of the accident. The patient had an abrasion on the right side of the face and complained of neck pain. He also had a fracture of the left femur. He was initially neurologically normal and was placed in a soft cervical collar and his femur was immobilized. A, An AP film of the upper cervical spine appears relatively normal. B, A cone-down lateral radiograph of the upper cervical spine reveals a fracture of the posterior arch of C1 (*arrowhead*). It also appears that the basion is slightly more posterior than would normally be seen. There is significant soft tissue swelling in the retropharyngeal space at C1 and C2. C, This lateral radiograph of the upper cervical spine reveals that the head is posteriorly displaced on the atlas. At this time the patient was in a soft cervical collar. He was experiencing problems with hypertension and paroxysmal atrial tachycardia and respiratory distress associated with a spastic quadriparesis. At this time the head-on-neck dislocation was appreciated and the patient was placed in skull 4.6 kg of traction. D, This lateral film of the upper cervical spine reveals that the occiput is now correctly located over the atlas but that there is moderate overdistraction. At this time the weight was reduced to 2.3 kg of traction. The patient's quadriparesis resolved over several hours and his spasticity subsided over approximately 6 weeks.

Illustration continued on following page

superior sagittal sinuses cephalad to the protuberance. A towel clip is then used to make a hole through the outer table and 20-gauge wire is looped through this hole and around the bony ridge. A second 20-gauge wire is passed around the arch of the atlas, and a third wire is passed through a drill hole in the base of the spinous process of the axis. Two curved corticocancel-

lous struts taken from the posterior iliac crest are prepared with three drill holes equal distances apart. The occiput is decorticated and the grafts are anchored in place on both sides of the spine by the wires. Additional cancellous bone graft is packed between the grafts. After meticulous hemostasis the wound is closed in layers.[61] In the series described by Wertheim

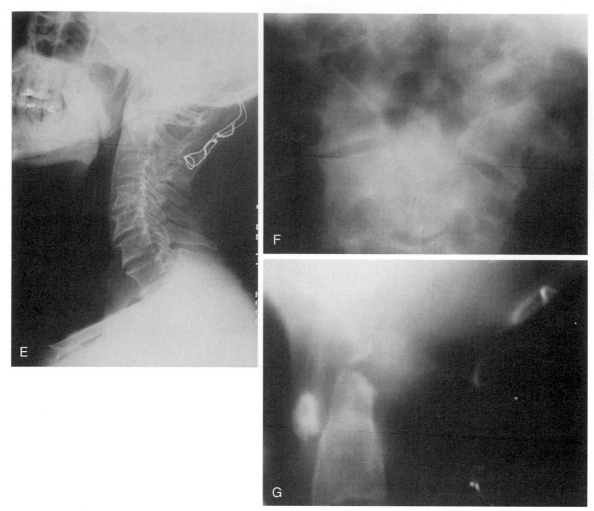

Figure 14–5 *Continued = E,* At 6 weeks after injury, a halo and body cast was applied to immobilize the patient's head on his neck. Twelve weeks after injury a posterior fusion from the occiput to C3 was performed with the iliac crest bone wired in place. This lateral radiograph was made 11 months after the fusion showing a solid fusion from the occiput to C3 with the head and cervical spine in their normal relationship. *F,* This AP tomogram obtained after fusion reveals that the tip of the odontoid process is avulsed in a type I odontoid fracture. The alar ligaments are presumably still attached to this piece of bone. *G,* This lateral tomogram made 10 weeks after fusion demonstrates avulsion of the apex of the odontoid process, which is a type I fracture. This probably includes the bone attachment of the alar ligaments. This film also shows that the relationship of the basion to the odontoid has been restored to normal and also shows that the posterior laminar line is now again normal.

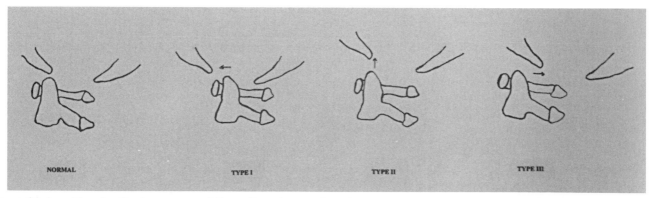

Figure 14–6 = The classification system of Traynelis and co-workers for occipitocervical subluxation and dislocation. (Redrawn from Traynelis VC, Marano GD, Dunker RO, et al: Traumatic atlanto-occipital dislocation. J Neurosurg 65:863–870, 1986.)

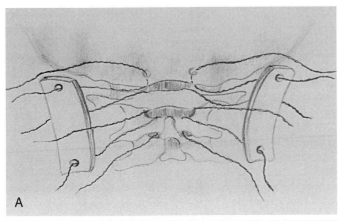

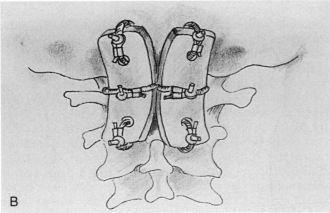

Figure 14–7 = *A* and *B*, These drawings represent the triple-wiring technique for occipitocervical fusion as originally described by Robinson and Southwick in 1960[47] and later reported by Starr and associates.[55]

and Bohlman, all 13 of their patients developed a solid fusion.

The technique described by Robinson and Southwick in 1960[47] has been used routinely by the senior author (F.J.E.) and has been reported by Starr and colleagues[55] (Fig. 14–7). The exposure is the same as described above. Burr holes are then placed on each side in the occiput 1 cm lateral to midline and 1 cm posterior to the foramen magnum. A Woodson elevator is passed through the burr hole toward the foramen magnum to separate the dura from the skull. A braided cable is then placed in the burr hole and brought out through the foramen magnum, and one cable is passed on each side of the skull. A third and a fourth cable are passed under the posterior arch of the atlas on each side, and a fifth and sixth cable are placed under the lamina of the axis, one on each side. The same type of thick corticocancellous iliac bone graft is obtained. Drill holes are placed in the bone graft at the cephalad and caudad end. The occipital cable is placed through the cephalad drill hole and secured to itself, the cable under C2 is placed through the caudad drill hole and secured to itself, and the cable under the posterior arch of C1 is passed over the graft and secured to itself on each side. If the patient's iliac crest bone is soft, then a cortical allograft plate of bone is utilized in the exact same fashion as described above to give structural

support. Combined with the soft autogenous bone graft which is placed underneath the cortical plate, this construct is quite stable. In the series of Starr and co-workers,[55] all 20 patients achieved a stable occipitocervical fusion and only one patient required revision surgery for a fractured graft.

When either of these techniques is utilized, the patient should be immobilized in a halo vest postoperatively until the fusion is solid. This will usually occur at approximately 3 months.

Occipitocervical Rod and Wire

A number of authors have recommended a modification of the posterior wiring technique where a 4- to 5-mm threaded Steinmann pin (or contoured rod) is wired to the occiput and the spinal laminae to be fused. In this technique two burr holes are drilled in the occiput 10 mm posterior to the foramen magnum. The dura is carefully dissected from the inner table of the occiput. Twenty-gauge double-stranded wires or braided cables are passed into the occipital burr holes and are brought out through the foramen magnum. Sublaminar or facet wires are passed inferiorly at the levels to be fused. The rod or pin is then contoured to the lordotic curve of the occipitocervical junction and fixed to the previously passed wires. If sublaminar wires are used they are positioned at the most lateral aspect of the laminae to provide the maximal surface for bony fusion. The occiput, facet joints, and posterior elements of the vertebrae to be fused are decorticated. A corticocancellous graft is then placed and the wound is closed in the standard fashion.[4, 20, 32, 45, 49, 54]

Occipitocervical Plating Technique

The operative approach is the same as that for the occipitocervical wiring technique. Once the exposure is complete the plate used is contoured to fit the occipitocervical junction with the head in neutral. The plate can either be a standard reconstruction plate, which is available with hole separations of 8 mm or 12 mm or a specially designed cervical plate. We prefer the reconstruction plates since they are always easily available and are relatively inexpensive.

This construct (Fig. 14–8) is designed around a transarticular C1–2 screw on each side because this is the strongest point of fixation in the cervical spine. This screw is inserted as the first screw on each side since it is the most difficult to place and has the most stringent requirements for the starting point location and screw orientation. This transarticular C1–2 screw placement was originally developed to provide stable fixation of the atlantoaxial joint from a posterior approach.[28] The pedicle of C2 is palpated with a blunt elevator to clearly define its borders. The C1–2 joint is identified with a Penfield elevator, and a small Steinmann pin is inserted into the atlas just above the C1–2 joint to safely retract the greater occipital nerve on each side. The starting point for screw placement of the C1–2 transarticular screw is 3 to 5 mm above the C2–3 facet joint, and it should be as medial as possible and still remain

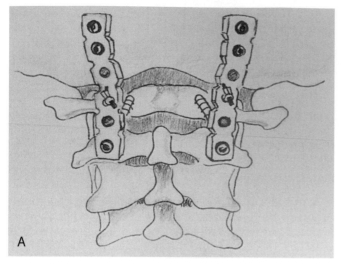

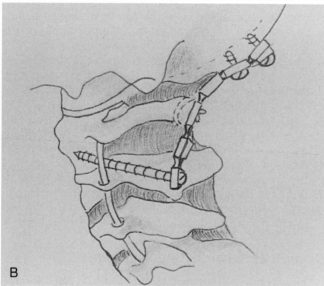

Figure 14–8 = *A* and *B,* These drawings represent AP and lateral views of the occipitocervical plating technique using C1–2 transarticular screws and titanium reconstruction plates with bicortical intracranial screws.

within the C2 pedicle. A lateral C-arm fluoroscopy image is used to help guide the placement of the screw and the surgeon aims exactly straight ahead (no medial or lateral angulation) and aims for the anterior arch of C1. The hole is drilled with a 2.5-mm bit and tapped in the appropriate fashion.[25–27] It should be noted that a CT scan obtained preoperatively will aid in defining the C1–2 anatomy and sagittal reconstruction through the C1 and C2 lateral masses and is most helpful in assessing the course of the screws. This is especially important because in about 10% to 15% of patients the location of the vertebral artery or the size of the C2 pedicle precludes the use of C1–2 transarticular screws.

If the fusion is to extend below C2, the lateral mass screws at the lower levels are placed at this time. The reader is referred to Chapter 22 for details concerning placement of lateral mass screws from C3 to C7.

The occipital screws are then placed in a bicortical fashion. Two screws can usually be placed into the occiput on each side. It is not uncommon for cerebrospinal fluid leakage to occur during placement of these screws, but simple insertion of the screw of the appropriate length appropriately seals the hole and prevents postoperative spinal fluid leakage. Using a drill guide with an accurate depth stop can often prevent this dural penetration from occurring. The placement of occipital screws in other locations has been optimized through the study of cadaver skulls.[16, 65] Although we do not use screws above the superior nuchal line, recent studies have shown that placing unicortical screws above the superior nuchal line may be performed safely.[65] Concern about intracranial venous sinus violation has prevented us from using this technique.

Although the plates and screws give a rigid fixation of the occiput to the cervical spine, the technique is not complete without adding a central fusion. This is done using the same techniques described above utilizing wires or cables to fix autologous corticocancellous bone grafts to the skull and to the cervical spine. The reader is referred to the above discussion for details.

Postoperatively, the patient is immobilized in a rigid cervical collar. If the fixation of the spine has been suboptimal, the patient is immobilized using a halo vest until the fusion is solid. The main difference between the simple wiring techniques and those techniques utilizing internal fixation is that a halo vest is always needed after simple wiring or cable techniques, and a rigid cervical collar will usually suffice after utlizing rigid internal fixation techniques (Fig. 14–9).

Results of Treatment of Occipitocervical Dislocation and Subluxation

The results depend on the severity of the initial injury and on the emergency and early hospital treatment. The senior author (F.J.E.) has treated five patients with this injury.[17, 38] The one patient who presented with an initial complete paralysis at the brain stem level died after 4 days. Of the two patients who presented with an incomplete quadriplegia, one recovered to normal function and one improved from 0–1/5 muscle strength and being respirator dependent acutely to 2–4/5 muscle strength and being ventilator-free after 8 years, but she is still wheelchair dependent. One patient presented with myelopathy, and he improved moderately. One patient was neurologically normal and remained normal at final follow-up.

OCCIPITAL CONDYLE FRACTURES

Occipital condyle fractures have been described and categorized by Anderson and Montesano.[3] Their type I fracture is an impacted occipital condyle fracture occurring as a result of axial loading of the skull on the atlas (Fig. 14–10). This may be associated with an incompetent alar ligament on the side of the fracture, but stability is provided by the contralateral alar ligament and the tectorial membrane.

Their type II fracture is an occipital condyle fracture associated with a basilar skull fracture. The mechanism

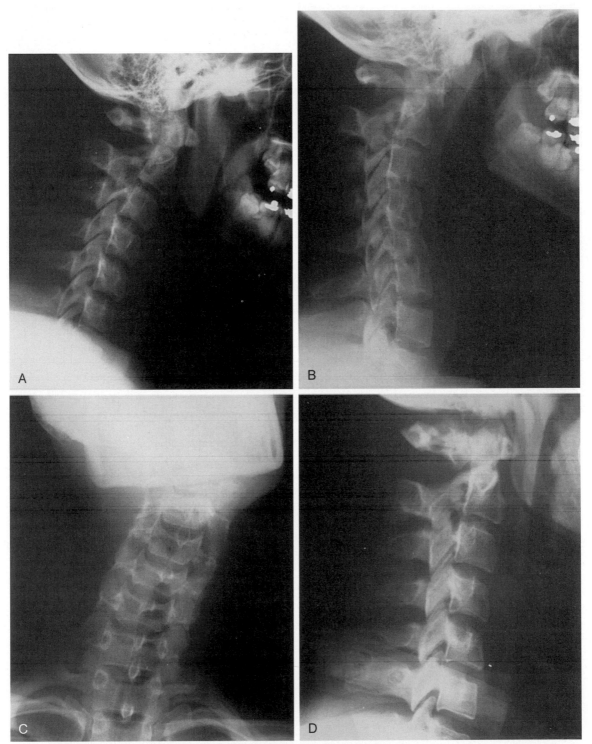

Figure 14–9 = This young man was involved in a motor vehicle accident with an unrecognized occipitocervical injury. *A,* The patient at the time of his original presentation to the emergency room had a tremendous amount of soft tissue swelling at the C3 level. No injury was diagnosed at this time and the patient was sent out of the emergency room in a collar. *B,* Lateral radiograph when the patient returned to the emergency room 10 days later. The soft tissue swelling is markedly reduced but his occiput is anteriorly displaced on his cervical spine. *C,* His severe torticollis can be appreciated on this AP film. *D,* In 5 lb of traction it can be seen that the patient's head is separating from his cervical spine.

Illustration continued on following page

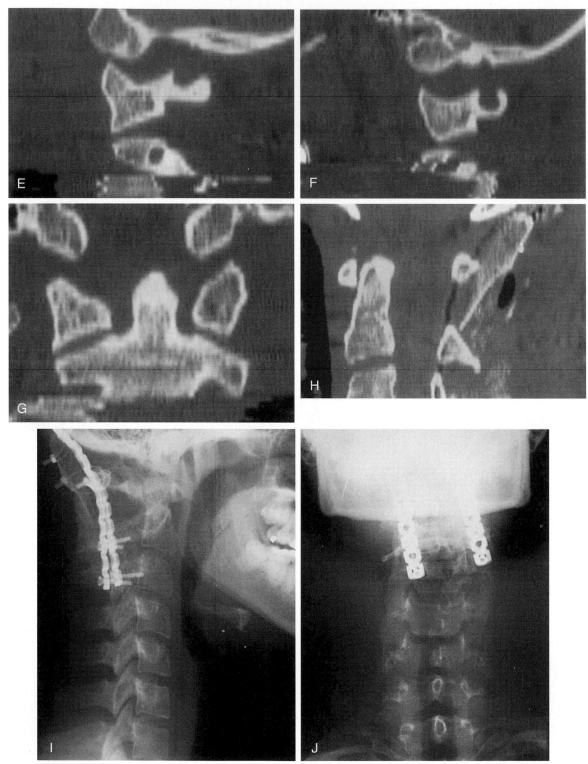

Figure 14–9 *Continued* = *E* and *F,* The CT scan reconstruction shows that the occipital condyles are distracted from the C1 lateral masses. On each side it can also be seen that the course of the vertebral artery precludes usual positioning for placement of C1–2 transarticular screws. *G,* This coronal CT reconstruction again shows the C1–2 distraction. *H,* Postoperatively, the large central bone graft can be seen extending from the base of the skull posteriorly down to the C2 spinous process and lamina. This type of structural graft is essential with or without the use of plates and screws. *I* and *J,* AP and lateral radiographs taken approximately 2 years after stabilization of the cervical spine reveal maintainence of good alignment and a solid posterior fusion from occiput to C3.

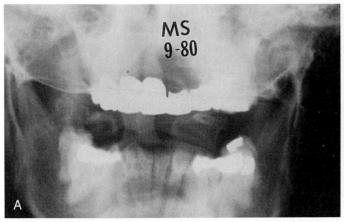
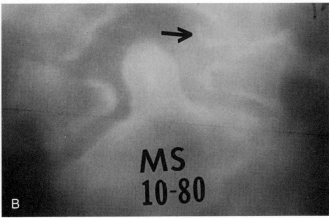

Figure 14–10 = This patient had fallen on his head, which applied an axial load to his occipitocervical junction. The patient complained of a persistent pain in his upper neck that was worse with moving his head and he also complained of persistent headaches. *A,* This attempt at an open-mouth view of the upper cervical spine reveals an asymmetry between the plane of the skull and the plane of the C2 vertebra. The head appears to be tipped toward one side. *B,* This AP tomogram of the occipitocervical junction reveals that the patient has sustained a type I impaction fracture of the occipital condyle and that the attachment of the alar ligament on that same side (*arrow*) has been fractured from the medial aspect of the occipital condyle. As a result one would expect some mild laxity of the alar ligament on that side, but, because of the mechanism of injury, it is reasonable to assume that the opposite alar ligament and the tectorial membrane are still intact. This patient was treated with a rigid collar for 8 weeks with gradual resolution of his pain.

is a direct blow to the skull. Stability is provided by the alar ligaments, which remain intact, and a normal tectorial membrane.

Their type III fracture is an avulsion fracture of the occipital condyle by the alar ligament. This may occur as a result of rotation or lateral bending or both. Once this injury has occurred, the tectorial membrane and the contralateral alar ligaments are loaded and if these also are weakened, significant occipitocervical instability may occur. This type of injury was discussed earlier in the section on occipitoatlantal dislocations (see Fig. 14–3).

The treatment for the type I and type II occipital condyle fracture is immobilization in a rigid collar for 6 to 8 weeks. The treatment for a type III fracture of the occipital condyle can range from immobilization in a rigid collar for 8 to 12 weeks, to halo immobilization, to posterior occipitocervical fusion if enough of the remaining bony and ligamentous restraints have been injured.

SUMMARY

The most important aspect of medical care for a patient with occipitocervical instability is the emergency and early hospital treatment. Recognition and prompt immobilization are essential to successful treatment. Most patients with occipitocervical subluxation or dislocation who survive will require a posterior occipitocervical fusion. Of those patients with type I or type II occipital condyle fractures, rigid collar immobilization usually will achieve a satisfactory result.

REFERENCES

1. Alker GH, Oh YS, Leslie FV, et al: Postmortem radiology of head and neck injuries in fatal traffic accidents. Radiology 114:611–617, 1975.
2. Anderson LD, D'Alonzo RT: Fractures of the odontoid process of the axis. J Bone Joint Surg Am 56:1663–1674, 1974.
3. Anderson PA, Montesano PX: Morphology and treatment of occipital condyle fractures. Spine 13:731–736, 1988.
4. Apostolides PJ, Dickman CA, Golfinos JG, et al: Threaded Steinmann pin fusion of the craniovertebral junction. Spine 21:1630–1637, 1996.
5. Apple JS, Kirks DR, Merten DF, et al: Cervical spine fractures and dislocations in children. Pediatr Radiol 17:45–49, 1987.
6. Banna M, Stevenson GW, Tumiel A: Unilateral atlantooccipital dislocation complicating an anomaly of the atlas. J Bone Joint Surg Am 65:5:685–687, 1983.
7. Bell HS: Paralysis of both arms from injury of the upper portion of the pyramidal decussations: "Cruciate paralysis." J Neurosurg 33:376–380, 1970.
8. Bivins HG, Ford S, Bezmalinovic Z, et al: The effect of axial traction during orotracheal intubation of the trauma victim with an unstable cervical spine. Ann Emerg Med 17:25–29, 1988.
9. Bohlman HH: Acute fractures and dislocations of the cervical spine: An analysis of 300 hospitalized patients and review of the literature. J Bone Joint Surg Am 61:1119–1142, 1979.
10. Bools JC, Rose BS: Traumatic atlantooccipital dislocation: Two cases with survival. Am J Neuroradiol 7:901–904, 1986.
11. Bucholz RW, Burkhead WZ: The pathological anatomy of fatal atlantooccipital dislocations. J Bone Joint Surg Am 61:248–250, 1979.
12. Cattell HS, Filtzer DL: Pseudosubluxation and other normal variations in the cervical spine in children: A study of 160 children. J Bone Joint Surg Am 47:1295–1309, 1964.
13. Clark CR, Igram CM, El-Khoury GY, et al: Radiographic evaluation of cervical spine injuries. Spine 13:742–747, 1988.
14. Davis D, Bohlman H, Walker AE, et al: The pathological findings in fatal craniospinal injuries. J Neurosurg 34:603–613, 1971.
15. Dublin AB, Marks WM, Weinstock D, et al: Traumatic dislocation of the atlanto-occipital articulartion (AOA) with short-term survival. J Neurosurg 52:541–546, 1980.
16. Ebraheim NA, Lu J, Bijani A, et al: An anatomic study of the thickness of the occipital bone: Implications for occipitocervical instrumentation. Spine 21:1725–1730, 1996.
17. Eismont FJ, Bohlman HH: Posterior atlanto-occipital dislocation with fractures of the atlas and odontoid process. J Bone Joint Surg Am 60:397–399, 1978.
18. Englander O: Non-traumatic occipito-atlanto-axial dislocation. Br J Radiol 15:341–345, 1942.
19. Evarts CM: Traumatic occipito-atlantal dislocation. J Bone Joint Surg Am 52:1653–1660, 1970.
20. Fehlings MG, Errico T, Cooper P, et al: Occipitocervical fusion

with a five-millimeter malleable rod and segmental fixation. Neurosurgery 32:198–208, 1993.

21. Fruin AH, Pirotte TP: Traumatic atlantooccipital dislocation. J Neurosurg 46:663–666, 1977.
22. Gabrielson TO, Maxwell JA: Traumatic atlanto-occipital dislocation—With case report of a patient who survived. AJR 97:624–629, 1966.
23. Georgopoulos G, Azzutillo PD, Lee MS: Occipito-atlantal instability in children. J Bone Joint Surg Am 69:429–436, 1987.
24. Gerlock AJ, Mirfakhraee M, Benzel EC: Computed tomography of traumatic atlanto-occipital dislocation. Neurosurgery 13:316–319, 1983.
25. Grob D, Dvorak J, Panjabi MM, et al: Posterior occipitocervical Fusion: A preliminary report of a new technique. Spine 16:17–24, 1991.
26. Grob D, Dvorak J, Panjabi MM, et al: The role of plate and screw fixation in occipitocervical fusion in rheumatoid arthritis. Spine 19:2545–2551, 1994.
27. Grob D, Jeanneret B, Aebi M, et al: Atlanto-axial fusion with transarticular screw fixation. J Bone Joint Surg Br 73:972–976, 1991.
28. Grob D, Magerl F: Unisegmental three dimensional stabilization of C1–C2: Report on a new surgical technique. Presented to the Annual Meeting of the Cervical Spine Research Society, Washington, DC, December 1987.
29. Grobovschek M, Scheibelbrander W: Atlanto-occipital dislocation. Neuroradiology 25:173–174, 1983.
30. Herzenberg JE, Hensinger RN, Dedrick DK, et al: Emergency transport and positioning of young children who have an injury of the cervical spine: The standard backboard may be hazardous. J Bone Joint Surg Am 71:15–22, 1989.
31. Hunter T: The spinal complications of ankylosing spondylitis. Semin Arthritis Rheum 19:172–182, 1989.
32. Itoh T, Tsuji H, Katoh Y, et al: Occipito-cervical fusion reinforced by Luque's segmental spinal instrumentation for rheumatoid diseases. Spine 13:1234–1238, 1988.
33. Kaufman RA, Carroll CD, Buncher CR: Atlantooccipital junction: Standards for measurement in normal children. Am J Neuroradiol 8:995–999, 1987.
34. Lee C, Woodring JH, Goldstein SJ, et al: Evaluation of traumatic atlantooccipital dislocations. Am J Neuroradiol 8:19–26, 1987.
35. Lesoin F, Blondel M, Dhellemmes P, et al: Post-traumatic atlantooccipital dislocation revealed by sudden cardiorespiratory arrest. Lancet 2:447–448, 1982.
36. Levine AM, Edwards CC: Traumatic lesions of the occipitoatlantoaxial complex. Clin Orthop 239:53–68, 1989.
37. Martel W: The occipito-atlanto-axial joints in rheumatoid arthritis and ankylosing spondylitis. AJR 86:223–240, 1961.
38. Montane I, Eismont FJ, Green BA: Traumatic occipitoatlantal dislocation. Spine 16:112–116, 1991.
39. Nielsen JM: A Textbook of Clinical Neurology, ed 3. New York, Hoeber, 1951, p 167.
40. Page CP, Story JL, Wissinger JP, et al: Traumatic atlantooccipital dislocation. J Neurosurg 39:394–397, 1973.
41. Pang D, Wilberger JE: Traumatic atlanto-occipital dislocation with survival: Case report and review. Neurosurgery 7:503–508, 1980.
42. Panjabi M, Dvorak J, Duranceau J, et al: Three dimensional movements of the upper cervical spine. Spine 13:726–730, 1988.
43. Powers B, Miller MD, Kramer RS, et al: Traumatic anterior atlanto-occipital dislocation. Neurosurgery 41:12–17, 1979.
44. Putnam WE, Stratton FT, Rohr RJ, et al: Traumatic atlanto-occipital dislocation: Value of the Powers ratio in diagnosis. J Am Orthop Assoc 86:798–804, 1986.
45. Ransford AO, Crockard HA, Pozo JL, et al: Craniocervical instability treated by contoured loop fixation. J Bone Joint Surg Br 68:173–177, 1986.
46. Redlund-Johnell I: Atlanto-occipital dislocation in rheumatoid arthritis. Acta Radiol Diagn 25:165–168, 1984.
47. Robinson RA, Southwick WO: Surgical approaches to the cervical spine. Instruct Course Lect 17:299–330, 1960.
48. Rockswold GL, Seljeskog EL: Traumatic atlantocranial dislocation with survival. Minn Med 62:151–152, 154, 1979.
49. Sakou T, Kawaida H, Morizino Y, et al: Occipitoatlantoaxial fusion utilizing a rectangular rod. Clin Orthop 239:136–144, 1989.
50. Scott EW, Haid RW, Peace D: Type I fractures of the odontoid process: Implications for atlanto-cranial instability. J Neurosurg 72:488–492, 1990.
51. Shapiro R, Youngberg AS, Rothman SLG: The differential diagnosis of traumatic lesions of the occipito-atlanto-axial segment. Radiol Clin North Am 11:505–525, 1973.
52. Shkrum MJ, Green RN, Nowak ES: Upper cervical trauma in motor vehicle collisions. J Forensic Sci 34:381–390, 1989.
53. Smith MD, Anderson PA: Occipital cervical fusion. Techniques Orthop 9:37–42, 1994.
54. Sonntag VK, Dickman CA: Craniocervical stabilization. Clin Neurosurg 40:243–272, 1993.
55. Starr J, Eismont FJ, Scuderi G: Posterior occipitocervical fusion for non-rheumatoid instability. Presented to the Annual Meeting of the Cervical Spine Research Society, Desert Springs, Calif, December 1992.
56. Tepper SL, Fligner CL, Reay DT: Atlanto-occipital disarticulation. Am J Forensic Med Pathol 11:193–197, 1990.
57. Traynelis VC, Marano GD, Dunker RO, et al: Traumatic atlanto-occipital dislocation. J Neurosurg 65:863–870, 1986.
58. Van Den Bout AH, Dommisse GF: Traumatic atlantooccipital dislocation. Spine 11:174–176, 1986.
59. Watridge CB, Orrison WW, Arnold H, et al: Lateral atlantooccipital dislocation: Case report. Neurosurgery 17:345–347, 1985.
60. Werne S: Studies in spontaneous atlas dislocation. Acta Orthop Scand Suppl 23:1–150, 1957.
61. Wertheim SB, Bohlman HH: Occipito-cervical fusion. Indications, techniques, and results in 13 patients. J Bone Joint Surg Am 69:833–836, 1987.
62. Wholey WH, Brauer AJ, Baker HL Jr: The lateral roentgenogram of the neck (with comments on the atlanto-odontoid-basion relationship). Radiology 71:350–356, 1958.
63. Wiesel SW, Rothman RH: Occipitoatlantal hypermobility. Spine 4:187, 1979.
64. Woodring JH, Selke AC, Duff DE: Traumatic atlanto-occipital dislocation with survival. AJR 137:21–24, 1981.
65. Zipnick RI, Merola AA, Gorup J, et al: Occipital morphology, an anatomic guide to internal fixation. Spine 21:1719–1724, 1996.

Fractures of the Atlas

Alan M. Levine

Fractures of the atlas form a particularly rare group of injuries that were not even described as an entity until 1822, when Sir Ashley Cooper, in a treatise on dislocations and fractures of the joints, described the first case.[8] Between 1822 and 1920, a period of almost 100 years, only 46 cases were subsequently reported. This prompted Geoffrey Jefferson to publish his noted report "Fracture of the Atlas Vertebra," in which he reviewed his experience of four cases as well as the 46 cases that had been previously reported in the literature. He very astutely analyzed the fracture and contributed a great deal to our knowledge of this interesting injury:

> Fractures of the atlas vertebra form one of those categories of rare accidents possessed of a considerable interest. . . . My first impression was that fracture of the atlas would be almost invariably followed by death. Greater knowledge of the subject, however, modified this opinion. No doubt, if the atlas were morphologically similar to other vertebrae death would be the common result of fracture. But the atlas presents so many peculiarities of shape, function, and relationship, that the accidents which may happen to it present many differences from those to which the other vertebrae are heir. The most interesting aspects of the question are the genesis of the atlas fracture, the mechanism by which it comes about and the displacement which follows.[25]

At that time, he correctly described the particular sites of fracture of the posterior as well as the anterior arch and, similarly, the appropriate mechanisms of injury. He recognized that the fracture of the posterior arch alone was the result of a hyperextension injury, whereas that of the four-part fracture resulted in spreading of the lateral masses by an axial loading fracture. He also provided full demonstrations of the schematics of the injury. In addition he felt that neurologic injury occurred less than 50% of the time and was less common in these injuries than in other types of cervical spine injury. Treatment was often complicated in this original series by "supplementary injury," which were frequently fractures of the dens. In the uncomplicated case, Jefferson recommended nonoperative treatment with the use of a Minerva plaster or a Lorenz bed.[25, 26] Subsequent improvements in radiologic imaging have made our awareness of this fracture considerably greater. Approximately 10% of all cervical spine fractures involve the atlas. The understanding of the various types of fractures and their instability has expanded with greater imaging techniques. However the most serious implications and problems with treatment have not remained with the fracture itself, but rather with injuries associated with the atlas fracture.

PATHOANATOMY

To fully appreciate the pathologic anatomy of fractures involving the atlas we must understand its critical position and the anatomic differences from other cervical vertebrae. The atlas forms a critical portion of what has been termed the *cervicocranium*, which refers to the mechanistic group involving the base of the skull, the atlas, and the axis. The atlas is a unique vertebra among the other cervical vertebrae in that it has no centrum, because its vertebral body is actually absorbed into the structure of the axis (dens). Instead, it has two large lateral masses that form the articulation with the occipital condyles and with the facet joints of C2. Both of these articulations lie on the anterolateral portions of the spinal canal. This is in a totally different position with reference to the weight-bearing axis and load transmission axis than the facet joints from C3 distally, which lie posterolateral to the spinal canal. The axis has, instead of a vertebral body, a very thick anterior arch that connects these two lateral masses (Fig. 15–1). Both articular surfaces are concave; those for the occipital condyles face upward and outward to support the condyles. The facet joints of the atlantoaxial joints are somewhat flatter than the atlanto-occipital joints and face downward and inward, thus transferring the force of the weight of the skull onto the superior articular facets of the axis. The vertebral arteries course up from C2 and cross the posterior arch just posterior to the edge of the facets. This groove for the vertebral artery lies just behind the lateral mass and thins the posterior arch at that location. Occasionally, accessory foramina are present, through which the vertebral artery may course.

An understanding of the embryology is critically important to appreciate the malformations that will occur in the atlas. Because the atlas does not have a vertebral body, its developmental anatomy is intrinsically tied to that of the axis. The caudal portion of the fourth occipital somite fuses to the cranial portion of C1 to form the end of the occiput. Instead of an intervertebral disc at this level, apical and alar ligaments are present that are associated with the dens and even perhaps with the terminal portion of the dens. The atlas in the early phases of development consists of

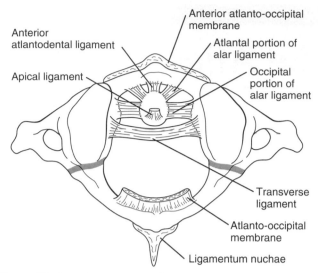

Figure 15–1 = This drawing of the atlas demonstrates many of the features that distinguish it from other cervical levels. Its articulations with the atlas and the occiput lie in the anterior third of the ring. A relatively thin area of the ring lies just posterior to the joint surface (*crosshatching*) as the vertebral artery passes across the superior surface of the ring at that point. The occipital membrane is in fact a thinned-out portion of the ligamentum flavum. All of the primary ligamentous structures, however, are also attached to the anterior third of the ring leaving the posterior portion of the ring isolated structurally from the more significant anterior portion. Even the anterior portion of the ring (residual body) is relatively thinner than the more anterolateral portions containing the joints and the ligamentous attachments. (Redrawn form Dvorak J, Panjabi MM: Functional anatomy of the alar ligaments. Spine 12:183, 1987.)

only the apical ossific nucleus, which subsequently forms the dens processes. Because no distinct centrum is present at C1, the caudal part of the C1 somite and the cranial portion of the C2 somite actually form the dens process, which is then incorporated into the vertebral body of C2. In C1 vertebra specifically, the anterior arch is formed from a dense band of tissue called the *hypochordal bow*, which extends around the anterior part of the vertebra. In the later phases of development, the hypochordal bow gives rise to the anterior longitudinal ligament. The cervical spine generally contains three ossific nuclei from which each vertebra forms, one in the body and one in each side of the neural arch. In the upper cervical spine they begin to ossify in approximately the second month of intrauterine life. Because the centrum of the atlas in fact forms the ossific nucleus of the dens there are only two centers, one in each lateral mass, from which the atlas forms. This accounts for the defects that generally will occur either in the central portion of the anterior arch or the central portion of the posterior arch of C1. This is different from lower cervical vertebrae, which have synchondrosis where each vertebral arch joins the ossific nuclei of the vertebral body, called the *neurocentral joint*. At the time of birth, both lateral masses and a portion of the arch, both anteriorly and posteriorly, have generally ossified. The ossification then continues along the posterior arches, usually with closure of the ring atlas by the third year of life. Ossific nuclei generally also form in the anterior portion of the ring, which

fuses with the lateral masses by approximately age 7 or 8 years. Three principal variations on this development pattern have been described[15, 16, 28] that commonly result in the majority of the anomalies. These include the following:

1. The body or the anterior arch of C1 is formed by two centers that fuse with each other and then with the lateral masses and posterior arches.[49]
2. The ossification center for the vertebral body may not appear, and the lateral masses continue forward and fuse with themselves.
3. The center for the vertebral body may not appear, and the lateral masses then fail to fuse, resulting in an anterior spondyloschisis[2, 38] (Fig. 15–2).

Failure of development and fusion posteriorly occurs much more frequently than do anterior defects (1.5% vs. 0.33%),[9, 42] although it has been thought that these failures of fusion are of little clinical significance.[39] With greater recognition of the fracture, however, they play a more significant role, especially in combined injuries. In pediatric fractures, these defects may indeed be the area of subsequent separation of the arch.[15] In the adult, these defects may be of extreme clinical significance, particularly when a C1–2 arthrodesis is indicated in the presence of a C2 fracture, but a significant nontraumatic defect is found in the posterior arch, precluding appropriate treatment. Thus, the anomalous development of C1 is clinically important both for recognition of failure patterns of the arch of C1 and for potential pitfalls in the treatment of injuries in the atlantoaxial complex.

Because no disc is present between the occiput and C1, the relationship of these two components is maintained in the normal circumstance by the substantial ligamentous mass connecting the two areas (Fig. 15–3). Similarly, the C1–2 joint relies on its ligamentous structure for integrity, also without an intervertebral disc. Beginning anteriorly, the anterior longitudinal ligament is a continuation of the ligament bridging the entire length of the spine, but it becomes somewhat thinner in the upper cervical spine. It attaches to the anterior portion of the body of C2 as well as to the anterior portion of the ring of C1 and then courses to the tubercle of the base of the skull. In part, the stability of the occipital-C1 joint is dependent on ligamentous

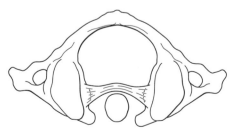

Figure 15–2 = Congenital absence of portions of the ring of C1 are relatively common anomalies that are more frequently appreciated on CT scan. The most common is failure of fusion of the posterior arch. However, an entire segment of the ring may be absent either posteriorly or anteriorly, as seen here; this is known as spondyloschisis.

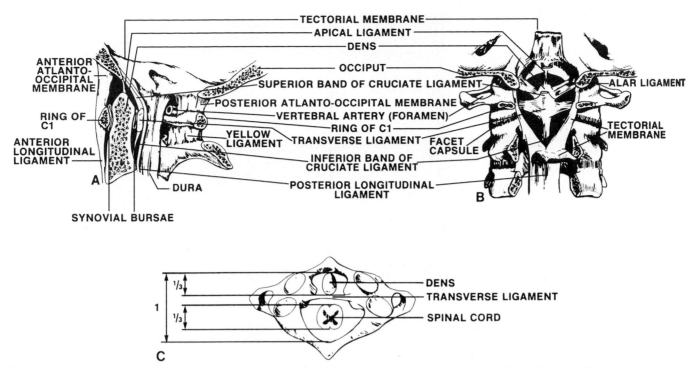

Figure 15–3 = Lateral (*A*) and coronal (*B*) views of the upper cervical spine demonstrate the vertical attachments of the occiput and atlas to C1. These include the anterior and posterior atlanto-occipital membrane as well as the posterior longitudinal ligaments, anterior longitudinal ligament, and the ligamentum flavum. Some of the ligamentous attachments run from the dens (C2) to the occiput, stabilizing but bypassing C1 (cruciate, alar, and apical ligaments). The axial view (*C*) shows Steele's rule of thirds of structures within the ring of C1. (From White AA, Panjabi MM: Clinical Biomechanics of the Spine. Philadelphia, JB Lippincott, 1988.)

attachments to the dens, which bypass the ring of C1. However, the atlanto-occipital ligament runs between the cephalad portion of the anterior ring of C1 and to the tubercle of C2, as previously mentioned, and may in fact be a continuation of the anterior longitudinal ligament. The posterior atlanto-occipital ligament or membrane connects the posterior ring of C1 to the posterior portion of the foramen magnum. This is generally a very thin ligament that does not offer a great deal of mechanical advantage. The alar and apical ligaments attached to the dens course in several directions. These clearly contribute to the stability of both the atlantoaxial and the atlanto-occipital joints, yet they bypass the atlas. They attach at the tip of the dens and course obliquely to the medial surfaces of the occipital condyles. The apical ligaments connect the tip of the dens to the anterior edge of the foramen magnum. Dvorak and co-workers demonstrated that in fact the alar ligaments contribute to limited axial rotation to the opposite side.[10] Transection of one alar ligament results in a 30% increase in axial rotation in the other direction. The transverse ligament is the most important structure in occiput C1–2 complex and extends from one condyle of the atlas to the opposite condyle of the atlas. This has both an ascending and descending branch; the ascending branch comes to the anterior edge of the foramen magnum and the descending branch to the body of C2. This one ligament is chiefly responsible for preventing anterior dislocation of C1 on C2. The ligamentum flavum is markedly attenuated in the upper cervical spine, but there are structures that are analogous to it. The posterior atlanto-occipital

membrane attaches the posterior portion of the ring of C1 and the posterior portion of the foramen magnum. The posterior atlantoaxial membrane attaches to the posterior portion of the ring of C1 and then down to the posterior ring of C2. The ligamentum flavum actually begins distal to that point, between C2 and C3.

Equally important for stability in the upper cervical spine are the various muscular attachments. Muscular attachments are also important as critical factors in the genesis of certain of the fractures seen at C1. The longus colli (the superior oblique portion) attaches to the anterior and inferior portion of the arch of C1. In addition, the rectus capitis lateralis traverses from the anterior portion of the transverse process of C1 to the lateral portion of the occiput. The rectus capitis medialis runs from the transverse process in a medial direction toward the anterior portion of the foramen magnum. Posteriorly, the cervical portion of the trapezius forms attachments to the posterior arch of the atlas. At a deeper level, the rectus capitis posterior minor traverses from the posterior portion of the ring of C1 to the occiput. Similarly, the superior oblique muscle traverses from the lateral aspect of the ring of the atlas to the posterior portion of the skull, and the inferior oblique muscle courses from C2 obliquely to the lateral aspect of the C1 ring.

CLASSIFICATION

The classification of injuries of C1 has evolved slowly. Instead of the evolution of a unified classifica-

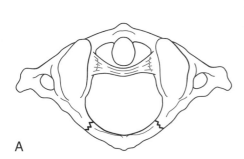

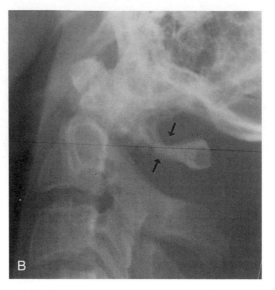

A

B

Figure 15–4 = Posterior arch fracture. Both the drawing (A) and the lateral radiograph (B, arrows) show the position of the posterior arch fracture. Often, on the lateral view, the fracture is difficult to visualize as it may be so close to the posterior edge of the facet as to be obscured by the overlying structures. In that case, the only evidence of fracture may be an angular deformity of the orientation of the posterior arch.

tion, multiple types of injuries involving C1 have been recognized progressively. The greatest advance in the ability to recognize injuries of the atlas occurred with the use of computed tomographic (CT) scanning. This allowed reasonably accurate delineation of the pathology of the ring, which had previously only been partially visualized with open-mouth and lateral roentgenograms and somewhat better visualized with the use of anteroposterior (AP) and lateral polycycloidal tomography. Initially, Jefferson identified two basic types of fractures: (1) isolated fractures of the posterior arch of the atlas and (2) fractures of both arches of the atlas. In addition to clinical experience with fractures in his own patients, he reviewed a case from the Manchester University Pathologic Museum and identified a two-part fracture, consisting of a fracture just anterior to the lateral mass on one side and another fracture posterior to the lateral mass on the same side. Jefferson's name, however, has become synonymous with the four-part fracture, consisting of two fractures in the anterior portion of the ring and two in the posterior portion of the ring. The question of the number of fractures of the ring of the atlas was raised

by Hays and Alker[20] in 1988. From both clinical and anatomic studies they identified two- and three-part fractures of the ring of the atlas. Segal and co-workers[50] identified six different fracture patterns, although some of them in fact overlap in terms of both anatomic and clinical criteria.

The classification for fractures of the atlas is derived from consideration of both the mechanism of injury and the clinical characteristics and treatment ramifications of these fractures. In fact, five different types of fractures have been demonstrated clinically. The most common injury is the posterior arch fracture (Fig. 15–4). This fracture generally occurs through the weakest portion of the posterior arch at the area of the junction of the posterior arch and the lateral masses, where the vertebral artery courses over the top of the posterior arch and the bone is at its thinnest. This injury has been well described by a number of authors.[33, 51, 53] The second type of injury is a fracture involving the lateral mass (Fig. 15–5). These have been called variously two-part or three-part fractures of the ring of C1. In fact, they involve a fracture just anterior to the lateral mass on one side and a fracture just posterior to the lateral mass

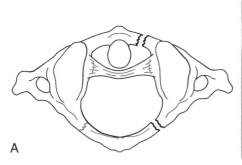

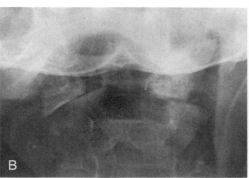

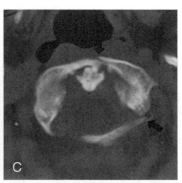

A

B

C

Figure 15–5 = Lateral mass fracture. This injury consists of one fracture just anterior to the joint surface and one just posterior to the surface (A), which in some cases may extend into the joint. A third fracture may also be present in the contralateral posterior arch. B, The typical finding on the open-mouth view is displacement of only one lateral mass of the C1 (with reference to C2) joint surface, whereas the other side has a normal anatomic relationship. In the extreme situation, one lateral mass may actually be displaced from its position between the occipital condyle and the lateral mass of C2. C, The CT scan is the optimal tool for defining the nature of the fracture (arrow).

(usually in the same position[3] as the posterior arch fracture) on the same side contralateral. Three-part fractures include a second fracture of the posterior arch as well.[20, 33, 35, 50] These fractures represent the same injury, as they result in the same degree of instability. Thus the treatment is the same whether the injury has two parts (fractures anterior and posterior to the lateral mass on one side) or three parts (with an additional contralateral posterior arch fracture). The third type of injury is the classic bursting injury of the ring of C1, which has been called the Jefferson fracture.[17, 18, 21, 23, 25, 26, 40, 43, 46, 60] This involves a four-part fracture to the ring, generally consisting of two fractures in the anterior arch and two fractures in the posterior arch, but it may occasionally consist of only one central fracture in the anterior arch (Fig. 15–6). The significant difference between this fracture and the lateral mass fracture is that the displacement of the lateral masses is relatively symmetrical, whereas in the lateral mass fracture it is quite asymmetrical only on the injured side. The fourth type of fracture is the horizontal fracture of the anterior arch of C1 (Fig. 15–7). This injury involves a transverse split in a horizontal direction through the anterior tubercle of C1, and is an avulsion fracture.[27, 47, 55] The final type of injury is the transverse process fracture of the atlas, which can be either unilateral or bilateral[7] (Fig. 15–8).

MECHANISMS OF INJURY

Fractures of the atlas have specific mechanisms of injury. Knowledge of these mechanisms is critically important for understanding both the resultant instability and the associated injuries. Fractures of the posterior arch of C1 have been thought to be the result of a hyperextension mechanism. This has been described as a hyperextension injury resulting in pinching of the posterior arch of C1 between the occiput and the ring of C2. In fact, however, White and Panjabi[57, 58] posited that the hyperextension mechanism caused fixation of the anterior portion of the ring of C1. This is the result of compression of the anterior arch against the dens, with similar compression of the C1–2 articulations. With this fixation, the occiput impinges against the posterior ring of C1, causing a bending moment. The cross-sectional moment of inertia is less resistant to bending at the area where the vertebral artery crosses the arch than it is further posterior in the arch. In addition, the forces are applied at the tip of the ring of C1, thus increasing the lever arm and also making the bending moment maximal at that location (Fig. 15–9). This mechanism of injury of hyperextension correlates well with the associated injuries seen frequently with posterior arch fractures. There is a very high association with other injuries known to result from hyperextension, such as C2 anterior teardrop fractures and type I traumatic spondylolisthesis of the axis.

The lateral mass fracture is an asymmetrical injury resulting from trauma to one side of the ring, which suggests a lateral bending and rotation mechanism. In the two-part fracture, the fracture line occurs just ante-rior and just posterior to the lateral mass, yielding displacement of the lateral mass without displacement of the entire ring of C1. This occurs as the result of a combined axial loading and lateral bending injury. Because the central portion of the anterior arch of C1 is thicker than the more lateral portions, the points of fracture are within the same location in the posterior arch and within the thinner areas of the anterior arch. Occasionally this will be accompanied by a second fracture on the contralateral side of the ring in the posterior arch, which would suggest that slight extension of the occiput must be present to result in bilateral posterior fractures in addition to the single asymmetrical anterior lateral mass fracture. The predominant mechanism, however, is that of axial loading with lateral bending. Indirect evidence of the mechanism is the asymmetrical instability with displacement of only one lateral mass, with the remainder of the ring left in normal configuration with reference to the C2 axis. This suggests isolated occiput and C1–2 capsular disruption resulting from "extravasation" of the affected lateral mass of C1. The concomitant fractures associated with this particular fracture similarly result from a lateral bending–axial loading mechanism and include pillar fractures and facet fractures of the lower cervical spine (Fig. 15–10).

The presumed mechanism of the Jefferson fracture was first described by Jefferson in 1920. The fracture is the result of axial compression, generally with a direct blow on the head either from diving or from an object falling on the head. The orientation of the condyles of the occiput are such that when driven distally by axial loading, they act in a wedge-like fashion, causing a splaying of the lateral masses with disruption of the ring (generally into four parts). It has been shown that the magnitude of disruption of the ligamentous structure is in fact related to the degree of splaying of the lateral masses. Spence and associates[54] have demonstrated in anatomic specimens that splaying of the lateral masses greater than 6.9 mm of combined right and left displacement is accompanied by transection of the transverse ligament. This mechanism of splaying of the lateral masses by axial compression is critically important for understanding the resultant instability of this injury. The rupture of the transverse ligament in this injury is not the same as the isolated transverse ligament rupture. In this particular injury, the alar and apical ligaments from the dens to the base of the skull are spared, as the injury to the transverse ligament occurs in axial compression, thus shortening the apical ligaments. In addition, because the injury results from axial compression, the degree of disruption of the capsules of the C1–2 joint is different than the pattern seen with a severe flexion transverse ligament rupture. In the transverse ligament rupture by a severe flexion force, not only is the transverse ligament ruptured, but so are the alar and apical ligaments and the anterior and posterior portions of the capsules of the C1–2 articulation. These ligaments are not disrupted in a pure axial loading injury; with splaying of the lateral masses, the anterior and posterior fibers of the capsules of the C1–2 articulation are spared. Although the trans-

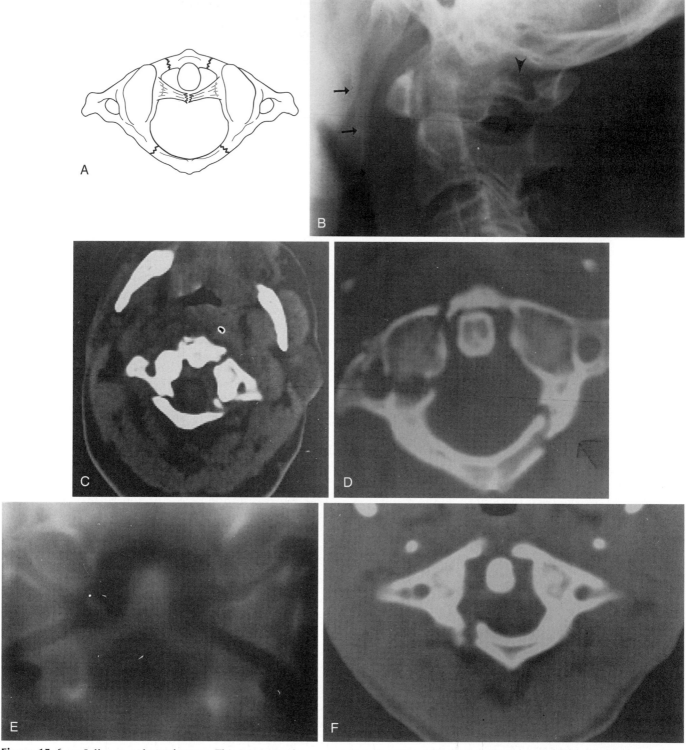

Figure 15–6 = Jefferson or burst fracture. This injury can have a number of various patterns, but the classic injury is described as a four-part fracture with two fractures in the anterior ring and two in the posterior portion (*A*). The lateral radiograph in this patient with a four-part fracture (*B*) simply shows a posterior arch fracture (*arrowhead*), but there is a greatly increased anterior soft tissue shadow (*arrows*) at the C1–2 level. The CT scan (*C*) shows the four-part fracture pattern with symmetrical displacement. Although some lateral mass fractures have a three-part pattern (two in the posterior arch and one in the anterior arch), this CT scan shows a three-part injury (*D*), and the open-mouth view (*E*) shows symmetrical spreading of the lateral masses. The difference between the two injuries is the variation in the ligamentous disruption that is associated with the injury. The three-part Jefferson fracture has symmetrical ligamentous disruption, whereas the lateral mass fracture has asymmetrical disruption; for the same total amount of spreading of the lateral masses, the true lateral mass fracture may be more unstable. *F,* Two-part injuries are seen with one fracture in the anterior arch and one in the posterior arch, usually more in the midline of each arch than is seen in the four- and three-part fractures.

Figure 15–7 = The drawing *A* shows the minimal involvement of the structure of C1. The anterior avulsion fracture from the tubercle of C1 is a stable injury and looks worse on the lateral radiograph (*B, arrow*) than it manifests clinically.

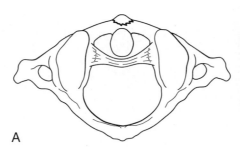

A

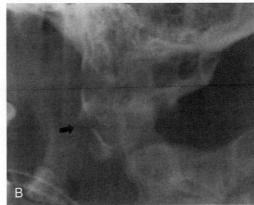

B

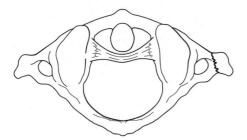

Figure 15–8 = Transverse process fracture. This fracture may be seen as either a unilateral or bilateral injury and is almost always discovered as an incidental finding on the CT scan while investigating another injury in the upper cervical spine.

Figure 15–9 = This drawing demonstrates the structural and biomechanical factors that contribute to the occurrence of C1 arch fractures. *A*, The midsagittal view shows how a force applied through the skull to cause hyperextension causes impingement of the base of the occiput on the posterior portion of the arch of C1, whereas the anterior portion of the ring is fixed by the dens and the large anterolateral joint surfaces. A bending moment is thus created at the point at which the vertebral artery crosses the arch. *B*, Structurally, that point has a lower moment of inertia to resist bending in the sagittal plane than the more posterior portions of the ring. The relative cross sections are shown in the drawing. (From White AA, Panjabi MM: Clinical Biomechanics of the Spine. Philadelphia, JB Lippincott, 1988.)

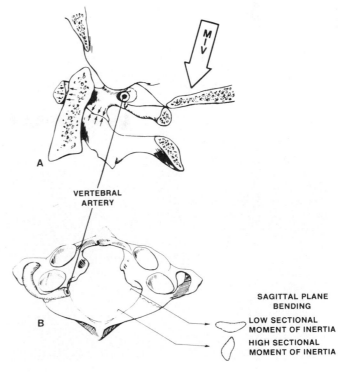

A

VERTEBRAL ARTERY

B

SAGITTAL PLANE BENDING

LOW SECTIONAL MOMENT OF INERTIA

HIGH SECTIONAL MOMENT OF INERTIA

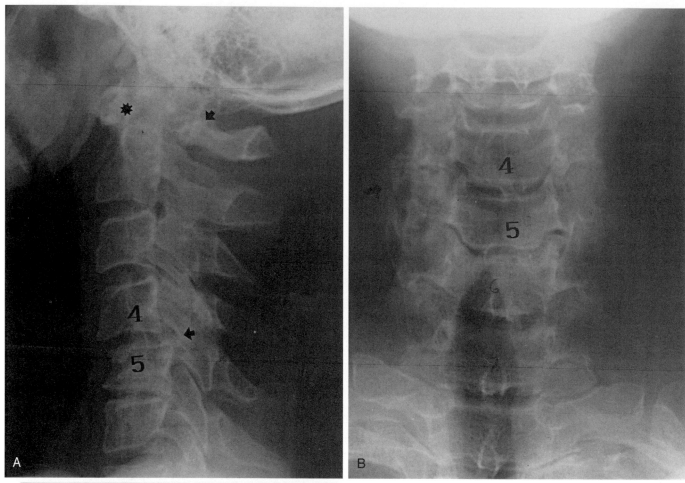

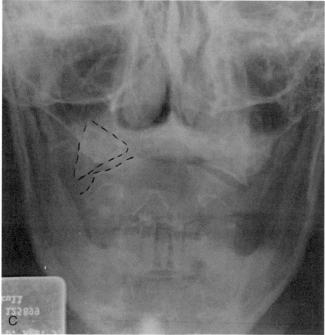

Figure 15–10 ═ This patient sustained an asymmetrical axial load to the head. The initial lateral radiographic findings (*A*) of both a C1 (*star, arrow*) and a C4–5 injury (*arrow*) are evident. The lateral film shows the posterior arch component of the lateral mass fracture, necessitating further examination at that level. It also demonstrates a 3-mm step-off at the C4–5 level, suggesting the presence of a facet injury. *B,* The open-mouth view shows displacement of only the right-side lateral mass of C1, thus confirming the diagnosis of a right lateral mass fracture. *C,* The anteroposterior radiograph centered at C4–5 shows horizontalization of the lateral mass at that level, also on the right side. Thus both injuries were the result of slight extension and axial load and lateral bending to the right side.

verse ligament is ruptured, the other secondary restraints to flexion are not disrupted. In fact, when healing takes place at the ring of C1, the anatomic relationships and length of the capsular fibers are restored to a relatively normal position. Then the capsular, alar, apical ligaments, anterior and posterior longitudinal ligaments act as restraints and resist flexion instability. Thus, the mechanism of injury of pure axial loading in the burst fracture bears a significant relationship to subsequent treatment dilemmas.

The mechanism of the fourth type of injury, transverse fracture of the atlas, is hyperextension resulting in an avulsion fracture. The superior oblique portion of the longus colli muscle inserts on the inferior portion of the anterior tubercle of the atlas. In a hyperextension injury of the neck, the ventral neck musculature may involuntarily contract in a defensive posture, causing an avulsion by the superior oblique portion of the longus colli and the anterior longitudinal ligament. This may be accompanied by other hyperextension injuries but as an isolated injury it is stable since no part of the articulation is affected. Understanding the mechanism is important, as is realizing that this injury is relatively stable and that it is not a true axial plane fracture through the dens, but rather an avulsion of the anterior portion.

The final type of injury is the transverse process fracture, most probably again a forced lateral flexion injury resulting in the contralateral avulsion fracture. This is an exceedingly rare injury, and insufficient clinical and experimental data exist to confirm the hypothesized mechanism of injury.

CLINICAL PRESENTATION AND RADIOLOGIC EVALUATION

Fractures of the atlas represent approximately 10% of all cervical spine injuries and approximately 2% of all spine injuries. They are most frequently seen in younger age groups (mean age, 30 years) and are most commonly the result of vehicular trauma. However, classic burst injuries may be associated with sports such as diving. Since these are rarely associated with neurologic deficit[1, 6, 34, 52] (which is directly related to the level of spinal trauma), patients commonly present with significant neck pain and a history of a fall or a blow to the head as a result of a motor vehicle accident. In polytrauma patients, the injuries are frequently associated with massive head injuries. Interesting other associated injuries at C1–2 (i.e., dens fractures) may result in neurologic deficit. An injury to C1 is frequently recognized on a lateral cervical radiograph taken at the time of admission and evaluation. Often, the fracture of the posterior arch (which can be isolated or one component of a more significant injury) is seen on initial radiograph. However, the more difficult problem is determining which patients have complex injuries and whether they also have associated cervical injuries. Two radiographic features help to determine whether the patient has an isolated posterior arch fracture, a more complicated ring fracture, or a combination of injuries. Patients with isolated posterior arch fractures commonly have evidence of an abnormality only on the lateral radiograph, which shows a defect in the posterior arch with either of the following: (1) a clearly visible defect or (2) distinctly abnormal orientation of the posterior arch. Patients with the latter finding should have an open-mouth view,[14, 19] which will help delineate either lateral mass fractures or Jefferson fractures, as the displacement of the lateral masses will be evident. However, not all patients with anterior arch fractures have significant displacement; thus the fracture may not be seen on an open-mouth roentgenogram. However, the open-mouth view used in combination with evaluation of the prevertebral soft tissue shadow on the lateral radiograph[35, 45, 56] helps to distinguish an isolated posterior arch fracture from either a complex atlas fracture or another associated anterior fracture, such as a dens fracture. Some fallacies have persisted about the use of the soft tissue shadow as a critical marker in that the appearance of the shadow is dependent on the time from injury and patient age. It may not be present in patients within the first hour after injury, but it usually develops within 6 hours. In addition the soft tissue shadow is unreliable in the child or the patient during significant inspiration, screaming, or uncontrollable behavior (which may be a problem in the head injury patient). Horizontal or anterior avulsion fractures are most frequently seen on the lateral radiograph, whereas transverse process fractures are seen on the open-mouth radiograph. In patients in whom either a complex atlas fracture or combined injuries are evident or suspected, the choice of the next radiographic evaluation technique is dependent on the data to be garnered. Patients with a suspected dens fracture, in combination with a possible posterior arch fracture, were previously best evaluated by AP and lateral hypercycloidal tomography. This both delineated the pathology of the dens fracture and clearly evaluated the anterior portion of the ring in the AP tomogram and the posterior portion of the ring in the lateral tomogram. Currently the use of CT scan[4] with two- and three-dimensional reconstructions is the standard method of evaluation for fractures of the atlas. For combined injuries of the upper cervical spine, such as dens and atlas fractures, axial cuts at 1.5- or 2-mm intervals must be combined with sagittal reconstructions for accurate visualization. Alternatively, 3-mm cuts with overlapping can be substituted. In patients suspected of having only a complex atlas fracture, the use of CT scans is accurate so long as the gantry is placed parallel to and along the exact same axis as the angle of the atlas when the patient is positioned in the scanner. Frequently the angle of the gantry and the angle of the atlas (with the patient's neck in slight extension) are divergent by as much as 30 degrees, thus yielding an inaccurate and confusing scan. In that situation, the axial cuts may obliterate fracture lines as a result of volume averaging. It is therefore necessary to angle the gantry so that the axial images are as close to parallel with the axis of the atlas as possible in order to have the highest resolution of the fracture anatomy.

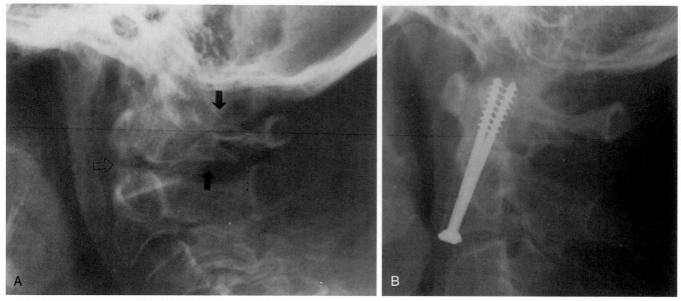

Figure 15–11 = *A,* This elderly patient sustained a combination of a posteriorly displaced dens fracture and a posterior arch fracture (*arrows*). Although reduction was achieved in traction, it was not able to be maintained in a halo vest. Thus operative stabilization was necessary. *B,* A direct osteosynthesis of the dens fracture was selected because the fracture of the posterior arch precluded a standard C1–2 arthrodesis.

ASSOCIATED INJURIES

Fractures of the atlas have an extremely high association with concurrent injuries of both the C1–2 complex and other areas. Of 86 patients with fractures of the atlas, 48% had additional fractures in the cervical spine, for a total of 55 additional fractures.[36] Two patients with posterior arch fractures also had thoracolumbar injuries. A very common association with fractures of the atlas are fractures of the dens[12, 37, 53] (Fig. 15–11). This is the single largest group of combined upper cervical spine injuries. Dens fractures can either be associated with posterior arch or with Jefferson fractures. A second very common group of injuries is the association of atlas fractures with traumatic spondylolisthesis of the axis. The majority of these are posterior arch fractures and type I traumatic spondylolisthesis of the axis, both of which are hyperextension injuries (Fig. 15–12). Posterior arch fractures can also be associated with anterior teardrop hyperextension injuries of C2. Finally, posterior arch fractures may be associated with other hyperextension or axial loading injuries in the lower cervical spine. Hyperextension injuries such as posterior arch fractures may be associated with laminar fractures in the lower cervical spine as well. The lateral mass fractures with asymmetrical lateral bending and axial loading are frequently associated with unilateral facet fractures or pillar fractures, located more distally in the cervical spine. Jefferson fractures that are axial loading injuries are frequently associated with burst fractures of the lower cervical spine. The incredibly high association of atlas fractures with other associated upper[31] and lower cervical spine injuries has a significant bearing on the treatment modalities for these particular injuries.

TREATMENT

Two major problems exist in the delineation of specific treatments for fractures of the atlas. The first is that few series have delineated treatment of these injuries in a significant number of patients.[11, 22, 29, 35, 50] This has hampered the ability to draw logical conclusions, as the majority of these injuries have been reported either as case reports or as very small series. The second

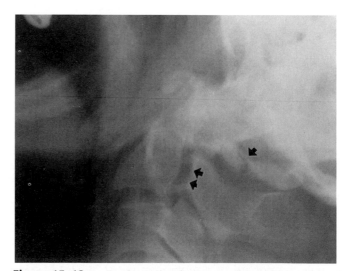

Figure 15–12 = As shown by the arrows this patient sustained both a type I traumatic spondylolisthesis of the axis as well as a posterior arch fracture. These injuries are both the result of a hyperextension and axial loading mechanism of injury. When these injuries occur individually, they are considered stable and can be treated with collar immobilization until union occurs. Thus this patient was also treated in a collar and went on to an uneventful union.

problem is the high incidence of concurrent injuries to both the upper and lower cervical spine. Often, the treatment of the patient is determined not by the atlas fracture but rather by the concurrent injury.

Treatment of fractures of the atlas covers a broad spectrum. Unfortunately, the treatment modalities applied to the various fractures of the atlas have not necessarily specifically addressed issues pertinent to the injuries themselves. As a result of the configuration of the atlas, surgical stabilization has not played a consistent role in the treatment of atlas fractures except in relation to C1–2 instability. The majority of treatment alternatives have been nonoperative, with treatment ranging from immobilization in a soft collar orthosis to a Minerva cast to a halo cast and vest. When the assumption has been made that the fracture has ruptured the transverse ligament and instability may be present, early C1–2 and occiput–C2 arthrodeses have been advocated.[1, 48] However, in treating fractures of the atlas, careful consideration must first be given to the nature of the injury and to its ramifications in terms of stability. Because neurologic deficit infrequently occurs with C1 fractures as a result of the expansion of the neural canal, decompression is rarely a problem. The second consideration is the restoration of normal anatomy both in relation to reestablishing the congruity of the atlanto-occipital and atlantoaxial joint surfaces and in achieving a union of the ring of C1. The relative importance of these two major considerations should determine the nature of the subsequent treatment.

Fractures of the posterior arch of the atlas constitute a significant proportion of atlas fractures seen. This injury is a stable injury that does not disrupt any significant ligamentous structures. Therefore, considerations of stability with this injury are not relevant, and the major considerations are related to the presence or absence of concomitant upper and lower cervical spine injuries as well as to the desire to achieve a union of the fracture. Because the displacement of posterior arch fractures is usually minimal, the union rates of posterior arch fractures are very high. Thus, the immobilization necessary to achieve such a result is minimal.

The major goal of treatment of isolated posterior arch fractures is to achieve patient comfort and protect the spine from further injury until union of the posterior arch occurs. Approximately 2 to 3 months are usually required until callus is evident at the junction sites. In patients with fractures of the posterior arch, however, the majority (approximately 50%) have additional injuries in the upper or lower cervical spine. Thus, treatment for the posterior arch fracture may indeed be significantly influenced by the presence of another injury or, more importantly, the treatment of the second injury may be influenced by the presence of the posterior arch fracture. Because fractures of the posterior arch of the atlas are predominantly hyperextension injuries, the injuries most commonly associated with them are posteriorly displaced dens fractures, type I traumatic spondylolisthesis of the axis, and extension-avulsion injuries in either the upper or the lower cervical spine. Additionally, spinous process

fractures of the lower cervical spine and laminar fractures may be associated with posterior arch fractures. The combination of a posterior arch fracture and a posteriorly displaced dens fracture presents an interesting treatment dilemma.

The criteria for treating type II posteriorly displaced dens fractures are based on the ability to achieve a reduction and to maintain that reduction as well as on the amount of initial displacement. Because a surgical option for treatment of dens fracture is a C1–2 arthrodesis, that option must be modified in the patient who has a posterior arch fracture associated with the dens fracture. The primary treatment for a patient with a posterior arch fracture and type II dens fracture would be reduction by traction and immobilization in a halo vest; the treatment would be directed at the displaced type II dens fracture instead of to the posterior arch fracture. Should the reduction of the type II dens fracture be difficult to obtain or maintain nonoperatively, nonstandard operative procedures need to be considered. Direct anterior dens screw osteosynthesis of the fracture is effective, with the posterior arch fracture then treated in its standard fashion in a collar. Alternatively, a C1–2 arthrodesis can be accomplished by the use of a posterior transarticular screw fixation with direct bone grafting of the C1–2 joint.

A second interesting dilemma is the posterior arch fracture combined with a type I traumatic spondylolisthesis of the axis. Again, both injuries result from a hyperextension mechanism. Both injuries taken individually are stable injuries. It has been well demonstrated that when simply treated with a collar, a type I traumatic spondylolisthesis has a very high union rate without any significant risk of displacement. This is similarly true for the posterior arch fracture. Although there might be a tendency to be more aggressive in treatment as a result of the presence of two injuries, the instability is no greater, and both heal adequately. Thus, treatment of two stable injuries, one of which is a posterior arch fracture of C1, can be accomplished with the most conservative method used for the two injuries. Treatment of posterior arch fractures is predominantly symptomatic to allow fracture healing, which is a predictable phenomenon because of the minimal displacement; the secondary goal is to treat concurrent injuries as needed.

For Jefferson and lateral mass fractures, treatment is determined on the basis of both the degree of instability and anatomic derangement. A smaller proportion of these patients have two significant cervical injuries; thus, treatment may be modified, although it is most often determined by the treatment of the C1 ring fracture. Treatment of ring fractures of C1 is related to the degree of displacement and the goal of treatment. The C1 lateral mass and Jefferson fractures can be divided into three groups, which are loosely correlated with the amount of energy and subsequent injury imparted to the C1 ring. These fractures can be (1) nondisplaced, (2) minimally displaced (up to 7 mm of total displacement), or (3) significantly displaced (>7 mm of displacement). Generally, initial documentation on CT scan or tomogram of fractures in both the anterior and

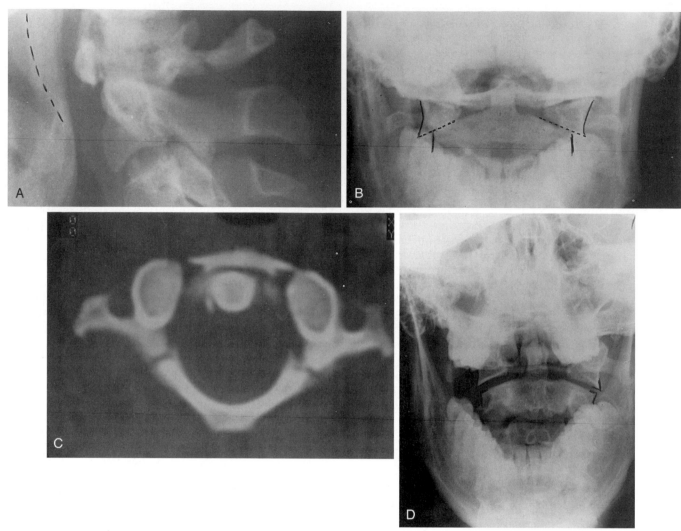

Figure 15–13 = *A,* The lateral radiograph shows a Jefferson fracture with evident posterior arch fractures and the anterior ring fracture inferred by the increased width of the anterior soft tissue shadow (*dotted line*). *B,* The open-mouth view shows symmetrical spreading of the lateral masses totaling 13 mm. This suggests that the transverse ligament has been ruptured by the splaying of the lateral masses during the injury, with the ligament failing in tension. *C,* The CT scan shows the standard four-part injury. *D,* When 30 lb of traction was gradually applied, a reduction of both lateral masses to an anatomic position was achieved within 48 hours of the time of injury.

posterior ring, but no displacement on an open-mouth view, indicates that little energy has been imparted to the ring; such injuries do not tend to displace secondarily. If no displacement whatsoever is seen on the open-mouth view, then treatment in either a halo vest or a cervical orthosis is an acceptable treatment and will yield a high rate of union with minimal morbidity. These injuries are uncommon, and most injuries fall into either the minimally displaced or the significantly displaced group. As demonstrated by Spence and associates,[54] patients with a combined displacement of more than 6.9 mm have sustained a rupture of the transverse ligament in a tension mode. They will, however, still have intact alar and apical ligaments as well as intact portions of facet capsules both anteriorly and posteriorly at C1–2. Because the incongruity is not significant, and because the rate of nonunion is acceptable (as the displacement of the fragments is insignificant), the goal of treatment of this minimally displaced injury is to attain union of the fracture. It is unnecessary to totally

reduce the injury, as the intact transverse ligament maintains the relevant relationship of the two lateral masses, and the incongruity of the joint is not massive. This injury is best treated in a halo vest, as studies have demonstrated that immobilization at the C1–2 joint is optimal in a halo as opposed to other types of orthoses. The surgeon must be cognizant of the fact that it is impossible to achieve a reduction of this fracture by use of a halo vest. The position of the halo with reference to the vest should be such that the neck is maximally straightened and lengthened in a resting position. This prevents a significant axial compression force from being applied to the fracture while the patient is upright. For patients with significantly displaced Jefferson fractures or lateral mass fractures (7 to 10 mm of total displacement) a different clinical scenario exists. These patients have sustained a rupture of the transverse ligament, and the displacement of the fragments can become quite significant. As demonstrated by Segal and associates,[50] nonunions of these

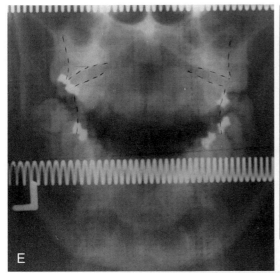

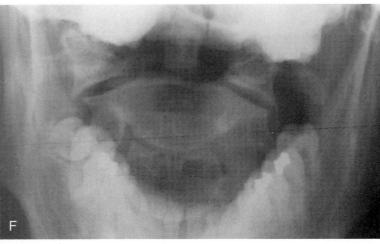

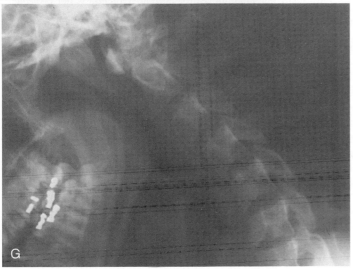

Figure 15–13 *Continued* = *E*, The patient was maintained in traction on a Stryker frame for 6 weeks and the reduction was unchanged throughout the entire period as verified by sequential open-mouth x-rays. At the end of 6 weeks, the traction was removed and an open-mouth view was taken in the supine position, with no change in the fracture reduction because preliminary callus formation had occurred in the reapposed fracture fragments. The patient was immobilized in a halo vest for another 6 weeks. *F*, At the end of that time, the vest was removed and an open-mouth view was taken, which again showed maintenance of the reduction. At the same time a flexion-extension view was taken to test the stability of the C1–2 segment. *G*, In flexion, minimal displacement (<3 mm) occurs, indicating restoration of stability without the need for arthrodesis.

injuries are more common than previously recognized. In addition, as the displacement becomes more significant, incongruity can become an important factor. Because the transverse ligament is not present, there is no structure in the significantly displaced fracture to maintain the relative relationship of one lateral mass to the other. Patients with this injury may therefore benefit from reduction of the fracture. As demonstrated by Han and co-workers[18] and Zimmerman and associates,[60] immediate immobilization in a halo vest does not achieve or maintain reduction of the lateral masses. Even with short-term traction in a halo vest for reduction, upon removal of the traction and placement in a halo vest, the fracture slips back to its original position. Because the primary mechanism of injury in these fractures is either axial loading or axial loading and lateral bending, axial traction is required to achieve reduction. Thus, constant axial traction is necessary for the reduction of the injury (Fig. 15–13). Patients with significant displacement can have axial traction applied through a halo ring in increments beginning at 10 lb and progressing as high as 40 lb as necessary to achieve full reduction of the ring on open-mouth view. Complete

symmetry of the C1–2 lateral masses must be achieved. Once the fracture has been fully reduced and the fragments brought in contact, approximately 4 to 6 weeks must pass before preliminary healing of the fracture is sufficient to allow immobilization of the patient in a halo vest without subsequent loss of reduction. The degree of healing can be assessed periodically by removing the traction from the halo and allowing the patient to lie in a supine position for 1 hour, after which an open-mouth radiograph is taken. If the reduction is maintained, then the patient can be mobilized in a halo vest, and if the reduction is lost, the traction can be replaced and the reduction regained and held until it is possible to remove the traction weight without loss of reduction. Immobilization in a halo vest for an additional 6 weeks will bring the total immobilization period to approximately 3 months. Alternatively, another approach can be taken for the patient with a severely displaced lateral mass or Jefferson fracture. Since it has been demonstrated that the reduction achieved with axial traction is lost with immediate mobilization, operative stabilization in the reduced position allows earlier mobilization. If the fracture is ana-

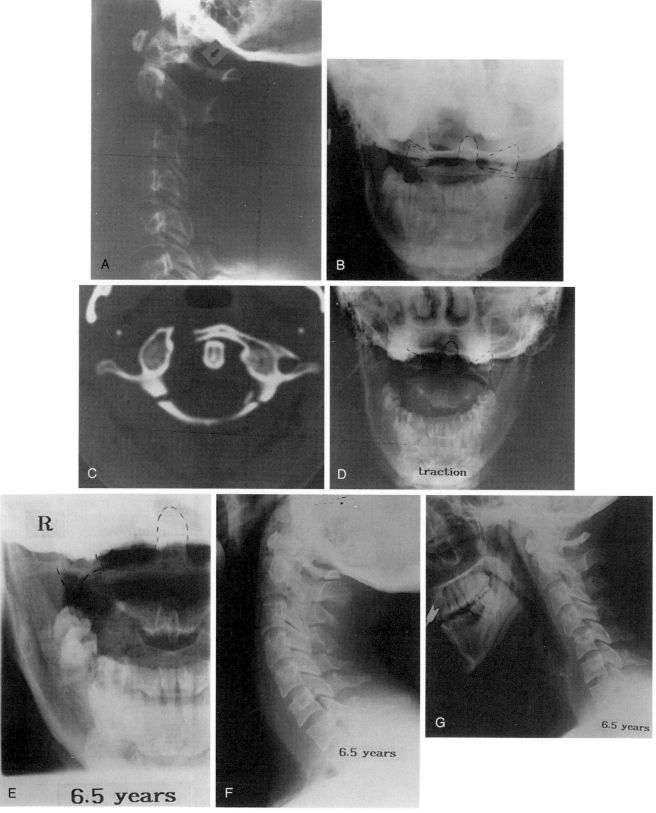

Figure 15–16 = This patient presented with a widely displaced fracture of the lateral mass. *A,* The initial lateral radiograph shows fractures involving the posterior arch on both sides *(arrow). B,* The initial open-mouth view is quite dramatic, showing very marked and asymmetrical displacement of one lateral mass almost to the point of dislocation. *C,* This is confirmed by the CT scan, on which a wide gap appears between the lateral mass and the anterior arch, with fractures in the posterior arch on both sides. *D,* The fracture was initially reduced with halo traction, but the patient refused to either remain in the hospital in traction or undergo any operative procedure. He therefore was taken out of traction after 3 days and discharged in a halo vest. The halo vest was removed after 3 months and the patient was lost to follow-up for the next 4 years. He returned after 4 years complaining of some neck pain, but again refused anything but nonoperative treatment. When he returned at 6½ years, the pain was so severe that he could no longer work and could not turn his head. *E,* The open-mouth view shows wide displacement of the lateral mass with sclerosis, loss of the joint space, and remodeling of the lateral mass of C1 to conform to the edge of the C2 joint surface. *F* and *G,* Flexion and extension views show that despite the displacement and obvious rupture of the transverse ligament, stability of the C1–2 segment exists.

of both in an anatomic position. However, failure to achieve a reduction of either injury in traction negates the relative value of the traction. The patient with an unreduced unilateral facet fracture might require operative stabilization of the unilateral facet fracture followed by prolonged traction for the C1 injury. However, incomplete reduction of the C1 injury may be acceptable because of the position of the fracture fragments, and prolonged traction for that injury is not necessary. Operative treatment of the lower cervical facet injury followed by immediate halo vest immobilization, accepting the less complete reduction of C1, may therefore be the appropriate treatment in that situation.

Finally, patients with avulsion fractures of either the anterior portion of the ring or the transverse processes are most frequently treated in a symptomatic fashion with collar immobilization. The incidence of these fractures is so small that long-term follow-up and results are currently not available.

RESULTS OF TREATMENT AND COMPLICATIONS

For patients with posterior arch fractures, the expected result is a union with minimal to no symptoms. In the group of patients with posterior arch fractures combined with other associated injuries, any residual symptoms are most commonly related to the other injury. Posterior arch fractures and traumatic spondylolisthesis of the axis (especially type I injuries) may proceed to secondary degenerative changes as a result of the destruction by compression of the C2–3 facet joint and require subsequent arthrodesis. This however is not a result of the posterior arch fracture but of the associated injuries. For patients with lateral mass and Jefferson fractures, the data on overall results are relatively clear. For patients treated in a halo vest with minimally displaced fractures, there is little tendency toward increased placement during treatment. Although there may be minimal increase of up to 2 mm, significant increased placement is rare. It is possible to achieve reduction, as documented in a series of patients treated with traction; mean total displacement was 12.3 mm and was reduced to 3.9 mm.[35] All of these patients subsequently underwent flexion-extension radiographs with no demonstrated instability. At follow-up, approximately 80% of patients had some residual neck pain, especially related to weather, but none needed secondary arthrodesis. However, nonunions occur in 17% of patients.[32] This is related to the amount of displacement; thus, displacement should clearly be minimized to prevent nonunion. Secondary progressive dural compression and myelopathy are possible with nonunion, and can occur in cases in which the fracture fragment directly impinges on the dural sac (Fig. 15–15). Most commonly, however, neurologic deficit is not a sequela of the injury itself, but it may be a sequela of associated injuries. Complications in the treatment of these injuries are relatively rare. Interestingly, the injury may be complicated by direct trauma to the greater occipital nerve.[59] Especially in older individuals, who are placed in a Yale brace or Philadelphia collar, the numbness over the occiput from greater occipital nerve injury can result in a decubitus ulcer over the occiput. Prior to application of a brace, the occipital sensation should be checked; if it is absent, halo vest management should be considered.

Complications of halo vest use for treatment are well documented and include loosening pins, bone erosion, skull perforation, and CSF leaks. Appropriate care of the halo vest and torquing of the pins is critical for normal mobility during its use.

Although the incidence is poorly documented because of the lack of long-term follow-up of this patient population, degenerative changes of incongruent joint surfaces are inevitable. In patients with severely displaced lateral mass and Jefferson fractures, if reduction is not achieved and maintained, both the occipito-atlantal and atlantoaxial joints are in jeopardy of rapid onset of degenerative changes. With lateral mass fractures, this may be asymmetrical (Fig. 15–16), whereas in Jefferson fractures it may be more bilateral. Early manifestations are pain with head rotation and occasionally on flexion-extension. Radiographic evidence of sclerosis and loss of joint space is later evident (see Fig. 15–16). If increased symptoms occur, occipitocervical fusion provides a solution to the pain.

Atlas fractures span a spectrum of injury and instability from trivial to significant. Treatment should be directed at appropriate goals, and more long-term follow-up is necessary in studying the implications of lateral mass and Jefferson fractures.

REFERENCES

1. Alker GJ, Oh YS, Leslie EV, et al: Post mortem radiology of head and neck injuries in fatal traffic accidents. Radiology 114:611–617, 1975.
2. Bailey DK: The normal cervical spine in infants and children. Radiology 59:712, 1952.
3. Barker EG, Krumpelman J, Long JM: Isolated fracture of the medial portion of the lateral mass of the atlas: A previously undescribed entity. AJR 126:1053–1058, 1976.
4. Baumgarten M, Mouradian W, Boger D, et al: Computed axial tomography in C1–C2 trauma. Spine 10:187–192, 1985.
5. Broom MJ, Krompinger WJ, Bond SD: Fracture of the atlantal arch causing atlanto-axial instability. J Bone Joint Surg Am 68:1289–1291, 1986.
6. Bucholz RW, Burkhead WZ: The pathological anatomy of fatal atlanto-occipital dislocations. J Bone Joint Surg Am 61:248–250, 1979.
7. Clyburn TA, Lionberger DR, Tullos HS: Bilateral fracture of the transverse process of the atlas. J Bone Joint Surg Am 64:948, 1982.
8. Cooper A: A Treatise on Dislocations and Fractures of the Joints. London, Longman, Hurst Rees, Orme Browne, E. Cox & Son, 1823, p 542.
9. Desgrey H, Gertag R, Cherrel P: Anomalies congenitales des arc de l'atles. J Radiol 48:819, 1960.
10. Dvorak J, Panjabi MM, Gerber M, et al: CT functional diagnostics of the rotatory instability of the upper cervical spine: I. Experimental study in cadavers. Spine 12:197, 1987.
11. Ersmark H, Kalen R: Injuries of the atlas and axis: A follow-up study of 85 axis and 10 atlas fractures. Clin Orthop Rel Res 217:257–260, 1987.
12. Esses S, Langer I, Gross A: Fracture of the atlas associated with fracture of the odontoid process. Injury 12:310, 1981.
13. Fielding JW, Cochran GVB, Lawsing JF, et al: Tears of the trans-

verse ligament of the atlas: A clinical and biomechanical study. J Bone Joint Surg Am 56:1683–1691, 1974.

14. Flournoy JG, Cone RO, Saldana JA, et al: Jefferson fracture: Presentation of a new diagnostic sign. Radiology 134:88, 1980.

15. Galindo MJ Jr, Francis WR: Atlantal fracture in a child through congenital anterior and posterior arch defects. Clin Orthop Rel Res 178:220–222, 1983.

16. Gehweiler JA Jr, Daffner RH, Roberts L Jr: Malformations of the alas vertebra simulating the Jefferson fracture. Am Roentgen Ray Soc 140:1083–1086, 1983.

17. Hamilton AR: Injuries of the atlanto-axial joint. J Bone Joint Surg Br 33:434–435, 1951.

18. Han SY, Witten DM, Mussleman JP: Jefferson fracture of the atlas. J Neurosurg 44:368–371, 1976.

19. Harris JH Jr: Acute injuries of the spine. Semin Roentgenol 13:53–68, 1978.

20. Hays, MB, Alker, GJ: Fractures of the atlas vertebra: The two-part burst fracture of Jefferson. Spine 13:601–603, 1988.

21. Hentzer L, Schalimtzek M: Fractures and subluxations of the atlas and axis. Acta Orthop Scand 42:251–258, 1971.

22. Highland TR, Salciccioli GG: Is immobilization adequate treatment of unstable burst fractures of the atlas? Clin Orthop 201:196–200, 1985.

23. Hinchey JJ, Bickel WH: Fracture of the atlas. Ann Surg 121:826, 1945.

24. Jeanneret B, Magerl F: Primary posterior fusion C1/2 in odontoid fractures: Indications, technique and results of transarticular screw fixation. J Spine Disord 5:464–475, 1992.

25. Jefferson G: Fracture of the atlas vertebra. Br J Surg 7:407, 1920.

26. Jefferson G: Fractures of the first cervical vertebra. Br Med J, July 30, 1927, pp 153–157.

27. Jevtich V: Horizontal fracture of the anterior arch of the atlas. J Bone Joint Surg Am 68:1094–1095, 1986.

28. Kattan KR: Two features of the atlas vertebra simulating fractures by tomography. Am Roentgen Ray Soc 132:963–965, 1979.

29. Kesterson L, Benzel E, Orrison W, et al: Evaluation and treatment of the atlas burst fractures. J Neurosurg 75:213–220, 1991.

30. Koch RA, Nickel VL: The halo vest: An evaluation of motion and forces across the neck. Spine 3:103, 1978.

31. Korres SD, Kosmides A, Andreakos K, et al: Fracture de Jefferson avec dislocation occipito-cervicale. Orthop Traumatol 1:77–79, 1991.

32. Levine AM: Avulsion of the transverse ligament associated with fracture of the atlas. Orthopedics 6:1467, 1983.

33. Levine AM, Edwards CC: Treatment of injuries in the C1-C2 complex. Orthop Clin North Am 17:31–44, 1986.

34. Levine AM, Edwards CC: Traumatic lesions of the occipitoatlantoaxial complex. Clin Orthop 239:53–68, 1989.

35. Levine AM, Edwards CC: Fractures of the atlas. J Bone Joint Surg Am 73:680–691, 1991.

36. Levine AM, Fischgrund J: Fractures of the C1-C2 complex: Concurrent injuries. Concurrent Spinal Injuries (in press).

37. Lipson SJ: Fractures of the atlas associated with fracture of the odontoid process and transverse ligament ruptures. J Bone Joint Surg Am 59:940–943, 1977.

38. Lipson SJ, Major J: Anteroposterior spondyloschises of the atlas revealed by computerized tomographic scanning. J Bone Joint Surg Am 60:1104, 1978.

39. Logan WW, Stuard ID: Absent Posterior Arch of the Atlas, Am J Roentgenol Radium Ther Nucl Med, 118:670, 1960.

40. Marlin AE, Williams GR, Lee JF: Jefferson fractures in children. J Neurosurg 58:277–279, 1983.

41. McGuire RA, Harkey HL: Unstable Jefferson's fracture treated with transarticular screws. Orthopedics 18:207–209, 1995.

42. McRae DL: The significance of abnormalities of the cervical spine. AJR 84:3, 1960.

43. Mixter SJ, Osgood RB: Traumatic lesions of the atlas and axis. Ann Surg 51:193–207, 1910.

44. O'Brien JJ, Butterfield WL, Gossling HR: Jefferson fracture with rupture of the transverse ligament: A case report. Clin Orthop Rel Res 126:135–138, 1977.

45. Penning L: Paravertebral hematoma in cervical spine injury: Incidence and etiologic significance. AJR 136:553–561, 1981.

46. Pierce DS, Barr JS: Fractures and dislocations at the base of the skull and upper cervical spine. In The Cervical Spine, ed 1. Philadelphia, JB Lippincott, 1983, pp 196–206.

47. Proubasta IR, Sancho RN, Alonso JR, et al: Horizontal fracture of the anterior arch of the atlas. Spine 12:615–618, 1987.

48. Schlicke LH: A rational approach to burst fractures of the atlas. Clin Orthop Rel Res 154:18–21, 1981.

49. Schneider RC, Livingston KE, Cave AJ, et al: Hangman's fracture of the cervical spine. J Neurosurg 22:121, 1965.

50. Segal LS, Grimm JO, Stauffer ES: Non-union of fractures of the atlas. J Bone Joint Surg Am 69:1423–1434, 1987.

51. Sherk HH, Nicholson JT: Fractures of the atlas. J Bone Joint Surg Am 52:1017–1024, 1970.

52. Sherk HH: Lesions of the atlas and axis. Clin Orthop Rel Res 109:33–41, 1975.

53. Sherk HH: Fracture of the atlas and odontoid process. Orthop Clin North Am 9:973–984, 1978.

54. Spence KF, Decker S, Sell KW: Bursting atlantal fracture associated with rupture of the transverse ligament. J Bone Joint Surg Am 52:543–549, 1970.

55. Stewart GC Jr, Gehweiler JA Jr, Laib RH, et al: Horizontal fracture of the anterior arch of the atlas. Radiology 122:349–352, 1977.

56. Templeton PA, Young JWR, Mirvis S, et al: The value of retropharyngeal soft tissue measurements in trauma of the adult cervical spine. Skeletal Radiol 30:1–7, 1987.

57. White AA III, Panjabi MM: The clinical biomechanics of the occipitoatlantoaxial complex. Orthop Clin North Am 9:867–878, 1978.

58. White AA III, Panjabi MM: Clinical Biomechanics of the Spine. Philadelphia, JB Lippincott, 1991.

59. Zielinski CJ, Gunther SF, Deeb Z: Cranial nerve palsies complicating Jefferson fracture. J Bone Joint Surg Am 64:1382–1384, 1982.

60. Zimmerman E, Grant J, Vise WM, et al: Treatment of Jefferson fracture with a halo apparatus. J Neurosurg 44:372–375, 1976.

Odontoid Fractures

Gregory D. Carlson ‖ *John G. Heller* ‖ *Jean-Jacques Abitbol*
Steven R. Garfin

Odontoid fractures, once thought to be rare injuries, constitute up to 18% of cervical spine fractures and dislocations.* Traditionally, these injuries have been frequently unrecognized, misdiagnosed, and not adequately treated, leading to pain and progressive neurologic deficit.[23] These problems can be traced to the complex anatomy of the craniocervical junction. This region provides the majority of the segmental axial rotation in the neck and relies on the integrity of the bone-ligament complex of the atlantoaxial articulation. This region is at risk in all age groups. Owing to the large head-to-body size in young children, more than 75% of cervical injuries occur in the craniocervical junction. Elderly people are at risk of falls and resultant osteoporotic odontoid fracture, whereas younger and middle-aged adults sustain high-velocity craniocervical trauma in motor vehicle accidents.

Type II odontoid fractures have traditionally been difficult to treat because of poor healing. Unlike type III fractures, which can be successfully managed in halo vest immobilization, nonunion rates for displaced type II fractures may approach 100%. Factors such as patient age, fracture displacement, and early fracture diagnosis and treatment have been recognized to significantly affect union rates. Now the conservative treatment of some type II fractures is recognized as primary surgical stabilization.

Recent innovations in internal fixation techniques have provided benefits of early immediate rigid fixation with either posterior atlantoaxial fusion or direct anterior fracture fixation with resultant preservation of cervical motion. As these techniques have been refined, the indications for, and relative contraindications to, their use have also become better understood. Similar to other areas of spine surgery, treatment of odontoid fractures has become more complex, requiring greater levels of training and experience to provide optimal care.

This chapter seeks to provide the reader with the basic pathophysiology of odontoid fractures. Treatment of these complex injuries requires a thorough understanding of the regional anatomy and mechanical support structures. Also, we provide a synthesis of recent advances in fracture fixation and stabilization procedures. The reader should always consider the level to which he is trained when considering new surgical techniques. For this reason, the traditional methods of posterior fusion are described and recommended for they are the standard by which other methods are judged.

ANATOMY

Ligament Support

The odontoid process is an important stabilizer of the atlantoaxial joint. The anterior arch of the atlas forms a gliding synovial articulation with the anterior facet of the odontoid, and functions as the primary restraint against extension at C1–2. Affixed to the tubercles on the lateral masses of the atlas, the transverse ligament traverses posterior to the odontoid process, securing the latter to the posterior facet of the anterior arch of the atlas (Fig. 16–1). This ligament provides the primary restraint to atlantoaxial flexion or anterior translation of the atlas.[35, 105] The normal joint space between the atlas and the odontoid does not exceed 3 mm between flexion and extension in the presence of an intact transverse ligament.[35]

The axis forms a unique articulation with the atlas.[16, 59, 103] Their respective articular facets permit rotation, accounting for nearly 50% of such motion in the cervical spine.[80] From the body of the axis, the odontoid process projects upward into the ring of the atlas. Its mean height is 14.4 mm,[89, 103] or nearly 40% of the total height of the axis. Under normal circumstances the odontoid remains in close contact with the anterior arch of the atlas, providing a stable articulation in flexion and extension while allowing a range of rotational motion in the atlantoaxial complex.[35, 80] The sagittal diameter of the atlas easily accommodates the odontoid process and the spinal cord.[89] Under normal circumstances, as observed by Steel,[101] the anteroposterior (AP) space available for the spinal cord is twice the sagittal diameter of the cord. Anatomically, one-third of the space available within the ring of C1 is taken up by the odontoid, one third by the spinal cord, and one third by compressible soft tissue. This generous allocation of space for the spinal cord helps explain the relatively low incidence of spinal cord injuries associated with odontoid fractures.[49, 50]

The most important secondary ligamentous stabilizers preventing anterior translation are the alar liga-

---

*References 6, 7, 22, 25, 30, 41, 49–51, 53, 62, 64, 81, 90, 95, and 104.

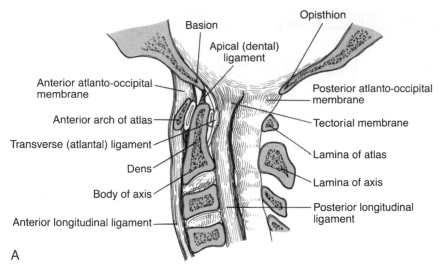

A

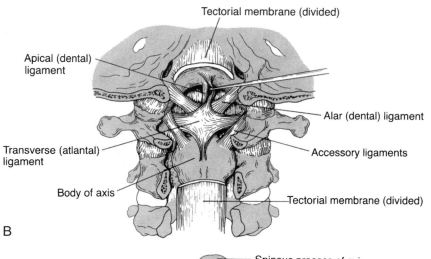

B

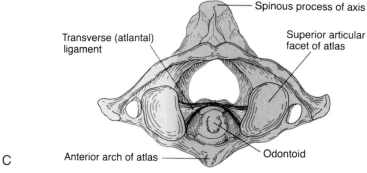

C

Figure 16–1 = Atlantoaxial ligamentous complex. *A,* Sagittal view of ligamentous anatomy. *B,* Coronal view of anatomy after resection of posterior elements. *C,* Axial view of atlantoaxial articulation. (From Jarrett PJ, Whitesides TE Jr: Injuries of the cervicocranium. *In* Browner BD, Jupiter JB, Levine AM, et al (eds): Skeletal Trauma: Fractures, Dislocations, Ligamentous Injuries, vol. 7. Philadelphia, WB Saunders, 1992, pp 666, 667.)

ments.[27, 28, 35, 72, 105] These paired ligaments arise from the medial aspect of the occipital condyles and lateral masses of the atlas. They insert broadly along the lateral portion of the odontoid. They restrict contralateral rotation and lateral bending of the atlas on the axis.[27, 28] The accessory ligaments arise from the lateral mass of C1 and insert into the base of the odontoid. They appear to play a role in the vascular supply to the dens.[90, 92] The apical ligament arises from the anterior rim of the foramen magnum and inserts into the tip of the odontoid. Together with the alar ligaments, the accessory and apical ligaments function as secondary stabilizers of the atlanto-dens complex.[27, 28, 35, 72] In

adults, no more than 3 mm of sagittal displacement between the posterior arch of C1 and the anterior odontoid process should be observed on standard lateral upper cervical spine radiographs. Displacement of 5 mm or more is consistent with rupture of the transverse ligament complex and clinical instability.[35, 72]

Osseous Structure

The osseous shape of C2 has a distinct anatomic structure that provides the intrinsic support of the highly mobile C1–2 complex (Fig. 16–2). The odontoid process serves as a rigid post resisting in AP C1–2

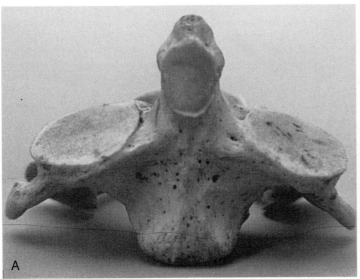 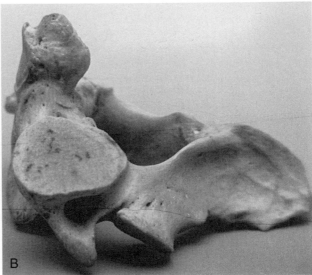

Figure 16–2 = *A* and *B*, Osseous anatomy of the dens. (From Heller JG, Alson MD, Schaffler MB, et al: Quantitative internal dens morphology. Spine 17:861, 1992.)

translation. In addition, it provides the center of rotation for C1–2 axial rotation (approximately 50% of the total axial rotation in the cervical spine).

Variations in odontoid process shape and longitudinal orientation to the body of C2 have been described. Morphometric anatomic studies of the odontoid have revealed the average height to range from 13.7 to 15.0 mm, with males showing slightly greater height than females.[89, 103, 106] Based on axial sections of the odontoid and on radiographic examination, Koebke[59] classified the shape of the odontoid and suggested that biomechanical stresses affected the kyphosis, lordosis, or straight orientation.

The osseous anatomy of the odontoid and its relationship to the body of C2 are of importance to the spine surgeon contemplating direct fracture fixation with bone screw techniques. Fracture fixation is usually accomplished with two 3.5- or 4.0-mm screws inserted caudocephalad through an anterior approach; however, for patients with smaller intraosseous constraints, 2.7-mm screws may be necessary. Measuring the cortical thickness at the base of the odontoid, Heller and coworkers[52] found the cortical thickness to be greatest in the transverse plane (Fig. 16–3). Though fractures most commonly occur at the base of the odontoid (type II), the minimum AP diameter of the odontoid corresponds to the midregion in contact with the transverse ligament. In morphometric studies of the C2 vertebrae in the extensive Hamann-Todd skeletal collection, Heller and co-authors found the average minimum internal AP and transverse diameters of the odontoid to be 6.2 and 4.5 mm, respectively. Males had slightly larger osseous dimensions than females.[52] Their data underscore the relative difficulty of accurate intraos-

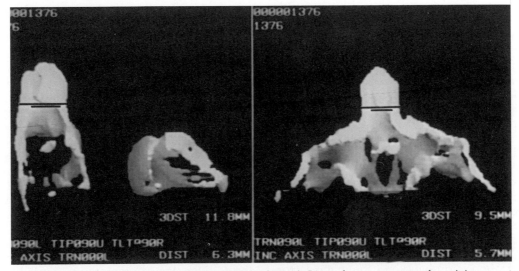

Figure 16–3 = Three-dimensional CT image of C2 through the odontoid. Lines drawn represent the minimum external and internal transverse diameters (see text). (From Heller JG, Alson MD, Schaffler MB, et al: Quantitative internal dens morphology. Spine 17:861, 1992.)

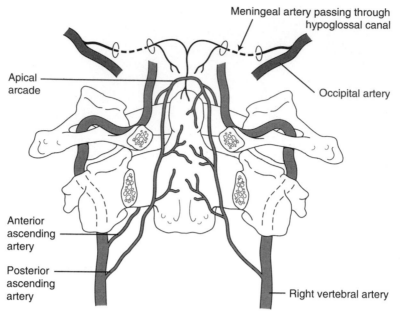

Meningeal artery passing through hypoglossal canal

Apical arcade

Occipital artery

Anterior ascending artery

Posterior ascending artery

Right vertebral artery

Figure 16–4 = Vascular anastomoses supplying the odontoid process. The odontoid receives its blood supply from the carotid and vertebral arteries.

seous screw placement in individuals with small odontoid processes.

VASCULARITY

The regional blood supply to the odontoid has been shown to be highly vascular, in contrast to early theories which posited avascularity to explain the high rates of fracture nonunion.[3, 79, 90–92] The carotid and vertebral arteries provide a rich blood supply to the odontoid through endosteal and ligamentous vessels (Fig. 16–4). Paired anterior ascending arteries branch from the anteromedial aspect of the ipsilateral vertebral artery and course cephalad on the anterior aspect of the dens to send perforators into the subchondral bone at the base of the dens. The ascending arteries have multiple points of anastomosis, and eventually join the posterior ascending arteries around the tip of the dens. The posterior ascending arteries originate from the posteromedial surface of the respective vertebral artery. The arteries course in the groove formed by the pedicle and body of the axis and supply branches to the apical regions, as well as the ligaments and soft tissues attached to the apex. The internal carotid artery also supplies the dens through horizontal arteries that anastomose around the apex of the dens and contribute to an apical vascular arcade. Additionally, the external carotid artery contributes through a branch of the ascending pharyngeal artery.

The dens has a rich blood supply inferiorly, around the base, as well as proximally. Although displacement of the odontoid process may temporarily attenuate the blood supply to the proximal fragment, studies suggest that devascularization is probably not the major factor contributing to nonunion of the odontoid process.[79]

EMBRYOLOGY

The anatomic development of the axis vertebra is a complex process and may provide a source of diagnostic dilemma for the most experienced physician. At birth the axis is composed of four primary ossification centers which are unfused and separated by synchondroses (Fig. 16–5). The pattern of synchondrosis in the AP plane forms an H configuration.[37] Proximally, the ossific nucleus of the dens forms a synchondrosis with the vertebral body well below the level of the superior articular facets. The neural arches make lateral contact with the body and dens through the neurocentral synchondrosis. Two secondary centers of ossification, which appear later, include the inferior epiphyseal ring apophysis of the axis body and the ossiculum terminale at the proximal tip of the dens, which has a V configuration.[8]

The odontoid process is formed in utero by the fusion of two adjacent independent ossification centers. This fusion starts during the fifth month following conception, and is complete by the seventh month. Occasionally, an incomplete fusion occurs which may produce a bifid dens, easily mistaken for a fracture.[37]

Before the age of 3 years, when fusion of the synchondroses occur, odontoid "fractures" extend through the cartilaginous portion of the growth plate. These end plates are caudal to the base of the odontoid and facet joints well within the body of C2. Ewald[33] has shown this region to be a true synchondrosis with a zone of endochondral ossification from both the body and the dens, as opposed to the process of ossification in the hypertrophied zone of cartilage of a true epiphyseal plate. A fracture through this area propagates through the weak horizontally oriented trabecular bone surrounding the endochondral growth plate.[76] Typical

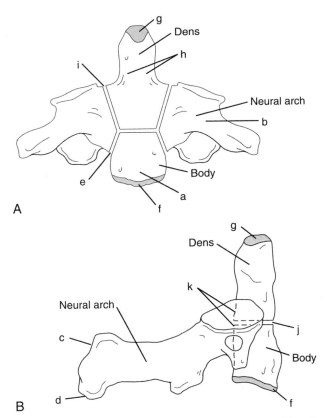

The neurocentral arches form posteriorly by 2 to 3 years of age and subsequently fuse the body and odontoid process by 3 to 6 years of age. The ossiculum terminale appears by 6 years of age and fuses to the odontoid by the age of 12 years.[8] The inferior ring apophysis appears at puberty and fuses to the body by the age of 25. The apical odontoid epiphysis is present by the age of 2 years and ossifies by 12 years of age. It is usually visualized on AP radiographs, and may appear with a radiolucent V at the tip of the odontoid.[8, 20] Knowledge of these growth plates, combined with the clinical history and evaluation, may help prevent an erroneous diagnosis of odontoid fractures in children.

CLASSIFICATION

Schatzker and associates[90] were the first to introduce a classification system for odontoid fractures. They classified fractures as "high" or "low" in relation to the attachment site of the accessory ligaments at the base of the dens. They observed in dogs that experimentally induced fractures of the dens above the accessory ligaments failed to unite, while fractures below the accessory ligaments showed a union rate of 100%.[91] However, when they applied this classification system to a study group of 37 patients with dens fractures, the level failed to be a helpful aid in predicting union.[90]

The anatomic level of injury has been shown to be a key factor in fracture healing and is the basis of the most widely used fracture classification.[2] In 1974, Anderson and D'Alonzo reported on 60 patients treated with odontoid fractures and described three levels of injury which corresponded to varying rates of healing (Fig. 16–6).[6] This classification remains the standard for early assessment and prognostication of potential fracture union.[1, 5, 7, 21, 22, 30, 49, 50, 51, 64, 81]

Type I fractures occur through the tip of the odontoid cephalad to the transverse ligament. The mechanism of injury may relate to severe rotational and lateral bending forces which cause avulsion of bone through the alar and apical ligaments.[26–28] Clinical association with occipitocervical dislocation has been reported.[29] However, in most clinical situations, type I injuries are "incidental" fractures and usually not associated with vertebral instability. However, a distraction injury must be ruled out before it can be assumed to be a relatively benign injury.

Type II injuries occur through the base of the odontoid, above the body of C2. These injuries are associated with the highest rates of nonunion. Reported nonunion rates range from 11%[49, 62] to 100%.[64] Significant variables affecting fracture union include patient age, fracture displacement (translation or angulation), and delay in diagnosis or institution of treatment. Distraction or comminution of the fracture site may also promote nonunion of type II fractures.[48, 85, 86]

Type III injuries propagate fracture through the body of C2 and have a larger fracture surface area of bleeding cancellous bone. This probably accounts for the relatively high union rates with immobilization, which may approach 100%.[49, 51, 98] However, Clark and White[22]

Figure 16–5 = Diagrams of embryologic development of the odontoid and body of C2. *A,* Anterior view. *B,* Lateral view. *(a)* One center (occasionally two) forms in the body by the fifth fetal month. *(b)* Neural arches appear bilaterally by the seventh fetal month. *(c)* The neural arches fuse posteriorly by the second or third year. *(d)* The spinous process is bifid and occasionally a secondary center is present in each tip. *(e)* The neurocentral synchondrosis fuses at 3 to 6 years. *(f)* The inferior epiphyseal ring appears at puberty and fuses at about 25 years. *(g)* "Summit" ossification center for the odontoid appears at 3 to 6 years and fuses with the odontoid by 12 years. *(h)* In the odontoid, two separate centers appear by the fifth fetal month and fuse with each other by the seventh fetal month. *(i)* The synchondrosis between the odontoid and the neural arch fuses at 3 to 6 years. *(k)* The posterior surface of the body and the odontoid. (Redrawn from Baily DK: The normal cervical spine in infants and children. Radiology 59:713, 1952.)

adult fracture patterns traverse the dens superior to facet joints, cephalad to the original growth plate region.

By the age of 7 years, fusion is usually complete and the only remaining evidence of a growth plate may be a small sclerotic line in the body of C2 visible on radiograph.[8] Bardeen in 1910 described a rudimentary island of cartilage in the body of the adult axis which can be demonstrated radiographically.[10] Plaut in 1938 also noted this finding and suggested that cartilage remnants could be found in a quarter of the population between the ages of 30 and 50 years.[82] These centers of ossification fuse at various periods in the child's life and can be confused with fractures, either acute or old.

The basilar odontoid cartilaginous plate is present at birth and begins to close by 3 years of age.[20] The basilar synchondrosis follows an irregular curved line within the body of the axis, and by the age of 12 years a sclerotic margin may be the only remaining remnant.

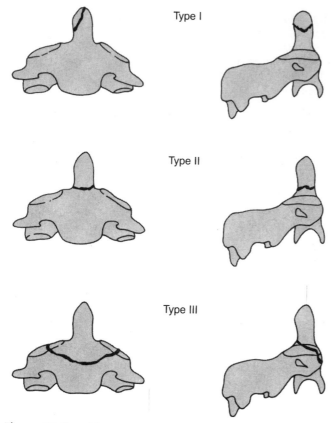

Type I

Type II

Type III

Figure 16–6 = Three types of odontoid fractures as seen in the anteroposterior and lateral planes. Type I is an oblique fracture through the upper part of the odontoid process itself. Type II is a fracture at the junction of the odontoid process with the vertebral body of the second cervical vertebra. Type III is really a fracture through the body of the atlas. (From Anderson LD, D'Alonzo RT: Fractures of the odontoid process of the axis. J Bone Joint Surg Am 56:1664, 1974.)

observed a higher rate of nonunion (13%) and malunion (15%) in type III injuries than previously reported. This underlines the need for careful assessment, early treatment, and proper fracture reduction and immobilization of type III injuries.

MECHANISM OF INJURY

Motor vehicle accidents and high-velocity trauma account for most injuries in the young adult population (age 16 to 34 years). Lower-velocity trauma, particularly falls, results in injury to older adults (age greater than 55 years) and children (age 0 to 15 years).[6, 7, 12, 21, 24, 25, 49, 64, 98] In the early 1900s, odontoid fractures were caused by falls and blows to the head.[12, 77] Later, motor vehicle accidents became the predominant cause of fractures, often concomitant with other injuries.[25, 49]

Various theories on the causes of odontoid fracture have suggested mechanisms such as avulsion, shear, compression, and lateral bending. Avulsion of the odontoid through stretched alar ligaments during hyperextension, hyperflexion, or extremes of rotation has been postulated as a cause of odontoid fractures.[4, 12, 13, 56, 109] Fritzche in 1912 produced fractures of the odon-

toid process imitating the forces involved in judicial hanging, suggesting avulsion through taut longitudinal ligaments.[12] However, Wusthoff found in cadaver specimens that the alar ligaments were loose in hyperextension.[109]

Several authors have experimentally produced odontoid fractures with lateral shear forces, which presumably act through the atlantal condyles, resulting in laterally displaced fractures.[2, 72] However, this model lacks clinical support.[53, 74, 90]

Most clinical cases of odontoid fractures occur through the base, leading investigators to postulate a pure AP shear mechanism of fracture.[90] Additionally, clinical findings of anterior and posterior fracture displacement are much more common than lateral displacement.[53, 74, 90] However, biomechanical studies displacing the atlas anteriorly on a fixed axis showed that in slow and rapid loading conditions the transverse ligament failed before odontoid failure. AP shear testing of the odontoid after ligament rupture showed the load to failure was never significantly less than the force that had been required to cause complete failure in all ligaments in the same specimen. In this testing mode, odontoid fracture did not typically occur through the base.[35] Other investigators have tested flexion, extension, lateral bend, and rotation-extension mechanisms without producing odontoid failure patterns consistent with clinical observation.[2, 72] These studies suggest a multifactorial mechanism of odontoid fracture involving axial compression, tension, AP flexion-extension, lateral bend, rotation, and shear forces.

PRESENTATION

As mentioned, motor vehicle accidents are the most common cause of adult odontoid fracture. Because the majority of these injuries are associated with high energy, it is not uncommon for the odontoid fracture to be initially undetected during the workup of more obvious injuries of the chest, abdomen, or other bone fractures. Facial trauma and altered mental status may mask the symptoms of upper cervical injury and delay diagnosis. Head injury associated with odontoid fracture may be high as 40% and complicates the initial assessment and treatment.[49, 51] A high level of suspicion should be entertained in any trauma victim with altered mental status, history of concussion, scalp lacerations, mandibular fracture, or other skull fracture. Since a high energy is required to fracture other vertebrae, high-velocity blunt trauma is a common denominator for chest and abdominal injuries and long bone fractures. Concern for an odontoid fracture should always be heightened when these injuries occur.

Children and older people incur odontoid fractures with low-velocity falls. Altered mental status in the old person is a common cause of diagnostic delay. Older people may fall; resultant gait disturbances and myelopathic findings are progressive and easily missed by caretakers.[23]

Eighteen percent of odontoid fractures present with other cervical spine injuries[49] (Fig. 16–7). Jefferson[57]

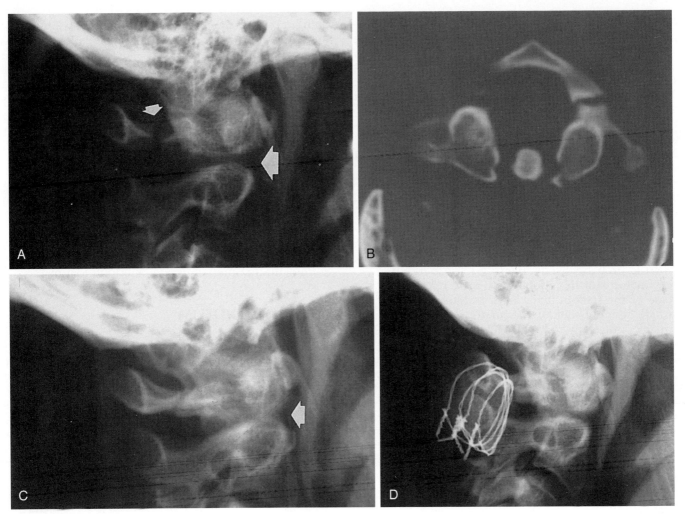

Figure 16–7 = Lateral radiograph *(A)* and CT scan *(B)* of a trauma patient with a type II odontoid fracture *(large arrow)* and concomitant arch fracture of the atlas *(small arrow)*. *C,* Halo vest treatment was instituted; 3 months post injury the atlas healed, but the odontoid fracture was ununited *(arrow)*. *D,* The fracture was stabilized with a modified Brooks-type fusion.

first noted the common association of atlas fractures with odontoid fractures and reported that 12 of 15 patients died within 5 weeks of injury. An increase in early mortality was also reported by Hanssen and Cabanela[51]: five of seven patients with combined atlas and type II odontoid fractures died shortly after trauma.

Symptomatic presentation may be limited even in the absence of altered consciousness. Pain referred to the head and neck region is a common complaint. Numbness and paresthesia in the distribution of the greater occipital nerve, as well as posterior cervical muscle spasms, should lead to closer investigation. Neurologic deficits, less common in fractures of the atlantoaxial complex than of the subaxial cervical spine, may present as complete quadriparesis or partial cord involvement. In a multicenter study by the Cervical Spine Research Society, 16 of 152 patients presented with neurologic deficits, including 11 quadriparetic, 3 hemiparetic, and 2 persons with Brown-Séquard syndrome.[22] Patients with posterior subluxation or displacement are at increased risk of cord injury, as well as higher mortality.[25] Lewallen and associates[61] reported a

higher risk for respiratory arrest in patients with posterior fracture displacement. Myelopathic symptoms such as spastic paresis, urinary and fecal incontinence, and dysphagia may be the initial presentation in otherwise undiagnosed odontoid fractures.[6, 23, 69, 77]

RADIOLOGY

Early fracture recognition is based on consistent application of high-quality radiographs in all suspected patients. A cervical spine trauma series is not complete without AP, lateral cervical, and open-mouth views. The majority of odontoid fractures are recognized on screening radiographs. Closed head injury, or other evidence of facial trauma, should prompt a search for cervical spine trauma.[49, 74] The prevertebral soft tissues should be examined, although prevertebral swelling may not be a common finding in isolated odontoid fractures. The pre-dens space or atlanto-dens interval (ADI) should be less than 3 mm in an adult and less than 4 mm in a child.[35, 37]

A V-shaped ADI is commonly found in normal

subjects. Monu and others[71] studied the ADI by measuring the angle between the posterior border of the anterior C1 ring and the anterior border of the dens in 202 normal lateral cervical spine radiographs. This space measured between 0 and 13 degrees in neutral position and 0 and 18 degrees in flexion, and was not a sign of injury or instability due to ligament rupture.[71] However, the ADI is an important radiographic indicator of the competence of the transverse atlantal ligament, which is the primary ligamentous stabilizer of the atlantoaxial joint.

Radiographic evaluation of the odontoid is often difficult due to the superimposition of shadows from the surrounding structures. Computed tomography (CT) allows excellent delineation of the three-dimensional anatomy of the odontoid and spinal canal. Conventional tomography or magnetic resonance imaging (MRI) is probably preferable to CT for identifying occult fractures of the odontoid, since CT images in the plane of the fracture may inadvertently miss the fracture. Sequential sagittal reformatting of CT images is possible, but many times lacks resolution.[11] The role of MRI in acute evaluation of the upper cervical spine is rapidly evolving. Some advantages include direct sagittal imaging, intramedullary spinal cord assessment, and excellent soft tissue resolution, including the transverse ligament.[66] CT scans are justified for preoperative planning of direct anterior screw fixation.[52] Preoperative CT of the odontoid may provide valuable information regarding the minimal internal bony diameter needed for direct anterior screw fixation.[52]

PEDIATRICS

Pediatric spine injuries make up less than 1% of all spine injuries. Owing to the large head-to-body size ratio in children, cervical spine injuries in children differ from those in adults. The fulcrum of injury is in the upper cervical spine in children compared to the lower subaxial spine in adults.[76, 96] Blockey and Purser[12] were the first to recognize that odontoid fractures in children less than 7 years of age were "different" from adult odontoid fractures. In children, the fracture line lies well below the level of the articular facets, as compared to the usual adult fracture pattern which is at or above the level of the facets (type II). These injuries are epiphyseal separations and heal well with external immobilization.[33, 96]

Odontoid fractures in young children, like those in older people, may be easily missed[20, 33, 37, 76, 84, 88, 94, 96] (Fig. 16–8). Seimon reported on two children less than 3 years of age who fell from heights as low as 61 cm and incurred odontoid fractures. The children complained of pain when moving from a sitting to a lying position, but when fully upright would play vigorously without complaint. Each child strongly resisted any attempt at extension of the neck and cried if passive assistance were not given when brought to either the erect or recumbent position.[94]

Sherk and associates,[96] in a review of 11 patients less than 7 years of age with odontoid fractures, found the injuries occurred as a result of either falls, motor vehicle accidents, or birth trauma. All fractures occurred through the cartilaginous plate and were displaced anteriorly. The cases were treated with reduction and bracing for 6 to 16 weeks. Healing occurred in all cases without growth disturbances or long-term sequelae.

Reduction and immobilization is the goal of early treatment.[84] Since the majority of fractures are anteriorly displaced, manipulative reduction usually involves an extension-type maneuver, placing the patient supine with the head extended until radiographic evidence of reduction is obtained. External immobilization in a halo vest or Minerva brace for 2 to 3 months is sufficient. Nonunion and avascular necrosis have not been reported in the younger age population, although some evidence suggests unrecognized fractures in young children may antecede os odontoideum.[93]

OS ODONTOIDEUM

Os odontoideum, a rounded, smooth ossicle, is found proximal to the base of the dens. It may be located either in the normal position of the odontoid process (orthotopic) or near the base of the occiput in the region of the foramen magnum (dystopic).[92] Firmly embedded within the transverse atlantoaxial ligament, it translates over the axis creating the potential risk of spinal cord injury. The usual radiographic findings demonstrate an ossified fragment with smooth, uniform margins separated from the axis, with a wide zone of radiolucency above the level of the superior facets of the axis (Fig. 16–9). The anterior arch of the atlas may also be hypertrophied.[36] The incidence of os odontoideum is unknown and presentation is relatively uncommon. It was first described by Giacomini in 1886.[43] A bony ossicle was observed within the ligaments extending from the occiput to the body of the axis in a postmortem examination of a patient with cretinism. This evidence, combined with the comparative anatomic features of other vertebrates, led early investigators and anatomists to suggest a developmental or congenital cause.[68, 107]

More recent evidence supports an acquired or post-traumatic cause of os odontoideum.[34, 36, 38, 39, 83, 93, 102] Although os odontoideum has been associated with Klippel-Feil syndrome, myelodysplasia, epiphyseal dysplasia, and Down's syndrome, the relatively low incidence of os odontoideum associated with congenital abnormalities argues against this.[107] Fielding and Griffin,[36] in the largest reported series of os odontoideum, presented nine patients with radiographically documented normal odontoid processes prior to the development of the os odontoideum. Schuler and others[93] documented the occurrence of os odontoideum in a 2-year-old and correlated it with a traumatic event.

Os odontoideum may present incidentally on a routine cervical spine series or with signs of spinal cord impingement associated with abnormal upper cervical spine motion. The atlantoaxial instability associated with os odontoideum usually necessitates operative

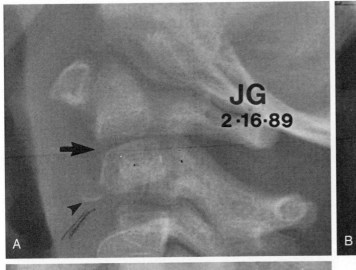

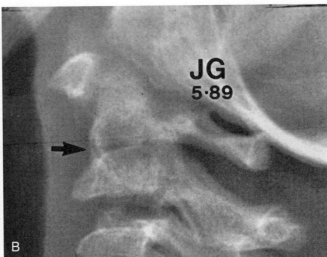

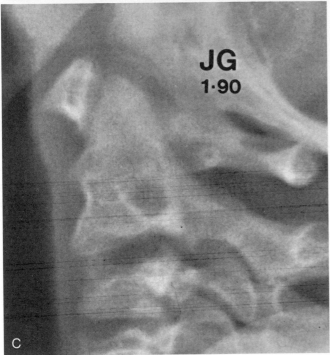

Figure 16–8 = Odontoid fracture sustained by a 2-year-old after a minor fall. The child cried vigorously when changed from supine to sitting, and supported his head with his hands. *A,* Lateral radiograph taken shortly after injury showing prevertebral soft tissue swelling, bone avulsed from the anterior inferior corner of the C2 body *(arrowhead),* and a neurocentral synchondrosis that seemed more apparent than normal *(arrow). B,* Lateral radiograph taken 3 months after injury showing osseous bridging of the anterior neurocentral synchondrosis *(arrow). C,* Lateral radiograph 1 year after injury revealing complete healing of the avulsion from the C2 body, normal soft tissue planes, and premature closure of the synchondrosis.

intervention to obtain stability. Posterior atlantoaxial fusion is the procedure of choice in these patients.

ADULT TREATMENT

Type I

Type I fractures occur through ligamentous avulsion of the tip of the odontoid. Clinically these injuries are often incidental and not usually associated with instability. In reviews of treatment, several recent studies have not included these injuries.[22, 25] Anderson and D'Alonzo[6] reported on two type I fractures which both healed without problems. Treatment usually involves external immobilization for symptomatic relief and a careful radiographic examination to rule out associated cervical spine fractures or dislocations. Even if union

does not occur, the clinical results are usually satisfactory and the patient asymptomatic. If the avulsion injury occurs in conjunction with a craniocervical distraction, then surgical stabilization of the level is necessary.

Type II

Type II fractures occur through the base of the odontoid process, distal to the entry site of the nutrient vessels. With nonoperative treatment, nonunion rates are consistently high and may approach 100% under certain circumstances (Fig. 16–10).* Variables of proven significance in fracture nonunion include displacement (translation or angulation), ability to achieve and maintain a reduction, patient age, and delayed diagnosis

---

*References 5–7, 12, 22, 25, 48–51, 64, 81, 91, 98, and 104.

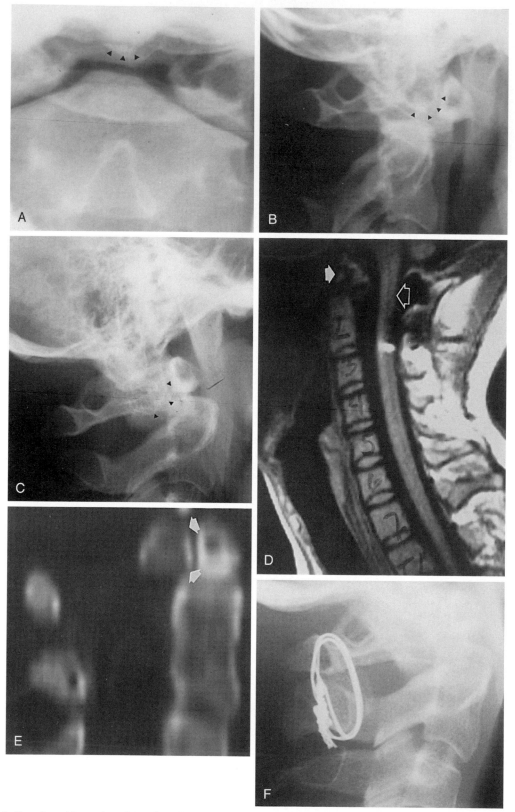

Figure 16–9 = *A,* Os odontoideum found incidentally in a 26-year-old man involved in a motor vehicle accident. The rounded, smooth ossicle *(arrowheads)* is proximal to the base of the dens and separated by a zone of radiolucency. *B* and *C,* Lateral flexion and extension radiographs demonstrate atlantoaxial instability which may result in neurologic compromise *(arrowheads* show ossicle). *D,* Magnetic resonance imaging reveals the position of the ossicle *(white arrow)* in relation to the spinal cord *(black arrow). E,* The lateral reconstruction view of this computed tomographic scan shows the malalignment of the os odontoideum *(arrows)* and its close relationship to the anterior arch of C1. *F,* Stabilization with posterior atlantoaxial fusion.

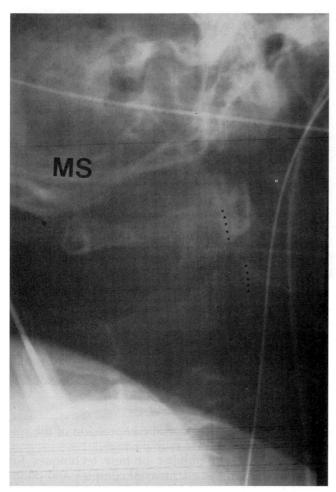

Figure 16–10 = Lateral radiograph of type II odontoid fracture in a trauma patient with 15 lb of traction. In this fracture, both the 5 mm of posterior displacement and the distraction of the fracture gap may predispose to fracture nonunion.

or treatment. Factors of probable significance include fracture comminution[48, 85] and distraction.[86] No single study in the literature documents all of these factors, thus perpetuating some controversy.

A strong case can be made relating the initial degree of fracture malalignment with nonunion rates. It has not been definitely shown that the direction of displacement has an independent influence; however, it is strongly suggested by several studies. Apuzzo and co-workers[7] noted all fracture dislocations greater than 4 mm were associated with a significant incidence of nonunion. Schatzker and colleagues[90] found nonunion in 72% of displaced fractures compared to 42% in nondisplaced fractures. Those with posterior displacement had higher nonunion rates. Hadley and co-authors[49] noted a 26% nonunion rate in all type I fractures, which increased to 67% with displacement greater than 6 mm. No association with direction was found.[49] However, Dunn and Seljeskog[25] found no increase in nonunion with anterior subluxation, while all posterior subluxations greater than 3 mm went on to nonunion. These authors recommended early posterior cervical fusion for patients over 65 years old with type II fractures and posterior displacement greater than 2 mm.[25] This

finding was corroborated by Hanssen and Cabanella[51] who found 50% nonunion in posterior displacement and 75% in those patients with greater than 5 mm of displacement. The Cervical Spine Research Society's multicenter study found an overall nonunion rate for type II fractures of 32%. Displacement of 5 mm or more and angulation of 10 degrees or more was significantly correlated with nonunion or malunion.[22]

Many authors have investigated older age as an independent variable in fracture union. Though a number of studies have demonstrated a statistically significant difference between age groups, the age categories have varied. Poorer union rates have been found for patients over 40,[7, 81] 55,[30] 60,[49, 90] 65,[25] and 70 years of age.[51] Clark and White[22] failed to note a significant difference between patients over or under 40 years of age.

Studies of type II fractures document especially poor union rates in patients with late diagnosis and treatment.[12] Frequent causes include a partial history and physical examination, particularly in multiple trauma patients, and incomplete initial radiographic evaluations.[25] Patients with systemic diseases such as rheumatoid arthritis, alcoholism, osteoarthritis, and osteoporosis frequently have late diagnosis.[24] Early posterior fusion has been advocated for patients presenting 7 to 14 days post injury.[24, 25]

The initial patient assessment is important to determine who is appropriate for nonoperative treatment, which should be reserved for early recognized injury in the young patient with minimal fracture displacement on screening radiographs. Immobilization of the upper cervical spine is difficult with standard external cervical orthoses. Halo vest immobilization provides the best means for early fracture stability. Skeletal traction should be kept to a minimum since small amounts of weight may significantly displace the fracture.[86] Successful nonoperative treatment is dependent on maintenance of a nondisplaced fracture alignment. The halo vest is not a fail-safe means of immobilization; unwanted distraction forces may cause loss of reduction.[58] Radiographic evaluation after patient mobilization should be routine (Fig. 16–11). Patients with unstable fracture patterns or those who lose initial reductions should be considered for surgery.

Operative stabilization, either posterior C1–2 fusion or anterior screw fixation, has been shown to be the treatment of choice for unstable type II fractures, those with displacement exceeding 4 mm or 10 degrees of angulation, comminuted fractures, and atypical oblique fractures in the coronal plane. Primary operative stabilization is indicated in (1) odontoid fractures associated with polytrauma, closed head injury, and spinal cord injury; (2) odontoid fractures in elderly and debilitated patients with accentuated thoracic kyphosis and limited cervical extension; (3) fractures in debilitated patients with altered mental status or difficult skin care problems requiring extended nursing support; (4) odontoid fractures with a concomitant unstable Jefferson fracture or comminution of the atlantoaxial joints; (5) pathologic fractures associated with osteomy-

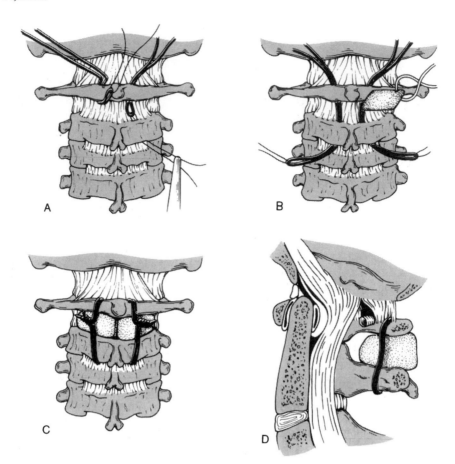

Figure 16–13 = *A,* The occipital nerves emerge through the interlaminar space between the atlas and the axis; the vertebral arteries are more lateral. With a midline approach, the arteries and nerves are fairly well protected by the neck muscles. *B,* On the left a suture is passed under the posterior arch of the atlas. On the right the suture is used to guide the wire under the arch of the atlas and the lamina of the atlas. *C,* The wires are now in place and lie anterior to the anterior portion of the atlantoaxial membrane, which was not removed during exposure of the posterior elements of the atlas and axis. On the right the graft, with edges beveled to fit in the interval between the atlas and axis, is being held with a towel clip. When wired in place, the beveled edges will be in contact with the arch of the atlas and the lamina of the m axis. *D,* The grafts are secured, and stability is maintained by the wires. (From Jarrett JP, Whitesides TE Jr: Injuries of the cervicocranium. *In* Browner BD, Jupiter JB, Levine AM, et al (eds): Skeletal Trauma: Fractures, Dislocations, and Ligamentous Injuries, vol 1. Philadelphia, WB Saunders, 1992, p 689.)

tion, including hypoglossal nerve irritation from excessive screw length, instability from lack of screws crossing the joint, and screw breakage. In this series the rate of pseudarthrosis was extremely low, 0.6%.[47]

Direct anterior screw fixation has the advantage of preservation of motion at C1–2 and early postoperative fracture stability.[15, 55] Clinical studies have shown this to be an efficacious technique in the experienced hands. Early results reported with this technique show a significant learning curve with major complications. With surgical familiarity and experience, later results revealed a significant improvement in patient outcomes.[1, 22]

Indications for direct anterior screw fixation include acute type II and "shallow" type III fractures. Both displaced and nondisplaced fractures are considered indications for anterior screw fixation due to the high incidence of nonunion in type II fractures. Patients with unstable posterior arch (C1) fractures are also good candidates. Relative contraindications are comminuted odontoid fractures, concomitant unstable C1 ring fractures,[56, 57] atypical oblique coronal plane fractures

which begin in the anteroinferior portion of the C2 vertebral body and then extend posteriorly and superiorly, fractures unreducible with closed manipulation, and nonunions with poor bone quality.[32]

Technical factors which prohibit screw alignment include older patients with thoracic kyphosis or limited cervical motion, short-necked patients with a prominent anterior chest wall structure, and fracture configurations where reduction can only be maintained with head flexion.

For anterior screw placement, patient positioning is critical. The head fixed with Gardner-Wells tongs or a halo is maximally extended without fracture displacement for surgical access (Fig. 16–17). A right-sided incision above the level of the cricoid cartilage facilitates exposure for the right-handed surgeon.[99] The sternal-mandibular distance should be maximized for K wire passage in the appropriate trajectory. This can be checked by placing a long K wire on the skin parallel to the trajectory of the intended screw. The retropharyngeal space is accessed through a standard Smith-Robinson approach. A K wire is started at the inferior

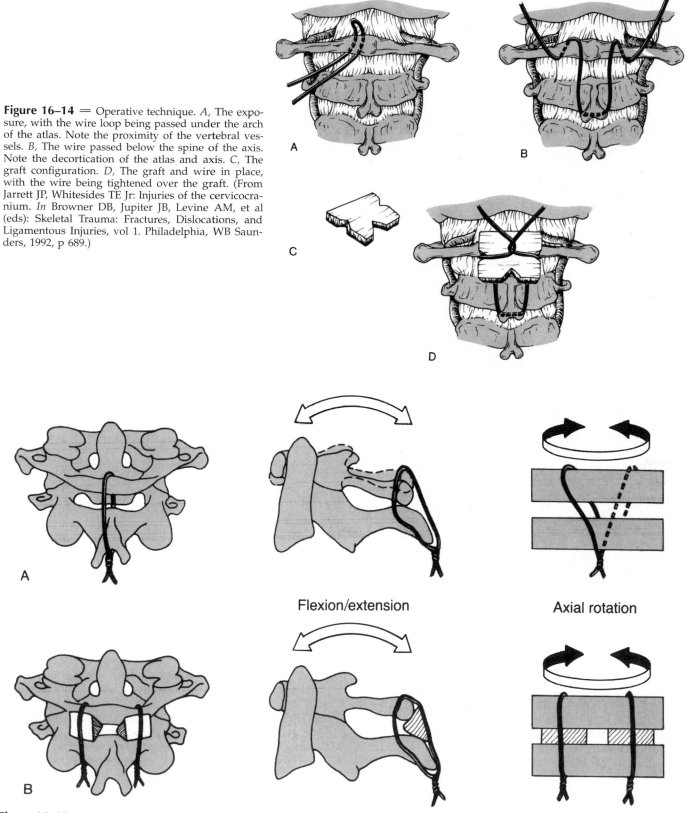

Figure 16–14 = Operative technique. *A,* The exposure, with the wire loop being passed under the arch of the atlas. Note the proximity of the vertebral vessels. *B,* The wire passed below the spine of the axis. Note the decortication of the atlas and axis. *C,* The graft configuration. *D,* The graft and wire in place, with the wire being tightened over the graft. (From Jarrett JP, Whitesides TE Jr: Injuries of the cervicocranium. *In* Browner DB, Jupiter JB, Levine AM, et al (eds): Skeletal Trauma: Fractures, Dislocations, and Ligamentous Injuries, vol 1. Philadelphia, WB Saunders, 1992, p 689.)

Flexion/extension

Axial rotation

Figure 16–15 = Biomechanical advantages of the Brooks construct. *A,* A single midline wiring. The construct would be relatively stable in flexion; in extension, however, there would be little stability because the two rings would readily approximate. In axial rotation there is nothing to resist the relative horizontal displacement between the ring of C1 and that of C2. *B,* With the Brooks construct there is stability in both flexion and extension. Flexion is restrained by tension in the circumferential wires, and extension is restrained by the bone graft, which serves as a buttressing block. Rotation is resisted by some combination of wire tension and bone block, but this time the mechanism is one of friction. The bone grafts compressed between the two posterior rings serve as friction blocks and offer stability against axial rotation. (From White AA III, Panjabi MM: Clinical Biomechanics of the Spine. Philadelphia, JB Lippincott, 1990.)

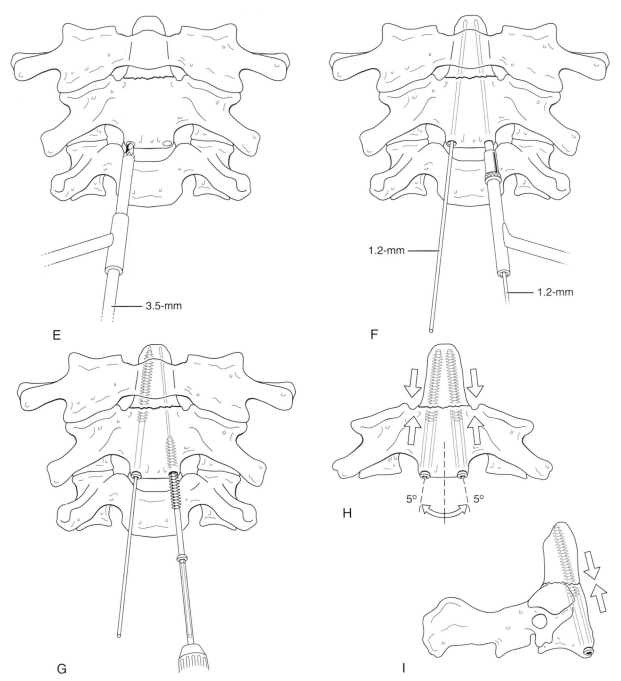

Figure 16–17 *Continued = E–G,* This can be accomplished with a cannulated set as well. *H* and *I,* Final screw fixation should have the screw slightly oblique toward the midline and optionally may perforate the cortex of the tip of the dens. Care should be taken to begin the screw on the undersurface and not the anterior surface of the C2 body to achieve the proper trajectory *(I).* (*A* redrawn from Grob D, Magerl F: Operative Stabilisirrung bei Frakturen von C1 and C2. Orthopade 16-48, 1987; *B–I* redrawn from Müller ME, Allgöwer M, Schneider R, et al (eds): Manual of Internal Fixation Techniques Recommended by the AO-ASIF Group, ed 3. Berlin, Springer-Verlag, 1991, pp 638–641.)

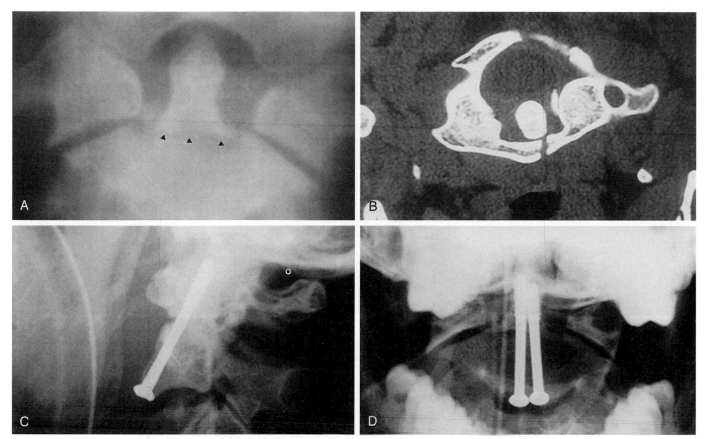

Figure 16–18 = *A* and *B,* Polytrauma patient presented with a type II odontoid fracture (*arrowheads* show fracture through base of odontoid), 4 mm of posterior displacement, and a concomitant C1 fracture with an intact transverse ligament. *C,* Through an anterior surgical approach fracture stabilization was accomplished with two smooth partially threaded pins started at the anterior inferior border of C2. *D,* The fracture is shown securely lagged with two 4.0-mm cannulated screws. The patient was immobilized in a Philadelphia collar.

authors recommend using 2.7-mm screws for smaller odontoid processes.[1, 32] The literature is clear that this technique should not be pursued by those casually associated with spine surgery who have not studied the techniques and contraindications. Complications of spinal cord injury, cranial nerve injury, and loss of fixation have been described and are directly related to early experience on the learning curve and inappropriate use of this technique.[1, 32, 70, 108]

Type III

Type III fractures are differentiated by extension of the fracture line into the body of C2. The incidence is less than half that of type II fractures. Like type II fractures, the exact mechanism of injury has not been completely elucidated. However, anterior displacement is more commonly seen, suggesting flexion-type forces.[22, 49, 72] Associated trauma, closed head injury, concomitant cervical spine fractures at other levels, and neurologic compromise are similar to the findings in type II fractures.[22, 49, 50, 51, 53] Type III fractures have consistently demonstrated a more favorable prognosis than type II injuries (see Fig. 16–12). Nonunion rates vary from 0% to 15%.* Reduction followed by halo

---

*References 5–7, 19, 22, 25, 30, 41, 49–51, 62, 64, 81, 86, 98, and 104.

immobilization is the mainstay of treatment (Fig. 16–19). Although the majority of these fractures heal with halo immobilization, Clark and White,[22] in a multicenter study, found a 15% malunion rate and a similar rate of nonunion. The poor results were associated with the use of cervical orthoses rather than halo vest immobilization.

CONCLUSIONS

1. Clinical suspicion and appropriate radiographic evaluation combine to facilitate early fracture treatment and improved long-term prognosis.
2. Pediatric (age 7 years or younger) odontoid fractures differ from adult fractures and usually heal with nonoperative treatment.
3. Type II fractures have an increased risk of progression to nonunion. Factors associated with susceptibility to nonunion include (1) lack of early recognition and treatment, (2) fracture displacement, (3) posterior displacement of 4 mm or greater, (4) unstable type II and type III fractures with redislocation, and (5) patient age.
4. Odontoid fracture nonunion is commonly associated with late progressive myelopathy and should be treated definitively rather than with "benign neglect."

69. Mixter SJ, Osgood RB: Traumatic lesions of the atlas and axis. Ann Surg 51:193, 1910.

70. Montesano PX, Anderson PA, Schlehr F, et al: Odontoid fractures treated by anterior odontoid screw fixation. Spine 16:S33, 1991.

71. Monu J, Bohrer SP, Howard G: Some upper cervical spine norms. Spine 12:515, 1987.

72. Mouradian WH, Fietti VG, Cochran GVB, et al: Fractures of the odontoid: A laboratory and clinical study of mechanisms. Orthop Clin North Am 9:985, 1978.

73. Müller ME, Allgöwer M, Schneider R, et al: Manual of Internal Fixation: Techniques Recommended by the AO-ASIF Group. Berlin, Springer-Verlag, 1991.

74. Nachemnson A: Fracture of the odontoid process of the axis. A clinical study based on 26 cases. Acta Orthop Scand 29:185, 1960.

75. Nakanishi T: Internal fixation of odontoid fracture [in Japanese]. Orthop Trauma Surg 23:399, 1980.

76. Ogden JA: Radiology of postnatal skeletal development XII. The second vertebra. Skeletal Radiol 12:169, 1984.

77. Osgood RB, Lund CC: Fractures of the odontoid process. N Engl J Med 198:2:61, 1928.

78. Paramore CG, Dickman CA, Sonntag VK: The anatomic suitability of the C1–C2 complex for posterior transarticular screw fixation. Presented to 23rd Annual Meeting of the Cervical Spine Research Society, Santa Fe, Nov 30–Dec 2, 1995, paper No. 20.

79. Parke WW: The vascular relations of the upper cervical vertebrae. Orthop Clin North Am 9:879, 1978.

80. Penning L, Wilmink JT: Rotation of the cervical spine. A CT study in normal subjects. Spine 12:732, 1987.

81. Pepin JW, Bourne RB, Hawkins RJ: Odontoid fractures, with special reference to the elderly patient. Clin Orthop 193:178, 1985.

82. Plaut HF: Fractures of the atlas resulting from automobile accidents. AJR 40:867, 1938.

83. Ricciardi JE, Kaufer H, Louis DS: Acquired os odontoideum following acute ligament injury. J Bone Joint Surg Am 58:410, 1976.

84. Ries MD, Ray S: Posterior displacement of an odontoid fracture in a child. Spine 11:1043, 1986.

85. Roy-Camille R, Saillant G, Marie-Anne S, et al: Prognosis elements in odontoid process fractures. Orthop Trans 4:45, 1980.

86. Ryan MD, Taylor TKF: Odontoid fractures. A rational approach to treatment. J Bone Joint Surg Br 64:416, 1982.

87. Sasso R, Doherty BJ, Crawford MJ, et al: Biomechanics of odontoid fracture fixation. Comparison of the one- and two-screw technique. Spine 18:1950, 1993.

88. Savader SJ, Martinez C, Murtagh FR: Odontoid fracture in a nine-month-old infant. Surg Neurol 24:529, 1985.

89. Schaffler MB, Alson MB, Heller JG, et al: Morphology of the dens: A quantitative study. Spine 17:738, 1992.

90. Schatzker J, Rorabeck CH, Waddell JP: Fractures of the dens (odontoid process). An analysis of thirty-seven cases. J Bone Joint Surg Br 53:392, 1971.

91. Schatzker J, Rorabeck CH, Waddell JP: Non-union of the odontoid process. Clin Orthop 108:127, 1975.

92. Schiff DCM, Parke WW,: The arterial supply of the odontoid process. J Bone Joint Surg Am 55:1450, 1973.

93. Schuler TC, Kurz L, Thompson DE, et al: Natural history of os odontoideum: A case report. J Pediatr Orthop 11:222, 1991.

94. Seimon LP: Fracture of the odontoid process in young children. J Bone Joint Surg Am 59:943, 1977.

95. Sherk HH: Fractures of the atlas and odontoid. Orthop Clin North Am 9:973, 1987.

96. Sherk HH, Nicholson JT, Chung SMK: Fractures of the odontoid process in young children. J Bone Joint Surg Am 60:921, 1978.

97. Sherk HH, Snyder BJ: An exceptional case analysis of posterior upper neck fusions. Orthop Trans 3:125, 1979.

98. Southwick WO: Current concepts review. Management of fractures of the dens (odontoid process). J Bone Joint Surg Am 62:482, 1980.

99. Southwick WO, Robinson RA: Surgical approaches to the vertebral bodies in the cervical and lumbar regions. J Bone Joint Surg Am 40:631, 1957.

100. Stauffer ES: Wiring techniques of the posterior cervical spine for the treatment of trauma. Orthopaedics 11:1543, 1988.

101. Steel HH: Anatomical and mechanical considerations of the atlantoaxial articulations. J Bone Joint Surg Am 50:1481, 1968.

102. Stillwell WT, Fielding JW: Acquired os odontoideum: A case report. Clin Orthop 135:71, 1978.

103. Tulsi RS: Some specific anatomical features of the atlas and axis: Dens, epitransverse process and articular facets. Aust N Z J Surg 48:570, 1978.

104. Wang G-J, Mabie KN, Whitehill R, et al: Nonsurgical management of odontoid fractures in adults. Spine 9:229, 1984.

105. White AA, Panjabi MM: The clinical biomechanics of the occipitoatlantoaxial complex. Orthop Clin North Am 9:867, 1978.

106. Williams P, Warwick R: Gray's Anatomy, ed 36. Philadelphia, WB Saunders, 1980.

107. Wollin DG: The os odontoideum. J Bone Joint Surg Am 45:1459, 1963.

108. Wörsdörfer O, Araud M, Neugebauer R: Problems of anterior screw fixation of odontoid process failures. Presented at the Second Common Meeting of the European and American Section of the Cervical Spine Research Society, Marseille, France, June 12–15, 1988.

109. Wusthoff R: Über die Luxations fraktur im unteren Kopfgelek, Atlas-Epistrophus-Gelenk. Dtsch 2 Chir 183:73, 1923.

CHAPTER 17

Atlantoaxial Rotatory Deformities

Bradford L. Currier

ANATOMY

The occipital condyles sit in the cup-shaped superior articular facets of the atlas. The orientation of the joints allows a large degree of rotation in the sagittal plane (flexion and extension) but only about 5 degrees of rotation to each side.[22] The inferior articular facets of the atlas and the superior facets of the axis are slightly convex. The geometry of these joints allows a great deal of motion at the expense of stability.[25] In addition to the facet joints, a synovial cavity exists between the anterior arch of the atlas and the dens and another between the dens and the transverse ligament. The C1–2 synovial joints may be isolated structures or have intercommunications.[12] Approximately 50% of the rotation of the cervical spine occurs at the C1–2 joint.[25] In a cadaver study performed by Dvorak and colleagues,[22] 32 degrees of rotation in each direction was possible when all ligamentous structures were intact. In a computed tomographic (CT) evaluation of normal adults, the mean rotation at C1–2 was approximately 43 degrees (range, 32 to 50 degrees).[20] On the basis of these data and on the CT evaluation of 43 patients with suspected rotatory instability, Dvorak and co-workers[20] concluded that more than 8 degrees of rotation at C0–1 or 56 degrees at C1–2 or a right-left difference of more than 5 degrees at C0–1 or 8 degrees at C1–2 represents hypermobility. Approximately 65 degrees of rotation is required for complete atlantoaxial rotatory dislocation.[12, 34, 55] Only minimal flexion, extension, and lateral bending occur at the atlantoaxial level.

The ligamentous structures of the occipitoatlantoaxial complex have been studied extensively (Fig. 17–1).[40] The cruciform ligament consists of the transverse ligament running horizontally and the longitudinal fasciculi oriented vertically. The transverse ligament arises from the medial aspect of each lateral mass of the atlas and passes behind the dens, which acts as a pivot point during rotation. The transverse ligament holds the dens in place and maintains the space available for the spinal cord behind the dens, especially during flexion.

The alar ligaments consist of two portions: one part extends between the sides of the dens and the occipital condyles, and the other portion connects the dens with the lateral masses of the atlas (Fig. 17–2).[21, 23] The alar ligaments are the primary restraints to axial rotation and side bending in the C0–2 complex, and accessory support is provided by the tectorial membrane, accessory atlantoaxial ligaments, and joint capsules.[21]

The capsular ligaments are loose coverings of the C1–2 facet joints that contain synovial fluid and function mechanically to limit rotation.[13] The greater occipital nerves are located in close approximation to the C1–2 capsules on each side.

Steel[70] demonstrated that the internal diameter of the ring of the atlas is approximately 3 cm; the spinal cord and odontoid each are about 1 cm in diameter. Thus, there is approximately 1 cm of "free space." This concept has become known as "Steel's rule of thirds," and it suggests that anterior displacement of the atlas on the axis exceeding 1 cm can damage the cord.[69, 70] The canal can be narrowed by rotation also. The dens is the pivot point for C1–2 rotation. It is located centrally in the coronal plane, but it is eccentrically placed in the sagittal plane. During rotation, the ring of C1 swings across the vertebral foramen of C2, narrowing the spinal canal.[12, 25] Coutts[12] noted that an average-sized canal is narrowed to 7 mm when C1 is rotated on C2 to the point of complete dislocation (65 degrees). He also recognized that when the transverse ligament is incompetent, allowing anterior shift of the atlas, less rotation is required to result in significant canal compromise. Fielding and Reddy[30] estimated that the combination of 7 mm of anterior atlantal shift and 50 degrees of rotation would lead to fatal cord compression.

Normally, the space between the odontoid and the anterior ring of C1 is small. This distance, called the atlantodental interval (ADI), measures up to 3 mm in adults[27, 70] and 4 mm[50, 70] or 4.5 mm[41] in children. Locke and others[50] described a normal, asymptomatic child with an ADI of 5 mm.

The vertebral arteries assume a tortuous course between the atlas and axis but are tethered in the foramen transversarium of each vertebra. Normal rotation does not impair the circulation in these vessels, but excessive atlantoaxial displacement, especially anteriorly, may compromise blood flow. Fielding and Hawkins[25, 28] and Schneider and Crosby[67] speculated that such vascular compromise could lead to brain stem or cerebellar infarction and death (Fig. 17–3).

A direct connection between the lymphatic drainage of the pharynx and the upper cervical spine was described in the 1930s,[3, 12] but the anatomic details of the connections were not understood until recently. Parke

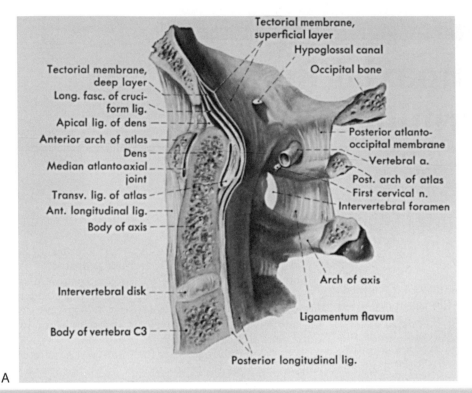

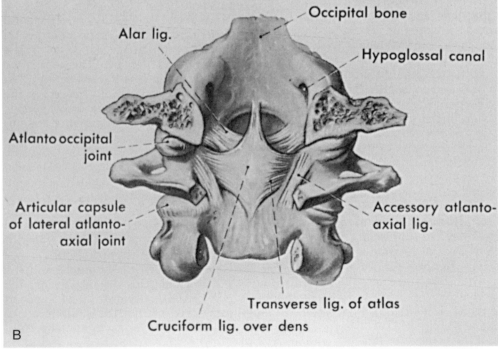

Figure 17–1 = *A*, Upper cervical spine and skull in median longitudinal section. *B*, Upper cervical spine and skull viewed from the posterior aspect after removal of the arches, the tectorial membrane, and the posterior longitudinal ligament. (From Hollinshead WH: Anatomy for Surgeons: The Back and Limbs, ed 3, vol 3. New York, Harper & Row, 1982.)

and colleagues[62] performed injection studies of the valveless epidural sinuses of human perinatal cadavers. They demonstrated retrograde filling of a series of veins that had numerous lymphatic anastomoses and appeared to drain the posterosuperior pharyngeal region. They called these the *pharyngovertebral veins* (Fig. 17–4).

BIOMECHANICS

The primary restraint to anterior atlantoaxial subluxation is the transverse ligament. In a biomechanical study, Fielding and associates[27] demonstrated that the ADI never exceeded 3 mm in adults before rupture of the transverse ligament. After rupture of the transverse ligament, the ADI measured 3 to 5 mm. They found that the alar ligaments are secondary restraints to forward displacement of the atlas, and when the ADI measured 10 to 12 mm, all restraints, including the alar ligaments, were ruptured. The tensile strength of the transverse ligament is greater than that of the alar ligaments.[23, 27] Fielding and co-workers[27] found that if the transverse ligament is ruptured, the alar ligaments

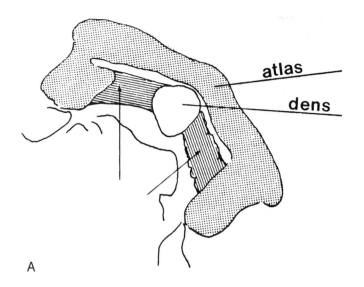

A

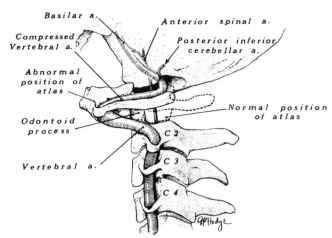

Figure 17–3 ═ Lateral view of the occipitocervical complex demonstrates compression of vertebral artery by atlantoaxial dislocation. The artery may be compressed at the C1 intervertebral foramen or the point at which the occipital condyle slides over the groove in the C1 lamina. (From Schneider RC, Crosby EC: Vascular insufficiency of brain stem and spinal cord in spinal trauma. Neurology 9:643, 1959.)

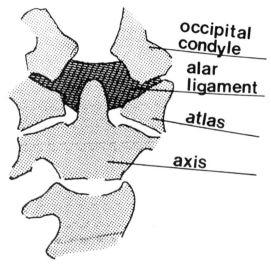

B

Figure 17–2 ═ Alar ligaments. *A*, Axial view with rotation of head to the left. *B*, Coronal view. (From Dvorak J, Panjabi M, Gerber M, et al: CT-functional diagnostics of the rotatory instability of the upper cervical spine: I. An experimental study on cadavers. Spine 12:197, 1987.)

the transverse diameter of the dens. The alar ligaments, therefore, cannot function as secondary restraints to further anterior C1–2 translation until all of the "free space" of the spinal canal at C1 has been occupied by the dens.[70] Coutts[12] found that the alar ligaments become taut and limit rotation beyond 45 degrees. If the head is tilted laterally, however, the distance between the occipital condyle and the dens is diminished and the alar ligament is relaxed, and rotation can continue up to 65 degrees.[7, 12]

Goel and others[34] showed that very small loads are required to produce large degrees of rotation at C0–2;

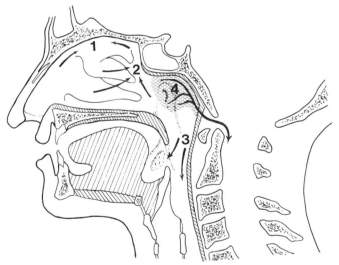

Figure 17–4 ═ Venous drainage of the nasal cavity, nasopharynx, and oral pharynx. The posterior nasopharyngeal region (*stippled area*, 4) drains by way of the pharyngovertebral veins through the pharyngobasilar fascia and anterior atlanto-occipital membrane to communicate with the periodontoidal plexus and epidural veins. (From Parke WW, Rothman RH, Brown MD: The pharyngovertebral veins: An anatomical rationale for Grisel's syndrome. J Bone Joint Surg Am 66:568, 1984.)

are inadequate to prevent further significant displacement when a force similar to that which caused transverse ligament rupture is applied.

The primary function of the alar ligaments is to prevent excessive rotation (see Fig. 17–2). The secondary restraints to rotation include the tectorial membrane, the accessory atlantoaxial ligaments, and the joint capsules (see Fig. 17–1).[21] Each alar ligament primarily limits rotation to the opposite side, but the ligaments do not work independently. Transection of either ligament results in a significant increase in rotation to both sides.[61] To allow a wide range of rotation, the alar ligaments must be lax in neutral rotation.[34, 60, 70, 81] The laxity of the alar ligaments necessary for rotation is taken up when the occiput and atlas move anteriorly relative to the odontoid, a distance equal to

this finding suggests that the neck muscles are the primary stabilizers in the physiologic range of motion. Axial torque increases after the first 20 degrees of rotation until the point of maximal resistance, which corresponds to complete rotatory dislocation of C1–2. Up until the point of dislocation, Goel and co-workers[34] found that both capsular ligaments and the alar ligament on the side opposite the rotation were only mildly stretched, and spontaneous reduction occurred after release of the rotational load. If the specimens were loaded well beyond that point, alar ligament avulsion and C1–2 capsular ligament rupture occurred, and spontaneous reduction did not occur. The transverse ligament and C0–1 capsular ligaments did not rupture even with maximal rotational loading.

Lateral flexion of the head is coupled with rotation of C2 such that the spinous process of C2 is deviated to the side opposite the direction of head tilt. This conjoined motion occurs as a result of the coronally oblique contour of the articular processes between C2 and C3. During lateral flexion, the inferior facet on the concave side glides downward and backward, whereas the facet on the convex side slides upward and forward, producing rotation as well as tilt.[25] Werne[81] found that when the head is tilted to one side, the opposite alar ligament becomes taut. With further attempts at lateral bending, the dens rotates and thereby tightens the other alar ligament. Motion is inhibited only after both alar ligaments are tight. These findings were confirmed by Panjabi and colleagues,[60] who also demonstrated that the alar ligaments limit flexion at both the C0–1 joints and the C1–2 joints. The alar ligaments are most taut and therefore most at risk of rupture when the head is rotated and flexed.[23]

The capsular ligaments have a secondary role in preventing excessive atlantoaxial rotation and lateral tilt. Disruption of the capsular ligaments alone should not lead to rotational dislocation.[13]

ATLANTOAXIAL ROTATORY DEFORMITY

The first reported case of atlantoaxial rotatory deformity (AARD) was described by Sir Charles Bell in 1830.[2] His patient suffered a dislocation of the atlas as a result of a deep ulcer involving the posterior pharynx that "destroyed the transverse ligament." Since that time, numerous names have been given to the condition, including rotatory dislocation of the atlas,[11] maladie de Grisel,[17] nontraumatic dislocation of the atlantoaxial joint,[3] spontaneous hyperemic dislocation of the atlas,[80] and atlantoaxial rotatory fixation,[28] to name a few. Although all of these disorders share certain radiographic and clinical features, the names proposed often represented an attempt to describe a subset of the condition or to help describe the suspected pathophysiology.

A spectrum of disorders can be considered AARDs. They may be classified anatomically by the degree of rotation or subluxation, clinically by the duration of disease or response to treatment, or by the cause of the condition.

Corner[11] suggested an anatomic classification of rotatory deformities. The term *atlantoaxial dislocation* should be reserved for the infrequent occurrence of complete dislocation of the C1–2 facet joints.[11, 33, 35, 43, 59] The more common situation involves a temporary or permanent rotational deformity of the C1–2 joints within their physiologic range of motion. Fielding and Hawkins[28] recommended that the term *atlantoaxial rotatory displacement* be used to describe the condition, rather than terms such as atlantoaxial rotatory subluxation, dislocation, or instability. The joints are not truly subluxated or dislocated, and unless there is concomitant transverse ligament laxity, there is no instability.

AARDs may also be classified by the degree of anterior translation of the atlas on the axis allowed by incompetence of the transverse ligament[28] or by the direction of rotation of the C1–2 joints.[3] These schemes are described in detail in the section on classification.

Rotatory deformities may be classified on the basis of the clinical course of the disease. Fielding and Hawkins[28] introduced the term *atlantoaxial rotatory fixation* to describe the condition in which the deformity is fixed and is refractory to nonoperative management. Patients with fixation may have C1–2 facet joints that are dislocated or held within the normal range of motion and may or may not have laxity of the transverse ligament. Rotatory fixation may follow an infection or trauma or have other causes. Fielding and Hawkins[28] stated that "the importance of recognizing atlantoaxial rotatory fixation lies in the fact that it may indicate a compromised atlantoaxial complex with the potential to cause neural damage or even death."

Etiology

The cause of AARDs is generally either an infection or a traumatic event, but the condition may also arise spontaneously or in association with other conditions. Isolated case reports have documented rotatory deformities caused by ankylosing spondylitis,[48] metastatic tumor,[83] generalized ligamentous laxity,[52, 87] eosinophilic granuloma[52] following a suboccipital craniotomy and C1–3 laminectomy,[75] and various other non-destabilizing procedures about the head and neck.[73, 84]

The cause in the case described by Bell[2] was a severe local infection. Many other physicians reported cases of AARD after infectious processes in the 100 years between Bell's report and Grisel's article in 1930.[36, 82] Desfosses[17] published a case report in the same year and called the condition "maladie de Grisel"; the eponym "Grisel's syndrome" has been in common usage since then. Watson Jones[80] noted that the infection need not be in the nasopharyngeal region, as suggested by Grisel. This fact has been confirmed by many authors who have described cases resulting from a wide variety of conditions, including upper respiratory infection, sinusitis, tonsillitis, otitis media, parotiditis, mastoiditis, acute rheumatic fever, and many others.[3, 5, 52, 54, 73, 82, 84, 85]

The first reported case of traumatic atlantoaxial rotatory dislocation was described by Buisson in 1852. A

16-year-old boy sustained a fatal neck injury when a cart fell on him. The autopsy revealed a complete anterior dislocation of the right atlantoaxial joint that narrowed the spinal canal by 50%.[11] In 1907, Corner[11] brought attention to Buisson's case and described 17 others previously reported in the literature and added two cases of his own. Some of the cases were diagnosed clinically without the benefit of radiographs because x-rays were not introduced until 1896, but eight of the cases were confirmed by autopsy to be dislocations. Corner noted that an injury of less severity could cause a rotatory subluxation, which would be distinguished from a dislocation only in the "quantity of its symptoms, not in their quality." He correctly surmised that subluxation ("displacement") would prove to be more common than dislocation.

Pathophysiology

The pathophysiology of AARDs is not well defined; there is a paucity of pathologic information because the vast majority of patients survive the condition. Rotatory deformities have been documented in all age groups from infancy to the seventh decade of life. There is a clear predilection for children and young adults regardless of cause.[28, 64, 73] In Corner's review of the literature,[11] traumatic C1–2 rotatory *dislocation* was more common in adults than in children, but he included many cases with associated upper cervical fractures. Isolated rotatory *dislocation* is an unusual injury in children and is very rare in adults.[11, 33, 35, 43, 59] Atlantoaxial rotatory *displacement* resulting from minor trauma is also much more common in children.[28, 64]

In two large reviews of the literature from the 1940s, more than three fourths of the patients with Grisel's syndrome were younger than 13 years.[73, 85] In 1969, Keuter[45] noted that the incidence of the condition in adults was increasing relative to that in children. Between 1981 and 1989, 11 patients with Grisel's syndrome were described in the North American literature; their average age was 17.5 years.[54] The widespread use of antibiotics for childhood infections may be responsible for the shift in age distribution.[54] The disease still primarily affects individuals younger than 30 years, in contrast to vertebral osteomyelitis, which is much more common in elderly persons.[14]

Parke and co-workers[62] noted that the age distribution may be partly explained by the fact that the peripharyngeal lymphoid tissue is hypertrophic in childhood. The adenoids are especially prone to inflammation in children and are located in the area drained by the pharyngovertebral venous plexus (see Fig. 17–4). This venous system provides an anatomic rationale for Grisel's syndrome because it allows a hematogenous route for peripharyngeal septic exudates to enter the periodontoidal venous plexus and suboccipital epidural sinuses. Parke and colleagues suggested that surgical trauma may enhance the transport of inflammatory products into the pharyngeal vertebral plexus; this possibility would explain the cases of Grisel's syndrome that occur after procedures such as tonsillectomy, adenoidectomy, or mastoidectomy.

Positioning of the patient for these procedures may also be a factor.[39, 72, 73, 84] Because upper respiratory tract infections are so much more common than Grisel's syndrome, Parke and associates theorized that affected children must have an anatomic predisposition to instability.

The upper cervical spine joints are much more mobile in children than in adults, and this trait is manifested by a greater ADI[41, 50, 70] and subaxial pseudosubluxation.[9] Kawabe and others[44] found that the facets of the axis in children are more steeply inclined in the coronal plane and are more curved in the sagittal plane than those of adults. Children with the greatest mobility would presumably be at higher risk for rotatory deformities.

There are many theories concerning the pathologic changes that occur as a result of periodontoidal inflammation and lead to the development and fixation of rotatory deformities. Wittek[86] suggested that an effusion develops in the C1–2 joints that stretches the facet capsules, and this stretching leads to excessive laxity. Coutts[12] implicated infolded inflammatory synovial fringes as the mechanism preventing reduction of the displaced joints. Grisel believed that muscle spasm was primarily responsible for the displacement.[36] Watson Jones[80] theorized that decalcification of the bone adjacent to the ligamentous attachments occurs secondary to inflammatory hyperemia and leads to ligamentous laxity. He claimed that the infection need not be in the nasopharyngeal region, as suggested by Grisel, and that any infection leading to hyperemia of the base of the skull could lead to the disorder. Hess and co-workers[39] suggested that reduction in the early stages of the disease is prevented by a combination of factors, including muscle spasm. Fielding and Hawkins[28] concluded that a combination of swollen capsular and synovial tissues and muscle spasm is responsible for blocking reduction in the early stages. If the deformity is not reduced, ligament and capsular contractures can occur, leading to atlantoaxial rotatory *fixation*. Wortzman and Dewar[88] proved that muscle spasm alone is not the mechanism that prevents reduction of rotatory displacement. They described four patients who underwent infiltration of local anesthetic into the C1–2 joints. The patients experienced pain relief with reduced muscle spasm and thus improvement in range of motion, but radiographs showed persistent C1–2 rotatory deformity.

Kawabe and co-workers[44] recently provided more information on the synovial fringes described by Coutts.[12] They identified meniscus-like synovial folds at the occipitoatlantal and lateral atlantoaxial joints in infant cadavers but not in adults (Fig. 17–5). Inflammation, infolding, or rupture of the folds into the joints was cited as the explanation for rotatory fixation. Atrophy of the synovial folds with advancing age may be another explanation for the age distribution of AARDs.

Infolding of the synovial folds into the C1–2 joints in association with muscle spasm and subsequent ligamentous contracture could also be the mechanism for persistent displacement in cases of traumatic AARD. Wortzman and Dewar[88] thought that tearing and in-

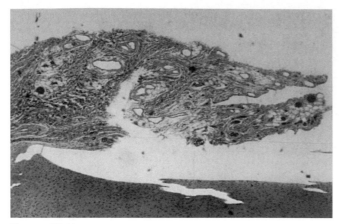

Figure 17–5 = High-power view of meniscus-like synovial fold found attached to the capsule of the lateral atlantoaxial joint in a 2-year-old girl. Note the rich blood supply. (From Kawabe N, Hirotani H, Tanaka O: Pathomechanism of atlantoaxial rotatory fixation in children. J Pediatr Orthop 9:569, 1989.)

vagination of the capsular ligaments of the atlantoaxial joints was the mechanism in traumatic cases of C1–2 rotatory deformity. Traumatic articular cartilage damage or facet fracture may also block reduction of the joints.[28] Locking of the facet joints may explain the fixation in cases of complete dislocation.[11, 33, 35, 43, 59] Rotatory hypermobility or instability may occur after trauma from irreversible stretching or rupture of the alar ligaments.[22]

In long-standing cases of atlantoaxial rotatory fixation, the C0–1 articulation may become hypermobile and rotate in the opposite direction from the C1–2 deformity; this change would allow for clinical improvement of the torticollis. Ono and colleagues[59] believed that children younger than 10 years have excessive C0–1 hypermobility, which may explain some cases of atlantoaxial rotatory fixation. In these children, attempts at reduction only increase the C0–1 counterrotation and do not alter the C1–2 deformity.

Clinical Findings

The typical patient with AARD is a child or young adult who presents with torticollis after minor trauma or an upper respiratory tract infection. The patient's head is rotated away from the anteriorly displaced C1–2 joint and tilted toward the involved side "like a bird with his head cocked listening for a worm."[88] He or she may be able to increase the deformity actively but cannot overcome the torticollis beyond the neutral position. Attempts to correct the deformity are painful.[3, 11, 28, 36, 64] The sternocleidomastoid on the side opposite the tilt may be in spasm, as if attempting to correct the deformity.[28, 36, 64] On palpation, the C2 spinous process may be prominent and deviated to the side to which the chin is pointed, as a result of the lateral tilt of the head[11, 25, 28] or possibly from counterrotation of C2 in an attempt to realign the head.[26, 73] This phenomenon is known as Sudeck's sign,[72] although it was described by Corner in 1907,[11] who also pointed out that the prominence of the C2 spinous process is due to

flexion and forward displacement of the head. Before the advent of x-rays, examination of the pharynx was an important part of the assessment. Corner noted that two prominences in the pharynx can be identified. The transverse process of the anteriorly rotated atlas can be palpated on one side and the lateral mass of the axis may be prominent on the other side if the corresponding lateral mass of the atlas is rotated posteriorly.

Neurologic involvement is fortunately uncommon. Although the condition is uncommon in older patients, they may be predisposed to neurologic compromise. Fielding and Hawkins[28] and Wilson and co-workers[85] each reported only one patient with a neural deficit, and both patients were older than 60 years. Occipital neuralgia may occur because the greater occipital nerve runs in close proximity to the C1–2 facet capsule.[3, 13, 28]

In long-standing cases of atlantoaxial rotatory fixation, facial flattening may occur. This feature was noted on presentation in 7 of 17 patients in the series of Fielding and Hawkins.[28]

With time, the torticollis may eventually resolve despite the persistence of the C1–2 rotatory deformity. This phenomenon was first described by Wortzman and Dewar,[88] who noted that the radiographic abnormality returned to normal in only 1 of 23 cases. They thought that the improvement in head position was due to compensation in the lower cervical spine. More recently, the compensatory rotation has been shown to occur primarily at the occipitoatlantal joint.[10, 28, 59] Adults have less capacity for occiput-C1 counterrotation and therefore may have persistent deformity.[59]

Goddard and others[33] described an association of atlantoaxial rotatory fixation with a fractured clavicle. The injuries all occurred from a fall onto the shoulder. Attention may have been directed at the clavicle fracture, leading to delayed recognition and treatment of the cervical deformity with resultant fixation.

Diagnostic Evaluation

Plain Radiography

Plain radiographs are difficult to interpret because of the rotation and tilt of the occiput-C2 complex. Just 10 years after the introduction of x-rays, Corner[11] noted the typical findings on a lateral radiograph. Because of C1–2 rotation, "the two lateral masses of the atlas . . . are seen laterally *en échelon*, obscuring the odontoid process." The two sides of the posterior arch of C1 are not superimposed on a lateral projection because of the tilt of C1.[3, 28] The transverse ligament may be incompetent, leading to a widened ADI. It is difficult to measure the ADI on plain radiographs; lateral tomograms[28] or a CT scan[31] is often necessary to assess this critical factor. The ADI normally measures up to 3 mm in adults[27, 70] and 4 mm[50, 70] or 4.5 mm[41] in children.

On the anteroposterior, open-mouth projection, the lateral mass of the atlas that is rotated anteriorly appears wider and closer to the midline than its counterpart on the opposite side (Fig. 17–6).[28, 88] Unfortunately, the odontoid-lateral mass relationship is frequently asymmetrical in normal individuals.[47, 63] The C1–2 joint

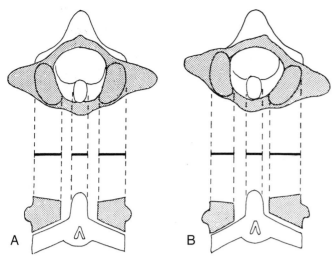

Figure 17–6 = Atlantoaxial joint, demonstrating view seen on CT scan compared with open-mouth odontoid radiograph. *A*, Neutral position. *B*, Rotation to right. With rotation, findings on open-mouth view include apparent approximation of the left atlantal articular mass to odontoid, increase in width of left atlantal articular mass, decreased width of the right atlantal articular mass, and a widened left and narrowed right atlantoaxial joint due to the slope of joints in the sagittal plane. (From Wortzman G, Dewar FP: Rotary fixation of the atlantoaxial joint: Rotational atlantoaxial subluxation. Radiology 90:479, 1968.)

spaces appear asymmetrical, often leading to a narrow joint space on one side and a widened space on the opposite side.[3, 28, 88] Occasionally, the facet joint on one side may be totally obscured from apparent overlapping.[3, 28] The change in height of the atlantoaxial facet

joints is due to the convex shape of the opposing joint surfaces. In neutral, the convex inferior facet of the atlas sits on the summit of the convex superior facet of the axis. With rotation, the facets articulate at their periphery, causing the atlas to assume a lower position; this leads to apparent narrowing or overlap of the joint (Fig. 17–7). The width of each joint space is dependent on whether one or both joints are subluxated. The spinous process of the axis may be rotated away from the side of the anteriorly displaced C1–2 facet joint (Sudeck's sign).[11, 72]

Sullivan[73] noted that unilateral posterior displacement of C1–2 is also possible, in which case the C2 spinous process is rotated toward the involved side. In contrast, when a normal individual rotates the head, the axis does not rotate until approximately 50% of the normal rotation of the neck has occurred. Beyond that point, C2 will normally rotate in the same direction as the occiput and atlas, placing the C2 spinous process on the side opposite the chin. Ironically, lateral flexion of the head causes more rotation of C2 than does pure rotation of the head. Because of coupled motion, the spinous process of the axis is rotated to the side opposite the direction of head tilt and tilted in the same direction.[25] Torticollis from any cause generally involves both rotation and head tilt, and therefore the axis will often be rotated in one direction and tilted in the other.[28]

Anteroposterior tomograms may demonstrate that the two lateral masses of the atlas are in different planes, and this finding leads to the false impression that one lateral mass is absent.[28]

Wortzman and Dewar[88] recommended obtaining an

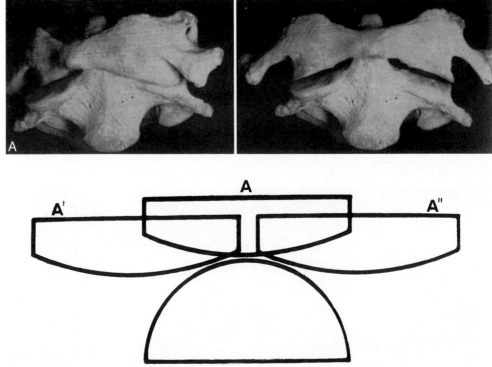

Figure 17–7 = Apparent decrease in atlantoaxial joint space during rotation. *A*, Decreased joint space is shown on left, and neutral position is shown on right. *B*, One atlantoaxial joint as seen from the side. The lower figure represents the convex superior facet of the axis. The upper figure represents the corresponding inferior facet of the atlas. A represents neutral, and A′ and A″ represent positions of rotation. (From Fielding JW: Cineroentgenography of the normal cervical spine. J Bone Joint Surg Am 39:1280, 1957.)

anteroposterior, open-mouth view with 10 to 15 degrees of rotation to each side. They claimed that the radiologic criteria for diagnosis of atlantoaxial rotatory *displacement* is "persistent asymmetry of the odontoid in its relation to the articular masses of the atlas, with this asymmetry not being correctable by rotation." Two studies have demonstrated, however, that normal individuals may have asymmetrical dens-C1 lateral mass relationships that do not correct with rotation.[47, 63] Because the technique is not always reliable, it should be used only if better studies are not available.

Cineroentgenography

Cineroentgenography in the lateral projection has been shown to be one of the best procedures for demonstrating atlantoaxial rotatory fixation.[25, 28] The atlas and axis are shown to move as a unit during attempted rotation. Since the advent of CT, this procedure has been performed infrequently.

Computed Tomography

CT may be helpful for differentiating cellulitis from an abscess in cases of Grisel's syndrome.[3] The alar and transverse ligaments can be visualized by CT, and thus it provides some information on the integrity of these structures.[16, 22] Plain CT scanning is an excellent means of demonstrating abnormal C1–2 relationships.[3, 22, 31, 59, 64, 65] Unless the C1–2 facet joints are dislocated, however, the rotational deformity seen on a static CT scan may represent simple head rotation in a normal individual because the joints are held within the physiologic range in most cases of AARD. Rinaldi and co-workers[65] were the first to recommend dynamic CT for the diagnosis of atlantoaxial rotatory fixation. Their first case in 1977 clearly showed rotational displacement of the atlantoaxial joint that did not change with head rotation to either side (Fig. 17–8). Many authors have confirmed that obtaining a CT scan in maximal head rotation to the left and maximal rotation to the right is the best means of demonstrating the condition.[10, 22, 46, 59, 64] CT may also be used to demonstrate compensatory occiput-C1 rotation or the unusual occurrence of simultaneous subluxation of both occiput-C1 and C1–2 joints.[10, 31, 59] The latter condition can be diagnosed with certainty only if the CT scan is obtained shortly after injury or onset of the condition because compensatory occiput-C1 rotation leading to some pseudoreduction is common.[59] Three-dimensional CT scans are capable of demonstrating the static

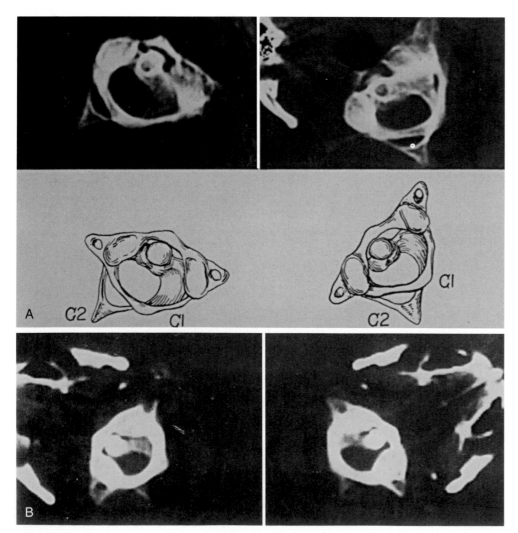

Figure 17–8 = Dynamic CT evaluation of the atlantoaxial joint. *A,* CT scan obtained on maximal head rotation with the face turned to the right (*upper left*). Maximal rotation with the face turned to the left (*upper right*). Note that the relative positions of C1 and C2 remain unchanged, a finding demonstrating fixation of rotational deformity. *Lower figures* are diagrammatic representations of the CT scans. *B,* Dynamic CT scan of a normal patient. *Left,* Maximum rotation with the face turned to the left. *Right,* Maximum rotation with the face turned to the right. Note that the relative positions of C1 and C2 change with rotation. (From Rinaldi I, Mullins WJ Jr, Delaney WF, et al: Computerized tomographic demonstration of rotational atlanto-axial fixation: Case report. J Neurosurg 50:115, 1979.)

Figure 17–9 = A 9-year-old girl with atlantoaxial rotatory deformity. Profuse bleeding developed 24 hours after a tonsillectomy, and repeated attempts at intubation were made. Postoperatively, she complained of painful torticollis. *A*, Plain CT scans demonstrate posterior displacement of the left atlantoaxial joint and anterior displacement of the right atlantoaxial joint. *B* and *C*, Three-dimensional CT scans demonstrate rotational displacement clearly but do not provide any additional information.

deformity very clearly (Fig. 17–9), but the expense of the examination is rarely justified. Three-dimensional CT has the same limitations as two-dimensional static CT in that normal head rotation cannot be differentiated from a fixed deformity.

Magnetic Resonance Imaging

Dickman and co-workers[18] recently reported success with direct visualization of the transverse ligament with magnetic resonance imaging (MRI). They evaluated 20 normal subjects and 14 patients with various upper cervical spine problems using gradient-echo MRI pulse sequences. They had pathologic correlation in one case of transverse ligament disruption and one patient with a normal ligament. The authors concluded that the MRI characteristics of a torn transverse ligament are similar to the findings of a torn cruciate ligament in the knee. The normal ligament has a homogeneous low signal intensity on gradient-echo images, whereas loss of continuity of the ligament with regions of high signal intensity characterize a tear.[18] The clinical significance as well as the sensitivity and specificity of these MRI findings will need to be evaluated in future studies.

Differential Diagnosis

A wide variety of conditions can cause torticollis (Table 17–1). A careful history, physical examination, and radiographic evaluation are necessary to differentiate AARDs from other nondystonic (see Table 17–1) and dystonic (Table 17–2) causes.[4, 8, 28, 53, 64, 71, 76]

Natural History

The natural history of AARDs is poorly documented because most reports and series in the literature describe patients who underwent some form of treatment. Some patients have a benign course with rapid, spontaneous resolution of symptoms.[59, 88] Alternatively, some patients continue to have symptomatic torticollis, a condition designated atlantoaxial rotatory *fixation* by Fielding and Hawkins.[28] In a group of 17 patients that they described who had this condition, two refused operation and were followed for 8 years; these patients allowed a limited understanding of the natural history of refractory cases.

The condition was unchanged in one of the children, with persistent torticollis and facial flattening. The other child was asymptomatic with a functional range of motion and no clinical deformity; however, the radiographic deformity persisted.

Persistent radiographic deformity despite clinical improvement has been described by others.[59, 88] Ono and associates[59] found that the clinical improvement in such cases resulted from compensatory occiput-C1 rotation and documented that the phenomenon is relatively common. They described 13 children younger than 13

rotatory fixation. The weight used is dependent on the age of the patient. They advised using about 3.5 kg in young children and up to 6.8 kg in adults. The weight may be increased in increments of 0.5 to 0.9 kg every 3 to 4 days until correction is achieved or up to an arbitrary limit of 6.8 kg in children and 9.1 kg in adults.

Wetzel and La Rocca[82] devised a protocol of postreduction immobilization based on the classification scheme of Fielding and Hawkins[28] and on a study of cervical orthoses by Johnson and others.[42] They recommended a cervical collar for type I deformities, a Philadelphia collar or sterno-occipitomental immobilizer for type II lesions, and a halo vest for type III lesions. Halos may be applied even in infants if a low-torque, multiple-pin technique is used.[58]

Fielding and Hawkins[28] advised immobilization for 3 months after reduction. Other authors recommend a period of 6 to 8 weeks[82] or until the patient has full pain-free range of motion.[64] After immobilization, flexion and extension radiographs should be obtained to rule out instability.

Manipulation

The role of manipulation in the management of nontraumatic AARDs is limited. Fielding and Hawkins[28] did not recommend the procedure for fixed deformities "because of the inherent dangers." Phillips and Hensinger[64] noted that the best candidates for manipulation are patients with torticollis of recent onset, but the procedure is riskier than reduction by bed rest or traction. If manipulation is elected, they recommended continuous neurologic monitoring.

There is a role for manipulation in cases of acute traumatic AARD.[7, 11, 24, 35, 43, 49] Levine and Edwards[49] recommend performing the manipulation with the patient awake using topical anesthetic in the posterior pharynx. Gentle traction is applied through a halo ring, and the skull and C1 are derotated. They note that the reduction is often accompanied by an audible "pop" and can be confirmed by palpation of the ring of C1 through the mouth. The spine may be immobilized in a halo vest if no fractures are present and the reduction is stable.[49] If the lateral mass of C1 reduces but snaps back into a subluxated or dislocated position, the deformity is considered unstable, and surgical intervention is required (Levine AM: Personal communication. August, 1995).

Sullivan described a procedure for manipulation under anesthesia of AARD cases caused by inflammatory conditions about the neck.[73] "The neck is hyperextended, its tilt and rotation exaggerated and as traction is applied to the head with countertraction to the shoulders, the head is slowly rotated toward the midline." He gave credit to Walton[78] for devising the method of reduction, although Walton's technique did not involve traction and was described for unilateral facet dislocations in the subaxial spine. Sullivan noted that the method was not always successful and could be dangerous in inexperienced hands or in the presence of a fracture or avulsion of the transverse ligament.

Fielding and Hawkins[28] described a 65-year-old woman in whom type III AARD developed when she yawned and twisted her neck. She was placed in traction, and after 10 days she turned her head in the direction of the deformity and died suddenly. An autopsy revealed that the cord was crushed from C1 as it displaced forward and rotated across the canal. On the basis of this case, Fielding and colleagues[28, 30] cautioned against increasing the deformity, because it may increase rotation with further narrowing of the canal.

Surgical Management

A surgical approach is advised for cases of AARD with spinal instability, for cases with neural involvement, or when conservative measures fail to achieve or maintain reduction (Fig. 17–11).[28, 49, 57] When surgery is indicated, a posterior C1–2 fusion is the procedure of choice. Preoperative traction should be attempted to reduce the deformity. If traction is unsuccessful, however, in situ C1–2 fusion may be performed.[28, 33, 64] Three factors should be considered when performing an in situ fusion. First, the passage of wires may be more dangerous because the canal will be narrowed with fixed atlantoaxial rotation.[11] Second, the final clinical result, although "acceptable," may not be as good as fusion after reduction.[33] Third, the improvement in torticollis is a consequence of compensatory occiput-C1 rotation.[59] Conceivably, the unphysiologic position of the C0–1 joints may place the patient at some increased risk during future traumatic episodes, and the long-term effects of C0–1 hypermobility are unknown. If a closed reduction is unsuccessful, open reduction is reasonable. A wire passed under the arch of C1 can be used to manually derotate the atlas. After the deformity is reduced, the wire may be used to maintain the alignment by incorporating it into a C1–2 fusion. If the joint is fractured, an oblique wire is passed from the anteriorly displaced side of the C1 arch to the spinous process of C2.[49]

The type of posterior C1–2 fusion performed is a matter of surgeon preference. In 1973, McGraw and Rusch[56] described a fusion method that is now commonly referred to as the *Gallie technique*. It consists of a rectangular corticocancellous iliac crest graft measuring 3 × 4 cm, which is secured to the back of the C1 ring and lamina of C2 (with a notch for the C2 spinous process) with a loop of wire passing beneath the ring of C1, under the C2 spinous process, and around the graft (Fig. 17–12). They reported excellent results in 14 of 15 patients treated with the technique and only one pseudarthrosis. Although Gallie is credited with the original description of the technique, his frequently quoted 1939 article[32] describes basic principles of management of cervical spine trauma, including skeletal traction and fusion for subaxial dislocations and fracture-dislocations, but it does not mention atlantoaxial arthrodesis.

Brooks and Jenkins[6] described a wedge compression method of C1–2 fusion in 1978. They recommended the use of two doubled 20-gauge wires passed beneath the arch of C1 and the lamina of C2 to secure two beveled, full-thickness iliac crest grafts in the interlami-

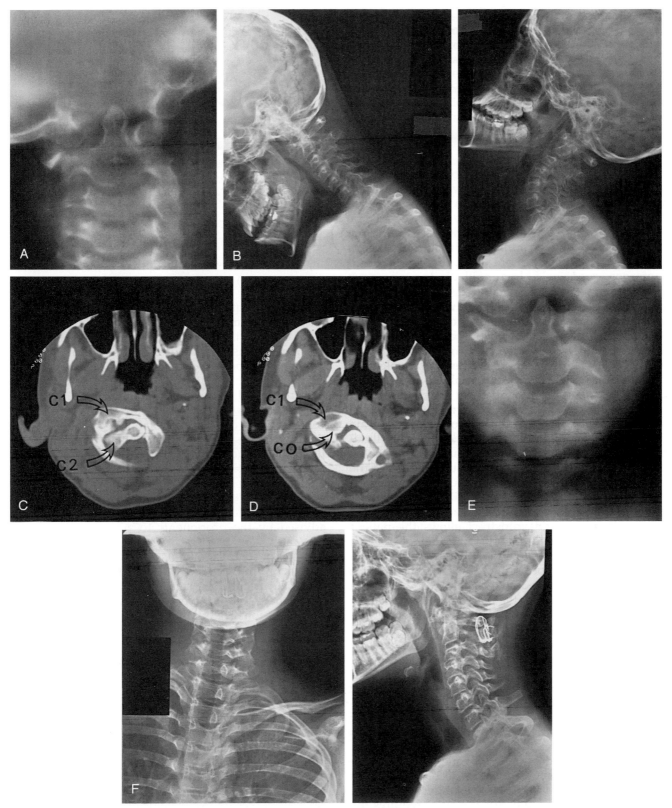

Figure 17–11 = A 12-year-old boy in whom atlantoaxial rotatory deformity developed after excision of a cholesteatoma of his right ear. His deformity was refractory to traction at home and 1 week of traction in the hospital. He presented 10 months after onset of torticollis. *A,* Anteroposterior tomogram demonstrates complete dislocation of the right atlantoaxial joint. *B,* Lateral flexion (*left*) and extension (*right*) radiographs demonstrate atlantoaxial rotatory deformity with widened atlantodental interval. *C,* Static CT scan demonstrates dislocation of right atlantoaxial joint and asymmetrical widening of the atlantodental interval. *D,* Static CT scan demonstrates subluxation of occiput-C1 joints, presumably from compensatory counterrotation of the occiput. *E,* Anteroposterior tomogram demonstrates partial reduction of the C1-2 joint after institution of skeletal traction. *F,* Anteroposterior (*left*) and lateral (*right*) radiographs obtained 6 weeks after C1–2 fusion. The fusion extended to C3 spontaneously. The patient had no complaints except neck stiffness and had marked improvement of torticollis.

Insufficiency of the Transverse Ligament

Lawrence T. Kurz ‖ *Harry Herkowitz*

Instability of the atlantoaxial joint may arise due to incompetence of the bony or soft tissue structures. Although abnormalities of the axis, atlas, or atlantoaxial articulation may be causative factors, this chapter focuses on atlantoaxial instability that is due solely to insufficiency of the transverse ligament.

Transverse ligament insufficiency may be post-traumatic, congenital, infectious, arthritic, or inflammatory. Isolated ruptures are reasonably infrequent, but may be seen in combination with other injuries. Consideration of the anatomic, biomechanical, and radiographic characteristics of the transverse ligament and the C1–2 articulation are critical to understanding this injury. Although other causes of transverse ligament insufficiency may be mentioned, the predominant intent here is the presentation and treatment of traumatic injuries.

ANATOMY

Anatomic studies[22] show that the transverse ligament itself is about 2 to 3 mm thick in its medial portion. This correlates well with findings on the computed tomographic (CT) scan.[3] The transverse ligament is separated from the posterior plane of the tectorial membrane by fatty tissues and from the posterior aspect of the odontoid by the cavity of the syndesmoaxoid joint between the anterior facet of the transverse ligament and the posterior surface of the odontoid process.

The transverse ligament is a part of the cruciform ligament, which itself represents only the middle of three layers of the posterior occipitoatlantoaxial ligament complex. The most posterior portion of the complex is the tectorial membrane. The next layer is the cruciform ligament, the transverse portion of which is the transverse ligament, attaching to the condyles of the axis (C2). The ascending portion of the cruciform ligament attaches to the anterior edge of the foramen magnum. The descending portion attaches to the body of C2. The most anterior layer of the complex consists of the apical and alar ligaments. The alar ligaments are paired structures attaching to the posterolateral surfaces of the tip of the odontoid and running obliquely to the medial aspects of the occipital condyles. The apical ligament connects the tip of the odontoid to the anterior edge of the foramen magnum.

The anteroposterior diameter of the C1 ring, which approximates 3 cm, can be divided into thirds, each with separate anatomic components.[41] The spinal cord and odontoid process each occupy almost 1 cm. The remaining one third is "free space" which allows for some degree of anterior displacement, without spinal cord compromise. Subluxations exceeding 1 cm may put the spinal cord in jeopardy. This danger of course is diminished if the odontoid process is fractured and moves forward with the anterior arch of C1. A hypoplastic or absent odontoid, such as that which occurs in os odontoideum, or in some congenital anomalies, also somewhat diminishes the risk of cord compression.[11] This is presumably due to less space being occupied by rigid structures adjacent to the spinal cord.

BIOMECHANICS

The transverse ligament is the strongest ligament of the cervico-occipital hinge. Resistance to anterior subluxation of C1 on C2 is afforded primarily by the transverse ligament, which is aided by the alar and capsular ligaments. The transverse ligament has no apparent role in providing resistance to posterior subluxation. That stability is rendered by abutment of the anterior ring of C1 on the odontoid.

Employing transverse loading of the transverse ligament, experimental studies on cadavers have revealed a number of important findings:[10] (1) An intact transverse ligament allows a maximum of 3 mm of anterior translation of C1 on C2; (2) failure of the transverse ligament usually occurs within a range of 3 to 5 mm of anterior translation; (3) failure is usually a sudden phenomenon, although the transverse ligament may fail progressively and slowly; (4) the majority of transverse ligaments fail midsubstance, although they may also fail at the ligament-bone junction; (5) in some patients the transverse ligament possesses very little strength, despite the lack of demonstrable local or systemic disease; and (6) there is no correlation between the strength of the transverse ligament and the patient's age.

Jackson[24] utilized flexion and extension radiographs to study the cervical spine of asymptomatic children and adults. In normal patients, maximum anterior translation of C1 on C2 was 4.0 mm in children and 2.5 mm in adults. This correlates well with experimental and clinical data presented by Fielding and others.[8, 10, 44]

RADIOLOGIC EVALUATION

The standard method for evaluating ruptures of the transverse ligament is by a lateral radiograph with the beam centered at the C2 level. The maximal normal atlantoaxial interval (ADI) is 3 mm in the adult and 5 mm in the child. In those patients in whom the lateral radiograph is taken in the supine position (as is customary in trauma victims) any subluxation may be reduced depending on the relationship of the size of the occiput to the size of the chest. Thus a child with a large head will be in a relatively flexed position and an adult with a large chest will be in a relatively extended position. If the patient is alert and conscious and neurologically intact, flexion-extension views will most often define the injury (Figs. 18–1 and 18–2). Care must be taken to examine the flexion-extension views carefully to ascertain that motion at adjacent levels is actually occurring. Often with this injury, the patient has significant protective paraspinal spasm and no motion occurs, thus invalidating the study. In that case either the paraspinal musculature can be injected with local anesthetic to decrease the protective spasm or the patient can be immobilized in a collar until the spasm diminishes (7 to 10 days) and an adequate study can be done. If the patient is neurologically compromised or not conscious, care must be taken to establish the diagnosis without compromising neural status. In a gradual controlled fashion, the head should be brought to a neutral position on a bolster, and a radiograph taken. This will often demonstrate the instability without significantly narrowing the spinal canal (Fig. 18–3A).

A CT scan (Fig. 18–3B) may also be helpful in assessing the competence of the ligament in comatose patients.

High-resolution CT scanning[3] shows that the mean density value of the transverse ligament is greater in its midportion than at its insertions into the atlas. This correlates well with the histologic structure of the transverse ligament which demonstrates layers of collagen that are thicker and more closely arranged in the central portion of the ligament than laterally, where the fibers fan out to attach to the atlas tubercles. CT also reveals a triangular space which is bounded by the dura posteriorly, the medial edge of the lateral mass of C1 laterally, and the lateral portion of the transverse ligament and tubercle anteriorly. This space normally contains fatty tissue and veins. These veins are probably part of the pharyngovertebral venous system, and may be associated with Grisel's syndrome.[35] The CT scan will occasionally demonstrate and differentiate an avulsion fracture of the ligament from the condyle as opposed to a midsubstance rupture.

Axial gradient-echo magnetic resonance images (MRI), angled parallel to the atlas, provide the best visualization of the transverse ligament. The ligament's high degree of contrast with surrounding structures permits it to be visualized consistently in normal subjects. Tears of the ligament appear as a loss of anatomic continuity of the ligament containing regions of high signal intensity compared with the homogeneous low signal intensity of the normal ligament on gradient-echo images.[5] Injuries have been demonstrated in the midportion of the ligament, and as an avulsion laterally at the site of bone insertion.[5]

ACUTE POST-TRAUMATIC INJURY

Survival after acute traumatic rupture of the transverse ligament is unusual, but has been reported.[6, 26, 45]

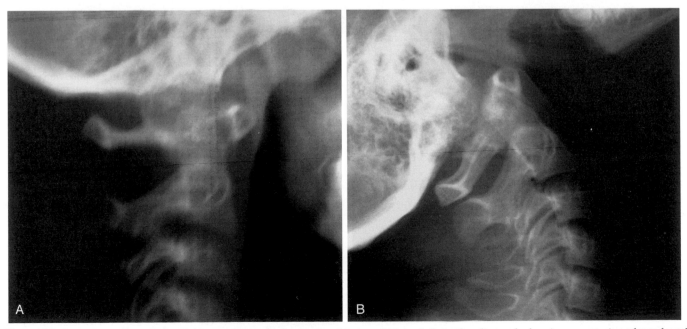

Figure 18–1 ═ Acute hyperflexion injury to the cervical spine in a 10-year-old boy. *A,* Lateral radiograph showing an anterior atlantodental interval (ADI) in flexion of 6 mm. *B,* Lateral view showing complete reduction of C1–2 subluxation in extension.

with an acute odontoid fracture obtained a solid arthrodesis.[25] Others have shown lesser rates of union with the Brooks[2] and Gallie[14] techniques. McGraw and Rusch,[30] in detailing Gallie's method of posterior C1–2 fusion, reported one nonunion in 15 patients. Fielding and associates reported that Gallie fusions resulted in nonunion in 1 of 46 patients. Schatzker and others[38] fared worse when treating 15 patients with odontoid fractures operatively with a Gallie-type procedure: 2 of the 15 fusions failed. Fried[13] reported an even higher rate of failed fusions after Gallie-type procedures on 10 patients with C1–2 fracture/dislocations. Brooks and Jenkins[2] reported 13 of 14 successful fusions with their wedge compression technique of C1–2 sublaminar wiring. Griswold and others[18] improved on this by modifying the Brooks method by using four sublaminar wires and double-twisting them. He believed that the added stability was a major factor in promoting solid fusion in 28 of 29 patients.

The use of posterior interlaminar clamps for C1–2 fixation was first described in 1982 by Roosen et al.[37] Its clinical stability and its ability to promote union is not well established. Furthermore, it requires intact posterior arches of C1 and C2, and has another disadvantage of being bulky enough to render less host bone of C1 and C2 available on which to place bone graft.

Biomechanical studies[19, 21] have shown that the transarticular screw fixation technique provides significantly higher stiffness than the Gallie[14] or Brooks[2] techniques. The main advantage of the transarticular screw fixation technique is not to make the Gallie fixation unnecessary (since a posterior arthrodesis is always added anyway), but to prevent postoperative translational movements which are responsible for the resubluxation seen with the Gallie and Brooks techniques, and to allow early mobilization without major external support. In point of fact, it is believed that the subsequent C1–2 movement following the Brooks- or Gallie-type procedures (but before posterior fusion occurs) is the offending agent in producing nonunions of fusions. Posterior C1–2 transarticular screw fixation is ideal for strongly stabilizing the articulation, thereby restricting movement and promoting solid fusion.

Chronic Post-Traumatic Insufficiency

Those patients with insufficiency of the transverse ligament due to congenital bony ankyloses at the occiput–C1 or C2–3 levels should be treated symptomatically. This lesion develops slowly and is chronic. Asymptomatic patients should have a posterior C1–2 arthrodesis if the anterior ADI is greater than 7 mm in flexion. Patients with progressive pain or neurologic symptoms whose anterior ADI in flexion is greater than 5 mm should undergo posterior C1–2 arthrodesis.

Congenital Insufficiency

Those patients with C1–2 instability due to transverse insufficiency, and not to aplasia or hypoplasia of the bony elements, are treated symptomatically. Those symptomatic patients with an anterior ADI of greater

than 5 mm should undergo posterior C1–2 arthrodesis. Asymptomatic patients with an anterior ADI greater than 7 mm in flexion should also be surgically fused. Although these recommendations are controversial, they at least address the patients with a "cord at risk."

REFERENCES

1. Bharucha EP, Dastur HM: Craniovertebral anomalies (a report of 40 cases). Brain 87:469–480, 1964.
2. Brooks A, Jenkins E: Atlanto-axial arthrodesis by the wedge compression method. J Bone Joint Surg Am 60:279–284, 1978.
3. Burguet JL, Sick H, Dirheimer Y, et al: CT of the main ligaments of the cervico-occipital hinge. Neuroradiology 27:112–118, 1985.
4. Curtis BH, Blank S, Fisher RL: Atlantoaxial dislocation in Down's syndrome. JAMA 205:464–465, 1968.
5. Dickman C, Mamourian A, Sonntag V, et al: Magnetic resonance imaging of the transverse atlantal ligament for the evaluation of atlantoaxial instability. J Neurosurg 75:221–227, 1991.
6. Dunbar HS, Ray BS: Chronic atlanto-axial dislocations with late neurologic manifestations. Surg Gynecol Obstet 113:757, 1961.
7. Dzenitis A: Spontaneous atlanto-axial dislocation in a mongoloid child with spinal cord compression. J Neurosurg 25:458–460, 1966.
8. Fielding JW: Normal and selected abnormal motion of the cervical spine from the second cervical vertebra to the seventh cervical vertebra based on cineroentgenography. J Bone Joint Surg Am 46:1779, 1964.
9. Fielding JW: The cervical spine in the child. Curr Pract Orthop Surg 5:31–55, 1973.
10. Fielding JW, Cochran GVB, Lawsing JF, et al: Tears of the transverse ligament of the atlas. J Bone Joint Surg Am 56:1683–1691, 1974.
11. Fielding JW, Hawkins RJ, Ratzan SA: Spine fusion for atlantoaxial instability. J Bone Joint Surg Am 58:400–407, 1976.
12. French HG, Burke SW, Whitecloud TS, et al: Chronic atlantoaxial instability in Down's syndrome. Orthop Trans 9:135, 1985.
13. Fried L: Atlanto-axial fracture-dislocations. Failure of posterior C1–C2 fusion. J Bone Joint Surg Br 55:490–496, 1973.
14. Gallie W: Fractures and dislocations of the cervical spine. Am J Surg 46:495–499, 1939.
15. Gonzalez TA, Vance M, Helpern M, et al: Legal Medicine: Pathology and Toxicology. New York, Appleton-Century-Crofts, 1940, p. 312.
16. Greenberg AD: Atlanto-axial dislocations. Brain 91:655–684, 1968.
17. Greene K, Dickman C, Marciano F, et al: Transverse atlantal ligament disruption associated with odontoid fractures. Spine 19:2307–2314, 1994.
18. Griswold D, Albright J, Schiffman E, et al: Atlanto-axial fusion for instability. J Bone Joint Surg Am 60:285–295, 1978.
19. Grob D, Crisco J, Panjabi M, et al: Biomechanical evaluation of the four different posterior atlanto-axial fixation techniques. Spine 17:480–490, 1992.
20. Hamilton AR: Injuries of the atlanto-axial joint. J Bone Joint Surg Br 33:434–435, 1951.
21. Hanson P, Montesano P, Sharkey N, et al: Anatomic and biomechanical assessment of transarticular screw fixation for atlantoaxial instability. Spine 16:1141–1145, 1991.
22. Hecker P: Appareil ligamenteux occipito-atloïdoaxoïdien: Étude d'anatomie comparée. Arch Anat Histol Embryol 1923.
23. Highland TR, Aronson DD: Traumatic rupture of the cervical transverse ligament in a child with a normal odontoid process. Spine 11:73–75, 1986.
24. Jackson H: The diagnosis of minimal atlanto-axial subluxation. Br J Radiol 23:672, 1950.
25. Jeanneret B, Magerl F: Primary posterior fusion of C1–2 in odontoid fractures: Indications, technique, and results of transarticular screw fixation. J Spinal Disord 5:464–475, 1992.
26. Krantz P: Isolated disruption of the transverse ligament of the atlas: An injury easily overlooked at post-mortem examination. Injury 12:168–170, 1980.
27. Levine A, Edwards C: Fractures of the atlas. J Bone Joint Surg Am 73:680–691, 1991.

28. Lipson SJ: Fractures of the atlas associated with fractures of the odontoid process and transverse ligament ruptures. J Bone Joint Surg Am 59:940–943, 1977.

29. Martel W, Tishler JM: Observations on the spine in mongoloidism. AJR 97:630–638, 1966.

30. McGraw R, Rusch R: Atlanto-axial arthrodesis. J Bone Joint Surg Br 55:392–405, 1971.

31. McRae DL: Bony abnormalities in the region of the foramen magnum: Correlation of the anatomic and neurologic findings. Acta Radiol 40:335–354, 1953.

32. McRae DL: The significance of abnormalities of the cervical spine. AJR 84:3–25, 1960.

33. McRae DL, Barnum AS: Occipitalization of the atlas. AJR 70:23–46, 1953.

34. O'Brien JJ, Butterfield WL, Grossling HR: Jefferson fracture with disruption of the transverse ligament. Clin Orthop 126:135–138, 1977.

35. Parke WW, Rothman RH, Brown MD: The pharyngovertebral veins: An anatomical rationale for Grisel's syndrome. J Bone Joint Surg Am 66:568–574, 1984.

36. Pennecot GF, Leonard P, DesGachons SP, et al: Traumatic ligamentous instability of the cervical spine in children. J Pediatr Orthop 4:339–345, 1984.

37. Roosen K, Trauschel A, Grote W: Posterior atlanto-axial fusion: A new compression clamp for laminar osteosynthesis. Arch Orthop Trauma Surg 100:27–31, 1982.

38. Schatzker J, Rorabeck C, Waddell J: Fractures of the dens. J Bone Joint Surg Br 53:392–405, 1971.

39. Spence KF, Decker S, Sell KW: Bursting atlantal fracture associated with rupture of the transverse ligament. J Bone Joint Surg Am 52:543–549, 1970.

40. Spitzer R, Rabinowitch JY, Wybar KC: A study of the abnormalities of the skull, teeth, and lenses in mongolism. Can Med Assoc J 84:567–572, 1961.

41. Steel HH: Anatomical and mechanical considerations of the atlanto-axial articulations. J Bone Joint Surg Am 50A:1481–1482, 1968.

42. von Torklus D, Gehle W: The Upper Cervical Spine. New York, Grune & Stratton, 1972.

43. Wackenheim A: Occipitalization of the ventral part and vertebralization of the dorsal part of the atlas with insufficiency of the transverse ligament. Neuroradiology 24:45–47, 1982.

44. Weissman BNW, Aliabadi P, Weinfeld MS, et al: Prognostic features of atlantoaxial subluxation in rheumatoid arthritis patients. Radiology 144:745–751, 1982.

45. Wigren A, Anici F: Traumatic atlanto-axial dislocation without neurological disorder. J Bone Joint Surg Am 55:642, 1973.

rupture of the posterior aspect of the disc. This must be differentiated from the type II injury for several reasons. First, with the flexion distraction mechanism of injury, the injury propagates from posterior to anterior along the disc, causing angulation without translation. Application of traction in this injury (because it has a distraction mechanism) will result in an increase in the deformity and the widening of the disc space. In some individuals, as the injury propagates from posterior to anterior by this flexion-distraction mechanism, the anterior longitudinal ligament will be ruptured in distraction. Should that occur, dramatic widening of the disc space can be seen with minimal application of weight. In addition to the characteristics of angulation out of proportion to translation, the obliquity of the fracture line in the neural arch and compression of the anterosuperior portion of the C3 vertebral body is rarely seen in type IIA injuries.

The fifth type of injury is the type III fracture, which combines facet injuries at the C2–3 facet levels with type I fractures of the neural arch. Multiple combinations of these injuries have been reported previously,[6, 7, 19, 20, 21] but the most common injury is a bipedicular fracture with a standard bilateral facet dislocation (Fig. 19–6). Other combinations occur that involve facet injuries; these include more oblique injuries with unilateral facet fracture dislocation combined with a contralateral neural arch fracture (Fig. 19–7). The critical feature in these injuries is that as a result of the neural arch fracture, the inferior facets of C2 are free-floating fragments, and if bilateral dislocation from C3 occurs, the fracture cannot be reduced by closed methods. The most logical mechanism of this injury is a flexion-distraction mechanism, which produces a bilateral facet dislocation, followed by a hyperextension injury, which causes the type I fracture of the pars. Were the fracture of the pars to occur first, it would then be impossible to dislocate the facet joint at C2–3, as it would no longer be connected to the cervicocranial segment. The usual methods for reduction of facet dislocations by application of traction are not applicable to this injury pattern. Traction applied to the skull by tongs will result in application of traction to the body of C2, but because the inferior facets are no longer connected as a result of the fracture of the pars, no force can be applied to them to achieve reduction of the C2–3 dislocation.

Finally, a group of fractures should be mentioned that are not truly hangman's fractures but that in fact result in spondylolisthesis of the axis (C2) over C3. These are bilaminar fractures of C2, which result in spondylolisthesis of C2 over C3 and bilateral facet fractures (Fig. 19–8). These injuries are similar to other bilateral facet fractures in the cervical spine and are dealt with in Chapter 22 (the chapter on facet injuries of the cervical spine). However, they need to be differentiated from other types of traumatic spondylolisthesis because of their instability and also because of

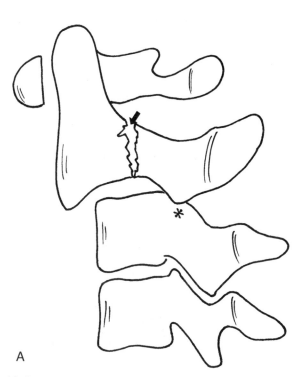
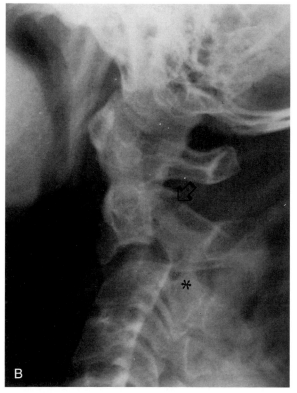

Figure 19–6 = *A* and *B*, Type III traumatic spondylolisthesis of the axis combines fractures of the neural arch with facet injuries at C2–3. The first type is a bilateral facet dislocation at C2–3 (*star*) with a type I hangman's fracture at the base of the body-pedicle junction (*arrowhead*). The mechanism most probably is initial flexion-distraction, which causes the dislocation, and then extension, which causes the traumatic spondylolisthesis. Reversing the mechanism would not permit the dislocation to occur, as the inferior facet of C2 would then be detached from the cervicocranium, which serves as the lever for the dislocation.

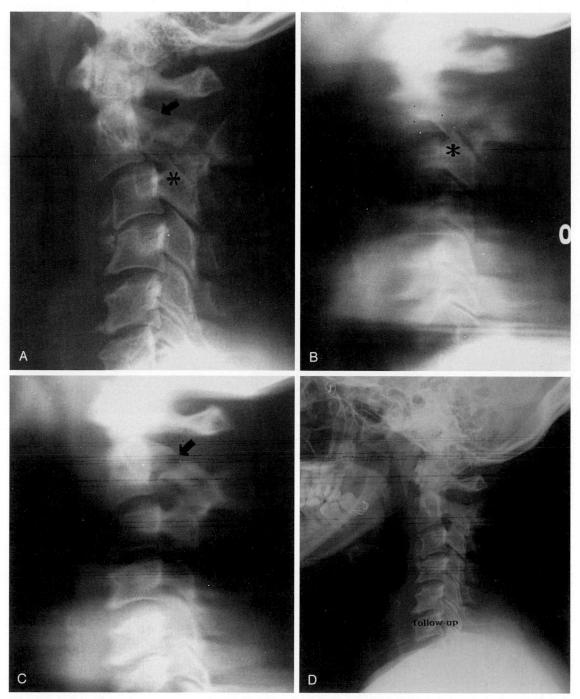

Figure 19–7 = This patient demonstrates one of the variants of the type III injury. *A,* The lateral radiograph shows the fracture through the right side of the pedicle (*arrow*) and with a dislocation of the left facet joint (*star*). *B,* The tomograms of the left side demonstrate the facet dislocation (*star*). *C,* The tomogram of the right side demonstrates the more standard fracture through the neural arch (*arrow*). *D,* The final lateral view shows the healed stable position.

the nature of the injury. As is true of other facet fractures, these are either flexion-distraction or, occasionally, shear injuries, which result in significant discal injury; therefore, the reduction of this injury may be complicated by herniation of the C2–3 disc. Additionally, because these fractures are grossly unstable, reduction and traction are not sufficient treatment, whereas in a severely displaced type II hangman's fracture, reduction and traction may be adequate (see later discussion).

RADIOGRAPHIC EVALUATION

On presentation in the emergency room or a trauma unit of a patient with a suspected hangman's fracture, the usual initial study is a lateral cervical spine radiograph, which is most commonly diagnostic in traumatic spondylolisthesis. In evaluating the lateral cervical spine radiograph, two factors must be taken into consideration. The first is the position of the patient during radiography, which is most commonly the su-

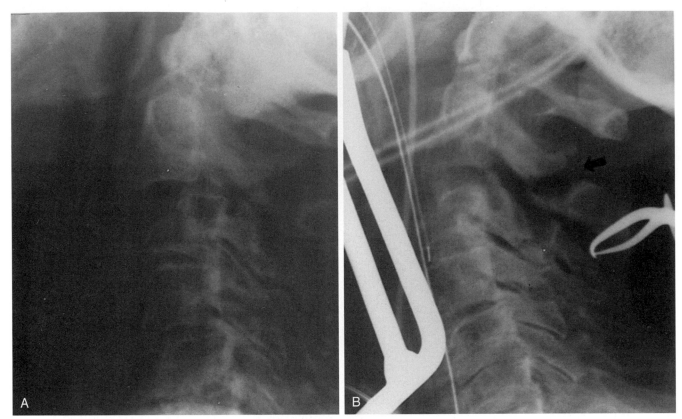

Figure 19–8 ═ *A*, This lateral radiograph of an elderly man involved in a motor vehicle accident demonstrates a traumatic spondylolisthesis at C2–3, which results from a bilateral facet fracture with fracture of the lamina at C2–3. The radiographic picture is similar to that of a traumatic spondylolisthesis with anterior compression to the body of C2 and translation of C2 over C3. *B*, This is easily reduced in traction, and the fracture line was clearly evident *(arrow)* preoperatively.

pine position. If the patient happens to have large shoulders, the neck will be in relative extension, and thus what may appear to be a type I traumatic spondylolisthesis of the axis may in fact be a type II lesion (Fig. 19–9). If the patient has a relatively large occiput and relatively small shoulders, the films will be taken at flexion, thus accentuating the deformity if it exists. Type IIA fractures generally are angulated and are reasonably evident on the lateral radiograph, irrespective of the patient's position. A true type III injury is also fairly evident, as the dislocation is usually easily seen in this particular injury. Type IA, or atypical hangman's fracture, is difficult to diagnose on a plain radiograph. There will be some suspicion that a fracture exists, but the fracture lines are not clearly seen because they are neither superimposed nor widely separated, and displacement in the form of angulation and translation is not evident. All patients with any type of traumatic spondylolisthesis should have an open-mouth and an anteroposterior (AP) radiograph in addition to the initial lateral film. This is meant to detect the presence of multiple fractures in the cervical spine that may occur in conjunction with traumatic spondylolisthesis. In patients who are neurologically intact and have what is thought to be type I traumatic spondylolisthesis, the next radiographic study that should be ordered is a *physician-supervised* flexion-extension lateral radiograph. To be a valid flexion/extension radiograph, it must show motion at adjacent normal

motion segments of the spine. If it does and if little or no motion is demonstrated at the fracture site, the workup for the type I injury is completed. For type IA injury (atypical hangman's fracture) or traumatic spondylolisthesis of the axis, a CT scan is the diagnostic study of choice. A CT scan will demonstrate the location of the breaks within the ring of C2. More important, it will demonstrate whether there an injury that goes through the vertebral foramen anteriorly. If the fracture pattern is such that it goes through the vertebral foramen, there is a risk of vertebral artery injury, and a digital subtraction angiogram or a magnetic resonance (MR) angiogram should be done to assess the flow in the vertebral artery on that side. This is especially true in the presence of evidence of any neurologic deficit that might be associated with a cerebral infarction based on the vertebral artery injury. In addition, the CT scan in patients with neurologic deficit can define the narrowing of the canal. For a patient with a suspected type II injury, either because of a displacement in angulation noted on the initial radiograph or because of the displacement noted on a flexion-extension film, no further studies are indicated. This is similarly true for type IIA injuries, which are most frequently evident on the initial study. However, for patients with both type II and IIA injuries who are going to be either placed in traction or a halo vest, sequential plain lateral radiographs need to be taken at indicated junctures during the treatment. In the ab-

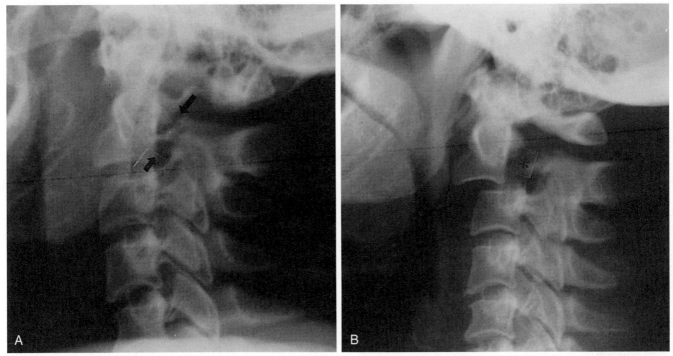

Figure 19–9 = This patient presented after a motor vehicle accident with what was initially thought to be a type I injury. *A,* The original radiograph was taken in the supine lateral position. Because of the patient's obesity, the neck was in an extended position, and although the fracture line was evident (*arrows*), the fracture was fully reduced. The patient was discharged in a collar and returned 2 weeks later for follow-up with marked displacement (*B*) and separation of the fracture (*star*).

sence of neurologic deficit, neither a CT scan nor an MRI is indicated. For patients with a type III fracture with a bilateral facet dislocation, both a CT and MRI are indicated. The CT scan should evaluate the bilateral facet dislocation component to ascertain whether the fractures are present in the facets and to aid in planning the surgical procedure. An MRI is indicated to look at the integrity of the C2–3 disc because the reduction of the dislocation must be done with the patient under anesthesia. In view of the association of disc hernia-tions with bilateral facet dislocations, if the dislocation cannot be reduced with the patient awake to signal any change in neurologic status, a preoperative MRI should be used to assess the disc. If no significant disc herniation is seen with a type III injury, the standard operative treatment can go forward.

The critical feature to observe in the radiologic evalu-ation of patients with traumatic spondylolisthesis of the axis is the presence of other fractures in both the upper and lower cervical spine. In a series of 335 patients with upper cervical spine fractures,[24] 15.2% had two or more fractures in the upper cervical spine and 22.7% had two or more anywhere in the cervical spine. There were 131 patients with traumatic spondy-lolisthesis of the axis in this group, of which 29 had other cervical spine fractures and 7 had thoracic or lumbar fractures. The second most common group of injuries with 12 patients was a combination of an atlas fracture with traumatic spondylolisthesis of the axis. Six of the 12 had type I injuries included traumatic spondylolisthesis of the axis (Fig. 19–10). Of those six, two had three upper cervical spine fractures, including

a type I traumatic spondylolisthesis, a posterior arch fracture of C1, and a hyperextension teardrop fracture of C2. The third most common group was a C2 exten-sion teardrop fracture and a type I traumatic spondy-lolisthesis of the axis. In addition, there were four patients with dens fractures and traumatic spondylolis-thesis of the axis. Therefore, in patients with traumatic spondylolisthesis of the axis, associated injuries should be considered both in the upper and lower cervical spine, and multiple injuries with similar mechanisms should be ruled out. In type I injuries, all hyperexten-sion injuries should be considered, especially in the upper cervical spine; in type II or IIA injuries, both hyperextension and flexion-distraction injuries should be considered; for type IA or atypical injuries, lateral bending injuries, such as fracture separations of the articular mass, should be considered.

NEUROLOGIC INJURY

In contradistinction to the true hangman's fracture, which results in death by either strangulation or trau-matic transection of the cord, traumatic spondylolis-thesis of the axis infrequently demonstrates neurologic deficit. Although these injuries are frequently accompa-nied by closed-head injuries, it is rare that neurologic deficit is related directly to the injury. In the largest series of traumatic spondylolisthesis that has been pub-lished, Francis and co-workers found that only 6.5% of the patients had neurologic deficit related to the injury.[9] With type I injuries, essentially no incidence of neuro-

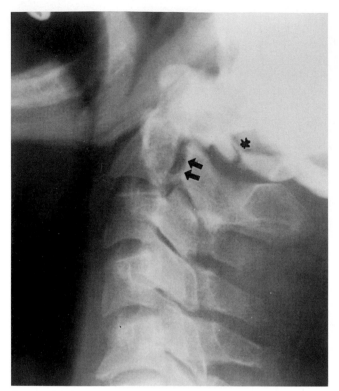

Figure 19-10 = Multiple injuries in the cervicocranial area are a fairly common phenomenon. Usually these injuries have a common mechanism. In this case, both the fracture of the posterior arch of C1 (*star*) and the type I traumatic spondylolisthesis of the axis (*arrows*) are the result of a hyperextension–axial load mechanism. Individually both injuries are stable and require only collar immobilization, and the two injuries together are no more unstable than either one alone.

logic deficit is seen in relation to the injury, although in a group of 15 patients with this type of injury, 5 had neurologic deficit. In three it was related to a closed-head injury, and the anterior cord syndrome and the central cord syndrome were each related to other major injuries.[19] Type IA, or atypical hangman's fracture, is believed to be accompanied by a higher incidence of neurologic deficit.[39] Two patients were found to have incomplete quadriplegia, which was thought to be the result of cord impingement by a fracture fragment with deformity of the canal from this atypical fracture pattern; one patient had minimal translation and angulation and one had significant translation and angulation. In addition, with type IA injury, when the fracture goes through the transverse foramen for the vertebral artery,[23] neurologic deficit may occur related to vertebral artery disruption. Type II injuries are occasionally associated with paraplegia, as demonstrated by Effendi and co-workers[7] and Levine and Edwards,[19] though again, in most type II injuries the neurologic deficit is usually related to the closed-head injuries and only infrequently to the level of injury. Type III injuries are more likely to demonstrate neurologic deficit, with three of five[19] demonstrating neurologic deficit related to the level of injury, including one patient with central cord syndrome, one with radiculopathy, and one with diffuse weakness. Two other patients had closed-head

injuries related to head trauma. In summary, neurologic deficit is infrequently associated with type I and II traumatic spondylolisthesis, but it is more commonly associated with type IA (atypical) and III injuries. The highest incidence with type III injuries results from the bilateral facet dislocation component.

TREATMENT

The purposes of a classification system of injury should be either to allow us to better understand the mechanism of injury and consequent instability or to subdivide the injuries in such a way that subgroups have specific and individual types of treatment. The treatment regimens for the various types of traumatic spondylolisthesis of the axis are easily associated with the various classification subgroups. The treatment range is from simple cervical immobilization in a collar, to halo traction and/or surgery followed by immobilization in an orthosis, to anteroposterior fusion. Early series related to the treatment of this injury were mixed and did not clearly identify treatment modalities. Some results were diametric opposites. For example, Schneider and others[35] successfully treated seven of eight patients with prolonged skeletal traction followed by immobilization in either a cast or brace. The one patient in that series with nonunion required an anterior C2–3 graft with fusion. Cornish,[4] at a similar time, condemned the use of traction and suggested C2–3 fusion for all patients with this type of fracture. He treated 11 patients with an anterior C2–3 arthrodesis and subsequent cervical immobilization and achieved a 100% fusion rate. However, his patients had a high complication rate, including three patients with Horner's syndrome and two with suboccipital pain and later degenerative changes. Anterior fusion remained a viable alternative and was documented to be effective in other series.[30] More recently, osteosynthesis of the fracture by direct screw fixation for either type III fractures or for widely displaced type II fractures was suggested by Roy-Camille and co-workers.[34] Caspar plate fixation for anterior C2–3 arthrodesis has been attempted but is technically very difficult.[41] Nonoperative treatment of this injury has varied dramatically from simple immobilization to prolonged treatment. Brashear and co-workers[2] and Seljeskog and Chou[36] suggested cervical traction for 6 weeks followed by 2 or 3 months of cervical immobilization in a Minerva cast. A large multicenter study[9] showed that satisfactory results could be achieved with either immediate immobilization (35 of 123 patients) or short-term traction with a mean of 8 days (45 of 123 patients). In that series, an additional 43 patients were treated for 6 weeks with traction. The overall union rate was 94.5% (16 of 123 patients), and the average time to union was 11.5 weeks. There was no correlation between the union of a fracture and the initial displacement or angulation, but it was that noted conservative treatment yielded a high incidence of union with no significant difference between the results of patients with early immobilization and prolonged halo traction. The treatment was not broken down by initial angulation and displacement (nor was residual displacement evaluated). This has prompted others to suggest that early immobilization[13] is the best method of treatment.

The first authors to really use a classification system to help identify methods of treatment were Effendi and colleagues,[7] who advocated bracing for type I fractures and halo immobilization for type II. They also suggested skeletal traction for 3 weeks for the more displaced type II fractures. Type III fractures, they thought, required closed manipulation of the dislocated facets and open reduction if unsuccessful.

Currently, however, there is good documentation of the rationale for treatment of traumatic spondylolisthesis of the axis based on the classification system that has been discussed previously. The treatment of traumatic spondylolisthesis is based on an understanding of the mechanisms of injury and the resultant instability from each mechanism. Optimal treatment can be selected on the basis of this fracture classification type, which takes into account mechanism and the degree of instability.[19, 22] Universally, type I fractures are considered to be stable by any criteria that can be invoked. The patient must have less than 3 degrees of translation and minimal angulation, both on static and flexion-extension radiographs. The extension force necessary for this mechanism of injury is such that little or no ligamentous destruction occurs. Because it has been shown that halo immobilization neither prevents toggle nor provides any more substantial immobilization at the C2–3 level than does a cervical collar,[18, 42, 43] a cervical orthosis yields the most reasonable immobilization with minimal complication. Prior to beginning immobilization in an orthosis, the patient must undergo *physician-supervised* flexion-extension radiography and demonstrate adequate movement of the remainder of their spine to prove that the injury is a type I fracture. Failures of treatment with increasing displacement of immobilization in type I fractures suggest that the injury was originally a type II fracture that was reduced on the supine lateral film and was not verified to be a type I fracture. Body habitus must be considered; immobilization in a collar may not be possible in patients who are extremely obese and have a very short neck, and halo immobilization might be considered.

In atypical or type IA fractures, an oblique fracture occurs through the body of C2 on one side and the pars or pedicle on the opposite side. The majority of these are stable injuries. Again, in the patient without neurologic deficit, flexion-extension radiographs should be done after completion of the CT scan. The majority of these injuries in patients who are neurologically intact without displacement on flexion-extension radiographs are stable injuries that can be treated with a cervical collar. Union will occur in a slightly displaced position (Fig. 19–11), and there will appear to be an elongation of the vertebral body, with anterior translation of approximately 2 to 3 mm. Because at least one portion of this fracture is through the cancellous portion of the C2 body, the union rate is extremely high and reduction does not need to be achieved. Occa-sionally a patient will have either neurologic deficit or a very unstable fracture, in which case traction may be necessary to achieve reduction of the fracture and the neural canal; this occurs less than 10% of the time. Essentially these fractures can be treated as a type I even though the mechanism and the fracture pattern are different than a type I fracture.

Type II fractures are subdivided into standard type II and IIA, which are treated very differently. Type II fractures are unstable.[19, 42] The degree of instability varies, but in all cases the dural sac should not be compressed by this type of fracture, because the neural canal is expanded by the fracture of the neural arch, rather than compressed (in contradistinction to other types of spinal fractures). Although it has been demonstrated that the neural arch fractures as a result of hyperextension and axial load force, the displacement of a type II fracture is a result of the flexion component. Therefore, the anatomic reduction of a type II fracture is achieved by using forces directly opposite to the ones that created the fracture deformity and displacement, that is, the flexion component and the compression component. Thus, the reduction of a severely displaced type II traumatic spondylolisthesis can be achieved by axial distraction (or traction) and slight hyperextension of the neck. However, if that traction is removed prior to achieving at least provisional union of the arch (at least 4 to 6 weeks), the reduction is generally lost. It has been demonstrated many times that if the fracture is reduced in halo traction and then the patient is immediately placed in a halo vest or cast, axial distraction is not maintained in this upright position. The spine is subjected to an element of either neutral force or axial compression, resulting in subsequent redisplacement of the fracture. Therefore, patients who have moderate degrees of displacement in angulation (less than 5 mm and less than 10 degrees of angulation), and in whom the displacement can be accepted, can be treated successfully with immediate immobilization in a halo vest. Two goals should be achieved in the treatment of such patients: First, the degree of residual angular deformity or kyphosis between C2–3 should be reduced to a point that it is not severe enough to require extreme hyperextension at the levels below to achieve a satisfactory alignment of the remainder of the spine. Compensatory hyperlordosis will lead to late pain and early degenerative disease at the facet joints adjacent to it. Second, the amount of displacement should be minimized because if the amount of displacement between the fracture fragments at the body-pedicle junction is significantly more than 5 mm, the rate of nonunion may be higher. Despite the fracture gap, a spontaneous anterior arthrodesis between C2 and C3 occurs in some of these patients. The anterior arthrodesis results from the destruction of the disc and bleeding as the anterior longitudinal ligament is stripped off the body of C3. Nonunion occurs in a small percentage because of the widely displaced fracture fragments. Therefore, in patients with more than 5 mm of translation and more than 10 to 15 degrees of angulation in whom the displacement cannot be accepted, there are two methods

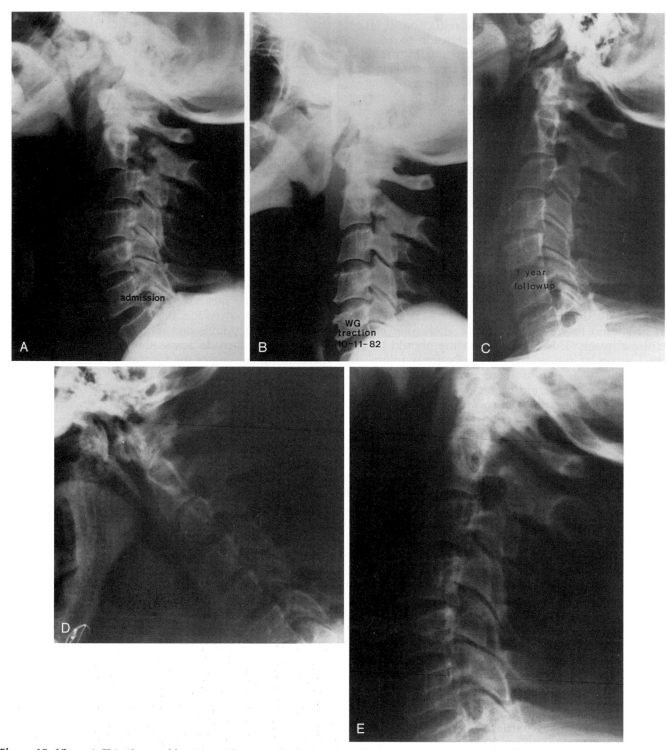

Figure 19–12 = *A,* This 63-year-old patient with a severely displaced type II traumatic spondylolisthesis of the axis had 12 mm of translation on the initial lateral radiograph. *B,* The patient was placed in halo traction (30 lb) with slight extension of the neck over a roll to achieve anatomic reduction in traction. The patient was maintained in traction for 6 weeks and then immobilized in a halo vest. *C,* On follow-up radiographs at 1 year, the patient demonstrates maintenance of reduction and healing of the traumatic spondylolisthesis of the axis in an anatomic position. *D* and *E,* Flexion-extension roentgenograms demonstrate the ultimate stability obtained.

ratio of angulation to translation, the absence of compression of the anterior portion of the C2 body, and the angulation of the fracture line define the type IIA fracture on admission radiograph. Any injury in which 10 lb of traction, applied to reduce the fracture, causes disc space widening will have to be considered a type

IIA fracture. Overall, however, this constitutes a small percentage (rarely more than 5%) of a larger group with traumatic spondylolisthesis. Because the fracture mechanism for type IIA injuries is flexion-distraction, their reduction is done by extension and compression. In this group of patients, we immediately apply a halo

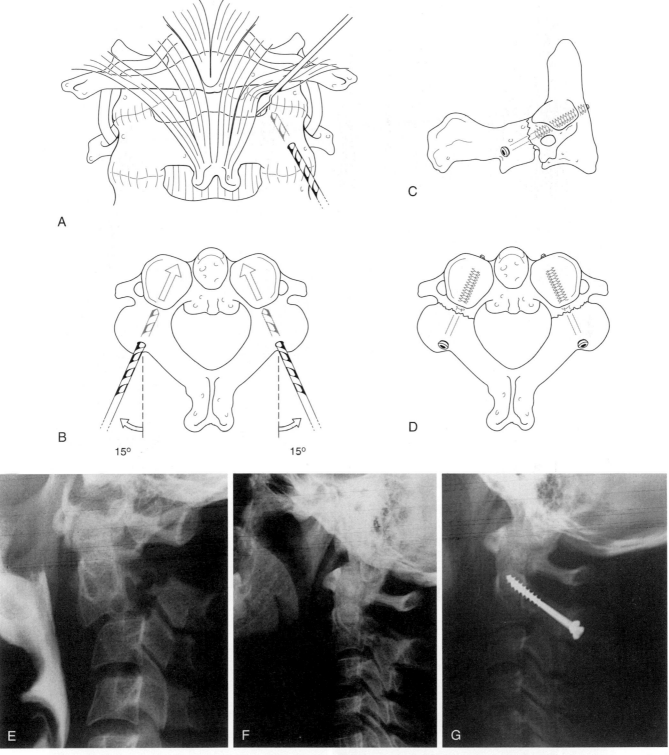

Figure 19–13 = *A,* The surgical technique for osteosynthesis of a traumatic spondylolisthesis of the axis. The procedure is done with the aid of biplanar image intensification so that the trajectory of the screws can be easily monitored. The initial portion of the dissection requires demonstration of the medial aspect of the pedicle of C2. The facet joint at C1–2 does not need to be disrupted, but dissection from posterior to anterior toward the facet will usually demonstrate the fracture of the pedicle. Prior to beginning screw insertion, care should be taken that the fracture is as reduced as possible and that a No. 4 Penfield elevator can be placed along the medial border of the pedicle for guidance. *B,* Orientation of the screws along the pedicle in an axial plane. Slight convergence of the screws is desirable. *C,* Orientation across the fracture line from the posterior fracture to the anterior fragment. A partially threaded screw is desirable with usually about 15 mm of thread and 20 mm of shank. The proximal fragment can be overdrilled and lagged to the anterior fragment. *D,* The final axial view. *E,* This patient sustained a displaced type II traumatic spondylolisthesis of the axis as well as other extremity and systemic injuries. As halo traction and bed rest were not an alternative, the patient was reduced in halo traction (*F*) and then direct screw fixation of the fracture was achieved (*G*).

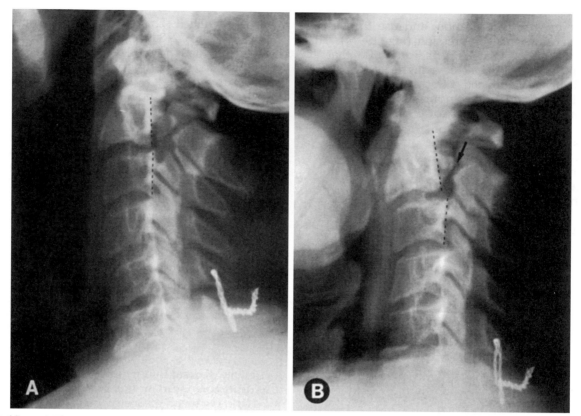

Figure 19–16 = *A,* This 41-year-old man sustained a type I traumatic spondylolisthesis of the axis 12 months before these flexion-extension radiographs were taken. *A,* The extension radiograph demonstrates full reduction of the deformity but with a lucent gap in the fracture line after 12 months of orthotic immobilization (*dotted line*). *B,* The flexion radiograph demonstrates both translation and angulation and widening of the gap in the fracture line (*arrow*) with sclerotic edges. The patient subsequently underwent arthrodesis for correction of nonunion. (From Levine AM, Rhyne AL: Traumatic spondylolisthesis of the axis. Semin Spine Surg 3:59, 1991.)

placement, either collar immobilization for the nondisplaced fracture or surgical intervention for the facet injury, followed by collar immobilization for the neural arch fracture, will yield an anatomic result. Care must be taken prior to embarking on surgical intervention to fully ascertain the nature of the injury. The surgeon should not confuse the spondylolisthesis or spondyloptosis of C2 over C3 resulting from a translational or shear injury with true traumatic spondylolisthesis. These generally do not contain a pars or pedicle fracture and are treated by more standard approaches. Occasionally, patients with significant translation and laminar and facet fractures require a C2–3 plate fixation. In this case, because there is no fracture of the anterior portion of the neural arch, a standard C2–3 plating can be achieved without concern about displacing the more anterior fracture.

RESULTS AND COMPLICATIONS

The treatment of type I injury, or minimally displaced traumatic spondylolisthesis of the axis, is accompanied by few complications and even fewer long-term problems. To date, no series have been published concerning the long-term (>5-year) follow-up of these injuries, although data are currently beginning to be available on our original series of patients.[19] However, the union rate of type I fractures, since the displacement is minimal, is approximately 98%. We have had only two cases of nonunion of a type I fracture (Fig. 19–16). Nonunions in this injury can be treated either by osteosynthesis with a pedicle screw across the fracture and compression or by C2–3 anterior arthrodesis. It is of note in treating type I fractures that they have a high rate of association with other fractures, including the fractures of the posterior arch of C1.[20, 21] Initial recognition of the multiple injuries is very important. It is also of note to realize that both the type I injury of spondylolisthesis of the axis and the posterior arch fracture of C1 are stable injuries, and either one alone requires collar immobilization for adequate treatment. The two combined also require collar immobilization for adequate treatment. A less frequently encountered combination is traumatic spondylolisthesis and a posteriorly displaced dens fracture, both resulting from hyperextension–axial load injuries. If the dens fracture is easily reduced or nondisplaced (since it is the more significant injury), it will require halo vest immobilization. The most common long-term problem of type I traumatic spondylolisthesis is the degeneration of the C2–3 facet joint. Because the mechanism of injury is hyperextension combined with axial loading, the C2–3 facets are oriented in such a direction that they will achieve significant loading during that injury. Approximately 10% of patients with this injury will have symp-

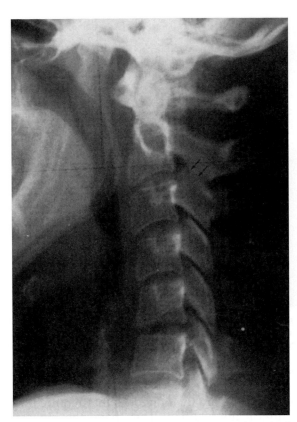

Figure 19–17 = This 27-year-old woman sustained a type I traumatic spondylolisthesis of the axis 3 years before these radiographs were taken. She healed in a completely anatomic position. However, she began to have both weather-related symptoms and intermittent pain, localized specifically to the upper cervical spine and reproduced with pressure over the C2 spinous process. On the flexion-extension radiograph, the patient is noted to have loss of the joint space at C2–3 (*arrows*), but she retains minimal motion at that level. (From Levine AM, Rhyne AL: Traumatic spondylolisthesis of the axis. Semin Spine Surg 3:58, 1991.)

toms and late degenerative changes at that level (Fig. 19–17). The majority have specific pain with pressure over the C2 spinous process, and symptoms are exacerbated by changes in weather. This phenomenon does not occur as frequently in type II fractures, because the majority of those patients experience spontaneous C2–3 ankylosis. Approximately 30% of patients with type I injuries who have mobile C2–3 joints have some degenerative symptoms.[14] In the long term, should symptoms become significant enough, they may require secondary arthrodesis.

Type IA injuries, or atypical hangman's fractures, fall into two groups. The first consists of patients who have an oblique fracture with minimal displacement, which is the majority of patients; their prognosis is similar to that of other patients with type I injuries. Fracture union is achieved approximately 98% of the time with minimal pain and no long-term problems. In collar immobilization or halo vest immobilization they maintain the initial position essentially completely. The second group consists of the few patients[23, 39] who have neurologic deficit as a result of this injury, but the follow-up again remains short, and the prognosis for this most recently defined type of injury remains incomplete.

Patients with type II traumatic spondylolisthesis of the axis occupy a wide spectrum. Many of the patients have head and other injuries in addition to the traumatic spondylolisthesis of the axis. However, as previously mentioned, few of them have neurologic deficit related to the injury, although all series report an incidence of neurologic deficit at the level of injury. Two possible long-term sequelae may result from these injuries:

1. Because the fracture fragments are displaced significantly and there may be a gap of 5 mm or more between the posterior and the anterior fragments, nonunion of that area is a significant possibility. However, approximately 70% of these patients develop anterior ankylosis of C2–3 anteriorly. The incidence of symptomatic nonunion is relatively low despite the radiographic evidence of no bony continuity across the arch posteriorly (Fig. 19–18). Rarely will a patient have both lack of bony continuity posteriorly and failure to develop ankylosis anteriorly. Although the numbers are very small, the patient with a moderately displaced fracture is somewhat more likely to go on to a symptomatic nonunion than one with a severely displaced fracture with marked destruction of the disc and the anterior portion of the body of C2.

2. A significant kyphotic defect, occurring locally at C2–3, is also possible. If the anterior portion of the C2 fragment is left angulated at 15 or more degrees, this will cause resultant local hyperextension at the occiput-C1–2 interval as well as below it. Patients can be symptomatic from the compensatory hyperextension. In addition, because a portion of the cervical extension motion is used to accommodate for the abnormal kyphosis, patients' ability to extend the neck will be proportionately decreased on physical examination, whereas flexion will be normal.

In the patient with a nonunion of C2–3 and widely displaced fracture fragments, posterior osteosynthesis is not possible as it is with the nonunited type I fracture. Nonunions of the type II fractures generally require an anterior C2–3 arthrodesis, which sometimes necessitates osteotomy of the inferior portion of the body of C2 to enter the C2–3 disc space. Again, because long-term results (>5 years) are not available in any series, the overall follow-up of patients with union and anatomic reduction is not statistically different from those with union in a displaced position.

Patients with type III injuries constitute a very small group. They have, in all series, a high rate of neurologic deficit because of the bilateral facet dislocation. Traditionally, all patients with high levels of quadriplegia have very poor long-term results. In the very small group of patients with either minimal or no neurologic deficit in whom an anatomic reduction can be achieved with arthrodesis, the long-term results are excellent. With the exception of the neurologic deficit and associated head injury that occur in essentially all patients, there are few other associated injuries.

Cervical Burst Fractures

Robert Benz ‖ *Jean-Jacques Abitbol* ‖ *Stephen Ozanne*
Steven R. Garfin

Burst fractures of the cervical spine are cervical body fractures produced primarily by axial compression forces. They have unique features as a result of cervical spine anatomy and a mechanism of injury which differentiates them from either compression fractures or teardrop fractures. Treatment options, which also differ significantly from other cervical injuries, will be discussed with an emphasis on anterior surgical techniques.

ANATOMY

The lower five cervical vertebrae have similar anatomy with a gradual increase in size cranial to caudal. The vertebral bodies are rectangular and have well-defined end plates. The width of the vertebral surfaces averages 17 mm from C2 through C6, and the depth averages 15 mm at these same levels.[72] At both posterolateral borders of the superior end plate are the uncinate processes. The uncinate processes extend from the posterior border of the vertebral body anteriorly one-half to two-thirds of the depth of the vertebral body and help resist translation in the coronal plane. This gives the vertebral body an overall concave superior end plate and a corresponding convex inferior end plate. This is in contradistinction to the coronal plane in which the superior end plate is slightly convex with a corresponding concave inferior end plate (Figs. 20–1 and 20–2).

The transverse processes are lateral projections from the vertebral body and consist of an anterior and posterior tubercle with an inferior sulcus for passage of the spinal nerve. The anterior tubercle of C6 is the most prominent and serves as a surgical landmark as the carotid tubercle. The transverse processes of the cervi-

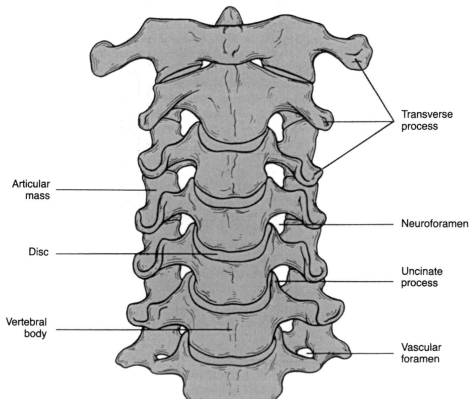

Figure 20–1 ═ This anterior view of the cervical spine demonstrates a number of pertinent features. All segments below C1–2 have a posterior lateral projection of the superior end plate, known as the uncinate process. The end plates are firmly fixed to the anulus fibrosus. The vertebral foramina are anterolateral to the neural canal. (From Bucholz RW: Lower cervical spine injuries. *In* Browner BD, Jupiter JB, Levine AM, et al (eds): Skeletal Trauma, vol 1. Philadelphia, WB Saunders, 1992, p 700.)

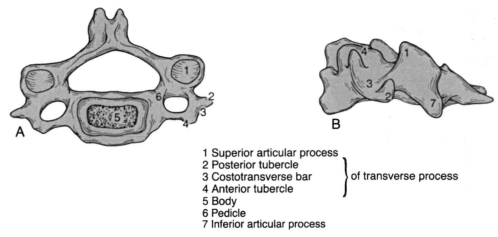

1 Superior articular process
2 Posterior tubercle
3 Costotransverse bar   } of transverse process
4 Anterior tubercle
5 Body
6 Pedicle
7 Inferior articular process

Figure 20–2 = This demonstrates a typical fifth cervical vertebra seen from above *(A)* and from the left side *(B)*. A number of important structures are delineated. The superior articular process is seen to be oblique and posterolateral to the neural canal *(1)*. The transverse process is composed of three portions: the posterior tubercle *(2)*, costotransverse bar *(3)*, and anterior tubercle *(4)*. The vertebral body *(5)* has posterolateral lips on the superior surface *(6)*, the uncinate processes. The inferior articular facet *(7)* parallels the superior articular facet. (From Bucholz RW: Lower cervical spine injuries. *In* Browner BD, Jupiter JB, Levine AM, et al (eds): Skeletal Trauma, vol 1. Philadelphia, WB Saunders, 1992, p 700.)

cal vertebrae possess vertebral foramina which contain the vertebral artery and venous system from C6 through C1. The vertebral artery passes anterior to the spinal nerve at each level. The cervical pedicles are short and broad, projecting posterolaterally from the vertebral body, and connect the body to the lateral masses. The angle of the pedicles in the sagittal plane relative to the body is approximately 45 degrees at C3 and gradually decreases to 30 degrees at C7. In the coronal plane, the pedicles range in angulation from 8 degrees inferiorly to 11 degrees superiorly. The superior and inferior facets are flat and are angled approximately 45 degrees in the coronal plane. Normal superior and inferior facets are covered with articular cartilage. The facet joints are covered with a loose capsule and possess a fibrocartilaginous meniscus of varying degrees.[3] The articulation between the vertebral bodies include the intervertebral disc, the uncinate processes, and the facet joints. This configuration allows flexion, extension, and lateral tilt. The normal range of flexion and extension motion decreases caudad. There is approximately 9 degrees of motion at each level in the coronal plane.[104] Lateral tilt is coupled with rotation. Each level of the subaxial cervical spine allows approximately 5 degrees of axial rotation.

The laminae of the cervical spine are relatively thin at C3 and gradually increase in thickness caudad. The lamina blend into the lateral masses, which are the areas of bone between the superior and inferior articular facets. The superoinferior interfacet distance has been shown to be 9 to 16 mm in the cervical spine.[4] The spinous processes of C3–5 are usually bifid and are also smaller than the more caudal ones. The C6–7 spinous processes are thicker and less often bifid. The cervical spinal canal has a triangular shape in the axial plane, with the lateral width greater than the anteroposterior depth throughout the cervical spine. Normal dimensions of the spinal canal are a sagittal depth of 17 to 18 mm at C3–6 and 15 mm at C7.[72]

The ligamentous attachments of the vertebrae include the anterior longitudinal ligament (ALL), the posterior longitudinal ligament (PLL), facet capsules, ligamenta flava, interspinous ligaments, and the supraspinous ligament (Fig. 20–3). The ALL originates as the anterior atlanto-occipital membrane and continues caudad to the sacrum. It has a more intimate attach-

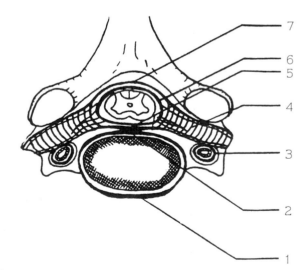

Figure 20–3 = Diagram of layers of the posterior longitudinal ligament. The posterior longitudinal ligament is double-layered, and the deep layer sends fibers to the anulus fibrosus and continues laterally to the intervertebral foramina. The anterior longitudinal ligament extends laterally to merge with the deep layer of the posterior longitudinal ligament in the region of the intervertebral foramina. The superficial or more dorsal layer of the posterior longitudinal ligament is adjacent to the dura mater and continues as a connective tissue membrane, which envelops the dura mater, nerve roots, and vertebral artery. *1*, Anterior longitudinal ligament; *2*, deep layer of the posterior longitudinal ligament; *3*, eparterial sheath; *4*, Epiradicular sheath; *5*, superficial layer of the posterior longitudinal ligament; *6*, dura mater; *7*, epidural membrane. (From An HS, Simpson JM (eds): Surgery of the Cervical Spine. Baltimore, Williams & Wilkins, 1994, p 13.)

76. Perret G, Greene J: Anterior interbody fusion in the treatment of cervical fracture dislocation. Arch Surg 96:530–539, 1968.

77. Petrie JG: Flexion injuries of the cervical spine. J Bone Joint Surg Am 46:1800–1806, 1964.

78. Rauschning W: Anatomy and Pathology of the Cervical Spine. *In* Frymoyer JW (ed): The Adult Spine. New York, Raven Press, 1991, pp 907–929.

79. Richman JD, Daniel TE, Anderson DD, et al: Biomechanical evaluation of cervical spine stabilization methods using a porcine model. Spine 20:2192–2197, 1995.

80. Ripa DR, Kowall MG, Meyer PR Jr, et al: Series of ninety-two traumatic cervical spine injuries stabilized with anterior ASIF plate fusion technique. Spine 16(suppl):S46–55, 1991.

81. Roaf R: A study of the mechanics of spinal injuries. J Bone Joint Surg Br 42:810–823, 1960.

82. Rogers WA: Fractures and dislocations of the cervical spine. J Bone Joint Surg Am 39:341–376, 1957.

83. Roy-Camille R, Saillant G, Edouard B: Posterior plate fixation of the lower cervical spine: A series of 274 cases. Orthop Trans 13:692, 1989.

84. Schaefer DM, Flanders A, Northrup BE, et al: Magnetic resonance imaging of acute cervical spine trauma. Correlation with severity of neurologic injury. Spine 14:1090–1095, 1989.

85. Schneider RC, Kahn EA: Chronic neurological sequelae of acute trauma to the spine and spinal cord, part I: The significance of the acute-flexion or "tear-drop" fracture-dislocation of the cervical spine. J Bone Joint Surg Am 38:985–997, 1956.

86. Schulte K, Clark CR, Goel VK: Kinematics of the cervical spine following discectomy and stabilization. Spine 14:1116–1121, 1989.

87. Stauffer ES: Management of spine fractures C3 to C7. Orthop Clin North Am 17:45–53, 1986.

88. Stauffer ES: Wiring techniques of the posterior cervical spine for the treatment of trauma. Orthopedics 11:1543–1548, 1988.

89. Stauffer ES: Subaxial injuries. Clin Orthop 239:30–39, 1989.

90. Stauffer ES, Kelly EG: Fracture-dislocations of the cervical spine. Instability and recurrent deformity following treatment by anterior interbody fusion. J Bone Joint Surg Am 59:45–48, 1977.

91. Stauffer ES, Rhoades ME: Surgical stabilization of the cervical spine after trauma. Arch Surg 111:652–657, 1976.

92. Suh PB, Kostuik JP, Esses SI: Anterior cervical plate fixation with the titanium hollow screw plate system. A preliminary report. Spine 15:1079–1081, 1990.

93. Sutterlin CE, McAfee PC, Warden KE, et al: A biomechanical evaluation of cervical spinal stabilization methods in a bovine model. Static and cyclical loading. Spine 13:795–802, 1988.

94. Tator CH: Early Management of Acute Spinal Cord Injury. New York, Raven Press, 1982.

95. Tew JM Jr., Mayfield FH: Complications of surgery of the anterior cervical spine. Clin Neurosurg 23:424–434, 1976.

96. Tracy PT, Wright RM, Hanigan WC: Magnetic resonance imaging of spinal injury. Spine 14:292–301, 1989.

97. Triggs KJ, Ballock RT, Lee TQ, et al: The effect of angled insertion on halo pin fixation. Spine 14:781–783, 1989.

98. Ulrich C, Woersdoerfer O, Kalff R, et al: Biomechanics of fixation systems to the cervical spine. Spine 16(suppl):S4–9, 1991.

99. Verbiest H: Anterolateral operations for fractures or dislocations of the cervical spine due to injuries or previous surgical interventions. Clin Neurosurg 20:334–366, 1973.

100. Webb JK, Broughton RB, McSweeney T, et al: Hidden flexion injury of the cervical spine. J Bone Joint Surg Br 58:322–327, 1976.

101. Weinshel S: Neurologic recovery in complete quadriplegia following cervical fusion. Othop Trans 13:207, 1989.

102. Weirich SD, Cotler HB, Narayana PA, et al: Histopathologic correlation of magnetic resonance imaging signal patterns in a spinal cord injury model. Spine 15:630–638, 1990.

103. White AA, Panjabi MM: Clinical Biomechanics of the Spine. Philadelphia, JB Lippincott, 1990.

104. White AA, Southwick WO, Panjabi MM: Clinical instability in the lower cervical spine: A review of past and current concepts. Spine 1:15–27, 1976.

105. White RJ, Yashon D: General care of cervical spine injuries. *In* Youmans JR (ed): Neurological Surgery. Philadelphia, WB Saunders, 1973.

106. Whitehill R, Richman JA, Glaser JA: Failure of immobilization of the cervical spine by the halo vest. A report of five cases. J Bone Joint Surg Am 68:326–332, 1986.

107. Whitley JE, Forsyth HF: The classification of cervical spine injuries. AJR 83:633–644, 1960.

108. Wilber RG, Peters JG, Likavec MJ: Surgical techniques in cervical spine surgery. *In* Errico TJ, Bauer RD, Waugh T (eds): Spinal Trauma. Philadelphia, JB Lippincott, 1990.

109. Willen J, Lindahl S, Irstam L, et al: The thoracolumbar crush fracture. An experimental study on instant axial dynamic loading: the resulting fracture type and its stability. Spine 9:624–631, 1984.

110. Wittenberg RH, Moeller J, Shea M, et al: Compressive strength of autologous and allogenous bone grafts for thoracolumbar and cervical spine fusion. Spine 15:1073–1078, 1990.

111. Yoganandan N, Sances A Jr, Pintar F, et al: Injury biomechanics of the human cervical column. Spine 15:1031–1039, 1990.

112. Young WF, Rosenwasser RH: An early comparative analysis of the use of fibular allograft versus autologous iliac crest graft for interbody fusion after anterior cervical discectomy. Spine 18:1123–1124, 1993.

113. Zdeblick TA, Ducker TB: The use of freeze-dried allograft bone for anterior cervical fusions. Orthop Trans 14:692, 1990.

114. Zdeblick TA, Wilson D, Cooke ME, et al: Anterior cervical discectomy and fusion. A comparison of techniques in an animal model. Spine 17(suppl):S418–426, 1992.

Teardrop Fractures of the Cervical Spine

Zaki G. Ibrahim ‖ *Jean-Jacques Abitbol* ‖ *Steven R. Garfin*

The term "tear-drop" fracture was coined in 1956 by Schneider and Kahn[75] to describe an acute flexion injury of the cervical spine that was characterized by compression of the involved vertebral body and displacement of the anteroinferior corner away from the remainder of the body:

This lesion is characterized by crushing of one vertebral body by the vertebral body superior to it in such a manner that the anterior part of the involved centrum is not only compressed but often is completely broken away from its major portion. In most of these cases, this fragment has resembled a drop of water dripping from the vertebral body and it has been associated with dire circumstances so frequently that the terms "tear-drop" and "acute-flexion" fracture-dislocation of the cervical spine seemed to describe the lesion and to suggest the mechanism of the injury.[75]

These authors recognized the devastating nature of the injury and documented the frequent association with severe neural injury. They correctly described the displacement of the inferior margin of the fractured vertebral body backward into the spinal canal as an important feature of the injury. However, their recommendations of early laminectomy and sectioning of the dentate ligaments to decompress the spinal cord have subsequently been shown to lead to increased deformity, pain, and potential neurologic deficit.[1, 10, 80]

Teardrop fractures of the cervical spine are often severe injuries which occur as a result of high-energy trauma. These fractures usually result from a combination of flexion and compression forces occurring when the neck is flexed and the top of the head strikes a solid object. Often, these fractures are the result of a fall from a height, a diving accident, or a motor vehicle accident.[13, 44, 49, 53, 60, 64, 74] The injury usually occurs in the lower cervical spine.[23, 27, 29, 63, 76] C5 is the most commonly involved vertebra.[17, 30, 46, 49, 52, 60, 64]

Since Schneider and Kahn's initial description of the injury, many authors have attempted to define the nature of instability associated with teardrop fractures and to recommend appropriate treatment measures.[6, 9, 16, 19, 42] Until recently, teardrop fractures were considered a variant of the more common compression fracture of the cervical spine.[7, 55] However, recent evidence suggests that the instability inherent in this injury justifies its categorization as a separate entity requiring special consideration of treatment options.[17, 20, 43]

This chapter provides a detailed discussion of the current understanding of teardrop fractures. The mechanism of injury, anatomic pattern of instability, radiographic evaluation, and treatment options are presented with respect to different authors' opinions. Special attention is given to evaluation and preservation of neural function.

ANATOMY

Discussion of the anatomy of the lower cervical spine is limited here because of detailed discussions in previous chapters. However, a number of important points deserve mention. The anatomy of the upper two cervical vertebrae is uniquely suited to support the occiput and allow rotation of the head. Because teardrop fractures do not occur in the upper two vertebrae, their anatomy will not be considered further. The anatomic characteristics of the lower five cervical vertebrae are remarkably similar, increasing somewhat in size from C3 to C7.

The cervical vertebral bodies are approximately half the size of those of the lumbar spine, reflecting the lighter loads borne by the cervical spine. In contrast to the three-joint spinal motion segment seen in the lumbar spine, the cervical spinal motion segment consists of a five-joint complex.[4, 67] In addition to the intervertebral disc and the paired posterior facet joints, a unique feature of the cervical spine is the two superior posterolateral extensions of the vertebral body known as the uncinate processes. These paired processes extend superiorly from the edges of the superior end plate, partially overlapping the disc above, creating a concavity on the superior end plates of C3–7. The uncinate processes together with the inferolateral margins of the superjacent vertebra form the neurocentral joints, or joints of Luschka.[67]

The transverse processes of the spinal vertebrae project directly laterally from the vertebral body and are composed of an anterior and posterior tubercle and an intervening groove which houses the exiting spinal nerve. Just medial and posterior to the anterior tubercle, but anterior to the spinal nerve, lies the transverse foramen, which surrounds the vertebral artery and venous system.[77]

The pedicles of the cervical vertebrae project posterolaterally from the vertebral body to the lateral mass, which consists of the superior and inferior facet joints. In contrast to the facet joints in the lumbar spine, those in the lower cervical spine are oriented in a coronal plane, angling from anterosuperior to posteroinferior at about 45 degrees in the sagittal plane. As a result of the morphology of the facet joints in combination with the presence of the uncinate processes, lateral flexion of the cervical spine is coupled with axial rotation.[87]

The ligaments of the cervical spine contribute significantly to stability.[84, 85] The intervertebral disc is composed of an outer, fibrous, anulus fibrosus and an inner nucleus pulposus. The discs are shaped to conform to the surface of the vertebral bodies; hence the superior surface of the disc is concave, and the inferior surface is convex in the coronal plane. The anulus fibrosus of the disc is tightly fixed to the cartilaginous end plates of the adjacent superior and inferior vertebral bodies. The outermost fibers of the disc anulus are contiguous with the anterior and posterior longitudinal ligaments. The ligamentum flavum of the cervical spine attaches to the anterior surface of the superior lamina, and to the superior margin of the inferior lamina. It extends laterally to the articular processes and contributes to the boundary of the intervertebral foramen. The interspinous ligament of the cervical spine is thin and less well developed than in the lumbar region. The ligamentum nuchae is an extension of the supraspinous ligament of the thoracolumbar spine. There is no separate supraspinous ligament in the cervical region.[67] It spans the cervical region from the occipital protuberance to C7. In addition to providing cervical stability, it functions as a fibroelastic septum for the attachment of adjacent paracervical muscles. The posterior ligaments of the cervical spine contribute more to stability in flexion than extension. The anterior ligaments contribute more to stability in extension than flexion[84] (Fig. 21–1).

The spinal canal in the cervical spine is triangular in shape with rounded corners. The width of the spinal canal is significantly greater than its depth at all levels. In the cervical spine, the proportion of space occupied by neural elements (spinal cord) to the space available for the cord is significantly greater than that in the lumbar spine. This characteristic places the cervical spinal cord at significantly greater risk from retropulsion of bone in the case of vertebral body fracture than the corresponding neural elements in the lumbar spine.[87]

The vascular anatomy of the spinal cord must be included in any discussion of cervical trauma with potential for neurologic loss. The major blood supply to the cervical cord and the cervical spine is the paired vertebral arteries, which originate from the subclavian arteries and usually enter the transverse foramen at C6, ascending through the transverse foramen of the upper cervical vertebra to C1, where they wind around the lateral masses and posterior arch of the atlas. The two vertebral arteries join together to form the basilar artery as they enter the foramen magnum. In the region of the foramen magnum, the vertebral arteries give off anterior branches which join together to form the single anterior spinal artery. This artery descends along the anterior aspect of the spinal cord, supplying the

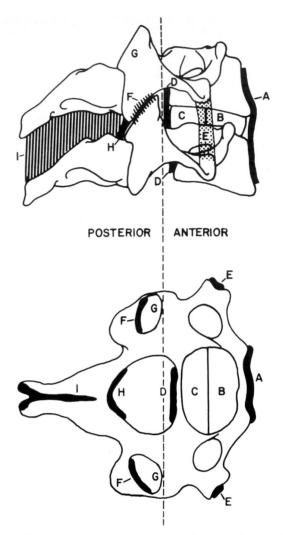

POSTERIOR | **ANTERIOR**

Figure 21–1 = Supporting ligaments of the cervical spine. *A*, ant. longitudinal lig.; *B*, ant. half of anulus fibrosus; *C*, post. half of anulus fibrosus; *D*, post. longitudinal lig.; *E*, costotransverse lig.; *F*, capsular ligaments of facet joints; *G*, articular facet; *H*, ligamentum flavum; *I*, interspinous and supraspinous ligaments. (From White AA, Johnson MR, Panjabi MM, et al: Biomechanical analysis of clinical stability in the cervical spine. Clin Orthop 109:85–96, 1975.)

majority of the spinal cord, with the exception of the posterior columns. The paired posterior spinal arteries are branches on the posterolateral aspect of the spinal cord which are derived from the posteroinferior cerebellar arteries. These arteries give rise to plexiform channels which are arranged transversely on the dorsum of the spinal cord. The paired posterior spinal arteries are the major source of blood supply for the posterior columns.

RADIOGRAPHIC CHARACTERISTICS

Schneider and Kahn[75] originally described the "teardrop" portion of the fracture (the anteroinferior portion of the vertebral body which fractures away from the centrum). These authors observed the frequent angular displacement of the posteroinferior margin into the spinal canal which was often associated with neurologic injury. However, they paid scant attention to other features of the teardrop injury and associated ligamentous instability.

Norton[64] and Rogers[69] found that in some instances the body of a cervical vertebra could be split in the frontal or sagittal plane into two or more major fragments. Norton theorized that these fractures were created by vertical forces applied to the cervical spine with the neck in different positions of flexion and extension. Both authors commented that posterior displacement of these fragments could have serious neurologic implications.

Scher[73] cautioned that the stability of the cervical spine after injury with a major flexion component is dependent upon the integrity of the posterior ligamentous complex. He encouraged examiners to look for evidence of injury to these structures. Signs which may indicate that a posterior ligamentous injury exists include (1) an increase in the interspinous process distance at the level of injury on the lateral radiograph; (2) loss of parallelism and subluxation at the apophyseal joints due to tearing of the joint capsules; (3) disruption of the intervertebral disc resulting in narrowing of the disc space; and (4) posterior displacement of the fractured vertebral body indicating disruption of the posterior longitudinal ligament (Fig. 21–2).

Kim and co-workers[49] also emphasized the importance of ligamentous disruption in their radiographic review of 45 patients with teardrop fractures. These investigators divided the cervical spine into an upper and lower column at the level of ligamentous disruption. They found that the upper column was displaced

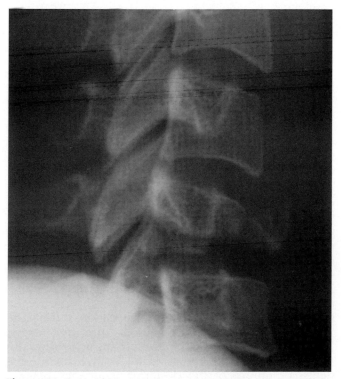

Figure 21–2 = Teardrop fractures of C5. There is posterior displacement of the C5 body and posteroinferior fragment, angulation of the C5–6 interspinous process space, and loss of parallelism of the C5–6 facet joint.

posteriorly relative to the lower column in 80% of cases. They believed that a characteristic feature of this injury, in addition to the displaced anterior fragment, is the displaced posterior fragment of the involved body. The disc space between the posterior fragment and the vertebral body below was narrowed in all 20 cases for which initial radiographs were available, although the disc space between the anterior fragment and the subjacent vertebral body was maintained. Of these cases, 18 (40%) showed widening of the interlaminar and interspinous spaces between the level of injury and the one below. In addition, in 12 (27%) cases, there was widening of the disc facet, and interlaminar and interspinous spaces on one of the serial lateral radiographs obtained after traction through tongs was applied. This study draws attention to the importance of attempting to determine the presence of ligamentous injury in the radiographic analysis of teardrop fractures, as this may greatly affect spinal stability.

A number of investigators have examined the occurrence of other fracture patterns which develop in this injury in addition to the anteroinferior teardrop fragment. Lee and colleagues[53] documented through the use of plain tomography and computed tomography (CT) scanning that 67% of teardrop fractures in their series had an associated sagittal vertical fracture of the vertebral body. This was the most commonly associated fracture accompanying the injury. In a separate paper,[52] the authors noted that a vertical radiolucent line projecting over the body, or cortical disruption of the end plates on the anteroposterior (AP) view, may be the only subtle finding(s) on plain radiographs to excite suspicion of a sagittal component of the fracture. Other authors[32, 60, 83] have verified that sagittal fractures occur in 44% to 60% of teardrop injuries and frequently may be missed on plain radiographs. Less commonly associated injuries include posterior arch fractures (pedicle or lamina) in 48% and articular mass fractures in 20%. Kim and associates[49] noted that in five of six cases with normal neurologic status, there were no sagittal body or laminar fractures. However, a sagittal body fracture was present in all but one of the 39 cases with complete or incomplete neurologic deficits (Fig. 21–3).

Because plain films often underestimate the degree of bony instability, and frequently do not provide a good assessment of neural canal compromise, further imaging is necessary to provide an adequate understanding of the fracture. Plain tomography has been shown in the past to be useful in delineating anatomy of the fracture pattern.[52, 53] However, the greater resolution of bony detail provided by CT and the ability to reconstruct the fracture pattern in the axial, sagittal, and coronal planes makes this technology the imaging study of choice for bony injuries of the cervical spine.[60] Plain radiographic studies remain the primary diagnostic evaluation and should direct the examiner's approach to further diagnostic investigation.[23]

MECHANISM OF INJURY

Fractures and dislocations in the lower cervical spine are usually the result of indirect forces originating in

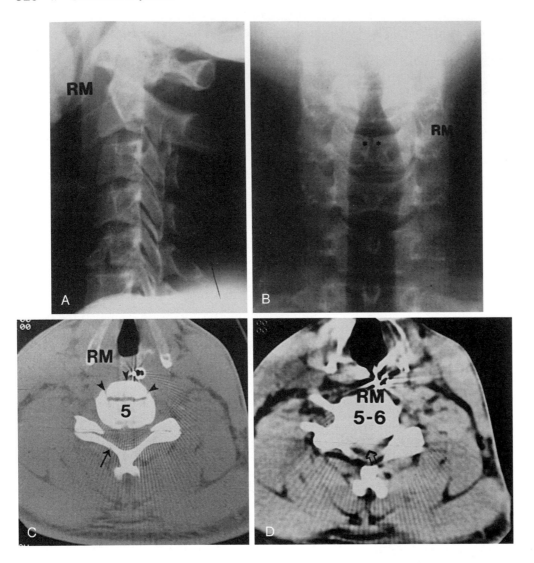

Figure 21–3 = Anteroposterior (A) and lateral (B) radiographs of a 39-year-old male victim of a motor vehicle accident who presented with a central cord syndrome. A vertical split in the C5 vertebral body is seen on the AP view with evidence of anterior compression on the lateral. C, Axial CT shows a C5 body fracture with a coronal component (below 5), and nondisplaced laminar fracture. D, A more caudal axial CT shows canal compromise caused by a retropulsed bone fragment.

the head and causing excessive axial loading along with components of flexion, extension, or rotational forces. The majority of these injuries result from being thrown headfirst against a solid object in a motor vehicle accident, diving headfirst and striking a solid object, or falling headfirst. As the head strikes a solid object and comes to a sudden stop, the inertial energy of the moving trunk and extremities is expended in the cervical spine, causing a buckling injury that results in tearing of the ligaments and an axial loading type of fracture of the vertebral body.[78]

The nature of the forces which result specifically in the teardrop fracture of the cervical spine have been studied by numerous examiners.[3, 14, 21, 43, 48, 53, 64, 73, 75] Schneider and Kahn[75] believed that the teardrop fracture is caused by acute flexion and vertical compression whereby the anterior portion of the vertebral body is compressed and fractured away from the remainder. Kewalramani and Taylor[48] suggested that the injury is caused by compression in an anteroposterior, as well as vertical, direction which allows "pinching off" of the anteroinferior angle of the vertebra. Norton[64] noted that teardrop injuries were produced by vertical forces applied to the cervical spine with the neck in various

positions of flexion as opposed to bursting fractures which involved a strong vertical force applied to a straightened neck.

Harris and co-workers[43] correctly realized that the injury seen on the radiograph was, in all probability, the result of multiple simultaneous forces with one vector predominant, rather than a single pure force. The authors went on to categorize the teardrop injury as a flexion injury, noting that in addition to the vertebral body fracture, the injury was characterized by complete disruption of all of the ligaments and the intervertebral disc at the level of injury, including the facet joint capsules.

Allen and co-authors described two types of flexion injuries—compression-flexion injuries (burst fractures and teardrop fractures) and distraction-flexion injuries (unilateral and bilateral facet dislocations). They divided compression-flexion injuries into five stages. Stage 1 lesions consist of blunting of the anterosuperior vertebral margin of the vertebral body with no evidence of failure of the posterior ligaments. Stage 2 lesions show obliquity of the anterior vertebral body and loss of some of the height of the anterior centrum. Thus, there is a "beak" appearance of the anteroinferior

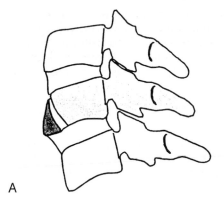

A

Stage III Flexion Compression

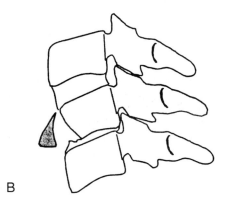

B

Stage IV Flexion Compression

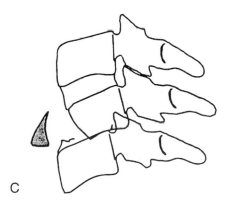

C

Stage V Flexion Compression

Figure 21–4 = Allen's compression-flexion injuries, stages III to V. *A,* The teardrop fragment first appears in a stage III injury. With further injury, there is posterior ligamentous disruption and retropulsion of the posteroinferior vertebral body into the spinal canal. *B,* Stage IV, less than 3 mm posterior displacement. *C,* Stage V, more than 3 mm posterior displacement. (From Allen BL: Recognition of injuries to the lower cervical spine. *In* Anderson LD, Clark CR (eds): The Cervical Spine. Philadelphia, JB Lippincott, 1989.)

vertebral body. With further force of injury, the beak is fractured and a stage 3 lesion develops. In this lesion, a fracture line passes obliquely from the anterior surface of the vertebral body through the inferior subchondral plate. A stage 4 lesion is similar to a stage 3 lesion with the addition of less than 3 mm of displacement of the posteroinferior margin into the neural canal.

Finally, in a stage 5 lesion, there is more significant retropulsion of bone into the canal, along with evidence of posterior ligament disruption. Thus, teardrop fractures would comprise those injuries in stages 3 to 5, with the majority of these injuries falling into stages 4 and 5 of compression-flexion injuries (Fig. 21–4).

Kim and co-workers[49] theorized that the anteroinferior margin of the involved vertebral body is fractured by shear stress with compressive loading and the major portion of the body is displaced backward into the spinal canal. The portion of the intervertebral disc between the major posterior fragment and the vertebral body below is disrupted while that portion between the smaller anterior fragment and the subjacent vertebra remains intact. The reciprocal distraction force that occurs in the posterior column of the spine results in disruption of the posterior ligamentous structures. Thus, the cervical spine is divided into an upper and a lower column at the level of injury. The line of injury separates the anterior and posterior body fragments, the disc space between the posterior fragment and the body below, the facet joint, and the interspinous space.

Torg and co-authors[83] described two types of fracture patterns associated with teardrop injuries in football players. The first pattern was an isolated fracture which was usually not associated with neurologic sequelae. The second pattern was a three-part, two-plane fracture in which there was an associated sagittal body fracture as well as a fracture of the posterior neural arch. Based on review of injury reports and hospital records, interviews with coaches, and stop-frame analysis of game films, the authors concluded that axial loading of the straightened cervical spine was the mechanism of injury in both types of teardrop fractures.[83]

It appears that the major vector of injury is axial compression with the spine in an attitude of flexion. In the earlier stages (Allen cervical fracture stages (CFS1 and CFS2) the force appears to be concentrated along the anterosuperior margin of the vertebral body. Resolution of this compressive force is achieved by the oblique fracture of the vertebral body (CFS3). In the majority of teardrop fractures (CFS4 and CFS5), there is an additional flexion injury vector which produces posterior ligamentous failure. The higher stages are associated with a greater force of injury and reflect a greater degree of instability. This is borne out by the neurologic picture in the 36 cases of compression-flexion injuries seen in the series of Allen and co-workers.[3] Complete spinal cord injury was present in 25% of CFS3 injuries, 38% of CFS4 injuries, and 91% of CFS5 injuries.

PATTERNS OF NEUROLOGIC DAMAGE

Frequently, teardrop fractures are associated with major neurologic deficits.* In the study of Lee and co-workers,[53] only 13% remained neurologically intact, while the majority (57%) became quadriplegic. Schnei-

---

*References 3, 7, 32, 42, 48, 49, 52, 53, 55, 64, 69, 73, 75, 83.

der and Kahn[75] and others[32, 42, 49, 73] noted a frequent association between teardrop fractures with retropulsion of bone and anterior spinal cord syndrome.

Anterior spinal cord syndrome is thought to be caused by compromise of the vascular supply of the anterior spinal artery by material from retropulsion, with resultant ischemia and cell death in the portion of the spinal cord is supplied primarily by this artery (anterior two thirds). Since the vascular supply to the posterior columns is usually spared, their function remains intact.[49, 73] A comprehensive review of anterior spinal cord syndrome was presented by Schneider in 1951.[72] This syndrome is characterized by immediate complete motor paralysis, hypoesthesia, and hypalgesia to a level consistent with the lesion with preservation of the sense of position, deep touch, and vibration. Other authors[32, 53] have documented the occurrence of central cord syndrome and Brown-Séquard syndrome with these injuries. Brown-Séquard syndrome is seen in those teardrop injuries with asymmetrical posterior displacement of one half of the sagittally split vertebral body.[32, 55]

Beatson[7] broadly categorized cervical spine injuries into three groups based on whether they had a bursting fracture of the vertebral body with displacement of the posteroinferior margin of the body into the spinal canal (group 1), anterior dislocation of one vertebral body on the subjacent body by less than one half of the anteroposterior depth of the body (group 2), or anterior dislocation of one vertebral body on the subjacent body by more than half of the anteroposterior depth of the body (group 3). He found that cord damage was a frequent complication of group 1 and group 3 injuries, but an infrequent complication of group 2 injuries. Many of the tetraplegic patients with group 1 injuries had some sensory sparing, but had complete motor paralysis below the level of the lesion (anterior cord syndrome), whereas the tetraplegics in groups 2 and 3 usually had complete sensory and motor loss.

Marar[55] analyzed 126 cases of cervical spine injuries with regard to the clinical patterns of neurologic damage and the radiographic patterns of skeletal injury. The author did not distinguish between vertebral burst fractures and teardrop fractures, classifying both under the broad category of compression injuries. Of the 22 patients with compression injuries, 16 had spinal cord damage. Of the 18 patients with complete spinal cord injuries, 10 had vertebral compression injuries and 8 had bilateral articular process dislocation. Four patients in this study had anterior spinal cord syndrome. All four had burst fractures of the vertebral body. Of the four patients who presented with a Brown-Séquard syndrome after injury, two patients had a unilateral articular process dislocation and two had burst injuries. In this article, all 16 patients with compression injuries and neurologic deficits had either complete injuries, anterior cord syndrome, or Brown-Séquard syndrome.

Indeed, severe neurologic damage is frequently seen as an unfortunate sequela of these devastating injuries. As may be seen from the previously cited work, it appears that the most common associated neurologic picture is that of a complete spinal cord injury followed by an anterior spinal cord syndrome. This implies that the usual mechanism of spinal cord injury in teardrop fractures is compression of the anterior portion of the spinal cord by retropulsion of fragments of the vertebral body. A complete spinal cord injury may result from high-energy displacement of the fractured fragments into the spinal canal. With lower-energy fractures, the anterior spinal cord is compromised, but the posterior columns are spared, resulting in anterior spinal cord syndrome. Brown-Séquard syndrome may uncommonly occur when there is asymmetrical posterior displacement of the fractured vertebral body fragments.

PATIENT EVALUATION

Teardrop fractures account for between 6% and 12% of reported cervical spine injuries. Common causes of severe cervical spinal injuries include motor vehicle accidents, falls from a height, and diving into shallow water.[3, 10, 34, 48, 64, 69, 78] A brief investigation at the accident scene and attempted reconstruction of the patient's injury mechanism should be conducted. Emergency medical stabilization takes precedence, but the cervical spine should be stabilized until an injury in this area is ruled out. If the patient has suffered a head injury, or is intoxicated or violent, cervical spine precautions should be applied in the field and maintained until spinal column injuries have been ruled out by radiographs. A high index of suspicion and increased vigilance for spinal stabilization prior to evacuation of a patient from a trauma scene are factors that are believed to have contributed to the recent decline in the percentage of complete spinal cord injuries.[34]

Upon arrival at the treating institution cervical immobilization is continued while standard emergency care is administered. Although a spinal cord injury is a catastrophic event and neurologic deterioration must be minimized, preservation of life takes precedence. Once the acute threat to life has been dispelled, a careful neurologic examination follows. In the case of suspected cervical spinal cord injury, the presence of function below the level of injury or of sacral sparing should be noted. A high-dose methylprednisolone spinal cord injury protocol (30 mg/kg of methylprednisolone over 1 hour followed by 5.4 mg/kg per hour for 23 hours) has been found to be beneficial in patients with spinal cord injuries, whether these injuries are complete or incomplete.[15]

A cervical hard collar remains in place while radiographs are obtained. In the severely injured patient, the limited examination of horizontal-beam lateral and anteroposterior (AP) projections is usually sufficient for evaluation of the acute problem. If possible, an open-mouth odontoid view should be obtained to visualize the atlantoaxial articulation in the frontal projection.[42] These three views make up the "three-view cervical trauma series." The routine addition of supine oblique views to this protocol has not been found to add additional diagnostic information.[31] However, these views may be helpful in the case of inadequate visualization of the cervicothoracic junction.[41] Of the three initial views obtained, the horizontal-beam lateral view is the "money" view, and should be made prior to application of head and upper extremity traction in order to avoid distracting an existing skeletal or soft tissue injury.[31]

The importance of obtaining images of the entire lower cervical spine and the upper portion of the first thoracic segment cannot be overemphasized. Kim and co-workers[49] and others[10, 52, 53] have documented the occurrence of adjacent segment injuries in up to 33% of cervical teardrop fractures. If the lower cervical spine is not adequately visualized, either a swimmer's[7] view or supine oblique projections may provide useful information about the cervicothoracic junction. Cervical traction for diagnostic radiographic purposes is contraindicated in the presence of an existing cervical spine injury.[42]

Often, a general idea about the degree of spinal instability may be inferred from the initial cervical spinal radiographs. White and colleagues[85] have defined clinical instability as the loss of the ability of the spine to maintain its premorbid patterns of motion without subsequent damage or irritation of the spinal medulla or nerve roots under physiologic loads, or the development in the spine of gross deformity or excessive pain. These authors considered the cervical spine unstable when any of the following conditions are present: (1) all of the anterior elements (the posterior longitudinal ligament and all the vertebral anatomic structures anterior to it) or all of the posterior elements (all vertebral anatomic structures posterior to the posterior longitudinal ligament) are destroyed or unable to function; (2) there is more than 3.5 mm of horizontal displacement of one vertebra in relation to an adjacent vertebra measured on lateral radiographs; or (3) there is more than 11 degrees of rotation compared with either adjacent vertebra measured on the lateral radiograph.[80, 81] Allen and co-authors drew a distinction between CFS3 lesions and CFS4 and CFS5 injuries because they felt that the displacement of the posteroinferior portion of the vertebral margin at the involved motion segment reflected a tension and shear minor injury vector through the posterior part of the anterior elements and the entirety of the posterior elements, while the displacement seen in CFS5 injuries (greater than 3 mm) denoted complete failure through the motion segment. Other signs of ligamentous instability include narrowing of the disc space, widening of the facet joints, and widening of the interlaminar and interspinous spaces between the level of injury and the one below.[49, 79]

The cervical trauma series should be carefully reviewed to assess the presence and degree of instability. Flexion and extension views should not routinely be obtained in the presence of instability.[3, 41] At the University of California, San Diego (UCSD), any teardrop fracture with known neurologic deficit, retropulsion of bone greater than 3 mm seen on the lateral view, or greater than 11 degrees of angulation to either adjacent segment, is considered an unstable fracture. Those patients who present with teardrop fractures but who do not have known neurologic deficits, greater than 3 mm of retropulsion of bone, or greater than 11 degrees of angulation, are considered to have stable injuries, and may continue to be immobilized in a hard collar as the remainder of the workup proceeds.

If an unstable fracture has been identified on plain films, Gardner-Wells skull tongs may be applied and skeletal-skull traction maintained with the patient on a kinetic treatment table.[34] Ten pounds of traction should initially be instituted. Weight is increased in 5-lb increments with serial radiographs after each 5-lb addition until the overall alignment of the cervical spine has been reconstituted. Aebi and associates[1] have demonstrated that patients who had a cervical spinal injury reduced within 6 hours of injury had a better rate of neurologic recovery than those in whom reduction was carried out after 6 hours. Care must be taken to avoid overdistraction of the injury through disrupted ligamentous structures.[49] A CT scan of the injured area is obtained at this point. Although CT is not indicated in every type of acute spinal injury, it is reasonably indicated in any injury resulting in neurologic deficit, in fractures of the posterior arch of the canal, and in every fracture with suspected retropulsion of posterior fragments.[23, 34, 42] Because of the frequent association of teardrop fractures with significant retropulsion of bone and disc material, fracture lines which may not be recognized on plain films, and the frequent association of neural deficits with these injuries, we believe that a CT scan is a necessary part of the diagnostic evaluation of both stable and unstable teardrop fractures.

Review of the CT scan may increase understanding of the teardrop fracture in a number of ways: (1) a sagittal split component of the vertebral body may be identified; (2) the degree of retropulsion of material into the spinal canal and spinal cord compromise may be quantitated; and (3) fractures of the posterior arch and adjacent segments, which may not have been seen on initial plain radiographs, may be identified.[7, 59, 60] Reformatting of the CT image in the sagittal or coronal plane allows appreciation of the three-dimensional characteristics of the fracture. Magnetic resonance imaging (MRI) may be helpful, as it is superior to the CT scan for visualization of injuries to discs, ligaments, and the spinal cord. However, its role is compromised by its limited ability to image cortical bone. Although the indications for MRI in cervical spinal trauma are expanding, we currently feel that MRI has only a limited place in the evaluation of acute cervical spinal injury.[42] Information gained from plain films and CT scan are sufficient to appreciate the nature of the instability and devise a treatment plan in most cases.

TREATMENT

The goal of cervical spinal injury management is to obtain a stable, healed cervical motion segment and to prevent further neurologic damage. At least three reasons exist for considering operative intervention for teardrop injuries. These include (1) restoring normal alignment, if this cannot be achieved by traction and closed reduction; (2) providing early stability to an unstable spine; and (3) decompression of neural structures for anticipated neurologic recovery.[78] The physician must consider how to best achieve both early and late stability, without unnecessarily jeopardizing the patient's neurologic status.

Patients Without Neural Deficit

Nonoperative treatment may be considered for patients with no neurologic deficit, in whom the teardrop fracture pattern is thought to be stable. A comminuted vertebral body fracture without posterior fracture, ligamentous disruption, facet dislocation, or neurologic injury will usually heal with symptomatic care and external orthotic immobilization. However, vertebral body fractures *and* posterior ligament disruption often result in an unstable injury.[78] Cheshire[20] has emphasized the difficulty in differentiating the true vertical compression injury, in which all surrounding ligaments are intact, from the flexion-compression injury, which is unstable by virtue of the disruption of the posterior ligament complex at the time of injury. Cheshire treated 63 "vertical compression" injuries nonoperatively with skull tongs and skeletal traction or a cervical collar. Three patients demonstrated instability on flexion-extension films taken at 12 weeks. Each of these patients was believed to have sustained a vertical compression injury while the neck was flexed and the flexion element had been missed in the early examination. One of these patients had a classic teardrop fracture as described by Schneider and Kahn.[75] Cheshire warned that teardrop fractures should be treated with suspicion and considered for early spinal fusion because of the likelihood of posterior ligamentous disruption.

Bohlman[10] reported 78 patients with cervical spine injuries treated nonoperatively and found a late instability rate of 42%. Twenty-one of the 33 patients (64%) with chronic instability had flexion injuries with disruption of the posterior elements.[10]

In contrast, Johnson and Cannon[46] treated 10 patients with acute teardrop fractures with skull traction, halo immobilization, or immobilization in a Minerva jacket. All patients had neurologic deficits and most had marked posterior displacement of the involved vertebra. One patient had significant functional recovery, and only one patient demonstrated persistent instability on flexion-extension films taken at 12 weeks' postinjury.

It appears that the most important factor in determining whether these injuries are amenable to nonoperative treatment is the integrity of the posterior ligamentous structures. Careful attention should be given to the appearance of the fractured vertebra on the lateral view and CT scan. The presence of posterior displacement of the fractured vertebral body, narrowing of the disc space, widening of the facet joints and the interspinous distance at the level of injury, and significant kyphosis should be noted. Allen and colleagues[3] observed that CFS4 (less than 3 mm displacement of the posteroinferior corner) and CFS5 lesions (greater than 3 mm displacement) suggest significant damage to the posterior ligamentous structures. White and colleagues[86] determined that the upper limit of physiologic angular displacement of the vertebrae in question is 11 degrees in relation to adjacent vertebrae. Angulation of greater than 11 degrees implies ligamentous instability in flexion. Spinal injuries with a ligamentous component heal less reliably than bony injuries.[7, 10, 20, 27, 34, 43, 75, 78–80]

In general, criteria for the nonoperative management of teardrop injuries include the following: (1) the patient should be neurologically intact; (2) there must be minimal displacement of the posteroinferior margin of the vertebral body into the canal (CFS1–CFS3 injuries) as seen on lateral radiograph and CT scan; (3) local kyphotic angulation of the involved vertebrae is less than 11 degrees greater than that of the adjacent segments; and (4) there is minimal (less than 1 to 2 mm) to no widening of the facet joints at the level of injury and the interspinous process distance must not be significantly greater than that of adjacent segments. These injuries may be satisfactorily immobilized in a hard collar for 12 weeks (Fig. 21–5). At the end of collar immobilization flexion-extension lateral radiographs should be obtained for evaluation of residual ligamentous instability. Those patients with persistent instability by the criteria of White and associates[84, 87] should be considered candidates for posterior cervical fusion.

In those patients who do not meet the above criteria for stability of the acute teardrop fracture, but remain without neurologic deficit, the patient should be considered for a two- or three-level posterior fusion with lateral mass plates. Roy-Camille and colleagues,[70, 71] as well as others,[5, 6, 28, 30, 45, 61, 63] have demonstrated success in the treatment of lower cervical spinal injuries using this technique, including the treatment of teardrop fractures. Other authors[2, 9, 16, 17, 35–38, 50, 65, 70, 81] have demonstrated excellent results with the use of anterior corpectomy and plating. Sutterlin and co-workers[82] and Coe and co-workers[25] have shown that anterior cervical plating is biomechanically inferior to posterior techniques in the treatment of simulated distraction-flexion injuries in a bovine model and a human cadaveric model, respectively. Because flexion is a major component of a teardrop injury, and because disruption of the posterior ligamentous structures which contribute to stability in flexion[84, 85] is a major determinant of cervical instability, reconstruction of the posterior tension band is important in treating unstable teardrop fractures without neurologic deficit. Cybulski and colleagues[26] have shown that posterior spinal fusion with wiring techniques is often not sufficient to prevent persistent instability in teardrop fractures. Lateral mass plates provide more rigid fixation of the cervical spine. Roy-Camille and co-workers[71] found that posterior plating resulted in a 92% increase in flexion load stability as compared to 33% for posterior wiring. Rarely is a subsequent anterior procedure necessary.

The Quadrangular Fragment Fracture

Favero and Van Peteghem[29] described a variation of a CFS5 lesion that responds poorly to posterior fusion

Figure 21–5 = This 19-year-old woman was involved in a diving accident and suffered a teardrop fracture of L5. Lateral (A) and AP (B) views show minimal posterior displacement of the posteroinferior corner of the fractured vertebra, minimal angulation relative to adjacent segments, and minimal posterior element separation. The injury was treated with hard-collar immobilization for 12 weeks and healed.

alone. They termed this lesion a "quadrangular fragment fracture." Four characteristics of this fracture were described: (1) an oblique vertebral body fracture line that passes from the anterior margin to the inferior end plate; (2) a significant degree of posterior subluxation of the cephalad vertebral body on the caudad vertebral body; (3) angular kyphosis at the level of injury; and (4) disruption of the disc and of both anterior and posterior ligament structures as indicated by an increased interspinous space and facet subluxation. Radiographically this lesion differs from a CFS5 lesion in that the latter has a smaller, more triangular bone fragment and less posterior ligament disruption. Instead of a posterior fusion *alone,* as might be considered for a teardrop injury, they recommended anterior decompression and strut grafting across two motion segments, with either external support in a halo vest or concomitant posterior stabilization and fusion (Fig. 21–6).

Patients with Neurologic Deficit

In those persons who present with a complete or incomplete neurologic deficit, radiographs usually reveal a markedly unstable teardrop fracture. These patients should have immediate application of Gardner-Wells tongs (or a halo ring), and attempted realignment of the spine in neutral. This is accomplished by careful addition of weight under radiographic control. Application of cervical traction creates tension in the posterior longitudinal ligament if it is intact, resulting in a force which aids in repositioning bone fragments.[40] Aebi and co-workers[1] have shown that attempted reduction of the cervical injury within 6 hours is more important for neurologic outcome than improved surgical technique. Care should be taken to avoid overdistraction. For preservation of spinal cord function, diastolic blood pressure should be maintained at or above 70 mm Hg.[33, 34]

Surgical management of teardrop fractures is indicated in most cases with neurologic deficit. Murphy and colleagues[62] have determined that patients with cervical fractures and spinal cord injuries treated with early surgical stabilization of the cervical column were hospitalized a mean of 21 fewer days than their nonsurgical counterparts and achieved their first therapeutic leave of absence from primary rehabilitation approximately 40 days sooner than patients stabilized nonsurgically. Johnson and Cannon[46] obtained "satisfactory" stability in 9 of 10 patients with teardrop fractures and neurologic injury who were treated nonoperatively. However, only one of these 10 patients had significant functional recovery. In contrast, rates of neurologic recovery appear improved in those patients who undergo surgical stabilization.[2, 6, 17, 28, 30, 63]

Controversy persists regarding the indications for anterior corpectomy and fusion vs. posterior stabilization in teardrop fractures with neurologic deficit. Anderson and associates,[6] Ebraheim and co-workers,[26] Fehlings and colleagues,[30] and Nazarian and Louis[63] have all reported excellent fusion rates and neurologic recovery with few complications in treating cervical spine injuries with posterior lateral mass plates and fusion. Beatson[7] and others[10] have described the importance of surgical stabilization to prevent further neurologic damage and increase the likelihood of recovery. Prior to the advent of the anterior cervical plate, it seemed that posterior stabilization was the recommended treatment, as opposed to anterior decompression and fusion (and frequently subsequent posterior wiring and fusion). Many authors[8, 9, 18, 80] reported that late instability was common when cervical trauma with posterior ligamentous disruption was treated with anterior interbody bone block or dowel fusion alone, even when halo immobilization was used.[86]

Most authors[2, 9, 10–12, 17, 35, 36, 68, 81] currently feel that in order to allow maximal opportunity for neurologic recovery, the spinal cord should be decompressed at

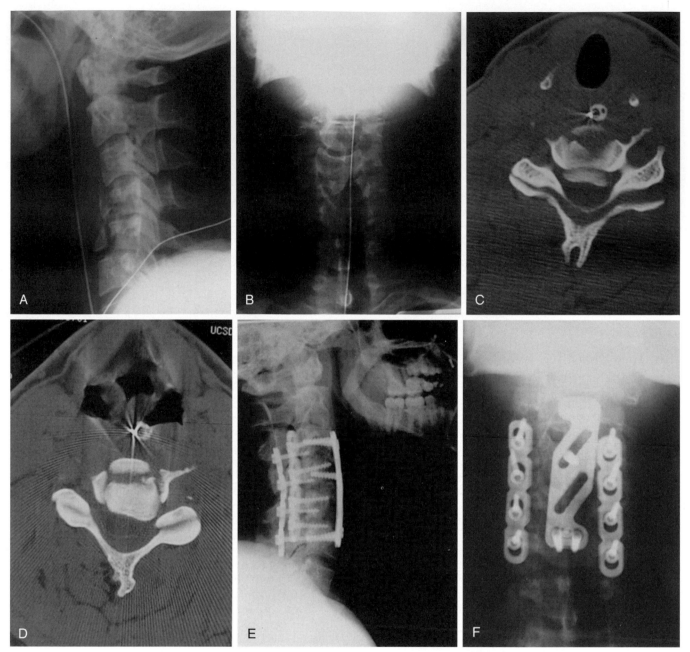

Figure 21–6 ═ This 22-year-old man sustained a two-level quadrangular fragment fracture after being hit by a car. He had complete quadriplegia. *A* and *B,* Note the characteristics of the injury. There are large anterior quadrangular fragments of C4 and C5. The presence of significant kyphosis and splaying of the spinous processes gives and indication of the marked instability of the injury. *C* and *D,* Axial CT images reveal marked retropulsion of bone. *E* and *F,* Due to the marked, multisegment instability of this injury, the patient underwent a staged anterior decompression and stabilization with allograft iliac crest and anterior Orion plate fixation, followed by posterior stabilization with lateral mass plates. One year after injury, he has regained partial use of his right arm.

its site of most significant compromise. In teardrop fractures this compression is nearly always anterior. Bohlman and Anderson[12] demonstrated significant motor improvement in 49 of 58 patients with cervical spinal fractures that were managed by anterior cervical decompression and arthrodesis an average of 13 months after injury. Bohlman and co-authors[12, 57] have recommended posterior stabilization followed by anterior decompression in those patients with anterior neurologic compromise and posterior ligamentous instability.

Cabanela and Ebersold[17] reported eight patients who had bursting teardrop fractures treated by decompressive vertebral corpectomy and anterior fusion with plate stabilization. The neurologic deficit was complete in five and incomplete in three patients. At an average follow-up of 3 years, all grafts were fully incorporated and all cervical columns were stable. All complete neurologic deficits remained complete, and all patients with incomplete deficits had significant recovery and were walking independently.

Aebi and co-workers[2] reported on 22 patients with

burst or teardrop fractures (of 86 total patients) who were treated with a partial or complete resection of the fractured body and bisegmental fusion and fixation with tricortical bone graft and plating with an anterior plate. There were no intraoperative complications. No patient with a neurologic deficit was made worse. No complete tetraplegia improved. Incomplete lesions improved, on average, one Frankel grade.

Ripa and associates[68] reported a series of 92 patients who underwent anterior decompression, tricortical inlay bone grafting, and the application of an anterior cervical plate for treatment of acute lower cervical spinal trauma. These authors had less than a 2% incidence of significant complications related to the use of anterior hardware, and a 99% fusion rate. Although they stated that in no patient did neurologic deterioration related to the use of anterior fixation occur, they did not specifically discuss the rate of neurologic improvement in their patients.

Garvey and colleagues[35] treated 14 patients with acute cervical spine fractures or dislocations and associated posterior ligamentous disruption with anterior decompressions, structural bone grafting, and stabilization with an anterior Caspar plate. There were no perioperative complications and no increased neurologic deficits. At 30 months' follow-up, all patients had solid anterior fusions and all were satisfied with the procedure. These authors criticized the biomechanical work of Coe and co-workers[25] and Sutterlin and co-workers[82] who concluded that Caspar anterior instrumentation does not restore enough flexural or axial compressive stability to obviate posterior stabilization. Garvey and colleagues pointed out that these tests were run without interposition of structural bone grafts, which provide significant reduction of motion in all load modalities.[77]

Others have reported success in treating these types of injuries with anterior decompression and stabilization with an anterior plate.[9, 16, 36–38, 50, 65, 81] With the exception of multiple segment injuries, anterior decompression with interposition strut grafting and anterior plating often provides adequate clinical stability to preclude a posterior procedure. Anterior and posterior stabilization is rarely necessary in single-level teardrop fractures, unless a quadrangular fracture is present.[28] In patients with fractures at more than one vertebral level, in whom a two- or three-level corpectomy is necessary, augmentation with a second-stage posterior cervical fusion and lateral mass plating should be considered (see Fig. 21–6)—or a halo applied for postoperative control.

Once traction has been applied to the patient's cervical spine, a lateral radiograph is obtained to assess realignment. Weight is carefully added in 5-lb increments until either realignment is obtained or there is mild (less than 1 mm) distraction of the disc space. If there is reduction of the posteroinferior corner of the fractured vertebra (less than 5 mm over the subjacent vertebra), an argument may be made for stabilization with posterior plates.[6, 28, 30, 63] If reduction is not obtained despite adequate cervical traction, the patient should undergo anterior cervical decompression and

strut fusion with three-level plating. Patients who undergo anterior or posterior fusion are immobilized in a hard collar for approximately 8 to 12 weeks.

THE TIMING OF SURGERY

The subject of how soon after injury the patient should undergo surgery is another area of controversy, especially in those patients with neurologic deficit. While many spinal surgeons believe that early surgical stabilization provides the best environment for neurologic recovery, this has not been proved by randomized, controlled studies. Immediate surgery under general anesthesia may be associated with greater surgical morbidity than treatment with closed traction during the first 24 to 48 hours because of the transient physiologic irregularities of the autonomic nervous system during spinal shock.[79] However, early surgery (3 to 5 days) offers several advantages over closed treatment. A more precise reduction can be achieved and bony or disc encroachment on the canal removed. In addition, early spinal stability may be achieved, protecting the spinal cord from further injury and allowing mobilization of the patient within a matter of days.[39]

Much of the literature associated with the timing of surgery after spinal fracture and neurologic injury deals with thoracolumbar injury. McAfee and co-workers[58] and Kaneda and co-workers,[47] despite reporting impressive rates of neurologic recovery after anterior decompression of thoracolumbar fractures, were unable to show a statistically significant association between the time from injury to neural decompression and subsequent motor recovery. On the other hand, Clohisy and associates,[24] in a review of 22 patients with incomplete neurologic deficits after fractures at the thoracolumbar junction, determined that early anterior decompression (less than 48 hours) was associated with improved rates of neurologic recovery when compared with late decompression (average, 61 days). As can be seen from these examples, the literature is, at best, inconsistent. Moreover, one may argue that injury to the lumbar spinal cord and cauda equina is not equivalent to injury in the cervical spine.

Bohlman and Anderson[12] reported their series of 58 patients who had anterior cervical decompression for neural deficit. Of the 42 patients who had decompression within 12 months after injury, 34 had a good or excellent result, compared with only 8 of 16 who had decompression more than 12 months after injury.

Marshall and co-authors[56] presented the results of a prospective drug randomization study of 283 spinal cord–injured patients of whom 14 deteriorated neurologically during acute hospital management. In 12 of the 14, the decline in neurologic function could be associated with a specific management event, and in 9 of these 12 the injury involved the cervical cord. The authors noted that each of the three patients with a cervical cord injury who deteriorated was operated on within the first 5 days. No such deterioration was observed following surgery performed from the sixth day on. They recommended that early surgery not be performed in the patient with cervical cord injury with the exception of those patients with incomplete injuries in whom progressive deterioration occurs. However, timing to surgery was not part of the randomization portion of the study and was based on surgeon preference and decision.

Krengel and colleagues[51] reviewed 38 patients with acute cervical spinal cord injuries requiring surgical stabilization. Group 1 consisted of 12 patients who underwent surgery within 72 hours of injury. Group 2 consisted of 26 patients who had surgery later than 72 hours following injury. They found that group 1 had a significantly greater improvement in Frankel grade than group 2 (one level per patient vs. one-half level per patient). Pulmonary complications were significantly fewer in group 1 than group 2, and there was a trend toward shorter acute hospitalization and mechanical ventilation in group 1 than group 2.

Schlegel and colleagues[74] reviewed 138 patients requiring operative decompression, reduction, and fixation of spinal injuries. Four subgroups were identified based on whether patients were victims of multitrauma or had isolated spinal injuries, and whether patients underwent spinal stabilization within 72 hours of injury. These authors' results indicated that in patients with multiple traumatic injuries and spinal fractures, those who underwent spinal stabilization within 72 hours of injury had a significantly lower rate of morbidity than those who underwent stabilization after 72 hours. No such association was noted in those who had isolated spinal trauma. Of those with neurologically involved cervical injuries, early surgical stabilization greatly reduced medical complications and morbidity regardless of whether the injury was isolated or a result of multitrauma. However, timing of surgical intervention did not appear to affect the function of neurologic improvement in any group.

At our institution (UCSD) the following protocol is observed. Upon documentation of neural deficit secondary to cervical spinal fracture or dislocation, the methylprednisolone trauma protocol is begun. Gardner-Wells tongs are placed and 10 lb of traction is initially applied. Traction is continued until satisfactory realignment is obtained or minor distraction at the injury site is detected radiographically. Further radiographic studies (CT scans) are obtained, and serial neurologic examinations are performed at 2-hour intervals for the first 24 hours. If acute neurologic deterioration is noted, the patient is immediately brought for further imaging (CT-myelogram or MRI). If an identifiable causative lesion is seen, the patient may be considered an urgent operative candidate. Otherwise, the patient's neurologic status is carefully monitored over several days until a plateau is reached. Once the patient is deemed medically stable and no further neurologic improvement is documented, the patient may undergo the indicated procedure. An effort is made to take the patient to the operating room earlier rather than later (3 to 5 days). However, if neurologic improvement continues during this time, or if the patient is unable to undergo the procedure secondary to compromised medical status, the procedure is delayed.

SUMMARY

Teardrop injuries are devastating injuries occurring in up to 12% of cervical spine injuries. They should be considered unstable, as evidenced by a high rate of associated spinal cord injury. The specific features of these lesions should be recognized in order to provide appropriate care. Unstable lesions and lesions with neurologic compromise benefit from surgical stabilization.

REFERENCES

1. Aebi M, Mohler J, Zach GA, et al: Indication, surgical technique, and results of 100 surgically-treated fractures and fracture-dislocations of the cervical spine. Clin Orthop 203:244–257, 1986.
2. Aebi M, Zuber K, Marchesi D: Treatment of cervical spine injuries with anterior plating. Indications, techniques, and results. Spine 16(suppl):S38–45, 1991.
3. Allen BL, Ferguson RL, Lehmann TR, et al: A mechanistic classification of closed, indirect fractures and dislocations of the lower cervical spine. Spine 7:1–27, 1982.
4. An HS: Anatomy of the cervical spine. In An SH, Simpson JM (eds): Surgery of the Cervical Spine. Baltimore, Williams & Wilkins, 1994.
5. An HS, Coppes MS: Posterior cervical fixation for fracture and degenerative disc disease. Clin Orthop 335:101–111, 1997.
6. Anderson PA, Henley MB, Grady MS, et al: Posterior cervical arthrodesis with AO reconstruction plates and bone graft. Spine 16(suppl):S72–79, 1991.
7. Beatson TR: Fractures and dislocations of the cervical spine. J Bone Joint Surg Br 45:21–35, 1963.
8. Bell GD, Bailey SI: Anterior cervical fusion for trauma. Clin Orthop 128:155–158, 1977.
9. Bohler J, Gaudernak T: Anterior plate stabilization for fracture-dislocations of the lower cervical spine. J Trauma 20:203–205, 1980.
10. Bohlman HH: Acute fractures and dislocations of the cervical spine: An analysis of three hundred hospitalized patients and review of the literature. J Bone and Joint Surg Am 61:1119–1142, 1979.
11. Bohlman HH: Pathology and current treatment concepts of cervical spine injuries. Instruct Course Lect 21:108–115, 1972.
12. Bohlman HH, Anderson PA: Anterior decompression and arthrodesis of the cervical spine: Long-term motor improvement. Part I—Improvement in incomplete traumatic quadriparesis. J Bone Joint Surg Am 74:671–682, 1992.
13. Bohlmann HA: Adult fractures and dislocations of the cervical spine. J Bone Joint Surg Am 61:1119, 1979.
14. Bozic KJ, Keyak JH, Skinner HB, et al: Three-dimensional finite element modeling of a cervical vertebra: An investigation of burst fracture mechanism. J Spinal Disord 7:102–110, 1994.
15. Bracken MB, Shepard MJ, Collins WF, et al: A randomized, controlled trial of methylprednisolone or naloxone in the treatment of acute spinal-cord injury: Results of the second national acute spinal cord injury study. N Engl J Med 322:1405–1411, 1990.
16. Bremer AM, Nguyen TQ: Internal metal plate fixation combined with anterior interbody fusion in cases of cervical spine injury. Neurosurgery 12:649–653, 1983.
17. Cabanela ME, Ebersold MJ: Anterior plate stabilization for bursting teardrop fractures of the cervical spine. Spine 13:888–891, 1988.
18. Capen DA, Garland DE, Waters RL: Surgical stabilization of the cervical spine. A comparative analysis of anterior and posterior spine fusions. Clin Orthop 196:229–237, 1985.
19. Caspar W: Anterior Cervical Fusion and Interbody Stabilization with the Trapezial Osteosynthetic Plate Technique. Tuttlingen, Germany, Aesculap-Werke, 1985.
20. Cheshire DJE: The stability of the cervical spine following the conservative treatment of fractures and fracture-dislocations. Paraplegia 7:193–203, 1969.

21. Chang DG, Tencer AF, Ching RP et al: Geometric changes in the cervical spinal canal during impact. Spine 19:973–980, 1994.
22. Ching RP, Watson NA, Carter JW, et al: The effect of post-injury spinal position on canal occlusion in a cervical spine burst fracture model. Spine 22:1710–1715, 1997.
23. Clark CR, Ingram CM, El-Khoury GY, et al: Radiographic evaluation of cervical spine injuries. Spine 13:742–747, 1988.
24. Clohisy JC, Akbarnia BA, Bucholz RD, et al: Neurologic recovery associated with anterior decompression of spine fractures at the thoracolumbar junction. Spine 17(suppl):S325–330, 1992.
25. Coe JD, Warden KD, Sutterlin CE, et al: Biomechanical evaluation of cervical spinal stabilization methods in a human cadaveric model. Spine 14:1122–1131, 1989.
26. Cybulski GR, Douglas RA, Meyer PR, et al: Complications in three-column cervical spine injuries requiring anterior-posterior stabilization. Spine 17:253–256, 1992.
27. Dorr LD, Harvey JP, Nickel BL: Clinical review of the early stability of spine injuries. Spine 7:545, 1982.
28. Ebraheim NA, Rupp RE, Savolaine ER, et al: Posterior plating of the cervical spine. J Spinal Disord 8:111–115, 1995.
29. Favero KJ, Van Peteghem PK: The quadrangular fragment fracture: Roentgenographic features and treatment protocol. Clin Orthop 239:40–46, 1989.
30. Fehlings MG, Cooper PR, Errico TJ: Posterior plates in the management of cervical instability: Long-term results in 44 patients. J Neurosurg 81:341–349, 1994.
31. Freemyer B, Knopp R, Piche J, et al: Comparison of five-view and three-views cervical spine series in the evaluation of patients with cervical trauma. Ann Emerg Med 18:818–821, 1989.
32. Fuentes JM, Bloncourt J, Vlahovitch B: La tear drop fracture: Contribution a l'étude du mécanisme et des lésions ostéo-disco-ligamentaires. Neurochirurgie 29:129–134, 1983.
33. Garfin SR, Katz MM: The vertebral column: Clinical aspects. In Nakum, AM, Melvin J (eds): The Biomechanics of Trauma. Norwalk, Conn, Appleton-Century-Crofts, 1985.
34. Garfin SR, Shackford SR, Marshall LF, et al: Care of the multiply injured patient with cervical spine injury. Clin Orthop 239:19–29, 1989.
35. Garvey TA, Eismont FJ, Roberti LJ: Anterior decompression, structural bone grafting, and Caspar plate stabilization for unstable cervical spine fractures and/or dislocations. Spine 17(suppl):S431–435, 1992.
36. Gassman J, Seligson D: The anterior cervical plate. Spine 8:700–707, 1983.
37. Goffin J: Subtotal cervical body replacement by c-shaped iliac crest graft, technical note. Acta Neurochir 84:68–70, 1987.
38. Goffin J, Van Loon J, Van Calenbergh F: Long-term results after anterior cervical fusion and osteosynthetic stabilization for fractures and/or dislocations of the cervical spine. J Spinal Disord 8:500–508, 1995.
39. Hamilton A, Webb JK: The role of anterior surgery for vertebral fractures with and without cord compression. Clin Orthop 300:79–89, 1994.
40. Harrington RM, Budorick T, Hoyt J, et al: Biomechanics of indirect reduction of bone retropulsed into the spinal canal in vertebral fracture. Spine 18:692–699, 1993.
41. Harris JH: The radiology of acute cervical spine trauma. Baltimore, Williams & Wilkins, 1978.
42. Harris JH: Radiographic evaluation of spinal trauma. Orthop Clin North Am 17:75–86, 1986.
43. Harris JH, Edeiken-Monroe B, Kopaniky DR: A practical classification of acute cervical spine injuries. Orthop Clin North Am 17:15–30, 1986.
44. Holdsworth F: Fractures, dislocations, and fracture-dislocations of the spine. J Bone Joint Surg Am 52:1534–1551, 1970.
45. Jeanneret B, Magerl F, Halterward E, et al: Posterior stabilization of the cervical spine with hook plates. Spine 16(suppl):S56–63, 1991.
46. Johnson JL, Cannon D: Nonoperative treatment of the acute tear-drop fracture of the cervical spine. Clin Orthop 168:108–112, 1982.
47. Kaneda K, Taneichi H, Abumi K, et al: Anterior decompression and stabilization with the Kaneda device for thoracolumbar burst fractures associated with neurological deficits. J Bone Joint Surg Am 79:69–83, 1997.
48. Kewalramani LS, Taylor RG: Injuries to the cervical spine from diving accidents. J Trauma 15:130–142, 1975.
49. Kim KS, Chen HH, Russel EJ, et al: Flexion teardrop fracture of the cervical spine: Radiographic characteristics. AJR 152:319–326, 1989.
50. Kostuik JP, Connolly PJ, Esses SI: Anterior cervical plate fixation with the titanium hollow screw plate system. Spine 18:1273–1278, 1993.
51. Krengel WF, Anderson PA, Yuan H, et al: Early versus delayed stabilization after cervical spinal cord injury. Orthop Trans 18:249–250, 1994.
52. Lee C, Kim KS, Rogers LF: Sagittal fracture of the cervical vertebral body. AJR 139:55–60, 1982.
53. Lee C, Kim KS, Rogers LF: Triangular cervical vertebral body fractures: Diagnostic significance. AJR 138:1123–1132, 1982.
54. Lindstrom A: Injuries in the cervical spine. Acta Chir Scandinav 1953; 106:212–223.
55. Marar BC, Orth MCH: The pattern of neurological damage as an aid to the diagnosis of the mechanism in cervical-spine injuries. J Bone Joint Surg Am 56:1648–1654, 1974.
56. Marshall LF, Knowlton S, Garfin SR, et al: Deterioration following spinal cord injury: A multicenter study. J Neurosurg 66:400–404, 1987.
57. McAfee PC, Bohlman HH: One-stage anterior cervical decompression and posterior stabilization with circumferential arhtrodesis. J Bone Joint Surg Am 71:78–88, 1989.
58. McAfee PC, Bohlman HH, Yuan HA: Anterior decompression of traumatic thoracolumbar fractures with incomplete neurological deficit using a retroperitoneal approach. J Bone Joint Surg Am 67:89–104, 1985.
59. Merianos P, Manousidis D, Samsonas P, et al: Injuries of the lower cervical spine associated with widening of the spinal canal. Injury 25:645–648, 1994.
60. Mori S, Ohira N, Ojima T, et al: Observation of tear-drop fracture dislocation of the cervical spine by computerized tomography. J Jpn Orthop Assoc 57:373–378, 1983.
61. Murphy MJ, Daniaux H, Southwick WO: Posterior cervical fusion with rigid internal fixation. Orthop Clin North Am 17:55–65, 1986.
62. Murphy KP, Opitz JL, Cabanela ME, et al: Cervical fractures and spinal cord injury: Outcome of surgical and nonsurgical management. Mayo Clin Proc 65:949–959, 1990.
63. Nazarian SM, Louis RP: Posterior internal fixation with screw plates in traumatic lesions of the cervical spine. Spine 16(suppl):S64–71, 1991.
64. Norton WL: Fractures and dislocations of the cervical spine. J Bone Joint Surg Am 44:115–139, 1962.
65. Oliveira JC: Anterior plate fixation of traumatic lesions of the lower cervical spine. Spine 12:324–329, 1987.
66. Rappoport LH, O'Leary PF: Cervical disc disease. In Bridwell KH, DeWald RL (eds): Spinal Surgery. Philadelphia, Lippincott-Raven, 1997.
67. Rauschning W: Anatomy and pathology of the cervical spine. In Frymoyer JW (ed): The Adult Spine. New York, Raven Press, 1997.
68. Ripa DR, Kowall MG, Meyer PR, et al: Series of ninety-two traumatic cervical spine injuries stabilized with anterior ASIF plate fusion technique. Spine 16(suppl):S46–55, 1991.
69. Rogers WA: Fractures and dislocations of the cervical spine. J Bone Joint Surg Am 39:341–376, 1957.
70. Roy-Camille R, Saillant G, Laville C, et al: Treatment of lower cervical spinal injuries—C3 to C7. Spine 17(suppl):S442–446, 1992.
71. Roy-Camille RR, Sailant G, Mazel C: Internal fixation of the unstable cervical spine by posterior osteosynthesis with plate and screws. In Cervical Spine Research Society (ed): The Cervical Spine, ed 2. Philadelphia, JB Lippincott, 1989, p 390.
72. Schneider RC: The syndrome of acute anterior spinal cord injury. J Neurosurg 8:360–367, 1951.
73. Scher AT: Tear-drop fractures of the cervical spine—Radiological features. S Afr Med J 6:355–356, 1982.
74. Schlegel J, Bayley J, Yuan H, et al: Timing of surgical decompression and fixation of acute spinal fractures. J Orthop Trauma 10:323–330, 1996.
75. Schneider RC, Kahn EA: Chronic neurological sequelae of acute trauma to the spine and spinal cord, part I: The significance of the acute-flexion or "tear-drop" fracture-dislocation of the cervical spine. J Bone Joint Surg Am 38:985–997, 1956.

76. Schulte K, Clark CR, Goel VK: Kinematics of the cervical spine following discectomy and stabilization. Spine 14:1116–1121, 1986.

77. Smith MD: Cervical spondylosis. *In* Bridwell KH, DeWald RL (eds): Spinal Surgery. Philadelphia, Lipincott-Raven, 1997.

78. Stauffer ES: Management of spine fractures C3 to C7. Orthop Clin North Am 17:45–53, 1986.

79. Stauffer ES: Subaxial Injuries. Clin Orthop 239:30–39, 1989.

80. Stauffer ES, Kelly EG: Fracture-dislocations of the cervical spine. J Bone Joint Surg Am 59:45–48, 1977.

81. Suh PB, Kostuik JP, Esses SI: Anterior cervical plate fixation with the titanium hollow screw plate system (THSP): A preliminary report. Orthop Trans 14:692–693, 1990.

82. Sutterlin CE, McAfee PC, Warden KE, et al: A biomechanical evaluation of cervical spinal stabilization methods in a bovine model, static and cyclical loading. Spine 13:795–802, 1988.

83. Torg JS, Pavlov H, O'Neill MJ, et al: The axial load teardrop fracture—A biomechanical, clinical, and roentgenographic analysis. Am J Sports Med 19:355–364, 1991.

84. White AA, Johnson RM, Panjabi MM, et al: Biomechanical analysis of clinical stability in the cervical spine. Clin Orthop 109:85–96, 1975.

85. White AA, Southwick WO, Panjabi MM: Clinical instability in the lower cervical spine—A review of past and current concepts. Spine 1:15–27, 1976.

86. Whitehill R, Richman JA, Glaser JA: Failure of immobilization of the cervical spine by the halo vest: A report of five cases. J Bone Joint Surg Am 68:326–332, 1986.

87. Whitley JE, Forsyth HF: The classification of cervical spine injuries. AJR 83:633–644, 1960.

CHAPTER 22

Facet Fractures and Dislocations

Alan M. Levine

Injuries involving the posterior articular pillar or facets of the vertebral elements can occur anywhere from C2 to L5–S1. However, the most common location for these injuries is in the cervical spine: C2–3 to C7–T1. The term *facet injury* encompasses a broad spectrum of pathologic entities. There has been considerable confusion concerning the differences between the different pathologic entities and the necessary treatment modalities for the various types of injuries.[1] Our ability to obtain radiographic images of these injuries has undergone a major advance since the early 1980s with the advent of improved techniques of tomography, as well as computed tomographic (CT) scan with three-dimensional (3D) reconstruction. Thus, the ability to differentiate these injuries precisely according to pathologic and mechanistic criteria has led to the ability to more specifically treat the resultant structural instability.

To appropriately apply treatment modalities to this range of cervical facet injuries, a clear understanding of the anatomic structures that contribute to the stability of the cervical spine is necessary. Although it is commonly felt that the anatomic configuration of the facet joints in the cervical spine contributes significantly to their stability, the role of the adjacent ligamentous structures, such as the posterior aspect of the disc, the joints of Luschka, the facet capsules, the interspinous ligaments, and the ligamentum flavum play significant roles in the stability, and therefore the resultant instability, of injuries affecting the facets. Facet joints of the upper cervical spine (levels cephalad to C2–3) are in the anterior portion of the vertebral ring and are completely different in their anatomic configuration than the joints of the lower cervical spine. The frequency of facet joint injuries of all types varies quite specifically with the level of injury. Therefore, injuries at C5–6 are most common with all types of facet injuries, followed by C4–5 and C6–7 injuries. Injuries at C3–4, C2–3, and C7–T1 are much less common. The injuries to the C2–3 facet joint are included with the following classifications despite the fact that C2 has a markedly different anatomic configuration than the remainder of the lower cervical spine joints. Those from C2–3 distally are in the posterior aspect of the ring and are inclined at an angle of 45 degrees from the vertical. In addition, these facet joints, which usually have an elliptical configuration of the articular surface, are either canted slightly medially or slightly laterally, depending on the individual vertebra. In the upper segments they are canted slightly medially, whereas in the lower segments they are canted slightly laterally as the transition is made into the thoracic spine. The actual area of the articular surface is approximately 1 cm^2. The proximity of the joint to other important structures is critical, especially in understanding the neurologic ramifications of injuries to this joint and in planning potential fixation techniques. The facet joint forms the posterior border of the neuroforamen with the anterior medial border of the foramen formed by the joint of Luschka. The vertebral artery lies directly anterior to the medial edge of the facet joint. The joint itself is an arthrodial joint with a synovial membrane and fibrous capsules. The volume of the joint is small, but its configuration can be demonstrated by direct injection of contrast medium. With the soft tissues removed, the posterior topographic anatomy of the facet joint becomes evident (Fig. 22–1). This is critical in understanding the rationale for correct placement of posterior wire in fixation and plating techniques. The spinous process–laminar junction is an important landmark, as it represents correct placement for wire fixation techniques at the point at which the spinous process begins to flare out into the lamina. The posterior aspect of the cervical spine has been described by Roy-Camille as being a hillock that represents the posterior aspect of the inferior facet, and with a valley separating the hillock from the lamina and the spinous process. Actually the posterior aspect of the facet joint is a dome-shaped area, measuring slightly less than a centimeter in mediolateral and inferosuperior dimension; a depression is just medial to it. The laminar facet junction is another critical landmark that is represented by a slight vertical depression at the junction of the lateral edge of the lamina and the medial edge of the facet. Just anterior to that point lies the vertebral artery. The posterior aspect of the inferior facet is a dome configuration. The exact center of the inferior facet joint is the high point of the dome. The posterior ligamentous complex, which includes this fibrous capsule, is critically important for the stability of the spine. The components of the posterior ligamentous complex include the supraspinous ligament, the intraspinous ligament, the ligamentum flavum in the mid-

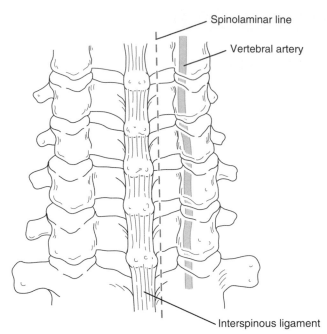

Figure 22–1 = This figure shows the topographic anatomy of the posterior aspect of the cervical spine. Proper positioning of wire constructs requires penetration of the posterior elements at the level of the spinolaminar line rather than in the spinous process. Proper screw placement uses the anatomy of the facet joint to avoid medial placement of the screw and penetration of the vertebral artery, which courses anterior to the medial half of the facet. The posterior aspect of the facet forms a little hillock, as described by Raymond Roy-Camille, with the valley on its medial side formed by the posterior aspect of the lamina.

line, and the fibrous capsules of the facet joints more laterally. Muscular origins include the multifidus as well as short and long rotators of the neck, which begin at the posterior tubercles of the transverse processes of the lower cervical spine and insert on the spinous processes. With most surgical approaches, these muscles are dissected subperiosteally, laterally over the facet joint. The most critical muscular insertions are those at the C2 spinous process.

As previously mentioned, there is a variation in motion noted in different levels of cervical spine. The upper cervical spine at C2–4 averages about 12 degrees of total flexion-extension motion, whereas the more mobile segments from C4–6 average approximately 20 degrees, decreasing to approximately 12 degrees at C6–7. Lateral bending averages approximately 6 degrees at each level and rotation varies from 0 degrees to as much as 10 degrees. A relationship has been noted between decrease in total motion and advancing age. In addition, as described by Lysell,[48] a coupled motion occurs with axial rotation and lateral bending. This is a result of the shape of the facet joints, and in the upper cervical spine 2 degrees of rotation occur for every 3 degrees of lateral bending, whereas in the lower cervical spine only 1 degree of rotation occurs for every 7.5 degrees of lateral bending. It is possible that the increased compliance to rotation with lateral bending may account for the fact that there are fewer unilateral facet fractures and dislocations in the upper cervical spine than in the lower cervical spine.

CLASSIFICATION OF INJURIES OF THE FACET JOINT

As mentioned in Chapter 9, the classification of injuries can be based on a number of different parameters. The most common, however, are anatomic-radiologic and mechanistic patterns of classification. For injuries of the cervical facets, these classifications merge together reasonably smoothly. Although the understanding of the mechanism of injury is incredibly important for establishing a surgical construct to maintain stability, classification of facet injuries is much more easily done on the basis of radiologic criteria. A radiologic classification, however, fails to take into account the progressive nature of the forces applied to the spine. Overall it is reasonably effective for classifying the injuries in order to understand the relative degree of instability and the mechanical constraints necessary to restabilize the spine. The ligamentous injuries of the cervical facets form a continuum based on a single mechanism of injury with varying degrees of application of force. The fractures of the facets and articular processes have differing but consistent mechanisms of injury. One of the earliest classifications of facet injuries was based predominantly on roentgenographic interpretation of both direct and indirect forces applied to the cervical spine. These included flexion, extension, rotation, and lateral bending.[80] The flexion injuries were further subdivided into distractive flexion and compressive flexion, initially by Braakman and Penning,[11] who were the first to suggest that unilateral facet fractures were distractive flexion injuries and that unilateral facet injuries dislocations also had an additional element of rotation. There have been disagreements concerning the mechanisms of these injuries, with some authors feeling that lateral flexion was a predominant injury[59] or that extension and bending contributed to facet injuries. The concept of a staged or progressive mechanism of injury and a classification was proposed by the AO group and for the spine was advocated by Allen and co-workers.[1] Although they divided the combination of distraction and flexion, "distractive flexion," into four stages, their reference was still the anatomic configuration noted radiographically. The subclassifications included stage 1 as facet subluxation, stage 2 as unilateral facet dislocation, stage 3 as bilateral facet dislocation with approximately 50% vertebral displacement, and stage 4 as an unstable or floating spine. The concept of compressive extension was felt to be somewhat hypothetical, but it could account for articular mass or fracture separations of the articular mass as noted by other authors. In each case, however, the mechanistic reference point was an anatomic configuration demonstrated radiographically.

A system more easily integrated into the treatment of cervical facet injuries is the descriptive classification. The phenomenon of facet injuries was first recognized by Malgaigne in 1855.[52] It was not, however, until the advent of radiography that the true descriptive classification of injuries of the facet joints became evident. Early description of cervical facet injuries mixed fracture dislocations and pure dislocations.[9, 21, 22, 27, 30, 60] The difference between unilateral and bilateral facet injuries was recognized in the 1950s by Roaf,[59, 60] Beatson,[5] and Rogers.[62] The descriptive classification as we know it today is a gradual accumulation of radiographic entities that we have slowly assimilated into a useful classification system. The earliest organized attempts at such a system can be credited to Roy-Camille and Judet in Garches, France, in 1970.[65, 66, 70] A number of authors in the 1960s contributed specific entities that began to coalesce into this classification system in the 1970s. These include the flexion injury with various degrees of unilateral and bilateral subluxation as described by Braakman and Penning[11] and the unilateral facet dislocation also described by Braakman and Vinken.[13] Thus, the initial attempts at classification by an anatomic system recognize both unilateral and bilateral cervical facet injuries. The recognition of unilateral and bilateral involvement of the articular processes and masses was initially based on the amount of displacement on the lateral radiograph as well as on visualization of the facets on oblique studies or *pillar views*. The injury of the individual facet process or mass was then also divided into either fractures or ligamentous injuries. As late as the 1980s, controversies still were present as to the significance of the fracture of the articular process.[36, 37] However, the ligamentous injuries could be divided into three stages, which have been named differently. These include subluxations, perched facets, and dislocations. Although the mechanism of the three injuries is the same, the extent of the disruption of the soft tissues is presumably related to the degree of anatomic displacement. The final group of injuries, either unilateral or bilateral, is the fractures. The most common injury is fracture of the superior articular facet. The next most common is fracture of the inferior articular facet, and the least common is a complex of injuries considered to be fracture separations of the articular mass.[46, 53, 65, 66] These three injuries most probably have different mechanisms of injury, but they are closely related in terms of the resultant instability, as are the appropriate treatment modalities.

FACET INJURIES AND MECHANISMS

This section discusses the specific facet injuries and fractures in detail. When dealing with facet injuries, they should initially be divided into bilateral facet injuries and unilateral facet injuries.[45] Bilateral facet injuries can then be divided into dislocations, which are predominantly ligamentous injuries and fractures.

Ligamentous Injuries

Although the ligamentous injuries of the cervical spine are, in fact, arrayed along a continuum, they can be artificially divided into three separate categories. The distinction is important for understanding the associated structural deficiencies as well as the critical features in treatment. The spectrum of ligamentous injuries runs from facet subluxations to "perched" fac-

ets to bilateral facet dislocations. Because these are flexion-distraction injuries, they form a spectrum from minor tearing, or "sprains," of supraspinous, interspinous, and facet capsules to complete disruption (with disruption of the disc) in the more severe variations of the injury. No clear demarcation fixes the amount of disruption that is truly pathologic. Often what are thought to be subluxated facets are indeed more severe disruptions that have simply fallen into a reduced position with extension of the neck. In addition, the ligamentous laxity is somewhat more significant in children, and therefore the delineation between pathologic characteristics and normal variants is even more difficult to ascertain. In the most minor degrees of injury (Fig. 22–2), the posterior ligaments are disrupted, but the disc remains relatively stable. The first type of injury is a bilateral facet subluxation. This is thought to be a flexion-distraction injury that represents a sprain of the posterior cervical ligamentous elements. Thus, there is a partial disruption of the intraspinous and supraspinous ligaments as well as partial disruption of the facet capsules. This is defined by a widening of the distance between the spinous processes, as compared to that of adjacent levels, on a flexion radiographic view. Such an injury, when seen on an extension view, will most commonly reduce completely into normal alignment; it may therefore be missed on an extended lateral screening view. The facet joints are subluxated superiorly and anteriorly on the flexion view. The inferior articular processes are subluxated superiorly and anteriorly with reference to the superior articular processes. This usually results in slight kyphosis (<10 degrees on a lateral radiograph). The oblique views also demonstrate this anterosuperior sliding of

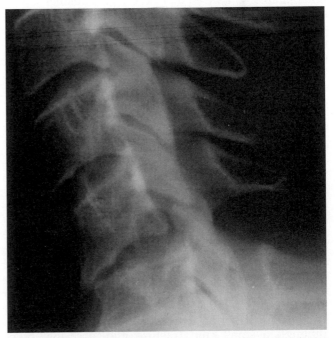

Figure 22–2 ═ This lateral radiograph of the cervical spine demonstrates bilateral subluxation at C5–6. Note the lack of rotation but the significant angulation and widening of the interval between the spinous processes posteriorly.

the facets. Generally, no further studies are necessary for this injury, although a magnetic resonance image (MRI) may, in extreme stages of the injury, show some slight discal disruption. In the acute phase of the injury, edema may also be visualized in the injured portion of the interspinous ligament on MRI. Because this is a bilateral injury, no rotational abnormalities are noted on any study. CT scan of such a lesion may demonstrate no pathology, as either the primary cuts are in a direction parallel to the disruption or the injury is fully reduced in the extended position.

The next stage in this injury is a bilateral "perched" facet. This is clearly an increase on the spectrum of injury from subluxation to full dislocation, although the mechanism is the same as the previously mentioned two injuries. In this injury the inferior articular process continues to slide superiorly and anteriorly until the inferior tip of the facet and the superior tip of the facet below come to rest one on the other. This results in significant kyphosis of the affected level, which often exceeds the kyphosis noted with a true bilateral facet dislocation. There is some translation noted on the lateral radiograph, but it is generally less than that noted with a bilateral facet dislocation. In addition, on the lateral radiograph, marked spreading of the distance between the adjacent spinous processes is noted. This "perching" can usually be clearly delineated on a lateral spine radiograph. The anteroposterior (AP) radiograph will not demonstrate any rotation, but it will demonstrate an increase in distance between the adjacent spinous processes. Again, CT scan and MRI will have little additional value in this injury, although MRI will most certainly demonstrate partial disruption of the involved disc. The injury involves essentially complete disruption of the intraspinous and supraspinous ligaments as well as of the facet capsules, and it also usually involves rupture of the ligamentum flavum and partial disruption of posterior anulus of the disc. On flexion-extension radiographs this injury generally does not show much motion, as the force between the tips of the facets may be considerable, with stretching of the ligamentous structures. The degree of disruption of the adjacent soft tissues is, in fact, generally comparable to that of a bilateral facet dislocation.

Bilateral facet dislocation is the terminal stage of a combination of flexion-distraction applied to the cervical spine, resulting in failure of the posterior ligamentous complex and disc. The percentage of cases with significant disc disruption is greater than 60%. The injury results in completion of the translation and distraction of the inferior facets so that they come to rest anterior to the superior facets of the lower level and lock in that position. This results in somewhat less angulation than is noted with a bilateral perched facet (approximately 10 degrees), but considerably more translation of the superior segment over the inferior segment (approximately 50% or 5 to 6 mm). Both the inferior and superior articular processes remain intact, although a small chip fracture may occasionally be evident (usually comprising less than 25% of the height of either the superior or inferior facet). The chip fracture, however, is not a significant component of the

injury. The injury is reasonably distinct on a lateral cervical spine radiograph. Translation and angulation are significant, but there is no rotational malalignment. On the lateral radiograph (Fig. 22–3) an overlap is often seen in the degree of translation and angulation between the unilateral and bilateral facet injuries. They can be differentiated on the lateral radiograph by the presence of rotational malalignment with unilateral facet injuries. The AP roentgenogram does not show findings significantly different from those of a bilateral perched facet, although the widening of the interspinous distances may not be as significant as with a bilateral perched facet. The injury can be further defined by a number of radiologic techniques, including oblique or pillar views (Fig. 22–4), which demonstrate the dislocation on both sides and may be useful in helping to differentiate a unilateral facet dislocation from a bilateral facet dislocation. In addition, a CT scan, although parallel to the plane of injury, demonstrates the juxtaposition of the superior and inferior articular processes. An MRI is much less helpful, but it will clearly define the obvious (i.e., disruption of the disc at the involved segment) and may be helpful in differentiating an extruded fragment in patients who are either neurologically intact or neurologically compromised. This severe translational deformity requires the complete disruption of the interspinous and supraspinous ligaments, facet capsules, ligamentum flavum, and a significant portion of the disc. This is a flexion instability, and solutions to the instability must contain a modality that serves at least as a tension band to resist flexion. In addition, in the more severe forms of the injury (bilateral facet dislocation) significant disruption of the disc occurs. This will result over time in the loss of height of the disc space by settling of the construct in injuries fixed by a pure tension-band method.

Unilateral ligamentous injuries are less common than their bilateral counterparts and are more difficult to deal with. All unilateral ligamentous injuries can be differentiated from their bilateral counterparts by the necessary rotational component that must exist in a unilateral injury. This rotational element is most easily demonstrated on a lateral cervical radiograph. The severity of the rotational deformity increases proportionately to the amount of disruption and translation of the facet. Thus, a unilateral subluxation will have less rotational abnormality than a unilateral dislocation. The rotational abnormality can best be demonstrated on a lateral radiograph by differences in the appearance of the vertebral bodies proximal and distal to the injury level. On one section of the spine the two lateral edges of the posterior aspect of the vertebral body will be superimposed, appearing as a single line. The other section of the spine will demonstrate a rotational abnormality where the two posterior edges of the cervical body do not overlap, thus appearing as two separate edges. In addition, the apparent translation of the vertebral body in this case is not real, and is only an apparent translation that is really a rotational abnormality. This results in an apparent foreshortening of one segment of the spine with reference to the other.

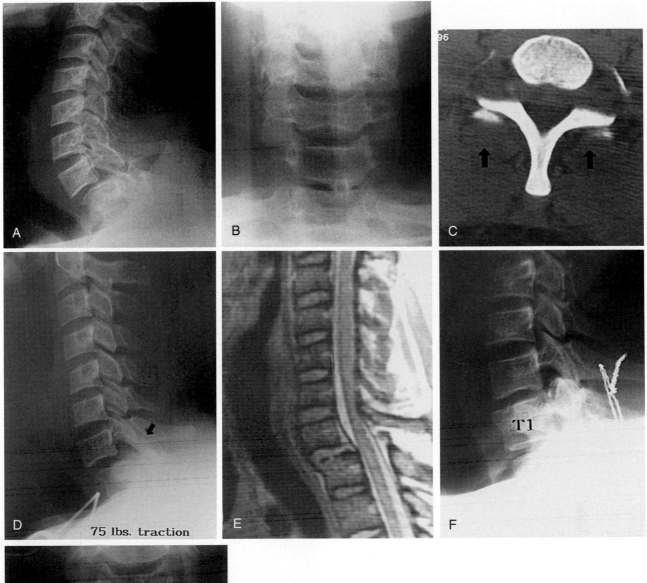

Figure 22–3 = This patient sustained a bilateral facet dislocation at C7–T1. *A*, The step-off, accompanied by slight kyphosis and narrowing of the disc space, is evident on the lateral radiograph. *B*, The AP radiograph demonstrated widening of the interspinous distance but no rotational abnormality. *C*, After the patient was placed in traction, a CT scan was obtained, which showed the dislocated facets (*arrows*) on the axial view. *D*, As a result of the patient's size and the distal position of the dislocation in the cervical spine, the dislocation could not be reduced using traction. *E*, An MRI was done because the facet dislocation would have to be reduced with the patient under anesthesia. No disc herniation was observed, but stripping of the posterior longitudinal ligament was evident. *F* and *G*, Using evoked potential monitoring, the reduction was accomplished operatively without removing any of the facets, and an intraspinous wire was selected to stabilize the injury. This technique was selected both because of the intrinsic rotational stability of the reduced facet dislocation and also because of the relatively poor fixation to the thin lateral mass of C7.

Thus on a lateral radiograph, one vertebral body of the pair involved in the injury appears longer than its counterpart, either above or below it. In addition, on an AP radiograph, malrotation of the spinous processes at the level of the injury will also be apparent. These three injuries, unilateral subluxation, unilateral perched facet, and unilateral dislocation, represent a progression of injury, as is the case with their bilateral

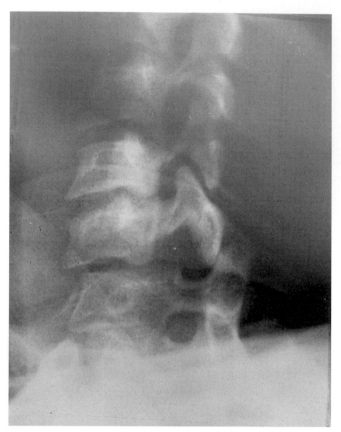

Figure 22–4 = Oblique radiograph demonstrates a bilateral facet dislocation at C6–7. Note that the intact inferior facet at C6 as well as the intact superior facet at C7 have been juxtaposed.

counterparts. Unilateral facet subluxations are extremely rare and are generally not visible in a resting radiograph. They are be demonstrated by flexion-extension radiographs; a rotational abnormality is induced on a flexion view. A unilateral perched facet is exceedingly uncommon, as most result in unilateral dislocations. The mechanism of all three of these injuries is a flexion-rotation and distraction injury. The most common of the three is a unilateral dislocation (Fig. 22–5). In this case, the inferior articular process slides up over the top of the superior process below and locks anterior to it. On a lateral radiograph this appears as an apparent translation of the superior level over the inferior affected level, generally with translation less than that noted in a bilateral facet dislocation (3 mm vs. 4 to 6 mm, or 25% vs. 50% translation). The exact pathologic lesion is often difficult to see, as the intact facet is superimposed on the injured facet and is therefore not apparent on a lateral radiograph. The rotational component, as previously described, is always present. This can be visualized on both AP and lateral radiographs. It may be possible to differentiate the injury on a CT scan, but it is best seen either on lateral tomography (to differentiate the intact from the injured facet) or on a 3D reconstruction (which allows excellent visualization of the dislocated facet). MRI is necessary infrequently, but it may be used to assess the injured disc. Unilateral dislocation injuries are rarely

associated with neurologic deficit, but extremely significant ligamentous disruption is necessary to achieve the dislocation. The mechanism is felt to be a combination of flexion, distraction, and simultaneous rotation, resulting in complete disruption of the facet capsule as well as attenuation of the interspinous ligament and partial disruption of the posterolateral corner of the disc, including the uncinate process of Luschka. It is interesting to note that the resultant instability after reduction is somewhat different than would be suggested by the sum of the ligamentous disruptions. If the facet is not removed in the reduction process, the resultant instability is a coupled flexion-rotation. In addition, understanding the nature of the disruption is important to comprehending the necessity for a reduction maneuver, as opposed to simple traction, to achieve reduction; this is discussed later in the chapter. Because the flexion and the rotation are a coupled motion, pure restriction of flexion in the case of intact facets after a dislocation results in spinal stability. In addition, to achieve the unilateral facet dislocation, discal disruption must occur, and that aspect of the

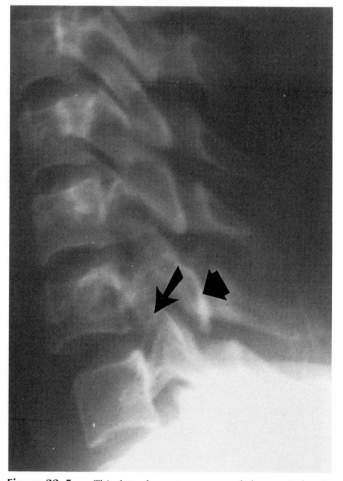

Figure 22–5 = This lateral roentgenogram of the cervical spine demonstrates a unilateral facet dislocation in a 19-year-old woman at the C6-7 level. Note the rotational deformity indicated by the apparent widening of the anteroposterior width of the C6 body with reference to the C7 body. In addition, the two facets at C6–7 are well visualized, and the normal inferior facet of C6 (*arrowhead*) can be differentiated from the dislocated inferior C6 facet (*arrow*).

injury should not be overlooked in evaluating the neurologic status.

Fractures of the Articular Components

Bilateral Facet Fractures

In contradistinction to the ligamentous injuries involving the articular facets and lateral masses, the facet fractures do not represent a continuum. They are distinct injuries, all with slightly different mechanisms of injury.[82] Bilateral facet fractures can be of several types. They are generally bilateral superior articular process fractures, bilateral inferior facet fractures, or combinations of the two.[67] Bilateral superior facet fractures (Fig. 22–6) are somewhat more common; they generally result from slight flexion and a translation or shearing injury in which the superior facets are broken off at the junction with the lamina. Depending on the degree of initial flexion, the location of the fracture may differ. If the shearing injury is severe, the posterior longitudinal ligament and the disc may be disrupted, and in the

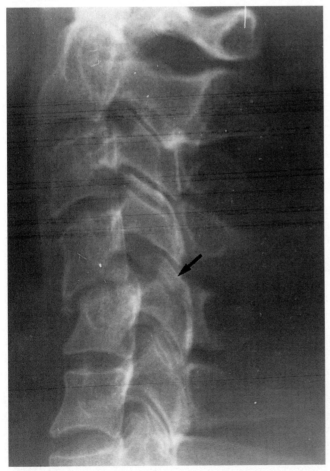

Figure 22–6 = This bilateral facet fracture at C4–5 in a 40-year-old woman demonstrates displacement and angulation similar to that shown in Figure 22–4. In addition, there is an absence of rotational deformity, demonstrated either by foreshortening of the affected bodies or by evidence of the biconcave nature of the posterior aspect of the body. The bilateral fractures of the superior facet of C5 are suggested (*arrow*) on the lateral radiograph but are best demonstrated on lateral tomography or by CT reconstructions.

most severe form of injury, total disruption of the disc occurs with marked instability. The degree of translation is related to the severity of injury. These injuries may be vertically unstable as well if significant shear has been imparted to the spine, so they may provide classic examples of the positive stretch test by the criteria of White and co-workers.[78] The second type of bilateral facet fracture is the bilateral inferior articular process fracture, in which slight flexion is imparted to the spine, but with less of a shear force. The inferior articular processes fracture either midway through the articular portion or in combination with laminar and spinous process fractures propagating up into the cancellous portion of the lamina. It is interesting to note that this fracture occurs with some frequency in the upper portion of the cervical spine (Fig. 22–7), and because of the widening of the canal that occurs with the laminar fractures, it may result in significant displacement and disruption of the disc with little or no neurologic deficit. The instability in both of the inferior and superior facet fractures without complete disc disruption is predominantly bidirectional rotation and anterior translation. Slight rotation can be visible if the two sides do not translate precisely to the same degree. These injuries may be differentiated from bilateral dislocations in that generally less angulation is visible than in bilateral dislocations. However, the translation may be significant if disc disruption is exaggerated. The mechanism of injury, as previously noted, is predominantly forward translation or shear, occasionally accompanied by slight flexion. Irrespective of the type of fracture (inferior vs. superior facet), the disruption is fairly similar. In both cases, the intraspinous and supraspinous ligaments are attenuated but are generally not completely disrupted. This may be accompanied by a bilaminar fracture or spinous process fracture. The facet capsule is not disrupted, as the injury usually occurs at either the superior or inferior limits of the capsule, with the facet complex instability occurring through the bony margin of the superior or inferior facet. The ligamentum flavum may be disrupted. The anulus is generally not as severely disrupted as in dislocations, as there is no little or no flexion component to the injury. Slight discal injury may occur, but generally without disruption of the anulus. As opposed to dislocations, the neurologic injury here is most prominently related to translation of the two vertebral segments and not the extrusion of disc material. Unlike those used in bilateral facet dislocations, constructs to stabilize this must be able to impart a resistance to translation, rather than purely to flexion. The final variant of bilateral facet injuries is a unilateral fracture combined with a contralateral dislocation (Fig. 22–8). This is the rarest of the bilateral facet injuries; it includes both flexion and rotational components and results in complex instability. The exact mechanism of injury is difficult to establish.

Unilateral Facet Fractures

Unilateral facet fractures are a diverse group that encompasses three major types of injury.

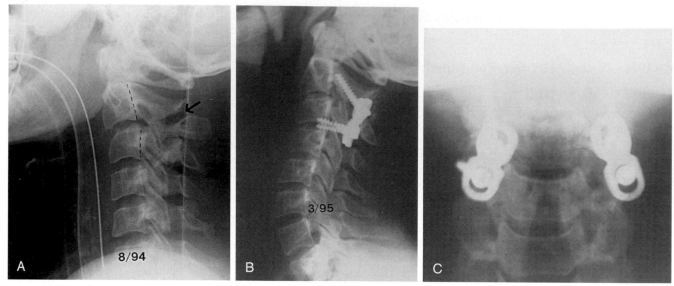

Figure 22–7 = *A,* The lateral radiograph shows fractures of the lamina and inferior facets of C2. This may be confused with type III traumatic spondylolisthesis of the axis, but it is an entirely different injury. Stabilization of this injury may be very difficult because it is rotationally unstable and cannot be fixed with an intraspinous wire. Because the inferior facets are involved, bilateral oblique wiring will also not suffice. Similarly, plating is difficult because there is no lateral mass of C2 to which to affix the upper level. *B* and *C,* Stabilization can be achieved with a plate construct, however, if the proximal screw in C2 is directed into the pedicle. A depth of 20 mm is usually sufficient to achieve solid fixation.

Superior Facet Fracture. The most common type of injury is a fracture of the superior articular process of the facet. This occurs in approximately 80% of all facet injuries (Fig. 22–9). The mechanism of injury is predominantly slight flexion and rotation with a minimal ligamentous component. The contralateral facet capsule is left intact, and a slight to moderate disruption of the intraspinous ligament is seen. Because the fracture generally occurs at the base of the superior articular facet, the components of the facet capsule that attach the inferior facet to the superior facet are left at least partially intact. If the superior facet fragment is translated into the neural foramen by injury, there are generally ligamentous attachments to the inferior facet. As with all rotational injuries, partial disruption of the disc occurs. The fractured facet fragment is often visible on lateral radiograph. The apparent translation is evident on lateral radiograph and is generally limited to between 4 and 4.5 mm. In fact, no true translation occurs, as this is a rotational instability, and the contralateral side remains aligned. This is often accompanied by angulation of approximately 5 to 7 degrees. The AP radiograph demonstrates the rotational deformity. As a result of the overlap of the affected and unaffected levels, the exact diagnosis is rarely evident on the initial radiograph. It is of note, however, that with this injury, placing the patient in traction with small amounts of weight (between 10 and 20 lb) results in a reduction of the unilateral facet fracture. This does not occur with the other injuries previously mentioned, and it may be helpful in differentiating a unilateral facet fracture from a dislocation. As with the bilateral facet fracture, because this injury is in the plane of the primary axial cuts of a CT scan, it is rarely well delineated on CT scanning; this requires 2D sagittal and parasagittal reconstructions, 3D reconstructions, or lateral tomography of the cervical spine. The nature of the instability is related to the fact that there is a fracture of the bony buttress, which is formed by the superior articular facet. There is generally attenuation of the intraspinous ligament with complete integrity of the contralateral capsule. The capsule of the involved facet is generally intact, and as a result, it carries the displaced fragment into the neural foramen with it. Most frequently, disruption of the posterior superior corner of the disc occurs.

Inferior Facet Fracture. As with the bilateral facet fractures, the second type of unilateral facet fracture is an inferior articular process fracture. Again, this is a flexion-rotation injury, and no significant evidence indicates how the forces are different so as to incur a superior facet fracture in one patient and an inferior facet fracture in another. The inferior articular process fractures usually occur at the base of the lamina, and some may penetrate up into the lamina and be associated with a more significant laminar fracture (Fig. 22–10). The ligamentous disruption is similar to the superior facet fractures, but the most significant component of the two injuries is the fracture of the buttress. In the case of the inferior facet fracture, the capsule is generally disrupted and the inferior facet often suffers a greenstick fracture posteriorly or it is a separate free fragment. The instability from this injury is purely rotational. Flexion instability is generally minimal. When axial traction is applied to the spine, an "unwinding" of the spine and a reduction of the deformity occur. Any constructs to stabilize the spine must take into account and counteract the rotational instability of vector.

Fracture Separation of the Articular Mass. The final type of fracture is the fracture separation of the articular mass.[45, 64] Its characteristic pattern (Fig. 22–11) is a

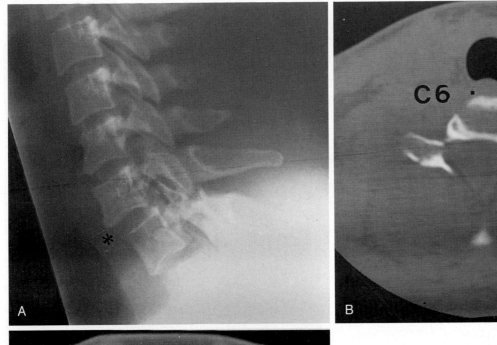

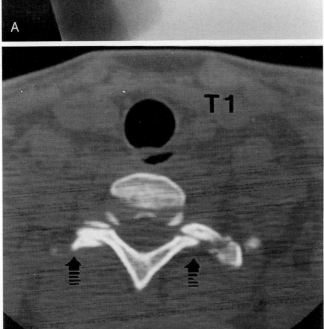

Figure 22–8 = *A*, This patient sustained injuries in a motor vehicle accident to both the C6–7 (*star*) and C7–T1 levels. *B*, The CT scan shows a fracture on one side at the upper level. *C*, The lower level demonstrates a dislocation on the left and a facet fracture on the right (*arrows*).

fracture through the pedicle and a longitudinal fracture through the lamina, parallel to the articular process on the same side. It occurs exceedingly infrequently as a bilateral injury and is most common as a unilateral injury. This injury, as opposed to the previous two types of facet fractures, is most probably an extension-rotation injury resulting in a fracture of the pedicle and a vertical fracture in the lamina. Associated with this are ligamentous injuries of the facet capsules, both above and below the fractures. Generally, one of the two (generally the lower) is significantly more unstable. Although the mechanism is different, the resultant instability is again rotational. This presents a unique problem, as the entire lateral mass is a free-floating fragment. The rotational instability cannot be stabilized

over a single level as the fixation into the free-floating lateral mass fragment will not result in a stable construct, and recurrent deformity can occur. Findings on lateral radiography are very similar to those seen in other unilateral facet injuries. There is evident rotation across the fracture segment with a difference in rotation noted by orientation of the vertebral bodies, as well as elongation and evident foreshortening of the two adjacent vertebral bodies across the injury segment. In addition, the lateral radiograph may show "horizontalization" of the lateral mass (Fig. 22–12), as it rotates after fracturing. The degrees of translation and angulation are similar to those seen with other unilateral facet fractures.[45] The AP radiograph will likewise show horizontalization of the lateral mass and may

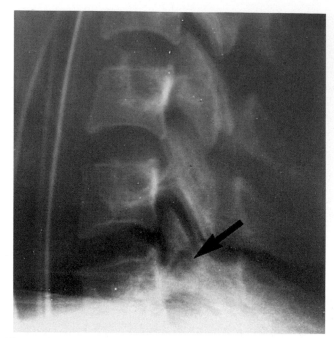

Figure 22–9 = A fracture of the superior facet of C7 is clearly visualized on this lateral radiograph (*arrow*). There is no associated deformity as it was reduced with 20 lb of traction.

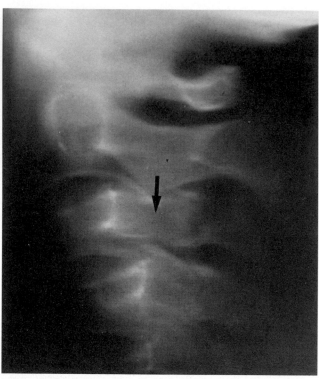

Figure 22–10 = This lateral tomogram shows a fracture of the inferior facet of C3. This injury is much less common than the fracture of the superior facet seen in Figure 22–9.

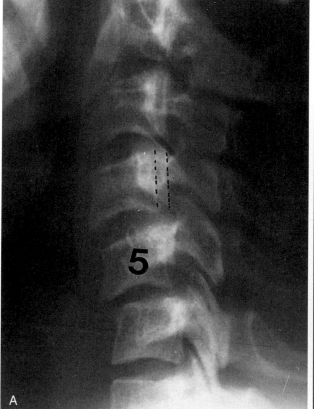

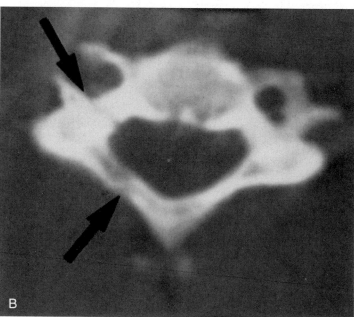

Figure 22–11 = This 19-year-old man was injured in a vehicle accident. *A*, The lateral radiograph demonstrates the unilateral facet fracture, which is a fracture separation of the articular mass of C5, and a rotational deformity at both C5–6 and C4–5. This is evident from the apparent elongation of the diameter of C5 with reference to C6 and also by the clear appearance of the two posterior edges of the concave vertebral body at C4. *B*, The CT scan demonstrates the characteristic pattern of a fracture separation of the articular mass, with *arrows* indicating one fracture through the pedicle and the second parallel to the spinous process in the lamina.

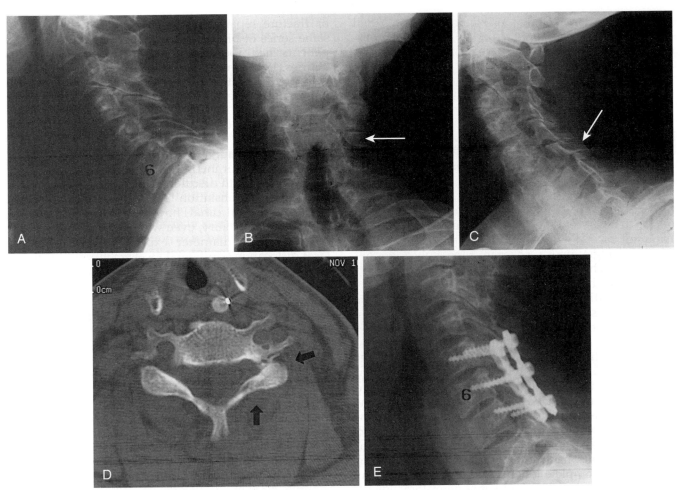

Figure 22–12 = This elderly woman sustained an extension and lateral bending injury in a motor vehicle accident and presented with neck pain and radiculopathy. *A*, The lateral radiograph showed a 4-mm step-off with the patient in an erect position. *B*, The AP x-ray shows foreshortening or horizontalization of the lateral mass (*arrow*), which is pathognomonic of a fracture-separation of the articular mass. *C*, The oblique or pillar view shows the horizontalization (*arrow*) more clearly than does the lateral view. Because the entire lateral mass is free-floating, as the spine collapses the orientation of the lateral mass changes. *D*, The two fracture lines in this injury are a vertical fracture in the lamina along the facet-laminar junction and a second fracture through the pedicle (*arrows*). Stabilization of this injury requires three-level plating. Because the fracture of the C6 lateral mass destabilizes both the C5–6 and the C6–7 joints on the affected side, the construct must involve C5–7. *E*, Plating only the C6–7 level will result in instability at the C5–6 level.

demonstrate the laminar fracture as well. The injury is best seen on CT scan, which demonstrates the characteristic pattern of the fracture through the pedicle, or through the foramen for the vertebral artery, with a second fracture line through the lamina, which frees and separates the entire lateral mass. This particular injury creates two levels of instability. Approximately three quarters of the noted instability is at the level of or below the fracture separation (at C5–6 for a C5 fracture separation) and approximately one quarter is at the level proximal to the fracture separation. However, stabilization of one level will result in instability at the second. Tomography and MRI are much less useful in this injury than in others. The disruption in this particular injury is purely bony. There is little attenuation of the interspinous ligament with little involvement of the contralateral posterior elements. However, the involved elements demonstrate a fracture line with only attenuation of the facet capsules on the affected side. Occasionally a true dislocation of one or both levels will result as well; more commonly the

levels are in their normal apposition, but a floating lateral mass is seen. The remainder of the instability results from the fracture of the bony elements anteriorly through the pedicle or through the foramen for the vertebral artery. Some discal involvement must also be evident to obtain the degree of apparent rotational translation.

Any of these injuries can occur in multiple combinations. Double-level unilateral facet fractures, double-level fracture separations of the articular mass, or alternate-level injuries can occur. In terms of instability, each of these injuries needs to be considered as a separate entity; if the total injury pattern is difficult to classify, then each individual injury can be considered as a separate unit and treated individually.

Neurologic Injury

The rate of occurrence and the severity of neurologic injury accompanying unilateral and bilateral cervical facet injuries is the result of a number of different

using a combination of axial traction, general anesthetic, and either a laminar spreader or Caspar cervical distractor. It is critical that the distractor be placed deeply into the disc space after complete discectomy and that the bodies be distracted enough to permit unlocking of the facets (Fig. 22–15A and B). Pressure can then be applied over the superior body and the distractor tipped superiorly to allow reduction to occur. At this point, a tricortical graft of 8 to 10 mm is placed in the disc space and a single-level anterior plate is used to stabilize the disrupted level (see Fig. 22–15D and E). If reduction cannot be achieved after the anterior discectomy, a Smith-Robinson–type graft is still

placed between the two involved vertebrae in the disc space and the anterior wound is closed. The patient is then flipped into the prone position on the Stryker frame and a posterior reduction and stabilization is done. If the graft displaces during the transition from supine to prone or during the operative procedure, a third procedure may be necessary to adequately position the anterior graft. Some authors think that anterior discectomy and reduction of the deformity from the anterior approach, irrespective of the condition of the disc, can be done routinely. Stabilization is then undertaken using an anterior graft and a plate. I believe that this is not the most reasonable alternative for treatment

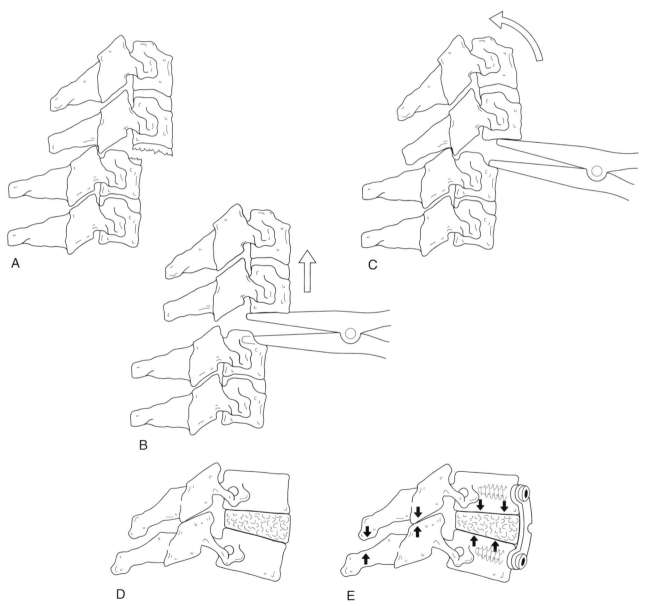

Figure 22–15 = Technique of anterior reduction of bilateral facet dislocation with a large disc extrusion. *A,* Complete discectomy is done initially to remove the extruded fragment within the canal. *B,* Either a laminar spreader or a Caspar distractor is placed deeply within the disc space and symmetrical distraction is applied to disengage the facets. Axial traction is also applied. Once the facets are disengaged, the superior body is pushed posteriorly while the distraction is released to achieve the reduction. *C,* The ability to achieve a reduction can be blocked by inserting the distractor into the anterior portion of the disc space, resulting in asymmetrical distraction. *D,* The tricortical graft is created in a routine fashion, with the exception that it is slightly tapered. *E,* The plate is then contoured slightly so that the graft is compressed and the posterior elements are not fixed in distraction, but rather they aid in the load-sharing with the anterior graft and hardware.

of a bilateral posterior facet injury that is chiefly a ligamentous injury in the posterior aspect of the spine. An anterior approach should be reserved only for cases in which discectomy is required to remove a large extruded fragment; this clearly represents a small segment of patients. An anterior approach compromises the remaining intact structure (i.e., the anterior longitudinal ligament) and therefore serves to further destabilize the spine. In addition, it requires an indirect reduction maneuver to reduce the dislocated posterior facets. It has also been shown that anterior plating is not as strong in resisting flexion as are posterior tension-band techniques.

Therefore, for the majority of bilateral facet injuries—both dislocations and fractures—the preferred approach is posterior. This approach can often be carried out for injuries as late as 6 weeks after trauma, assuming that the reduction of the deformity can be achieved initially by the use of traction. Should a reduction of deformity not be achievable by the use of traction on an older injury, a combined anterior and posterior approach may also be necessary. The surgical stabilization used for the facet injuries should take into account any deforming forces and instabilities caused by the trauma. In a patient with a bilateral facet dislocation, the predominant instability (flexion-distraction) can be counteracted easily by the use of a posterior tension-band technique, assuming that both facets are intact, there is no rotational instability, and no derotational force needs to be applied. Therefore, the most commonly used techniques are Roger interspinous wiring, a Bohlman triple-wire, and posterior cervical plating across one level. These should be accompanied by an arthrodesis in all cases. The simplest technique is posterior interspinous wiring (Fig. 22–16). For all patients undergoing this procedure, the positioning is critically important. Because many patients are already in traction with Gardner-Wells tongs, it is perhaps easiest to do the surgery on a Stryker frame. The patient is placed in appropriate traction; a face plate, which is a part of the Stryker frame, is placed in position so as to cause neither extensive lordosis of the cervical spine nor either flexion or extension of the head, and the patient is flipped into the prone position after awake nasotracheal intubation. The patient's neurologic status is then checked, and while in the prone position, the positioning of the neck is done and anesthesia induced. The position of the neck is checked by a lateral radiograph. Care must be taken that the reduction has remained and that excessive lordosis or straightening of the spine has not occurred. This can usually be maintained with approximately 20 to 25 lb of longitudinal pull. Visualization of the lower part of the cervical spine is done by taping the shoulders. Care must be taken that the tape is placed across the entire width of the shoulder and not just out to the distal part of the clavicle. This will prevent excessive pull on the brachial plexus and resultant brachial plexus injuries. In addition, pressure should not be applied via the arms, but through longitudinal traction on the entire shoulder girdle. With the patient in a correct position, the patient is then pre-pared and draped, leaving a small area for bone graft harvesting.

Alternately, the patient can be positioned (if not already in Gardner-Wells tongs or a halo) in a Mayfield headrest with three-pin positioner (see Fig. 22–16B). The patient can also be positioned (see Fig. 22–16A) by simply attaching the Mayfield headrest to a halo that is already in position should traction not be necessary. After injecting the skin with epinephrine (diluted 1:100,000) to diminish bleeding, exposure should be directly in the midline. The midline plane should be avascular, with the dissection taken down to the tips of the spinous processes. Subperiosteal dissection is done at the presumed level, but ligament is not removed, nor are the facet capsules damaged, before a lateral radiograph is taken to ascertain the position. Care should be taken to maintain the interspinous ligament unless it is completely disrupted, and only the facet capsules at the indicated levels are removed. Care should also be taken not to strip additional portions of the spine, as this may cause spontaneous fusion in the cervical spine. The remainder of the technique for interspinous wiring is described in detail in Figure 22–16. The technique is applicable currently for facet injuries with no element of rotational instability, and the main goal of surgery is to block flexion with a tension-band construct (see Fig. 22–3).

An alternate technique for treatment of this injury is a bilateral lateral mass plating. Plating of the lateral masses was originally introduced by Roy-Camille in the late 1960s using 14-mm screws and Vitallium plates.[65, 66] The technique of screw placement has been modified several times. It has gained popularity in North America since the late 1980s. Its advantages are additional stability at the time of fixation, less loss of reduction, decreased postoperative immobilization, and the implied advantage that the end point of fixation does not require compression of the interspace, which contains an injured disc. Using interspinous wiring, the tension band is tightened until either the spinous processes abut or until the wire tension "feels" appropriate, which may result in significant compression of the disc space. However, the plate fixation technique allows reduction of the relationship of the two levels but does not require tightening as an end point. The relationship achieved by traction can be maintained by appropriate screw placement. It also allows fixation in the absence of the spinous process and lamina. The original technique for screw placement described by Roy-Camille involves angling the screw approximately 10 degrees laterally and perpendicular to the plane of the facet joint, beginning directly in the middle of the facet so that the screw is bicortical but directly anterior just above the lower uninvolved joint. The modification of the technique by Magerl and co-workers[51] involved angling the screw approximately 30 degrees superiorly so that it is parallel to the articular surface of the superior facet. The starting point is slightly medial to the center of the facet joint, and the screw trajectory is angled laterally approximately 30 degrees to avoid the vertebral artery and to achieve the longest possible screw path within the bone. The

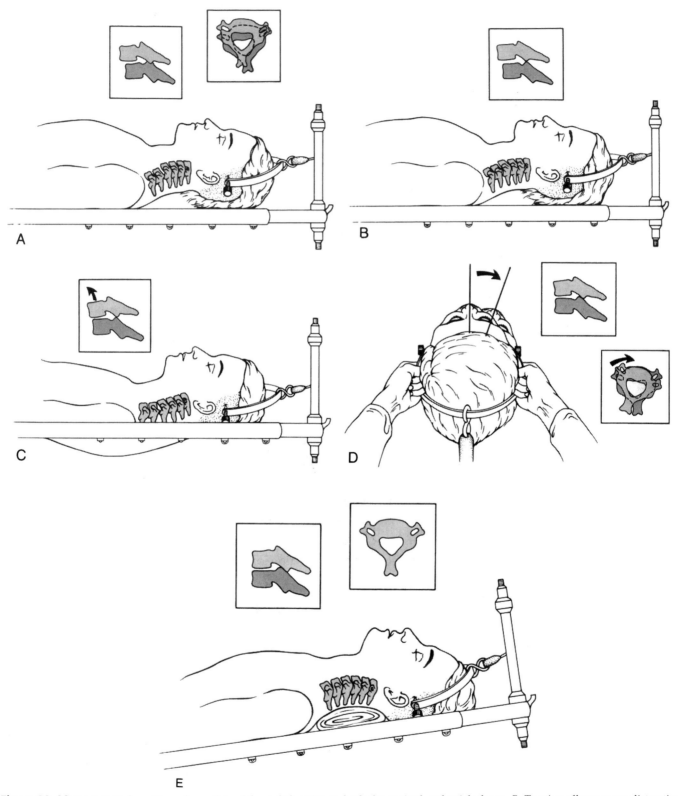

Figure 22–20 = *A,* Initial position of a unilateral facet dislocation in both the sagittal and axial planes. *B,* Traction allows some distraction but not reduction. *C,* Flexion of the neck increases the distraction but the dislocation remains. *D,* Lateral tilt away from the side of dislocation unlocks the dislocation. *E,* Extension and return of the neck to the neutral position completes the reduction. (From Bucholz RW: Lower cervical spine injuries. *In* Browner BD, Jupiter JB, Levine AM, et al (eds): Skeletal Trauma: Fractures, Dislocations, Ligamentous Injuries, vol 1. Philadelphia, WB Saunders, 1992, p 638.)

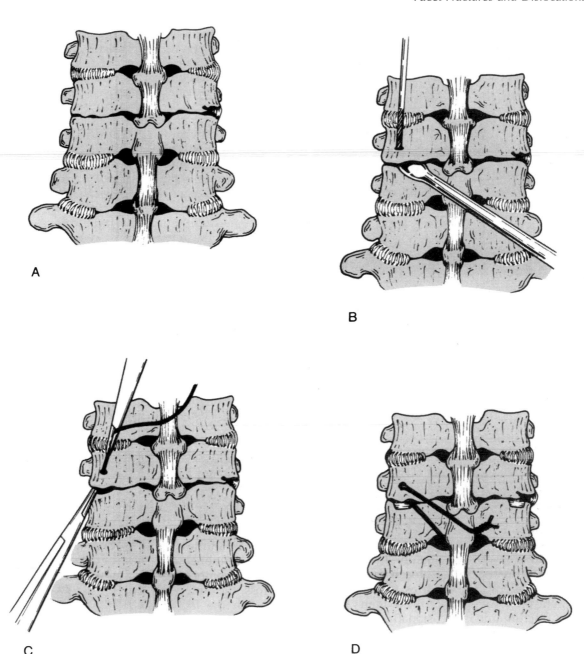

A

B

C

D

Figure 22–21 = Oblique wiring technique. Oblique wiring is most often utilized for a unilateral facet fracture when the superior facet of the inferior level is fractured. Most **unilateral** facet dislocations can be stabilized by an interspinous wire once the facet dislocation is reduced. Should reduction of the dislocation **require** compromise of the superior facet of the inferior level, an oblique wire may be used. The surgical approach is similar to that for interspinous wiring, with the patient placed in traction in a prone position, most commonly with Gardner-Wells tongs on a Stryker frame. A **midline** exposure is accomplished, and the level is checked using a marker and radiographic control. The exposure is carried out to the tips of the facets, and care is taken to expose only the facet at the level of injury. The facet capsules are generally totally disrupted on the fractured side and intact on the uninjured side. In addition, the interspinous ligament is usually present but somewhat attenuated. *A,* After removing all soft tissue at the appropriate level, a Penfield elevator is placed within the joint after all cartilage has been removed from the joint surfaces with a small curette. Using a hand drill and a ³⁄₃₂-in drill bit, a hole is made in the center of the facet and is directed perpendicular and slightly **inferior** and medial to the facet joint. *B,* A 20-gauge wire or a braided 22-gauge wire is passed through the facet joint from superior to inferior and grasped using a needle holder. *C,* The small cancellous plugs are placed into the facet joints to preserve height and promote fusion, and the wire is place around the spinous process of the lower level. It is progressively tightened and radiographs are taken until anatomic reduction is achieved. *D,* Generally, 1 mm of overreduction is desired so that the reduction is anatomic when the patient is immobilized. (From Bucholz RW: Lower cervical spine injuries. *In* Browner BD, Jupiter JB, Levine AM, et al (eds): Skeletal Trauma: Fractures, Dislocations, Ligamentous Injuries, vol 1. Philadelphia, WB Saunders, 1992, p 717.)

require immobilization of two vertebrae and one interspace, whereas for fracture separation of the articular mass, three vertebrae and two interspaces are involved.

Fractures of the superior articular facet with intact spinous process and lamina can be dealt with by the oblique wiring technique[29] (see Figs. 22–21 and 22–22). As with bilateral injuries, this is most easily done while

pediatric patients seen with spinal cord injury were found to have no radiographic abnormality.[71] It is likely that this occurs as a result of the unique anatomy and physiologic differences inherent in the spine of the skeletally immature. Several authors have published larger series regarding these patients.[35, 71, 80] The absence of radiographic findings is one contributing factor to a patient's injury being underrecognized, but it does not seem to be the most important contributor. Orenstein et al.[69] found that it is the clinician's failure to obtain films or to recognize existing radiographic abnormalities, commonly at the cervicothoracic junction or at the occiput–C1–2 motion segments, that usually results in diagnostic error. They found nine patients (12%) with abnormalities not appreciated on initial readings of plain films or in patients who failed to have adequate immediate radiographic examinations. In this group, only one patient, however, had neurologic deficit. Based on 50 pediatric patients with cervical injuries, Dietrich and co-workers[22] also reported a 10% error in the initial reading of radiographs where fracture or subluxations were eventually found to be present. The clinician must beware of this pitfall above all others.

Several important characteristics of the immature spine may account for the normal radiographic appearance in the face of high-energy injuries that have rendered the patient neurologically impaired. The first of these is the greater tissue compliance or elasticity seen in ligaments and joint capsules of children, which may allow for transient subluxations without gross mechanical failure. This laxity was described by Cattell and others[16] in their description of pseudosubluxation in children based on a review of 160 normal subjects. Secondly, the planes of the cervical facets in children are more horizontal and thus possess greater mobility but less stability.[71] Finally and most important, as demonstrated by Aufderman[2] in his elegant pathologic study of 12 children, catastrophic failure in the immature spine nearly always occurs through the cartilaginous end plate (see Fig. 23–4). The end plate or physis is the weak link in the child and fractures through it are not uncommonly missed unless they are complete and seen on stress radiographs. Consider the analogy of the distal femoral physeal fracture in the child where stress films help to differentiate it from significant ligamentous injury more commonly seen in the adult.

In patients with SCIWORA, however, even stress radiographs of the neck may be normal. This in part may be related to patient compliance or protective splinting, but may also be due to incomplete mechanical failure. It may also suggest that complete physeal failure contributes to only a portion of these clinical presentations. Pang and Wilberger,[71] in their comprehensive treatise on this subject, described 24 patients with SCIWORA seen over 20 years at the Children's Hospital of Pittsburgh. Eighteen of the patients had voluntary flexion-extension films done acutely and none revealed an abnormality. All 24 eventually received dynamic films and only one patient had radiographic instability. With MRI it may be possible in the future to detect a majority of these injuries of the cartilaginous end plate and determine the role that

they might have played in allowing for neurologic compromise.

In Pang and Wilberger's series hyperextension alone was the presumed mechanism of injury in 10 of 24 patients. Seven of the 10 patients were more than 8 years old. The majority of the lesions involved the lower cervical cord (C5–8 root level), while the five cases of upper cord injury were in the minority and only seen in children under 8 years of age. The younger children with upper cord injuries seemed to have an increased likelihood of serious injury in general. Corroborating physical signs such as chin lacerations, mandibular fractures, facial injuries, and frontal skull injuries were commonly seen to support a hyperextension injury. Overall, 58% sustained a complete or serious cord injury and the final outcome did not seem to be affected significantly by age or treatment.[71]

Management of these patients begins with neutral cervical immobilization in the field and the hospital until screening radiographs can be performed. To accomplish this, the small child and infant may require a roll to be placed under his or her shoulders to compensate for the disproportionately large size of the head. Associated basic life and trauma resuscitations take priority over all further workup. Avoidance of both cord edema and hypotension may be critical to maintaining cord perfusion pressures. Most authors consider administering high-dose corticosteroids.[11] Dynamic radiographs and MRI should be performed as early as feasible. Definitive management of the spine may require no more than the use of a secure rigid collar. Those patients with demonstrable instability will be more safely immobilized in a halo device or with cervical arthrodesis if the halo will complicate the patient's rehabilitation. Follow-up dynamic radiographs are mandatory in all patients. Evolving neurologic deficits were reported in one half of Pang and Wilberger's patients and this mandates emergency reevaluation.[71] Subsequent management is controversial, yet consideration should be given to decompression and fusion if a structural lesion is found. Laminectomy alone in the pediatric spine renders the patient prone to the eventual development of kyphosis and, in general, is contraindicated. The progression of neurologic deficit may be related, however, to occult instability and reinjury, or to evolving edema, hemorrhage, or watershed infarction in the absence of obvious epidural hematoma.[71] The management of these patients may be primarily medical and supportive.

WHIPLASH (ACCELERATION-DECELERATION INJURY TO THE CERVICAL SPINE)

Whiplash injuries, or acceleration-deceleration injuries of the neck, have been commonly referred to as cervical sprains. Although some whiplash injuries may indeed represent minor ligamentous injuries of the ALL experienced under tension, the syndrome likely represents a constellation of injuries rarely dramatically evident at initial or follow-up examination. The foundations of

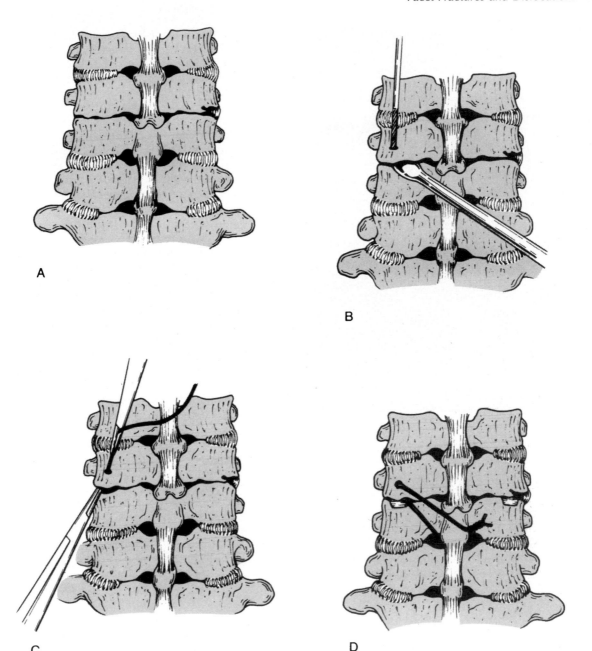

Figure 22–21 = Oblique wiring technique. Oblique wiring is most often utilized for a unilateral facet fracture when the superior facet of the inferior level is fractured. Most unilateral facet dislocations can be stabilized by an interspinous wire once the facet dislocation is reduced. Should reduction of the dislocation require compromise of the superior facet of the inferior level, an oblique wire may be used. The surgical approach is similar to that for interspinous wiring, with the patient placed in traction in a prone position, most commonly with Gardner-Wells tongs on a Stryker frame. A midline exposure is accomplished, and the level is checked using a marker and radiographic control. The exposure is carried out to the tips of the facets, and care is taken to expose only the facet at the level of injury. The facet capsules are generally totally disrupted on the fractured side and intact on the uninjured side. In addition, the interspinous ligament is usually present but somewhat attenuated. *A,* After removing all soft tissue at the appropriate level, a Penfield elevator is placed within the joint after all cartilage has been removed from the joint surfaces with a small curette. Using a hand drill and a ³⁄₃₂-in drill bit, a hole is made in the center of the facet and is directed perpendicular and slightly inferior and medial to the facet joint. *B,* A 20-gauge wire or a braided 22-gauge wire is passed through the facet joint from superior to inferior and grasped using a needle holder. *C,* The small cancellous plugs are placed into the facet joints to preserve height and promote fusion, and the wire is place around the spinous process of the lower level. It is progressively tightened and radiographs are taken until anatomic reduction is achieved. *D,* Generally, 1 mm of overreduction is desired so that the reduction is anatomic when the patient is immobilized. (From Bucholz RW: Lower cervical spine injuries. *In* Browner BD, Jupiter JB, Levine AM, et al (eds): Skeletal Trauma: Fractures, Dislocations, Ligamentous Injuries, vol 1. Philadelphia, WB Saunders, 1992, p 717.)

require immobilization of two vertebrae and one interspace, whereas for fracture separation of the articular mass, three vertebrae and two interspaces are involved.

Fractures of the superior articular facet with intact spinous process and lamina can be dealt with by the oblique wiring technique[29] (see Figs. 22–21 and 22–22). As with bilateral injuries, this is most easily done while

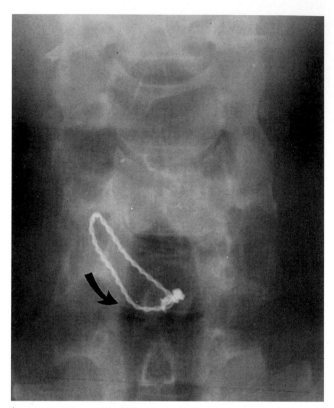

Figure 22–22 ═ This AP radiograph demonstrates an oblique wire fixation. This technique allows the correction of rotational deformities by providing an oblique tension band from the inferior facet on the involved side to the spinous process of the inferior level. By tightening the oblique wire, correction and stabilization of the rotational deformity are possible.

the patient is held in traction with Gardner-Wells tongs on a Stryker frame. Reduction and traction should be done by lateral radiograph before the operative procedure is performed. The approach is much the same as that for bilateral facet injuries. Generally, little will be apparent on visualization of the injury, except the transverse fracture line is occasionally evident after remnants of the facet capsule are removed. The inferior facet and lamina and the spinous process must not be damaged, because the passage of the oblique wire requires a relatively intact facet joint. The cartilage is removed from the facet joint and the joint is opened using a small Penfield elevator, which protects the superior articular facet as well as the nerve root. Using either a 3/32-in drill or a burr tip, a hole is made in the center of the inferior articular facet at the level above, angled slightly inferiorly and medially to allow passage of the wire. A braided 22-gauge stainless steel wire[75] is made using a hand drill and then passed through the hole in the inferior facet. With the facet held open, the tip of the wire is curved so that it can be picked up using a hemostat as it passes through the inferior facet and above the superior facet. It is then gently pushed through the facet pulling at the same time in an attempt to avoid sawing through the inferior articular process.

The upper limb is then passed through the interspinous ligament above the spinous process of the lower

level, and the inferior limb is passed beneath the interspinous ligament at the inferior end of the lower level. The graft is attained from the iliac crest, and a small plate of cancellous bone is put into the decorticated facet joint. Wires are then tightened around the opposite side of the spinous process until the fracture is anatomically reduced. The traction weights are removed to prevent overtightening of the wire, and the fracture reduction is then visualized on a lateral radiograph. The radiograph should demonstrate overreduction by 1 mm, so that when any soft tissues caught in the wire undergo necrosis in the postoperative period, the reduction will be maintained. The same technique can be used for an inferior facet fracture if a significant portion of the inferior facet remains, so that there is sufficient bone area to pass the wire, or it can be extended up to the uninvolved level above with the use of cervical plating. The graft is placed on the decorticated lamina on both involved levels.

Single-level cervical plating is easily used for reduction and stabilization of unilateral superior facet injury (Figs. 22–23 and 22–24). The technique is modified from that discussed previously for bilateral facet dislocations and fractures. The angle of screw insertion on the injured side must be carefully considered. The Roy-Camille technique is generally applicable in this instance, whereas if the Magerl technique is used, the angle of the inferior screw on the injured side will need to be decreased to avoid penetration into the fracture site. In all cases, the uninjured side should be instrumented first. The application of the plate along the posterior aspect of the contralateral (uninjured) side will allow stabilization and easy reduction. The injured side is then is instrumented secondarily.

Inferior articular process fractures present a slightly different and less common problem. Here the injury is again rotational, and the fragment is posterior, usually with a component of the fracture being transverse across the anterior facet with a vertical component through the facet laminar junction. If fragments are totally broken off they can be taken out and used for graft; this does not in any way enhance or detract from the stability. The fracture fragment does not in any way affect the neural foramen, although the rotational instability induced by the fracture does compromise the foramen. The problem in this case is obtaining sufficient purchase in the remaining portion of the facet at the level above to limit the length of the arthrodesis and stabilization to a single vertebral pair and one interspace. This is very difficult to do using oblique wiring, because the purchase site for the wire is the inferior facet. This is one of the cases in which a lateral mass plating can save a level over a wiring technique. In addition, in cases in which the presence of laminar and/or spinous process fractures would preclude the use of the Bohlman triple-wire technique, or oblique wiring, the use of lateral mass plating can conserve levels and allow the stabilization to be restricted to the injured segment. Again, the fractures are reduced as previously noted for superior facet fractures using traction. If sufficient facet remains to pass a wire through at the injured level, an oblique wire can be used. It is

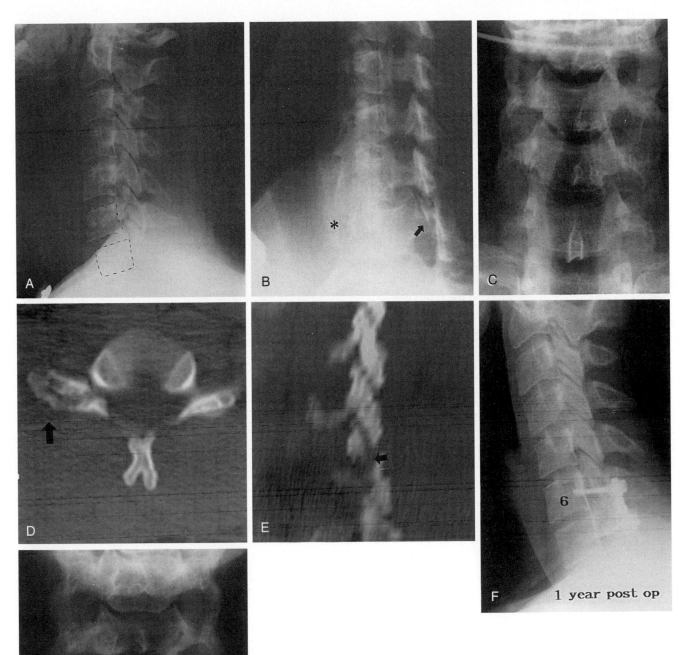

Figure 22–23 = This patient was involved in a motor vehicle accident; he struck his head on the windshield and sustained a right C6–7 facet fracture with C7 radicular signs and symptoms and a 3-mm step-off. *A*, He was placed in traction and had almost a complete reduction with 25 lb. *B*, The initial oblique view shows the step-off (*star*) and superior facet fracture (*arrow*). *C*, The AP view shows the rotational malalignment between the C6 and C7 spinous processes. *D*, The axial cut on the CT scan does not clearly show the nature of the fracture line, but the parasagittal reconstruction (*E*) clearly shows the superior facet fracture (*arrows*). *F* and *G*, The patient underwent a single-level plating and was noted to have a traumatic root sleeve dural tear at the time of surgery. He underwent a single-level plating (C6–7), and 1 year later he was neurologically intact with an anatomic reduction.

not recommended to go to the interspace above (which is involved), as was previously recommended,[28, 34, 47] just to secure fixation. In the case of the fractured inferior facet, a plate can be used, and the position of

the superior screw can be modified to achieve adequate fixation. A direction more consistent with the Magerl technique may be indicated in such a case, to allow the upper screw to achieve purchase in the undisturbed

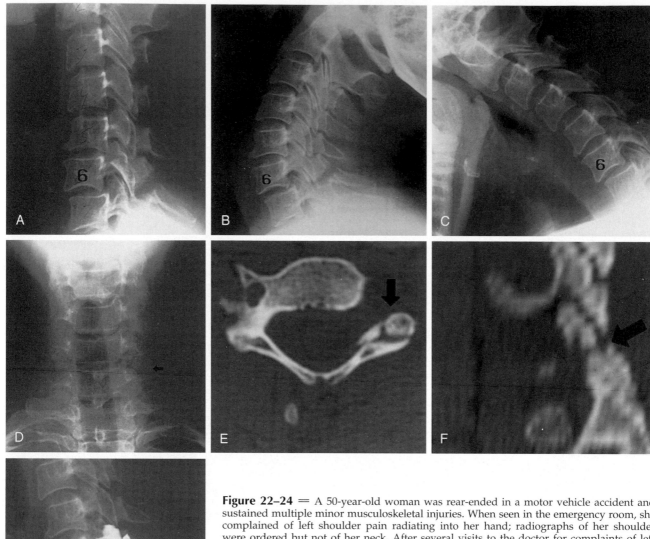

Figure 22–24 = A 50-year-old woman was rear-ended in a motor vehicle accident and sustained multiple minor musculoskeletal injuries. When seen in the emergency room, she complained of left shoulder pain radiating into her hand; radiographs of her shoulder were ordered but not of her neck. After several visits to the doctor for complaints of left arm pain and numbness, she was seen by an orthopedic surgeon and noted to have significant weakness in her left biceps, triceps, and intrinsic muscles. A step-off was noted between C6–7 on a lateral (*A*) and on flexion-extension (*B* and *C*) radiographs. *D,* The AP view showed the vertical component of the fracture in the superior facet (*arrow*). This was also clearly seen (*arrow*) on the axial section of the CT scan (*E*), although the true nature of the fracture and the displacement is best seen on the parasagittal reconstruction (*F, arrow*). *G,* The patient underwent a C6–7 plating, but due to the thin lateral mass and poor fixation at C7, it was extended to T1. The patient achieved anatomic alignment and full neurologic recovery.

portion of the facet (Fig. 22–25). This may require angling of the upper screw in a more cephalad direction to achieve adequate purchase, and it may also require the use of a longer screw. It is important to note that when any of these facet injuries involve the C2–3 facet, the upper screw cannot be placed in the lateral mass, as the lateral mass of C2 is not sufficient to achieve screw fixation. Screws in C2 need to be placed down in the pedicle of C2 (see Fig. 22–7), which is described in Chapter 19.

The final type of unilateral facet fracture is a fracture separation of the lateral mass; this is an extension-rotation injury with fractures of the pedicle and lamina on one side, which leaves the entire lateral mass floating freely. It thus involves both inferior and superior facet stability at one level and disrupts two consecutive facet joints, which results in two levels of instability. Although the lower level usually demonstrates the rotational abnormality, stabilization of only the lower level[46] generally results in less than anatomic reduction postoperatively and the presence of a step-off and/or kyphosis at the level above. Because the pedicle and lamina are both fractured and constitute a free fragment, the injury may be difficult to stabilize. Although a technique has been described that uses a transpedicular screw for direct osteosynthesis of the fracture,[42]

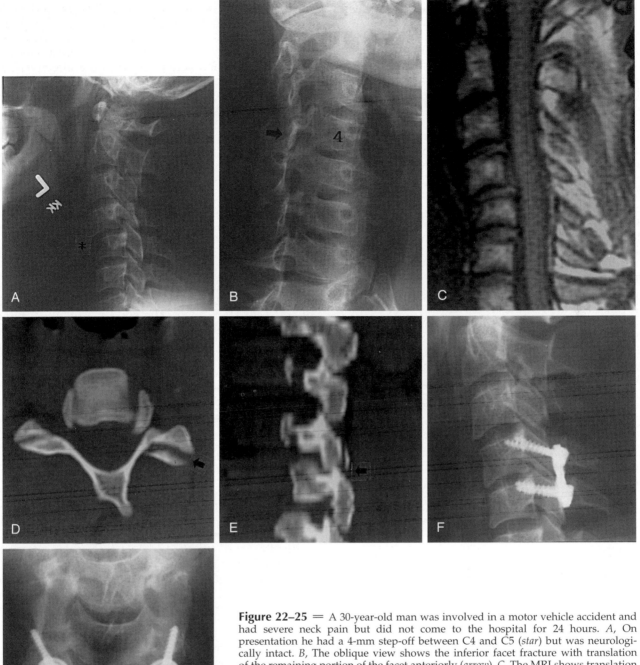

Figure 22–25 = A 30-year-old man was involved in a motor vehicle accident and had severe neck pain but did not come to the hospital for 24 hours. *A,* On presentation he had a 4-mm step-off between C4 and C5 (*star*) but was neurologically intact. *B,* The oblique view shows the inferior facet fracture with translation of the remaining portion of the facet anteriorly (*arrow*). *C,* The MRI shows translation but no significant disc disruption. *D,* The axial CT scan cuts show widening of the C4–5 facet joint (*arrow*) and the rotational abnormality. *E,* The parasagittal reconstruction shows the true nature of the fracture and the displacement (*arrow*). *F* and *G,* The patient underwent one-level plating (C4–5) with the screw placement modified by increasing the angle of insertion to miss the fracture and to increase the purchase in the fractured lateral mass at C4.

it has not been widely used, primarily owing to the extremely small size of the midcervical pedicles. This technique may, however, have applicability for C7. Modifications of lateral mass plating to allow adequate treatment of this particular injury involve three-level plating. Most wiring techniques will not achieve adequate stability, although a Bohlman triple-wire technique can be considered for this injury if the spinous processes of the lamina are intact (except at the injured level). It will not, however, achieve reduction of either of the lateral masses; therefore, patients with radiculopathy may not have full decompression of the injured root. Modifications of facet plating include a three-level stabilization arthrodesis (see Fig. 22–12). Again, the uninjured side should be instrumented first after the patient is placed in traction and the fracture is apparently reduced. However, on surgical exposure of the area, the lateral mass commonly remains rotated out of plane. It can easily be pushed back into the correct orientation using a Penfield elevator, but by plating the contralateral side, reduction and stabilization of the injured side are easier to accomplish. When doing a three-hole plating, it is possible to drill all three holes, making sure that the starting points are in a straight line and directly in the center of the articular mass. The screws are placed in the usual manner, and the plate is tightened down into position on that side. When drilling the holes on the injured side, the superior and inferior facets are easily drilled. They are drilled in a standard fashion, centered over the lateral mass 10 degrees superior and 10 degrees lateral. The lateral mass at the middle level, which is free-floating, must be stabilized using a Penfield level and drilled with a high-speed power drill to keep from damaging the roots. The fragment can be drilled in either of two orientations: (1) 10 degrees superior and 10 degrees lateral, which is the standard fashion, or (2) across the lower facet, with the intention of stabilizing the fragment. In the second case, it is drilled 10 degrees lateral and approximately 15 degrees inferior, so that the screw crosses the inferior facet joint. The plate is placed in the standard fashion: securing the superior and inferior screws first, placing them 50% of the way down; securing the middle screw next, and placing it approximately 50% of the way down; then advancing all three simultaneously, to complete the reduction (Fig. 22–26).

RESULTS

Reduction and Stabilization

There has been a great deal of controversy about the treatment of facet injuries because of the mixed results seen with early reports of treatment. A few more recent long-term series have reported outcomes of patients undergoing operative and nonoperative treatment of facet injuries.[7, 8, 35, 43, 68, 71, 81] Two major questions can be answered by such series: What is the effectiveness of nonoperative reduction and treatment with reference to restoration of alignment and stability? And can operative reduction and stabilization be successful according to the same evaluation parameters? Unfortunately, many of the series have combined all types of facet injuries (i.e., unilateral and bilateral dislocations and fractures), and because these are really quite separate injuries with significantly different instabilities and problems, it is difficult to garner any useful information from the combined series. A number of basic questions have been raised. The first involves the use of closed reductions in treatment of facet injuries. The use of rapid reduction using traction of facet injuries has yielded results that vary widely. Closed reduction has been achieved in anywhere from 40% to 80% of cases, depending on the method and the amount of weight used.[7, 8, 19, 20, 35, 44, 58, 68, 81] The accuracy of assessment of patients who achieve and maintain an anatomic closed reduction is partially dependent on accurate classification of the injury. However, two factors certainly influence the efficacy of the reduction. The first is the location of the dislocation. More proximal dislocations reduce more predictably than do distal dislocations.[44] Second, owing to the significant difference in degree of disruption of the soft tissues, the chance of achieving a closed reduction with a bilateral facet dislocation is at least 80%, whereas the chance of reduction with a unilateral facet dislocation is only 50%. Another feature that can be gleaned from these studies is the rate of spontaneous arthrodesis and of a stable closed result of nonoperative treatment. For many years, placement in a halo vest was considered adequate treatment for reduction and traction of bilateral facet dislocation. This rarely achieves an anatomic result,[18] and what is more important, the morbidity of halo vest use in a simple bilateral facet dislocation is clearly higher than that with a simple interspinous wire or plating fol-

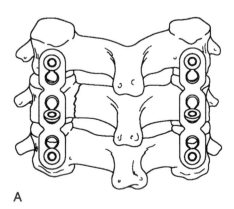
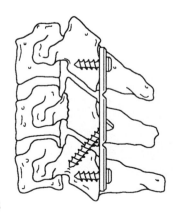

A   B

Figure 22–26 = A and B, An alternative technique for fixation of fracture-separations of the lateral mass is to achieve direct fixation of the free-floating fragment. Plate fixation of the contralateral side is first done using standard screw placement over three levels. On the affected side, the entire lateral mass is free-floating, and thus the central screw is placed obliquely to directly secure it to the matching joint surface below.

lowed by collar immobilization.[21] This is especially true in the patient with neurologic injury. Closed reduction of unilateral facet dislocations have been effective in 40% to 70% of patients with this particular injury, because of the relative lack of ligamentous disruption. For unilateral facet fractures, however, Rorabeck and co-workers,[64] Beyer and Cabanela and others[7, 8] and Shapiro[68] showed that the patients who were treated nonoperatively had a higher incidence of pain and deformity than did those treated operatively; many required secondary operative procedures. The results of operative stabilization, irrespective of the type of surgery, demonstrate a very high union rate and excellent restoration of anatomic alignment if the proper type of construct is used to counteract the deforming forces. Clearly, Levine and associates[46] have shown that for very difficult, unstable injuries, such as fracture separations of the articular mass, cervical plating offers a very effective modality with a relatively low complication rate, assuming that the principles of adequate stabilization are heeded.

Neurologic Injury

Recovery from neurologic injury can be separated into two categories: cord and root injuries. Patients with only radicular signs and symptoms from unilateral facet fractures generally show an extremely high rate of recovery, as these injuries often result from compression of the root at the time of injury, and adequate decompression can be achieved in almost all cases. Patients with bilateral facet dislocations and complete injuries, essentially show no recovery because of the high-energy nature of the injury. Those with complete neurologic injury show excellent recovery. It is important to realize that patients with bilateral facet injuries should achieve a nerve root recovery one level distal to the level of the injury. Thus in a C5–6 facet dislocation, at least the C6 root, and sometimes the C7 root, should demonstrate recovery. Lack of recovery in this case may be related to severe discal injury, and decompression of the disc may yield recovery at the adjacent roots rather than at the cord level, which may have a significant effect on the patient's overall functional status.

COMPLICATIONS

Complications related to the treatment of facet injuries fall into several categories. The first and probably the most problematic is the failure to diagnose injuries; this is common in unilateral facet injuries. Frequently, the patient who sustains an injury in a motor vehicle accident has contusions, lacerations, and multiple neck complaints. Because the initial screening radiographs are often taken in a supine position, as the patient is brought in on a spine board, the injury may indeed be in a reduced position and therefore be missed. In addition, the step-offs are usually not dramatic; they are often less than 4 mm but are frequently as little as 1 to 2 mm. Thus, the rotational abnormality

is not seen by the examining physician. After an initial reading of a negative x-ray and a diagnosis of simple neck strain, the patient is subsequently immobilized in a cervical collar and sent home, after which he or she experiences increased instability and, frequently, onset of radicular pain. The initial radiographs, both AP and lateral, should be checked carefully for any rotational abnormalities, and although no step-off is visible, the patient should have a CT scan on the basis of any rotational abnormality that is noted. In addition, any patient with radicular signs and symptoms should be assumed to have a unilateral facet fracture until proven otherwise.

A second type of complication is related to the use of excessive weight (>70 lb) in attempting to reduce the fracture. Care should be taken, especially initially, to verify that the injury is not a circumferential disruption, which could cause unnecessary stretching of the cord and additional neurologic deficit. Although it has been shown by Cotler and co-workers[20] that weights up to 140 lb can be used safely in the hands of experienced surgeons treating spinal injury, this is not the norm. Care should be taken to apply weight appropriately and to use appropriate maneuvers to reduce the injury; the physician should not rely solely on stretching to achieve reduction.

The next type of complication is loss of reduction, which is a frequently encountered phenomenon in both unilateral and bilateral facet dislocations in the cervical spine. It has been shown that the application of a halo vest will not control rotation well in the midcervical spine, nor will it prevent "snaking" of the cervical spine as the patient applies axial loading forces to the spine.[56] Control of the cervical spine is fixed only at the skull, with very loose control of the thoracic spine; thus, toggling occurs in rotational deformities when the patient sits up and lies down or walks up and down stairs. It has been reported by Whitehill and others[79] that unilateral facet injuries often lose reduction in a halo vest; therefore, these injuries should not be treated nonoperatively in a halo vest. Bucholz and Cheung[15] reported 125 cases of cervical trauma treated in a halo vest, including 9 of 20 patients with facet injuries who lost reduction in the halo vest. Sears and Fazl[71] reported a series of 70 patients with facet injuries treated in a halo vest. Only 44% achieved stability with that method of treatment, and half of those had a poor anatomic result. Of injuries without facet involvement, 70% treated in a halo vest had a satisfactory result. Anderson and co-workers[2] showed that the halo vest does not prevent motion at the fracture site when patients are moved from a supine to an erect position. The halo vest has no additional holding power over a semirigid collar in a nondisplaced fracture. Bilateral facet dislocations should not be treated with a halo vest. The reported incidence of redislocation, nonanatomic alignment, and the morbidity probably exceeds that of a one-level arthrodesis. Operative stabilization after either reduction in traction or operative reduction of bilateral facet dislocations has been shown to be a highly effective and predictable means of treatment.[81]

The next type of complication involves increasing

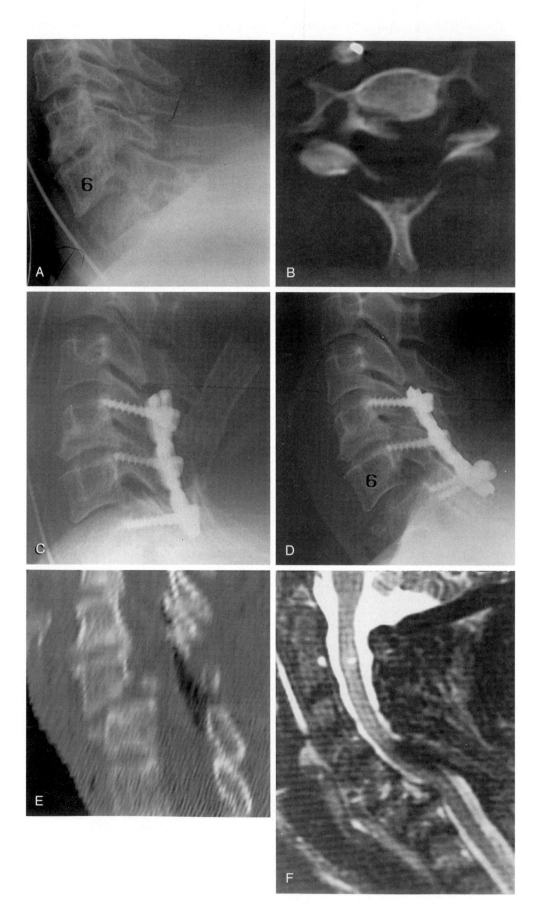

Figure 22–27 = This patient was involved in a motor vehicle accident and sustained multiple injuries, including a severe closed-head injury, a left C6–7 facet fracture, and a right-sided dislocation at the same level. As the patient awoke from the head injury it was apparent that she had severe radicular involvement, which was worse on the left than the right. *A,* The fractures reduced partially in traction, but the severe nature of the injury is best appreciated on the axial views of the CT scan *(B).* *C,* A portion of the fractured left lamina and facet were removed and a plate was placed from C5 to C7. *D,* Within 8 weeks it was evident that the fixation at C7 was inadequate, as shown by screw pullout and loss of fixation. In addition, the patient continued to have significant numbness and weakness in both arms and hands. Repeat CT scan *(E)* and MRI *(F)* revealed an angular deformity with compression of the dural sac. After removal of the hardware, reduction was accomplished and the patient underwent plating from C5–T1, with maintenance of reduction and recovery of neural function by 1 year.

neurologic deficit in the course of reduction and treatment. Marshall and colleagues[53a] have reported a 4% increase in neurologic deficit during the course of treatment of spinal injuries at spinal injury centers. This has also been confirmed by Arena and others[3] initially and by other authors subsequently[49, 50, 61] with specific reference to facet injuries. All cases of neural deficit occurred after reduction of severely displaced unilateral and bilateral facet injuries, with the increasing deficit as a result of disc extrusion. This results in part from a lack of understanding of the pathologic characteristics of the injury. None of these are pure bony injuries, and all involve some degree of disruption of the disc. However, disc extrusion is a relatively rare phenomenon. All closed reduction should be done with the patient awake and only slightly sedated, so that the neurologic function can be monitored at all times. Any patient who exhibits change in function or paresthesias, or in whom reduction is difficult, should have an MRI before treatment proceeds, to verify that this is not one of the rare patients with significant disc extrusion. Second, fixation of the injuries should minimize compression of the interspace, which can occur with wire fixation. Despite the nature of the discal injury, if reduction is achievable with the patient awake in traction or with manipulation; if the interspace can be held at height, especially with techniques such as cervical plating (without the significant compression of the interspaces that sometimes occurs with overtightening of tension-band wiring); then neurologic status should be maintained.

The final group of complications is related to the surgical treatment of these injuries. With the use of lateral mass plates, new and different complications have begun to appear. Heller and co-workers[39] reported a 6% incidence of root injury and a 0.2% incidence of facet violation in 654 screw placements. Screw loosening occurs in approximately 1% of cases, and hardware failure in a similar number. Because the C7 lateral mass is anatomically less substantial than the other cervical levels, purchase is more tenuous, and failure may result more frequently at that level (Fig. 22–27). Removing portions of the lateral mass to achieve reduction may in fact destabilize the injury more, and cause hardware failure. If the screw purchase is suboptimal at the C7 level, extension to T1 will increase the stability of fixation.

Injuries to the facets in the cervical spine encompass a very broad spectrum of injuries: bilateral and unilateral fractures and dislocations in various patterns. These represent less of a spectrum of injury than a group of injuries to a specific anatomic structure. The effective treatment really requires a precise understanding of the pathologic characteristics, the mechanism of injury, and the resultant instabilities. The final result depends on having a critical appreciation of which treatment modalities can effectively control the resultant instability in each particular injury pattern.

REFERENCES

1. Allen BL, Ferguson RL, Lehmann TR, et al: A mechanistic classification of closed, indirect fractures and dislocations of the lower cervical spine. Spine 7:1–27, 1982.
2. Anderson PA, Budorick TE, Easton KB, et al: Failure of the halo-vest to prevent in-vivo motion in patients with injured cervical spines. Spine 16(suppl):501–505, 1991.
3. Arena MJ, Eismont FJ, Green BA: Intravertebral disc extrusion associated with cervical facet subluxation and dislocation. J Bone Joint Surg Am 72:43, 1988.
4. Babcock JL: Cervical spine injuries. Arch Surg 111:646–651, 1976.
5. Beatson TR: Fractures and dislocations of the cervical spine. J Bone Joint Surg Br 45:21, 1963.
6. Berrington NR, vanStaden JF, Willers JG, et al: Cervical intervertebral disc prolapse associated with traumatic facet dislocations. Surg Neurol 40:395–399, 1993.
7. Beyer CA, Cabanela ME, Berquist TH: Unilateral facet dislocations and fracture-dislocations of the cervical spine. J Bone Joint Surg Br 73:977–981, 1991.
8. Beyer CA, Cabanela ME: Unilateral facet dislocations and fracture-dislocations of the cervical spine: A review. Orthopedics 15:311–315, 1992.
9. Bohler L: Die Technick der Knachenbruchbehandung, eds 12 and 13. Vierk Auflage Wein, Wilhem Maudrich, 1933.
10. Bohlman HH: Acute Fractures and dislocations of the cervical spine: An analysis of 300 hospitalized patients and review of the literature. J Bone Joint Surg Am 61:1119–1142, 1979.
11. Braakman R, Penning L: The hyperflexion sprain of the cervical spine. Radiol Clin Biol 37:309–320, 1968.
12. Braakman R, Vinken PJ: Old luxations of the lower cervical spine. J Bone Joint Surg Br 50:52–60, 1968.
13. Braakman R, Vinken, PJ: Unilateral facet interlocking in the lower cervical spine. J Bone Joint Surg Br 49:249–257, 1967.
14. Brav EA Miller JA, Bouzard WC: Traumatic dislocation of the cervical spine: Army experience and results. J Trauma 3:569–582, 1963.
15. Bucholz RD, Cheung KC: Halo vest versus spinal fusion for cervical injury: Evidence from an outcome study. J Neurosurg 70:884–892, 1989.
16. Burke DC, Berryman D: The place of closed manipulation in the management of flexion-rotation dislocations of the cervical spine. J Bone Joint Surg Br 53:165–182, 1971.
17. Chang DG, Tencer AF, Ching RP, et al: Geometric changes in the cervical spinal canal during impact. Spine 18:973–980, 1994.
18. Clark CR, Wessels, WE Jr: Unilateral cervical facet fracture-dislocation. Surg Rounds Orthop, Aug 1987, pp 15–19.
19. Cotler HB, Miller LS, DeLucia FA, et al: Closed reduction of cervical spine dislocations. Clin Orthop 214:185–199, 1987.
20. Cotler JM, Herbison GJ, Nasuti JF, et al: Closed reduction of traumatic cervical spine dislocations using traction weights up to 140 pounds. Spine 18:386–390, 1993.
21. Crooks F, Birkett AN: Fractures and dislocations of the cervical spine. Br J Surg 31:252, 1944.
22. Crutchfield WG: Treatment of injuries of the cervical spine. J Bone Joint Surg 20:696, 1935.
23. Crutchfield WG: Fracture dislocations of cervical spine: Further observations on the treatment of fracture dislocations of the cervical spine with skeletal traction. Surg Gynecol Obstet 63:513–517, 1936.
24. Crutchfield WG: Skeletal traction in treatment of injuries to the cervical spine. JAMA 155:29–32, 1954.
25. De Oliveira JC: Anterior reduction of interlocking facets in the lower cervical spine. Spine 4:195–202, 1979.
26. Doran SE, Papadopoulos SM, Ducker TB, et al: Magnetic resonance imaging documentation of coexistent traumatic locked facets of the cervical spine and disk herniation. J Neurosurg 79:341–345, 1993.
27. Durbin FC: Fracture-dislocations of the cervical spine. J Bone Joint Surg Br 39:23–38, 1957.
28. Edwards CC, Matz SO, Levine AM: The oblique wiring technique for rotational injuries of the cervical spine. Orthop Trans 9:142, 1985.
29. Edwards CC, Matz SO, Levine AM: The oblique wiring technique for rotational injuries of the cervical spine. Orthop Trans 10:455, 1986.
30. Ellis VH: Injuries of the cervical vertebrae. Proc R Soc Med 54:367, 1946.
31. Evans DK: Reduction of cervical dislocations. J Bone Joint Surg Br 43:552–555, 1961.

32. Forsyth HF, Alexander E, Davis C Jr, et al: The advantages of early spine fusion in the treatment of fracture-dislocation of the cervical spine J Bone Joint Surg Am 41:17–36, 1959.

33. Fried LC: Cervical spinal cord injury during skeletal traction. JAMA 229:181–183, 1974.

34. Gillick A, Levine AM: Posterior cervical stabilization techniques in facet and oblique wiring. In Garfin SR, Northrup B (eds): Surgery for Spinal Cord Injuries. New York, Raven, 1993, pp 105–112.

35. Hadley MN, Fitzpatrick BC, Sonntag VKH, et al: Facet Fracture-Dislocation Injuries of the Cervical Spine. Neurosurgery 30:661–666, 1992.

36. Harris JH, Edeiken-Monroe B: The Radiology of Acute Cervical Spine Trauma. Baltimore, Williams & Wilkins, 1987.

37. Harris JH Jr, Edeiken-Monroe B, Kopaniky DR: A practical classification of acute cervical spine injuries. Orthop Clin North Am 17:15–30, 1986.

38. Heller JG, Carlson GD, Abitbol J-J, et al: Anatomic comparison of the Roy-Camille and Magerl techniques for screw placement in the lower cervical spine. Spine 16:S552–S557, 1991.

39. Heller JG, Silcox DH, Sutterlin CE: Complications of posterior cervical plating. Spine 20:2442–2448, 1995.

40. Horlyck E, Rahbek M: Cervical spine injuries. Acta Orthop Scand 45:845–853, 1974.

41. Jacobs B: Cervical fractures and dislocations (C3-7). Clin Orthop 109:20–32, 1975.

42. Jeanneret B, Gebhard JS, Magerl F: Transpedicular screw fixation of articular mass fracture-separation: Results of an anatomical study and operative technique. J Spinal Disord 7:222–229, 1994.

43. Jonsson HC, Cesarini K, Petren-Mallmin M, et al: Locking screw-plate fixation of cervical spine fractures with and without ancillary posterior plating. Arch Orthop Trauma Surg 111:1–12, 1991.

44. Lee AS, MacLean JCB, Newton DA: Rapid traction for reduction of cervical spine dislocations. J Bone Joint Surg Br 76:352–356, 1994.

45. Levine AM, White JB, Edwards CC: Facet injuries in the cervical spine. Orthop Trans 11:1, 1987.

46. Levine AM, Mazel C, Roy-Camille R: Management of fracture separations of the articular mass using posterior cervical plating. Spine 17:447–454, 1992.

47. Levine AM: Facet injuries in the cervical spine, In Camins MB, O'Leary PF (eds): Disorders of the Cervical Spine. Baltimore, Williams & Wilkins, 1992, pp 293–302.

48. Lysell E: Motion in the cervical spine: An experimental study on autopsy specimens. Orthop Scand Suppl, vol 123, 1969.

49. Mahale YJ, Silver JR: Progressive paralysis after bilateral facet dislocation of the cervical spine. J Bone Joint Surg Br 74:219–223, 1992.

50. Mahale YJ, Silver JR, Henderson NJ: Neurological complications of the reduction of cervical spine dislocations. J Bone Joint Surg Br 75:403–409, 1993.

51. Magerl F, Grob D, Seemann P: Stable dorsal fusion of the cervical spine C2-T1 using hook plates. In Kehr P, Weidner A (eds): Cervical Spine. New York, Springer-Verlag, 1987, p 217.

52. Malgaigne JF: Traite des Fractures et des Luxations: Tome 2. Des Luxations. Paris, JB Bailliere, 1855.

53. Marie-Anne S: Les fractures separation des massifs articulaires du rachis cervical inferieur. In Roy-Camille R (ed): Leres Journees d'Orthopedie de la Pitie. Paris, Masson, 1979.

53a. Marshall LF, Knowlton S, Garfin SR, et al: Deterioration following spinal cord injury. J Neurosurg 66:400–404, 1987.

54. Miller LS, Cotler HB, DeLucia FA, et al: Biomechanical analysis of cervical distraction. Spine 12:831–837, 1987.

55. Pait TG, McAllister PV, Kaufman HH: Quadrant anatomy of the articular pillars (lateral cervical mass) of the cervical spine. J Neurosurg 82:1011–1014, 1995.

56. Perry J: The halo in spinal abnormalities: Practical factors and avoidance of complications. Orthop Clin North Am 3:69–80, 1972.

57. Rizzolo SJ, Piazza MR, Cotler JM, et al: Intervertbral disc injury complicating cervical spine trauma. Spine 16:187–189, 1991.

58. Rizzolo SJ, Vaccaro AR, Cotler JM: Cervical spine trauma. Spine 19:2288–2298, 1994.

59. Roaf R: A study of the mechanics of spinal injury. J Bone Joint Surg Br 42:810, 1960.

60. Roaf R: Lateral flexion injuries of the cervical spine. J Bone Joint Surg Br 45:36–38, 1963.

61. Robertson PA, Ryan MD: Neurologic deterioration after reduction of cervical subluxation: Mechanical compression by disc tissue. J Bone Joint Surg Br 74:224–227, 1992.

62. Rogers WA: Treatment of fracture-dislocation of the cervical spine. J Bone Joint Surg 24:245–258, 1942.

63. Rogers WA: Fractures and dislocations of the cervical spine: An end result study. J Bone Joint Surg 39:341–376, 1957.

64. Rorabeck CH, Rock MG, Hawkins RJ, et al: Unilateral facet dislocation of the cervical spine: An analysis of the results of treatment in 26 patients. Spine 12:23–27, 1987.

65. Roy-Camille R, Mazel G, Saillant G: Les fractures-separation du massif articulaire. In Roy-Camille R (ed): Rachis Cervical Inferieur: Sixiemes Journees D'Orthopedie de la Pitie. Paris, Masson, 1988, pp 104–107.

66. Roy-Camille R, Mazel G, Edourard B: Luxations et luxations-fractures. In Roy-Camille R (ed): Rachis Cervical Inferieur: Sixiemes Journees D'Orthopedie de la Pitie. Paris, Masson, 1988, pp 94–103.

67. Shanmuganathan, K, Mirvis SE, Levine AM: Rotational injury of cervical facets: CT analysis of fracture patterns with implications for management and neurologic outcome. AJR 163:1165–1169, 1994.

68. Shapiro SA: Management of unilateral locked facet of the cervical spine. Neurosurgery 33:832–837, 1993.

69. Scher AT: The value of the anteroposterior radiograph in hidden fractures and dislocations of the lower cervical spine: A case report. S Afr Med J 55:221–224, 1979.

70. Scher AT: Articular pillar fractures of the cervical spine. S Afr Med J 19:968–969, 1981.

71. Sears W, Fazl M: Prediction of stability of cervical spine fracture managed in the halo vest and indications for surgical intervention. J Neurosurg 72:426–432, 1990.

72. Sim E: Vertical facet splitting: A special variant of rotary dislocations of the cervical spine. J Neurosurg 82:239–243, 1995.

73. Star AM, Jones AA, Cotler JM, et al: Immediate closed reduction of cervical spine dislocations using traction. Spine 15:1068–1072, 1990.

74. Stauffer S: Management of spine fractures C3-C7. Orthop Clin North Am 17:45, 1986.

75. Taitesman JP, Sohn S: Tensile strength of wire reinforced bone cervical and treated stainless steel wire. J Bone Joint Surg Am 59:419–424, 1977.

76. Tribus CB: Cervical disk herniation in association with traumatic facet dislocation. Tech Orthop 9:5–7, 1994.

77. Webb JK, Broughton RBK, McSweeney T, et al: Hidden flexion injury of the cervical spine. J Bone Joint Surg Br 58:322–327, 1976.

78. White AA, Johnson RM, Panjabi MM, et al: Biomechanical analysis of clinical stability in the cervical spine. Clin Orthop 109:85–96, 1975.

79. Whitehill R, Richmann JA, Glaser JA: Failure of immobilization of the cervical spine by halo vest. J Bone Joint Surg Am 68:326, 1986.

80. Whitley JE, Forsyth HF: The classification of cervical spine injuries. AJR 83:633–644, 1960.

81. Wolf A, Levi L, Mirvis S, et al: Operative management of bilateral facet dislocation. J Neurosurg 75:883–890, 1991.

82. Woodring JH, Goldstein SJ: Fractures of the articular processes of the cervical spine. AJR 139:341–344, 1982.

Hyperextension Injuries of the Cervical Spine

Gregory S. McDowell || *Frank P. Cammisa, Jr.* || *Frank J. Eismont*

Hyperextension injuries of the cervical spine have long been regarded as less significant contributors to the overall incidence of spine lesions acquired traumatically, and yet this mechanism clearly has been demonstrated to play a role in a variety of pathologic entities. These include:

1. Atlanto-occipital dislocations
2. Fractures of the posterior arch of C1
3. Dens fractures
4. Hangman's fractures
5. Extension teardrop injuries
6. Anterior longitudinal ligament or disc disruptions
7. Central cord syndromes in spondylotic, stenotic, or ankylosed spines
8. Spinal cord injury without radiographic abnormality (SCIWORA)
9. Whiplash
10. Complex high-velocity fracture-dislocations

For the purpose of this chapter we address only the lesions of the subaxial spine[5-10] as the others have been discussed elsewhere in this book. We attempt to better clarify the common biomechanics, while emphasizing the varied etiology, presentation, evaluation, and treatment of these interesting injuries.

ETIOLOGY, EPIDEMIOLOGY, AND PATHOMECHANICS OF HYPEREXTENSION INJURIES

When the cervical spine is subjected to supraphysiologic hyperextension moments, either secondary to a direct blow to the forehead or through acceleration mechanisms such as seen in whiplash, it may fail subtly or quite dramatically. In part, the mode of failure can be attributed to variations in head position and the forces applied. The mode of failure will also be affected to a great extent by the age-dependent anatomic characteristics of the individual. The pediatric spine will fail differently from the middle-aged or elderly spine, or the spine affected by advanced spondylosis, stenosis, or ankylosing conditions. No single classification scheme for cervical injury explains the diversity seen in radiographic and clinical findings. Whitehill's review[108] of classification schemes relating to subaxial

fractures in the adult discusses taking each individual case through a so-called injury analysis which combines the mechanistic elements of six injury categories affecting Holdsworth's two-column spine and the biomechanical force vectors involved. For the purposes of this chapter, we have adopted a scheme which relies on commonly used descriptive terms for hyperextension injuries.

The function of the spine is to transmit physiologic loads, to allow for controlled active and constrained passive motion, and to protect the neural elements. The lordotic subaxial spine allows for flexibility, postural balance, and shock absorption with both disc and facet joints sharing in carrying compressive load.[74] This anatomy, however, can be the site of stress concentration in traumatic hyperextension given the high stiffness and large moment of inertia attributed to the thoracic spine below and the head above.

Which loads and patterns of loading in hyperextension are excessive and when is motion abnormally large either in translation or angulation such that it might permit injury to the cord or cervical nerve roots? White and Panjabi and their co-workers[107] were the first to look at this from a sound biomechanical perspective. They subscribed to a practical definition of stability. *Instability* is defined as the loss of the spine's ability under physiologic loads to maintain normal relationships to avoid neural injury. This can be expanded to include avoidance of deficit progression, incapacitating deformity, or intractable pain. Ultimately, their cadaveric testing model in which they sectioned constraining soft tissues from anterior to posterior and subjected spines to hyperextension loads allowed for the definition of more objective radiographic criteria for impending instability. Their results demonstrated remarkably small increments of change in angular and translational displacement until the posterior longitudinal ligament was sectioned, at which time catastrophic failure ensued without warning. No motion segments were observed to fail that exhibited less than 2.7 mm of linear translation or 10.7 degrees of angular displacement. These values subsequently served as guidelines for the development of White's instability diagnostic checklist[107] (Table 23–1). The checklist should serve as a guide for the experienced interpreter. However, problems can arise in its use, as noted by Whitehill.[108] Recently more detailed anatomic scoring

Table 23–1 = **GUIDELINES FOR THE EVALUATION OF CLINICAL STABILITY OF THE ADULT CERVICAL SPINE**

Any one of the following three are indicative of instability or potential instability:
1. All the anterior or all the posterior elements are destroyed
2. There is >3.5 mm of anterolisthesis and retrolisthesis on resting lateral or flexion-extension films
3. There is >11 degrees of angular deformity as compared to either adjacent motion segment on resting lateral or flexion-extension films

Adapted from White AA III, Johnson RM, Panjabi MM, et al: Biomechanical analysis of clinical stability in the cervical spine. Clin Orthop 109:85–96, 1975.

methods have been proposed based on modern three-dimensional imaging modalities.[64]

Shono and others[92] were able to demonstrate that with hyperextension in immature calf spines, predictable anterior avulsion fractures, and anterior longitudinal ligament and disc disruptions, as well as posterior element fractures in compression, are seen. This conclusion was supported by the work of White and co-workers in elderly cadaveric spines.[107] These investigators' experimental findings corroborate several good postmortem pathologic studies which elucidate the variety of typical hyperextension injuries seen.[27, 57, 46]

These injuries are not uncommon. Kiwerski[48] described a series of 1687 patients with cervical spine injury treated in Poland over 23 years. Twenty-six percent of these patients had a hyperextension mechanism. The average age of the patients with an extension injury was 53 years. Twenty-five percent had complete spinal cord lesions, 61% had incomplete lesions, and 13% were without neurologic deficit. Lesions were more commonly seen from C5 to T1 (n = 177), but the 120 hyperextension lesions from C1–3 represented 68% of all injuries at these levels. Interestingly, other authors have noted that C5–6 is a common site for hyperextension injury, a fact attributed to its high underlying mobility.[19] The outcome with extension injuries as a whole was better than that with flexion or axial load injuries, with 61% demonstrating improvement neurologically. Mortality, however, was high (21%), a fact that may be attributed to the advanced age of the patients as a whole.

Meyer wrote of the experience at Northwestern University's Spine Injury Center over 27 years with 1626 patients sustaining cervical spine fractures.[62] Of these, 532 (33%) were due to hyperextension, second only to the frequency of flexion injuries. Twenty-six percent of the patients had complete spinal cord lesions, 35% had incomplete lesions, and 39% had neurologic deficit. Bohlman's series of 300 hospitalized patients over 22 years included a number with presumed hyperextension injury, though a complete definition of mechanism is limited by the author's description of the lesions.[9] Similarly, Holdsworth's series includes descriptions of classic hyperextension injuries.[39] Burke[13] and Forsythe,[27] among others, have published specifically on hyperextension injuries, further elaborating their diverse characteristics and unique subtypes. We will discuss each subtype in more detail, but first it will be useful to elaborate on the clinical and radiographic evaluation of these patients.

CLINICAL AND RADIOGRAPHIC ASSESSMENT

The clinical and radiographic assessment of persons presenting with neck pain or neurologic symptoms following hyperextension injury should be thorough. It begins with a careful history. A review of the patient's past medical history, including any history of previous trauma, is important. Should the patient be presenting acutely, it may be appropriate for a full trauma evaluation to be performed with careful attention being paid to cervical immobilization throughout. The physical examination must include a detailed neurologic and skeletal examination. It is imperative that the clinician search for occult signs of closed head injury, orbital or facial fractures, cranial nerve injuries, and injury to soft tissue structures of the neck, including the musculature, larynx, esophagus, and great vessels, all of which have been noted to be injured with hyperextension.

The radiographic evaluation must include a full trauma series including anteroposterior (AP), lateral, oblique, and lateral swimmer's views (when needed), as well as an open-mouth odontoid view. The plain film criteria for instability were described by White[107] and included in his criteria for clinical instability. The finding of a prevertebral hematoma is highly suggestive of a cervical spine injury and this can certainly include those with a hyperextension injury. A retropharyngeal space measuring greater than 5.0 mm as measured in front of C3 or a retrotracheal distance greater than 15 to 18 mm as measured in front of C6 is abnormal. Penning[76] described large increases (up to 12.3 mm) above the upper limit of normal in prevertebral soft tissue measurements following hyperextension injury. Changes were most readily seen from C1–4 in the retropharyngeal space, regardless of injury location. Furthermore, he defined the upper limits of normal for prevertebral space measurement in 50 noninjury patients. Longitudinal follow-up of these hematomas revealed rapid decreases in size over 1 week and near normalcy typically within 2 to 3 weeks. Thus, the prevertebral hematoma should be considered a significant red flag for acute or subacute hyperextension injuries. Scher[86] has described additional plain film radiographic findings which are highly suggestive of hyperextension injury. These include small triangular avulsion fractures from the anteroinferior edge of a vertebral body (Fig. 23–1), disc space widening, fractures of the posterior elements without obvious anterior column bony abnormalities (Fig. 23–2), and retrolisthesis of a cranial-on-caudal vertebral body.[86]

If the radiographs of patients with neck pain are cleared of obvious fracture, subluxation, and angulation (i.e., gross instability) by a qualified radiologist or knowledgeable physician, lateral flexion-extension radiographs should routinely be obtained. Commonly, the dynamic films are also normal. Recently Wang and associates[104] reported finding only one positive study

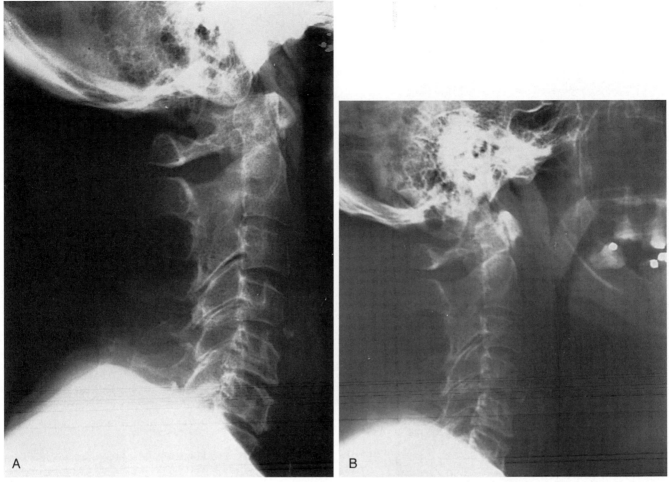

Figure 23–1 = This patient presented to the emergency room following a motor vehicle accident. She had significant facial lacerations and ecchymosis and she complained of some mild neck pain. No tenderness to palpation was noted posteriorly. *A,* The lateral cervical spine radiograph shows diffuse spondylosis consistent with her age, and the anterior aspect of the C4 vertebral body gives an excellent demonstration of a "teardrop fracture" of the anteroinferior portion of the vertebral body. This is consistent with a significant hyperextension injury. There is some slight rotation of the anterior fragment and we can also see that there is no sclerosis at the site of fracture indicating that this is a new injury. The soft tissue swelling measures 8 mm in front of C3. Anything more than 5 mm is abnormal and consistent with a new injury. *B,* This radiograph taken 1 day later shows an increase in the soft tissue swelling to 16 mm. The patient was neurologically normal and flexion-extension views did not show evidence of instability so she was immobilized for 6 weeks in a rigid collar.

in 290 patients in an emergency room setting. If these tests are normal but a high index of suspicion remains, the dynamic radiographs should be repeated within the first week, and if necessary at 2 weeks when muscular splinting may have resolved, allowing for recognition of occult instabilities. In the interim, the patient should be maintained in a rigid collar.

Linear tomography, computed tomography (CT), myelography, and magnetic resonance imaging (MRI) all have roles as imaging modalities to assist the clinician in recognizing occult injury to soft tissue or bony elements of the cervical spine. More than any other single modality except conventional radiography, MRI has emerged as a tool invaluable in diagnosing hyperextension injuries of the cervical spine. Recent data reported by Benzel and others[8] as well as by Davis and co-workers[21] suggests that MRI may be able to detect an alarmingly high percentage of trauma patients with significant occult disc, ligament, or soft tissue abnormalities. In their report of 130 patients with MRIs fol-

lowing trauma and having had normal radiographs, 50 of 130 patients had recognizable injuries of soft tissue or both, or disc. Goldberg and colleagues[29] have also stated that MRI is particularly helpful in recognizing and aiding in treatment decisions for patients with hyperextension injury. They noted that MRI allowed the clinician to correctly recognize occult injuries of the longitudinal ligaments, discs, and posterior elements (whether bony, capsular, or ligamentous), as well as contusion injuries of the cord, stenosis of the spinal canal, and associated soft tissue injuries of the anterior neck. The study by Schaefer and others[81] of 57 patients with cervical spine injuries revealed that MRI may not always detect cord injury, but when it does it is often able to distinguish between intramedullary hematoma (group I), edema involving more than one motion segment (group II), and edema involving one motion segment (group III). These diagnoses will often aid the clinician in prognosticating final motor outcome. The median percentage motor recovery for the three groups

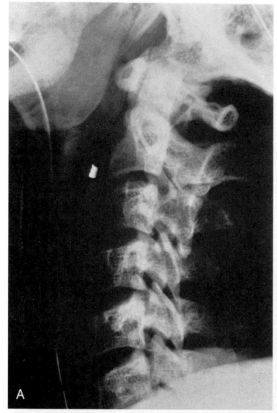

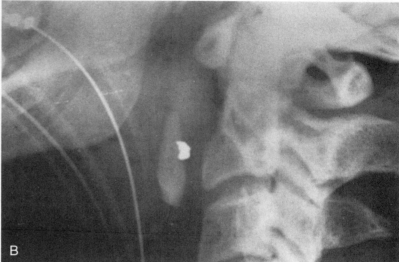

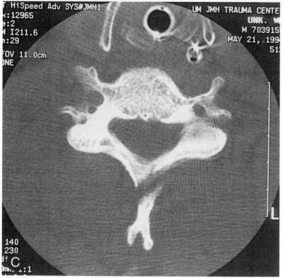

Figure 23–2 = This patient was brought to the emergency room following a motor vehicle accident in which he sustained significant trauma to his face. He had multiple comminuted fractures of the mandible and had significant respiratory distress which required intubation. He was neurologically normal but he did have neck pain with palpation in the lower cervical spine. *A*, This lateral cervical spine radiograph shows normal alignment of the spine but there is inadequate visualization of the lower cervical spine. The patient was immobilized awaiting further evaluation. What appears to be a foreign body is seen in the retropharyngeal area anterior to the C2–3 disc. *B*, A cone-down radiograph reveals that this foreign body was actually a tooth that had broken loose at the time of the mandibular fractures. Care was taken to remove this prior to extubation. *C*, This CT scan clearly shows a fracture of the spinous process of C6. This is consistent with the facial injuries and a cervical spine hyperextension injury. Once extubated, flexion-extension films revealed no significant instability and the patient was immobilized in a rigid collar for 6 weeks.

was, respectively, 9%, 41%, and 72% at a mean follow-up of 8 months. Ultimately, the MRI should be an invaluable tool in assisting the clinician in decisions regarding surgical management.

Interventional techniques such as diagnostic and therapeutic facet and nerve root blocks as well as cervical discography may help to better evaluate patients with subtle clinical presentations or ongoing pain in the face of a "normal workup." The risks of cervical discography and studies describing its lower predictive value make its widespread usefulness controversial.[20] As discussed by McLain,[60] however, the zygapophyseal joint is a structure noted to be innervated with mecha-

noreceptors and, as Barnsley and colleagues[6] have pointed out, zygapophyseal joint pain may well be the most common basis for chronic pain following injuries such as whiplash (54% prevalence). They described its diagnosis with double-blind controlled diagnostic blocks of medial branches of the cervical dorsal rami that supply the target joint. The patients' response to some of these interventional techniques, coupled with sound clinical judgment, may help aid the clinician in predicting their potential response to cervical arthrodesis. More recently, the use of a diagnostic external fixator was described for the same purpose.[72]

Prompt recognition and the maintenance of a high

index of suspicion for occult lesions will aid in the appropriate diagnosis and treatment of acute cervical hyperextension injuries. The patient who presents with subacute or chronic symptoms that persist in the face of an initially negative screening examination should be fully evaluated to ensure that a treatable lesion does not exist. We now discuss specific hyperextension injuries.

HYPEREXTENSION TEARDROP FRACTURES

Reports of *hyperextension* teardrop fractures of the cervical spine are few in the literature,[27, 28, 52, 53, 65] whereas there are several series reporting larger numbers of patients with *flexion* teardrop fractures.[45, 87, 103] The differences between these two entities in regard to mechanism, and radiographic and clinical findings, as well as treatment and outcome, differ substantially. Failure to recognize one in relation to the other could result in inappropriate treatment.

In distinction, the flexion teardrop fracture was first described by Schneider and Kahn in 1956.[87] Later series of larger numbers of patients described their occurrence in football players sustaining axial loads on their helmets with their necks slightly flexed (n = 45), and in patients involved in diving and vehicular accidents or falls (n = 55).[45, 103] The characteristic radiographic features of the flexion-axial load injury are an antero-inferior avulsion fracture and a sagittal midbody fracture occurring at the C4–6 level in association with posterior laminar fractures[45, 103] (Fig. 23–3). The triangular fragment remains aligned with the anterior margin of the spine.[53] Significant neurologic injury and quadriplegia are common, with 45 of 55 patients in the series of Torg and others[103] and 39 of 45 patients in the series of Kim and colleagues[45] presenting as such. Prognosis for neurologic recovery is grim. Definitive management of these injuries has been poorly addressed in the literature, but may require anterior decompression with circumferential fusion in order to attain decompression and stability. In contradistinction to this, the extension teardrop fracture constituted a larger percentage, 65%, (13 of 20 patients), with hyperextension injury reported in 1986[65] and has only recently been more adequately evaluated by Levine and Lutz.[53] The characteristic radiographic feature is a small teardrop fragment, thought to be avulsed via its attachments to Sharpey's fibers of the anulus (see Fig. 23–1), which may be malrotated 35 degrees from its resting position.[53] Commonly occurring at C2, and sometimes associated with a vacuum disc or disc space widening,[65] the soft tissue component of the injury can be defined on MRI.[32] Posterior element fractures may occur, but the midsagittal body fracture is absent. Neurologic injury was reported as rare by Levine and Lutz,[53] though central cord syndromes were not uncommonly noted by Monroe and associates.[65] Dynamic radiographic evidence of instability was rare, with only 4 of 24 patients demonstrating it in Levine and Lutz's series.[53] The majority of these patients are best managed conservatively in an external cervical orthosis, and most go on to stability uneventfully without surgical arthrodesis. In Levine and Lutz's series, 21 of 24 patients achieved bony union and 2 of 24 achieved stable fibrous union at a mean follow-up of 2.5 years.[53]

ANTERIOR LONGITUDINAL LIGAMENT AND DISC DISRUPTIONS

Just as hyperextension injuries may involve failure of bone anteriorly at ligamentous attachment sites, ligament itself and disc may fail in tension producing a primarily soft tissue injury. The radiographic presentation may vary from subtle to dramatic. Taylor and Blackwood[100] described the interesting case of a 31-year-old Scottish miner who in 1948 had fallen downstairs on his face and was rendered completely quadriplegic. Their discussion reveals the frustrations associated with negative plain radiographic and myelographic assessment of this patient whose stormy course was complicated by ascending paresis and eventual death. Their anatomic dissection of the postmortem pathologic findings is quite instructive. It demonstrates a pure anterior longitudinal ligament (ALL) and disc disruption with associated intramedullary hemorrhage and edema of the cord. The deformity reduces unrecognizably in flexion. The authors remind us to maintain patients' necks in neutrality, avoiding extension in those who may have suspected hyperextension-induced insufficiencies of the ALL and disc.

Few reports appear in the literature about this lesion, but many suspect that it may have been an unrecognized cause of spinal cord injuries in patients without spondylosis, stenosis, or other recognized plain film injuries to the spine (Fig. 23–4). Loading rates of ligaments, noted for their viscoelastic properties, have been implicated as determining sites of failure (whether at the bony site of attachment or in midsubstance).[59, 90] The rate, as well as the mechanism, of loading may ultimately play a role. In the final analysis, the weakest link again in the chain will fail first, a property determined undoubtedly by the tissue characteristics of the individual. In cadaveric preparations if the ALL is severed and a hyperextension moment is placed on the spine, the intervertebral disc will rupture allowing for retrolisthesis of the body above. Marar[57] showed that subtle retrolisthesis may be a helpful clue to recognizing hyperextension induced-disc injury in the spine. Additionally, Marar described tension failure through bone of the midvertebral body in four senile pathologic dissections and confirmed in elderly cadavers experimentally that with hyperextension a pure bony failure can occur. The ultimate determinant of site of failure again seems to be age and tissue dependent.

The definitive management of patients with ALL or disc disruptions has not been clarified, yet it remains logical that this condition represents a significant instability. The nonsurgical approach would be mandating 3 months of rigid halo immobilization followed by flexion-extension films to determine stability. If unstable, surgical intervention would be warranted. Surgically, anterior cervical discectomy and fusion possibly supplemented with instrumentation could be done.

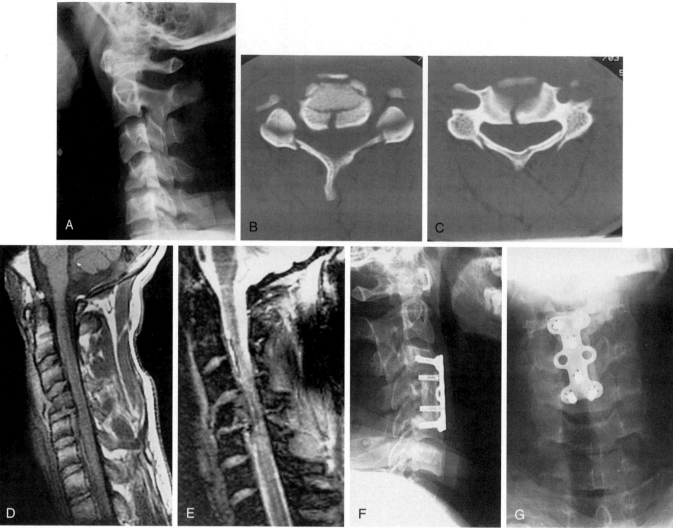

Figure 23–3 = This young man was injured tackling in a high-school football game. He was completely quadriplegic after the accident. *A,* The initial lateral cervical spine radiograph shows a typical flexion axial loading injury, which is often associated with significant vertebral body fractures, posterior soft tissue injuries and fractures, and retrolisthesis of the vertebral body into the spinal canal. Unfortunately, this type of fracture also has been termed a "teardrop fracture." This is clearly not a cervical hyperextension injury and is often associated with severe neurologic deficit, as was seen in this patient. *B* and *C,* These sequential CT sections show the significant intrusion into the spinal canal as well as the fractures involving the posterior portion of the vertebral body. Many cases also have fractured laminae, as shown here. *D* and *E,* These sagittal MRI scans (T1- and T2-weighted images) clearly demonstrate the intrusion into the spinal canal by the C4 vertebral body. At this time the patient is in traction. *F* and *G,* These postoperative films were taken at 2 months following the injury. The anterior corpectomy with spinal canal decompression and bone grafting and plating was done on the day of the injury because the neural compression could not be relieved in any other way. The patient has good strength in his biceps and in his wrist extensors but has no triceps function at 7 months following the accident.

The indication for posterior decompression in the face of hematoma or edema must be considered individually, and weighed against the risks of further destabilization. Studies relating to the outcome of surgical management are not available at this time.

HYPEREXTENSION IN SPONDYLOTIC, STENOTIC, OR ANKYLOSED SPINES

Hyperextension Injuries in Ankylosing Spondylitis

The evaluation and treatment of hyperextension injuries to the cervical spine in patients with ankylos-ing spondylitis (AS) poses significant challenges to the clinician. Algorithms in management which are ordinarily applied to patients with cervical injury require modification. Clinical suspicion must remain particularly high for occult injury and the acute and definitive management must be modified in consideration of the patient's underlying abnormalities of bone and soft tissue. The propensity for associated vascular and neural injury and preexisting abnormalities of alignment further compound the decision-making process. In general, exceptional precaution and a commitment to conservatism should be the cornerstone of care, while surgery should be reserved for the exceptional case. Patients with diffuse idiopathic skeletal hyperostosis (DISH) may also sustain fractures in association with

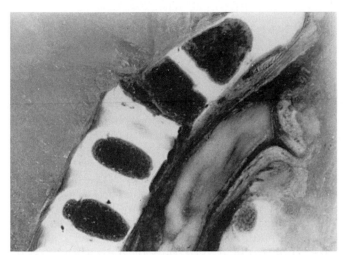

Figure 23–4 = This cryomicrotome section was made through the cervical spine of a young child who had presented with a high-level complete quadriplegia. This is a hyperextension-type injury and the disruption is through the end plate at the bottom of the vertebral body. This is often the anatomic appearance of those cases presenting with spinal cord injury without radiographic abnormality (SCIWORA). (Courtesy of Dr. Jose Becerra, Miami.)

hyperextension injuries. Although more rarely reported in the literature than AS, extension is a more common mechanism than flexion in creating complex skeletal and severe neurologic injury in such patients. Twelve of 14 fractures recently reported[63] occurred at either C5–6 or C6–7. Many patients benefited from surgical reduction, fusion, and instrumentation.

AS, originally described by Marie and Strümpell in 1897 and 1898, is an inflammatory seronegative spondyloarthropathy which may begin with general inflammation and a radiographic picture of osteopenia, but progress to painless ossification of the spine. More commonly seen in males, its incidence in the general population is roughly 2/1000. The disease is characterized by bilateral sacroiliitis and the formation of stiff joints by the consolidation of the articular surfaces.[5] Spine flexibility and chest expansion are reduced. This is typically seen in a patient with an elevated erythrocyte sedimentation rate (ESR) who is rheumatoid factor (RF)– and antinuclear antibody (ANA)–negative but HLA-B27-positive (90% of patients with AS). The disease process is that of an enthesopathy with inflammatory changes occurring in joint capsules and ligaments resulting in syndesmophyte formation and eventual ankylosis. Systemic involvement is commonly seen, especially uveitis.[5]

Seventy-five percent of patients with AS in whom the duration of disease is 16 years or more[109] develop cervical ankylosis. This ankylosis creates a cylinder of bone about the spinal cord which is rigid, brittle, and osteoporotic. When stressed, therefore, a tremendous lever arm exists for fracture initiation. It is not surprising that these patients present in their fifth and sixth decades, commonly after falls or vehicular accidents, with unstable spine fractures ranging from the occult to the catastrophic[26, 30, 37, 66, 70] (Fig. 23–5). Occasionally the patient will present after trivial or no injury at all

with a presumed stress fracture. Longitudinal studies of patients with AS sometimes minimize cervical fractures as a significant cause of morbidity and mortality. However, several authors have published series warning of their propensity to occur and urging aggressive assessment and cautious treatment. Other hyperextension injuries, such as odontoid fractures, may be prone to occur in patients with AS and cervical flexion deformities and have been reported.[43] Bohlman's series of 300 cervical injuries described 8 patients with AS, 7 of whom had neurologic deficits.[9] Four of these had significant epidural hematomas, a complication not seen in the 292 other patients. Murray and Persellin[66] reviewed the literature on fractures in AS in 1981 and added 8 additional patients from their own experience to present a total of 83 patients, 77 of whom were male. Their review suggests that hyperextension is clearly the most common mechanism of injury whether it be by direct blow on the forehead or rebound hyperextension through the deformed spine. The most common site of fracture in patients with AS is the cervical spine or at the cervicothoracic junction (75%).[41] The most common presentation is a fracture through the calcified intervertebral disc (70%), most often C5–6 or C6–7, though the fracture can also occur through the body,

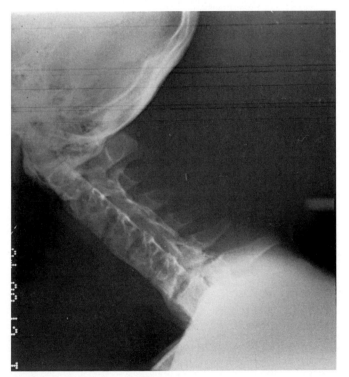

Figure 23–5 = This middle-aged man had ankylosing spondylitis but had a functional alignment of his spine. He had not had any significant spine pain for several years. He was in a motor vehicle accident, however, several months before this radiograph was taken. The lateral view shows that the patient has a very straight cervical spine. Also, between C6 and C7 there is a lucent line through the disc space and through the facet joints which cannot be seen at any other level. This was a fracture which had not been recognized at the time of the accident and we can see that some kyphosis and subluxation is beginning to develop at this level. This patient later developed a chin-on-chest deformity which required cervical osteotomy to improve his daily function.

commonly its cranial portion.[31, 66] The prognosis for the latter site of injury may be somewhat worse than for those that occur through calcified disc.

The patient may present with unsuspected injury and neck pain alone or with a painful flexion deformity. Pain should not be attributed to arthritis, even after trivial injury. Simmons cautioned that it is those with neck pain and no deformity who may be presenting with acute or subacute fracture, a condition which left untreated may well progress to a chin-on-chest deformity.[91]

Significant morbidity and mortality are the rule with these fractures. Ultimately, one third of these patients die in the face of injury, while 22% to 45% persist with significant neurologic morbidity, initially present in greater than one half.[66, 106] Disturbingly, Murray and Persellin[66] observed a trend that death has been noted to be more common in the group treated surgically (45%) than in the group treated nonsurgically (29%). However, this was a retrospective review of the literature in which the treatment groups were not matched for injury severity. It has, however, influenced the choice of initial and definitive care.

The early management of the patient consists in having a high index of suspicion for the injury. Rescue squad personnel must be attentive to the need to place a patient's head in the "normal" resting position for immobilization. This requires communication with the patient and his or her family and modification of protocols regarding field collar immobilization. The physician should continue to observe these precautions and should avoid the use of traction in extension or neutral positioning. Excessive traction may actually overdistract or malalign the spine.[78] Some authors recommend the immediate placement of a halo cast or custom halo vest in the patient's normal resting posture.

The radiographic evaluation may be complicated by distortion of normal anatomy and lack of displacement on plain films. Plain films and tomography, if needed, should alert the physician to the diagnosis. Most authors suggest utilizing reformatted CT to generate orthogonal images (coronal and sagittal) to avoid missing transverse (axial plane) vertebral fractures and to better evaluate the cervicothoracic junction.[24, 25, 34] MRI may also be helpful, but CT is thought likely to be adequate given the bony transformation of soft tissue. Dynamic radiographs should not be necessary and may well be hazardous. Throughout the evaluation, extreme caution with positioning and careful supervision of the procedures must be observed.

With few exceptions, definitive management of the patient is usually nonsurgical. Some authors argue for initial traction prior to extended management in a halo cast or vest. One must remember that a patient with AS has lungs that are less compliant with restricted intercostal motion and which may be further restricted by the cast or vest. Rarely, with halo cast or vest immobilization, a fracture may become redisplaced. Halo cast or vest immobilization alone, however, has allowed most patients to heal solidly without incident. Sherk[91] suggested that 4 months is required for safe healing. He attempted to restore the normal chin-to-brow vertical angle.[91] At present the indications for surgery should be limited to the patient in whom reduction has failed, who has significant canal compromise with neurologic impairment, or who has ascending paralysis due to epidural hematoma.[91, 106] These patients may require combined decompressions and instrumented fusion. Appropriate aftercare may still require the use of a halo cast given bone quality. Few believe there is an indication to use the fracture as an occasion to correct a chin-on-chest deformity if this deformity was present before the injury.[34]

In summary, significant hyperextension injuries to the cervical spine in patients with AS are easily missed unless one maintains a high level of suspicion. Cautious evaluation and immobilization are indicated, each of which should be performed with respect to the patient's pre-injury cervical alignment. Routine in-line traction may be harmful by creating a hyperextension bending moment or overdistracting the spine. The complication of epidural hematoma must be watched for and assessed carefully in patients with changing neurologic deficits.

Hyperextension Injuries in Congenital Cervical Stenosis

Hyperextension injuries in young persons with congenital cervical stenosis present an increased risk for spinal cord injuries as compared to similar injuries in patients with normal cervical canal size (Fig. 23–6).

Figure 23–6 = This patient had sustained a hyperextension injury to the cervical spine several months earlier. He had a myelopathy and was treated at another institution with a two-level anterior cervical discectomy and fusion. His myelopathy improved to a moderate degree, but he was still too severely impaired to return to work. He also had severe problems with pain radiating into his flank and right lower extremity. A and B, These cervical radiographs show that the cervical spine is fixed in satisfactory alignment. A very mild lordosis is present. The sagittal canal diameter measures 13 mm at C4–5 and 12 mm at C5–6 as measured on these films. C, This postmyelogram CT scan performed after the anterior cervical decompression and fusion reveals that there is still significant stenosis present at the C5–6 level. D, This midsagittal T2-weighted MRI scan was performed after two-level anterior cervical decompression and fusion. The spinal canal is still quite tight at the C5–6 level. In addition, a change in the signal intensity within the spinal cord at this level is seen. This is consistent with significant myelomalacia. E, This transverse MRI scan reveals the same narrowing of the spinal canal at the C5–6 level. F, This lateral film was taken after a posterior cervical laminoplasty was performed from C3 through C6. The patient's lordosis above and below the fusion has improved compared with his preoperative state. G and H, These postoperative CT scans were obtained at the level of the previous anterior decompression and fusion. It can be seen that the hinge side of the laminoplasty is healed. Allograft bone was placed at the C3, C4, and C6 levels to hold the laminoplasty open. This also is healing well. The size of the spinal canal is obviously significantly increased. I, This midsagittal T2-weighted MRI can was obtained 4 months after the posterior cervical laminoplasty. There is now copious room for the spinal cord. The small area of myelomalacia can still be seen within the spinal cord at the C5–6 level. At this time the patient's myelopathy is significantly improved and his pain is markedly improved. He is functioning and doing physical work.

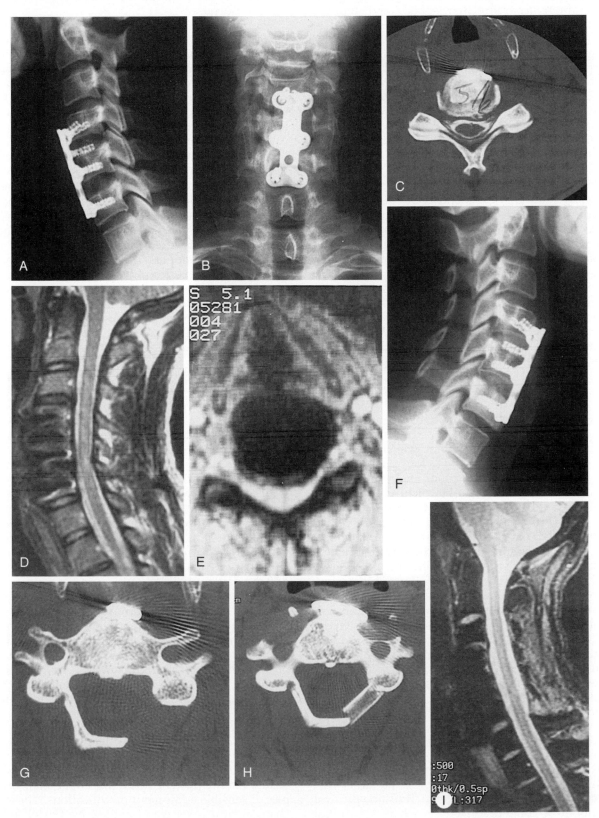

Figure 23–6 = *See legend on opposite page*

An increasingly large body of literature concerning younger patients with sports-related injuries supports this contention. Sports-related spinal cord injuries, however, likely constitute a small (2%) proportion of all patients seen with spinal cord injury.[3] Additionally, athletic injuries are thought to be more commonly seen with hyperflexion or axial loading. Patients with neuropraxia, however, may have a higher incidence of hyperextension injuries.[102] Because of the personal impact of these occasionally devastating injuries on the young person and the medicolegal implications relating to physician permission for return to sports after a transient neurologic injury, we devote further attention to this clinical entity.

Hinck and co-workers[36] originally described the picture of congenital cervical stenosis in 1962. More recently, Torg and others[102] described transient quadriplegia in football players with congenital stenosis. This study complements a growing body of literature on congenital stenotic patients sustaining hyperextension injuries in football, rugby, bodysurfing, and other sports.[3, 17, 23, 49, 67, 84, 96] Additional published reviews emphasize that patients with postsurgical, post-traumatic, and congenitally fused vertebrae are also at risk of spinal cord injury with hyperextension.[82, 102] This likely is a result of hypermobility or secondary degenerative arthrosis developing above or below a fused motion segment.[82]

Torg and associates[102] described the typical presentation of a young male athlete sustaining a hyperextension cervical injury with an acute transient neuropraxia of the cervical cord. Generally, the neuropraxia consists of burning dysesthesias and motor weakness, lasting 10 to 15 minutes but occasionally as long as 2 days. The athlete commonly has had no prodromal symptoms or history of previous injury.[102] This picture of transient quadriplegia or the milder form of central cord dysfunction known as "burning hands" syndrome[58] must be distinguished on the field from the athlete presenting with unilateral upper extremity neurologic dysfunction known as the "burner" or "prolonged burner," which represents a traction or direct blow injury to the brachial plexus or cervical nerve root(s).[94]

Commonly, plain films are normal after transient quadriplegia. However, Torg and co-workers[102] described 32 patients with neuropraxia in their study, 17 of whom were noted to have normal x-ray films, but who otherwise met criteria for congenital spinal stenosis. Seventeen of 32 patients were also thought to have hyperextension as the mechanism for their injuries. The plain radiographic criteria for stenosis as described by Pavlov is when the ratio of sagittal spinal canal diameter divided by the vertebral body is less than 0.80, as compared to a normal of 0.98 in controls.[102] This technique avoids errors in measurements of sagittal spinal canal diameters referable to variations in target distances of radiographic equipment. Traditionally, we have thought of congenital stenosis when AP sagittal diameters measure less than 14 mm, as measured from the midposterior aspect of the body to the spinolaminar line. The normal diameter is 17 to 18 mm as measured at a target distance of 6 ft. Quantitative CT

scanning has also given us guidelines for diagnosing cervical stenosis, though it is not commonly employed for that purpose.[95]

The incidence of transient quadriplegia as reported by Torg and co-workers[101] was 1.3/10,000 in a 1984 survey of 503 NCAA (National Collegiate Athletic Association) football programs. This contrasts with 6.0/10,000 for four-extremity paresthesias.[102] Speer and Bassett[94] reported an incidence of 5 to 10/100 for prolonged "burners" and a 4-year career incidence of up to 50% for burners in varsity collegiate football players.

Taylor[99] demonstrated in cadavers with myelography that infoldings of the ligamentum flavum occur with hyperextension resulting in 30% narrowing of the thecal canal outline. Brieg[12] demonstrated that the spinal cord actually thickens as tension is released on it and its dural investments, with shortening as might be seen in hyperextension injuries. This further reduces the potential free space constituting a safe zone for impingement.[12] Penning[75] described a "pincer effect" which in hyperextension bending squeezes the spinal cord between the posteroinferior portion of the vertebral body and the subjacent posterior elements. Additionally, hyperextension causes the posterior longitudinal ligament (PLL) and the ligamentum flavum to actually thicken secondary to stress relaxation.[102] These pathomechanical factors help explain why, in persons with congenitally stenotic canals, neurologic injury might occur with greater frequency.

What should the clinician do after recognition of this injury pattern? Clearly, in the field, a patient presenting with neuropraxia must be carefully stabilized and removed promptly from the playing field for a complete neurologic and musculoskeletal examination including radiographs, dynamic radiographs, and in some instances MRI. Clinical evaluation alone may be insufficient even for patients presenting solely with pain. The need for a cervical CT scan and myelography will vary, but is strongly advocated by some as an excellent way of evaluating congenital stenosis.[49] Any associated instabilities or neural compression will need to be addressed as required.

Most authors agree that patients with congenital stenosis and transient neuropraxia should be advised to discontinue participation in contact sports and high-risk activities. However, the data of Torg and associates[102] do not indicate that these persons are predisposed to more severe injuries with permanent sequelae should they choose to return.[3, 84] Some believe the presence of congenital stenosis alone should potentially preclude participation in contact sports.[49]

The role of the clinician should be expanded to assist in prevention through protective equipment modification, training, and rule changes. The addition of shoulder and neck rolls, modifications in facemasks, and changes in the posterior trim lines of helmets are examples of sensible equipment modifications. These biomechanical principles were studied by Carter and Frankel[15] in their evaluation of hyperextension injuries in football players using free body diagrams of helmeted cervical spines. Training programs emphasizing neck strengthening serve as additional prevention. Rule

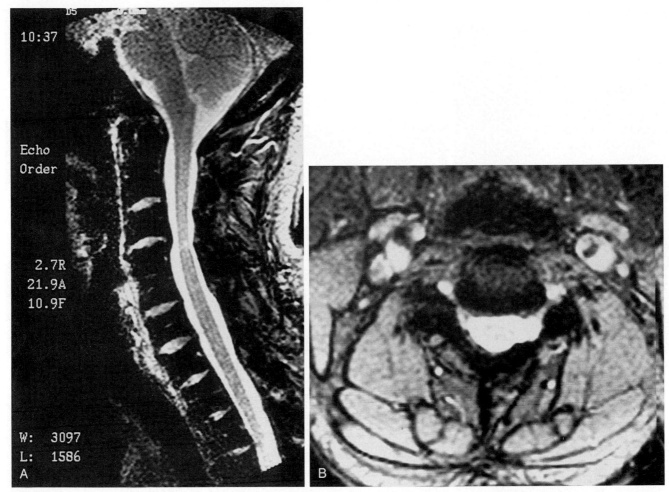

Figure 23–7 = This patient had severe congenital stenosis and injured himself as a teenager while diving. He had sustained a hyperextension injury with severe quadriparesis. In addition to the cervical stenosis, he also had a congenital fusion of C4–5. After he failed to improve significantly within a few weeks, he was taken to surgery and underwent a posterior cervical laminoplasty. *A,* This midsagittal T2-weighted MRI scan was obtained 6 years after the laminoplasty. The patient has had nearly complete resolution of his central cord syndrome. The area of myelomalacia can still be seen within the spinal cord at the C3–4 level which is the presumed site of the original injury. At this time there is copious room for the spinal cord and the narrowest level remains the C3–4 level. *B,* This T2-weighted transverse section was taken through the tightest level at C3–4. There is more than adequate room around the spinal cord. At 4 months after surgery, the patient can be cleared for return to full activities with no restrictions.

changes regarding spearing (1976) and existing rules regarding facemasking address risky tackling techniques. At present the clinician's role must be to recognize, treat, and appropriately advise the player with congenital stenosis or previous hyperextension injury who participates in high-risk activities (Fig. 23–7).

Hyperextension Injuries in Spondylotic Stenosis

Like patients with congenital stenosis, those with cervical spondylosis and stenosis have significant risk of neurologic injury with hyperextension. In middle-aged and elderly patients, minor hyperextension injuries may result in serious damage to the spinal cord[85] (Fig. 23–8). Disc space narrowing and collapse, hypertrophic degenerative facet changes, hypertrophic and infolded ligamentum flavum, and posterior end-plate osteophyte formation all result in significant re-

duction in the space available for the cord. Soft tissues, which are less compliant and therefore more likely to fail under hyperextension loading, include the ALL, disc, PLL, and perineural vascular structures.

A common presentation is that of an elderly person who has struck his forehead, either in a fall or vehicular accident, and who demonstrates findings of a central cord syndrome. Misdiagnosis is frequent in this group of patients.[9] The reasons for this are multifactorial, including (1) the subtleties of diagnosis in mild central cord lesions, (2) inadequate radiographs, (3) radiographs which appear strikingly normal except for spondylosis, (4) failure to recognize occult or subtle radiographic findings suggestive of significant hyperextension injury, and (5) impaired patient-physician communication secondary to advanced age or closed head injury. Prevertebral hematomas are not uncommonly seen and may be massive. Both Smith and others[93] and Howcraft and Jenkins[40] presented case reports of elderly patients with near-fatal asphyxia in the face

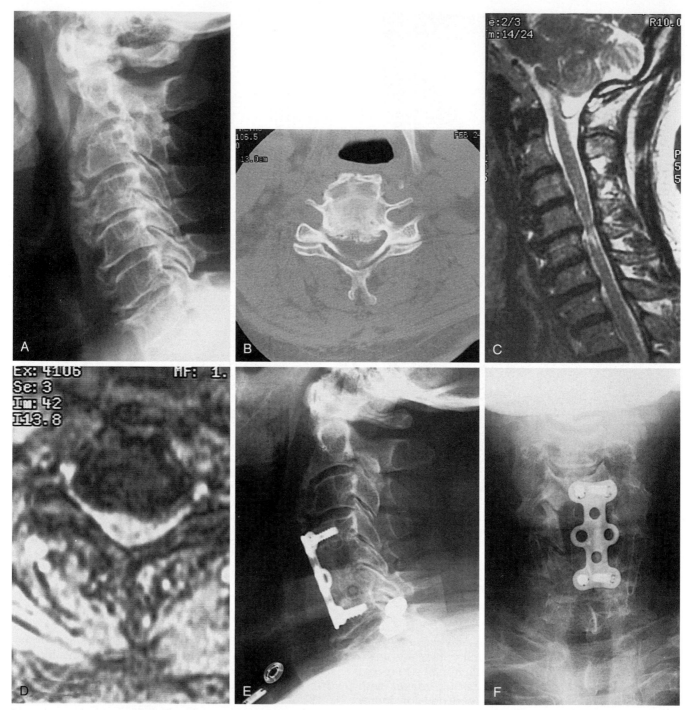

Figure 23–8 = This man had undergone a general surgical procedure in the supine position 5 years prior to this. He awakened after that surgery with severe pain radiating into his left shoulder. This pain persisted over the following 5 years and slowly seemed to be worsening. *A,* The lateral radiograph reveals significant cervical spondylosis. In addition to the obvious anterior osteophytes, the patient also has significant posterior osteophytes protruding into the spinal canal. *B,* This CT scan transverse section reveals that marked spinal stenosis is present at the C4–5 level. *C,* This midsagittal MRI scan reveals the very marked stenosis present at C4–5 and reveals the obvious myelomalacia within the spinal cord behind the C5 vertebral body. *D,* This transverse MRI scan reveals the large osteophytes protruding into the spinal canal at the C4–5 level and this clearly demonstrates the extent of spinal stenosis. *E* and *F,* The patient was treated with an anterior corpectomy of C5 with removal of the inferior one half of C4 and the superior one quarter of C6 and this was replaced with autogenous bone graft and plates and screws. Following surgery the patient noted an improvement in his left arm pain. It is not possible to tell how much of his left arm pain, which was a dysesthetic type of pain, was due to the damage present within the spinal cord vs. the compression of the C5 nerve root.

of this lesion prior to evacuation of the hematomas and tracheostomy.

Other associated soft tissue lesions reported in the anterior neck include esophageal perforation with the potential for life-threatening mediastinitis, a complication reported by several authors.[1, 51] Additionally, retropharyngeal abscess with airway obstruction and tetraplegia has been described in the elderly with hy-

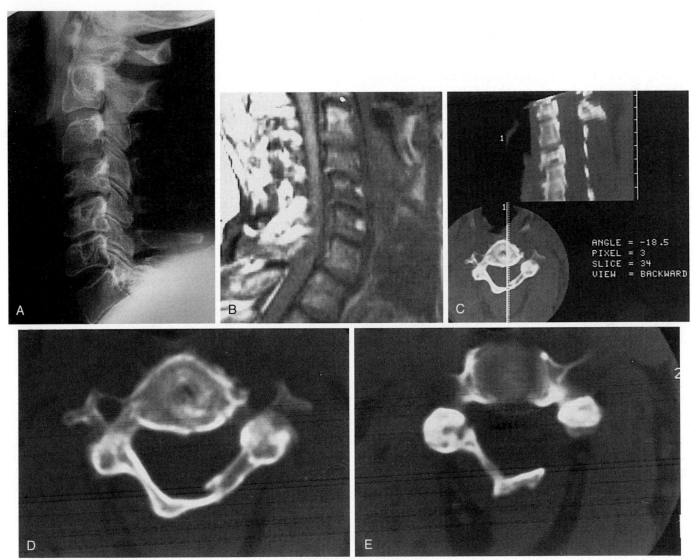

Figure 23–9 = This elderly man had sustained a minor hyperextension injury to his neck and developed a severe central cord syndrome. His hand function was most involved and his leg weakness was severe enough to prevent ambulation even with assistance. The patient failed to show significant improvement with conservative treatment. *A,* This lateral radiograph reveals moderate spondylosis and mild cervical lordosis. *B,* This midsagittal T1-weighted MRI scan shows severe cervical stenosis present from C4–5 down to C7–T1. *C,* The patient was treated with a cervical laminoplasty from C3 through C7. The midsagittal reconstruction reveals how the spinal canal diameter has been markedly improved. *D* and *E,* These transverse CT sections reveal how the spinal canal diameter has been improved. The hinge side of the laminoplasty is well healed and the bone graft is incorporating well. Bone grafts were placed at the C3, C5, and C7 levels and the intervening levels are adequately held open. This patient regained ability to ambulate with no aid or assistance and even his hand function improved significantly. The laminoplasty is an ideal procedure for those patients who would otherwise require three- and four-level anterior cervical decompressions.

perextension.[79] Traumatic dissection of the extracranial internal carotid artery when hyperextension is combined with lateral bending was described by Stringer and Kelly[97] in six patients.

The evaluation of older patients with hyperextension injury requires a high index of suspicion. Particular attention should be paid to the detection of associated injuries. Dynamic films as well as CT and MRI may be particularly important. Detailed neurologic examination will result in recognition of deficit. The care of the elderly spinal cord–injured patient will ultimately require a team approach and anticipation of a prolonged period of rehabilitation. Most patients with central cord lesions will walk, but upper extremity deficits are likely to persist. The need for decompression or stabilization, or both, must be individualized (Fig. 23–9). Many patients, however, will not benefit neurologically from decompression.

SPINAL CORD INJURY WITHOUT RADIOGRAPHIC ABNORMALITY (SCIWORA)

In the child who sustains a hyperextension injury to the cervical spine, injury to the spinal cord may occur in the absence of any abnormal findings on plain radiographs. In a recent review of the literature, 75 of 199 pediatric patients seen with spinal cord injury were found to have no radiographic abnormality.[71] It is likely that this occurs as a result of the unique anatomy and physiologic differences inherent in the spine of the skeletally immature. Several authors have published larger series regarding these patients.[35, 71, 80] The absence of radiographic findings is one contributing factor to a patient's injury being underrecognized, but it does not seem to be the most important contributor. Orenstein et al.[69] found that it is the clinician's failure to obtain films or to recognize existing radiographic abnormalities, commonly at the cervicothoracic junction or at the occiput–C1–2 motion segments, that usually results in diagnostic error. They found nine patients (12%) with abnormalities not appreciated on initial readings of plain films or in patients who failed to have adequate immediate radiographic examinations. In this group, only one patient, however, had neurologic deficit. Based on 50 pediatric patients with cervical injuries, Dietrich and co-workers[22] also reported a 10% error in the initial reading of radiographs where fracture or subluxations were eventually found to be present. The clinician must beware of this pitfall above all others.

Several important characteristics of the immature spine may account for the normal radiographic appearance in the face of high-energy injuries that have rendered the patient neurologically impaired. The first of these is the greater tissue compliance or elasticity seen in ligaments and joint capsules of children, which may allow for transient subluxations without gross mechanical failure. This laxity was described by Cattell and others[16] in their description of pseudosubluxation in children based on a review of 160 normal subjects. Secondly, the planes of the cervical facets in children are more horizontal and thus possess greater mobility but less stability.[71] Finally and most important, as demonstrated by Aufderman[2] in his elegant pathologic study of 12 children, catastrophic failure in the immature spine nearly always occurs through the cartilaginous end plate (see Fig. 23–4). The end plate or physis is the weak link in the child and fractures through it are not uncommonly missed unless they are complete and seen on stress radiographs. Consider the analogy of the distal femoral physeal fracture in the child where stress films help to differentiate it from significant ligamentous injury more commonly seen in the adult.

In patients with SCIWORA, however, even stress radiographs of the neck may be normal. This in part may be related to patient compliance or protective splinting, but may also be due to incomplete mechanical failure. It may also suggest that complete physeal failure contributes to only a portion of these clinical presentations. Pang and Wilberger,[71] in their comprehensive treatise on this subject, described 24 patients with SCIWORA seen over 20 years at the Children's Hospital of Pittsburgh. Eighteen of the patients had voluntary flexion-extension films done acutely and none revealed an abnormality. All 24 eventually received dynamic films and only one patient had radiographic instability. With MRI it may be possible in the future to detect a majority of these injuries of the cartilaginous end plate and determine the role that

they might have played in allowing for neurologic compromise.

In Pang and Wilberger's series hyperextension alone was the presumed mechanism of injury in 10 of 24 patients. Seven of the 10 patients were more than 8 years old. The majority of the lesions involved the lower cervical cord (C5–8 root level), while the five cases of upper cord injury were in the minority and only seen in children under 8 years of age. The younger children with upper cord injuries seemed to have an increased likelihood of serious injury in general. Corroborating physical signs such as chin lacerations, mandibular fractures, facial injuries, and frontal skull injuries were commonly seen to support a hyperextension injury. Overall, 58% sustained a complete or serious cord injury and the final outcome did not seem to be affected significantly by age or treatment.[71]

Management of these patients begins with neutral cervical immobilization in the field and the hospital until screening radiographs can be performed. To accomplish this, the small child and infant may require a roll to be placed under his or her shoulders to compensate for the disproportionately large size of the head. Associated basic life and trauma resuscitations take priority over all further workup. Avoidance of both cord edema and hypotension may be critical to maintaining cord perfusion pressures. Most authors consider administering high-dose corticosteroids.[11] Dynamic radiographs and MRI should be performed as early as feasible. Definitive management of the spine may require no more than the use of a secure rigid collar. Those patients with demonstrable instability will be more safely immobilized in a halo device or with cervical arthrodesis if the halo will complicate the patient's rehabilitation. Follow-up dynamic radiographs are mandatory in all patients. Evolving neurologic deficits were reported in one half of Pang and Wilberger's patients and this mandates emergency re-evaluation.[71] Subsequent management is controversial, yet consideration should be given to decompression and fusion if a structural lesion is found. Laminectomy alone in the pediatric spine renders the patient prone to the eventual development of kyphosis and, in general, is contraindicated. The progression of neurologic deficit may be related, however, to occult instability and reinjury, or to evolving edema, hemorrhage, or watershed infarction in the absence of obvious epidural hematoma.[71] The management of these patients may be primarily medical and supportive.

WHIPLASH (ACCELERATION-DECELERATION INJURY TO THE CERVICAL SPINE)

Whiplash injuries, or acceleration-deceleration injuries of the neck, have been commonly referred to as cervical sprains. Although some whiplash injuries may indeed represent minor ligamentous injuries of the ALL experienced under tension, the syndrome likely represents a constellation of injuries rarely dramatically evident at initial or follow-up examination. The foundations of the syndrome appear to be an injury of both the anterior and posterior column soft tissue structures. There is as well a plethora of potential associated injuries of the head and neck. The approach to patients with whiplash must be to methodically search for underlying pathologic changes that can cause persistent symptoms.

A large body of literature has been written on this topic. For the purposes of this chapter we discuss first the experimental studies relating to the mode of injury and then the clinical presentation, evaluation, treatment options, and outcome.

Basic experimentation as it relates to whiplash has centered on defining the biomechanical forces seen in acceleration injuries and the resultant diverse injury patterns. In 1955, Severy and associates[89] reported on the photometric and biomechanical evaluation of controlled low-speed rear-end collisions using human subjects and models. The seats in the vehicles tested were without headrests and the subjects were unrestrained. The magnitudes of head acceleration were far greater than that of vehicle acceleration. At 10 mph, 11 G was seen by the driver and 122 degrees of neck extension was noted with subsequent rebound flexion.[89] Out of this work grew an interest in automobile seat and restraint design changes which have attempted to lower the incidence of neck injury in vehicular accidents. The use of headrests, however, has not uniformly been shown statistically to reduce the incidence of whiplash,[68] which may be in part due to theft design or positioning. Most would agree, however, that properly positioned headrests are of benefit.

The collision severity clearly influences peak translational and angular accelerations. Williams[110] reported that for a 12 G impact, head horizontal acceleration climbs to greater than 50 G for a period of approximately 40 msec. Higher impacts (20 G) clearly exceed the tensile strength of the cervical spine's soft tissue and bony structures.[110]

Macnab[55] reviewed his clinical experience and discussed experimental work relating to monkeys sustaining various degrees of hyperextension injury. The pathologic findings included sternocleidomastoid, longus colli, esophageal, ALL, and disc lesions with retropharyngeal hematomas, findings which might help explain many of the clinical complaints of the whiplash patient. The author did not address possible compression injuries of the posterior column or associated head injuries.[55] Posterior capsular and cartilaginous injuries are common, however, and these experimental changes were reviewed by LaRocca.[50] Recent work by Barnsley and co-workers[6] suggests that the facet joint may be the first site of "contact" in hyperextension and that the zygapophyseal joints are likely to be one of the most important sources of segmental pain generation in whiplash. Additionally, Hohl[38] has shown that the zygapophyseal joints as well as the intervertebral discs develop an incidence (39%) of degenerative changes within the first decade after whiplash that is six times higher than normal.

A variety of hemodynamic, behavioral, and biochemical disturbances have been reported to occur in rats after whiplash injury, specifically disturbances in postural regulation of blood flow and variations in brain neurotransmitter levels. Associated learning impairment and overaggressive behaviors were also observed.[10] Additionally, subcortical electroencephalographic (EEG) changes have been seen in monkeys following whiplash.[54]

Clinical series reporting manifestations of whiplash describe a number of features which are summarized by LaRocca.[50] The principal symptoms are neck pain and stiffness reported in 97% to 100% and 78% to 95% of patients respectively. Forty percent to 72% complained of significant headaches, often occipital. At least one third of patients had shoulder or arm pain.[38, 56, 73] Many patients (40% to 60%) related psychological distress including irritability, insomnia, and anxiety. Some complained of dysphagia, visual blurring, tinnitus, and vertigo, the first perhaps related to retropharyngeal hematoma or occult esophageal injury and the latter three to vertebral artery spasm.[42] The literature contains reports of esophageal injury,[1, 79, 98] sternocleidomastoid rupture,[88] temporomandibular joint arthritis,[33, 105] vestibular injury,[18] thoracic outlet syndrome,[14] and cerebral or ocular injury[44, 47] in association with whiplash, which may be responsible for generating further occult symptoms.

Physical findings may reveal decreased range of motion and point tenderness while objective neurologic signs are rarely found. Radiographs are typically normal. However, 20 of 146 radiographs in Hohl's series[38] revealed a "sharp reversal of lordosis" which may have been indicative of occult disc, capsular, or mild ligamentous injuries. Interestingly, 60% of these patients went on to develop significant degenerative changes at the same level of the mild kyphosis, which was seen to be commonly C4–5 or C5–6.[38] Dynamic radiographs, though important to obtain, rarely add information in whiplash. MRI and invasive diagnostic procedures, such as discography and diagnostic facet blocks, may help to better localize the site of symptomatic injury (Fig. 23–10).

Treatment of whiplash can be challenging and frustrating for the patient and physician alike. The overlay of secondary gain seen with unsettled litigation can further complicate an already clouded clinical presentation. Claims of personal injury are filed in a high percentage of cases.[50] Interestingly, however, Macnab reported that 45% of patients continued to have some symptoms 2 years or more after settlement. He described these symptoms as "nuisance-like" rather than "significantly disabling."[55] Hohl also stated that only 38% of patients were asymptomatic at 5-year follow-up if settlement was achieved more than 18 months post injury.[38] Pearce maintained that despite this, 79% of his 100 patients returned to work by 1 month and 94% by 1 year.[73]

Treatment modalities most commonly utilized include the use of soft collar support, rest, analgesics, and physical therapy. Two prospective trials done in Europe have helped to better our understanding of treatment. The blinded study of age- and sex-matched patients by Mealy and colleagues[61] revealed that the

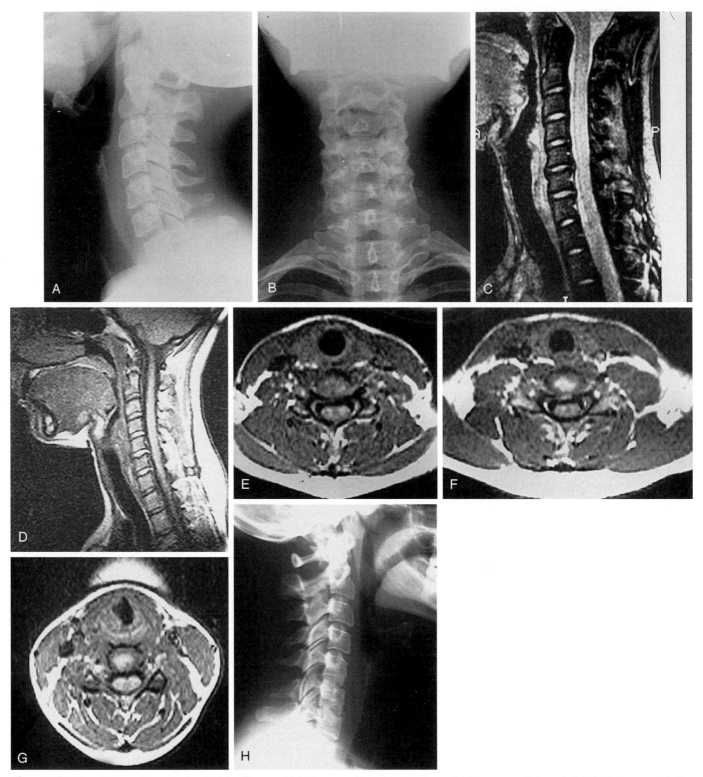

Figure 23–10 = This patient sustained a significant whiplash type of injury when her vehicle was struck from behind while stopped. She had severe and unremitting neck pain, extension into the shoulders bilaterally, and upper extremity symptoms resembling somatic referred pain. Her pain was worse on the left side than the right side. She also had persistent headaches. These symptoms were still present and severe 6 months after injury. *A* and *B*, These radiographs were taken the day of the accident and are normal. They show only very minor arthritic changes and these are most noticeable at C5–6. *C*, This midsagittal T2-weighted image obtained 3 weeks after injury reveals a disc bulge present at C5–6 and C6–7. At C5–6 it is possible that there is also a small extruded disc fragment. *D*, At 6 months after injury, when there had been no improvement in the symptoms, this patient was evaluated with discography at C4–5, C5–6, and C6–7. Gadolinium was injected in the disc space for later contrast evaluation on MRI scan. This right sagittal MRI scan reveals protrusion of the discs at C5–6 and C6–7 into the spinal canal. *E*, This transverse T1-weighted MRI scan was obtained after injection of the disc at C5–6. The injection recreated the patient's neck and shoulder pain. This study shows that the disc herniation at this level is quite small. *F*, This transverse T1-weighted image at C6–7 shows the gadolinium clearly within the disc space and a broad posterior midline contained herniation. Injection at this level caused moderate neck pain. *G*, This transverse MRI scan shows the gadolinium within the C4–5 disc space and a posterior transverse fissure, but injection at this level provoked no symptoms. *H*, The patient was treated with a two-level anterior cervical discectomy and fusion and this film was taken 2 months postoperatively. The fusion is not yet solid, but her symptoms have significantly improved. This includes the headache, neck pain, shoulder pain, and arm symptoms. Eight months after surgery the fusion was solid and symptoms were almost completely resolved.

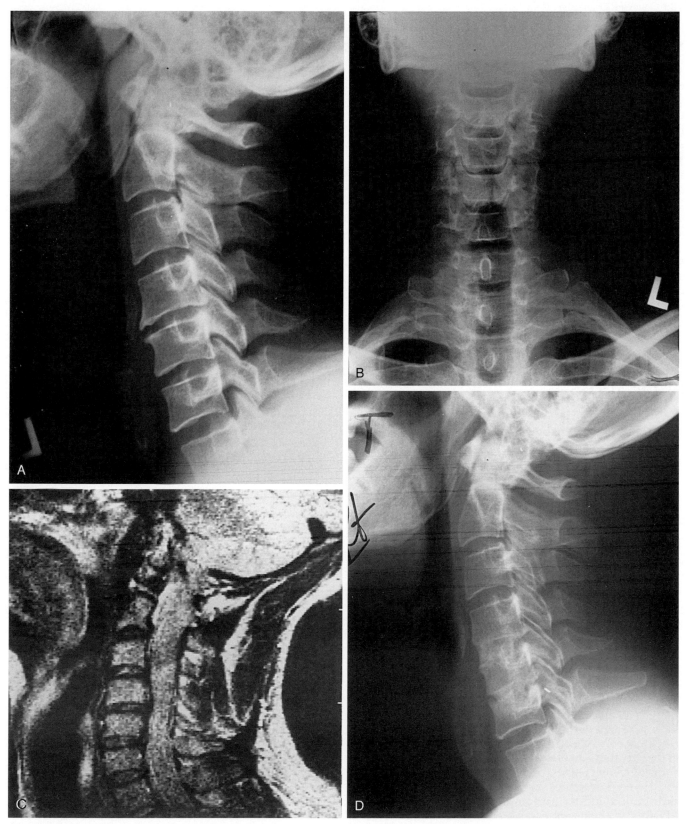

Figure 23–11 = This patient was involved in a motor vehicle accident and sustained a presumed hyperextension injury of the neck. Following this accident, he had a 3-year history of severe pain at the base of the neck and interscapular region with radiation into both shoulders. He also had somatic referred symptoms into his left arm. His symptoms were markedly worsened with any activity. There was no improvement of his symptoms over this period. He had stopped all of his activities except for his work. *A* and *B*, These radiographs were taken immediately after the motor vehicle accident. Arthritic changes are seen at C4–5 but these are mild. The AP film also shows the markedly hypertrophic and arthritic joints of Lushka at the C4–5 level. *C*, This midsagittal MRI scan reveals the arthritic changes within the spine at C4–5, but otherwise does not show any significant abnormality. *D*, Discography was performed and found to be completely painless at C3–4 and C6–7. Injection at C4–5 reproduced most of the patient's symptoms and C5–6 was painful but to a lesser degree. He was treated with an anterior cervical discectomy and fusion at C4–5 and C5–6 and was then able to return to all of his normal activities with no persistent symptoms. This film was taken 7 months postoperatively. At 3½ years after surgery he is still doing well.

subgroup treated with early mobilization and a supervised physical therapy program of stretching, heat, and ice improved pain scores and mobility above that of rest and soft collar use alone. Pennie and Agambar's[74] work contradicts that of Mealy and others.[61] They advocated the use of a molded rigid collar in slight flexion for best pain relief. Recent work suggests that therapeutic and diagnostic facet injections may be of some distinct benefit to patients, as discussed previously. The role of selective cervical arthrodesis in patients with substantial segmental dysfunction has not yet been clearly established, but may be appropriate for those with significant disability beyond 1 to 2 years and supporting studies that suggest segmental instability or arthrosis (Fig. 23–11). It is hoped that MRI and perhaps invasive techniques will help to guide the clinician in the future. Prevention remains the mainstay of effective treatment at this time.

COMPLEX HIGH-ENERGY HYPEREXTENSION FRACTURE-DISLOCATIONS

Dislocation of the cervical spine is a rare manifestation of hyperextension injury. Some authors have grouped significant failures of the anterior column in tension without associated subluxations together with this lesion. Hyperextension fracture-dislocations present characteristically with failure of the anterior column in tension and the posterior column via facet dislocation or posterior element fracture.[28, 32, 65] The latter is a dramatic presentation ultimately representing three-column instability, the likes of which are not seen in other hyperextension injuries. In reality, combined mechanisms with initial hyperflexion in rapid deceleration injuries may be responsible for allowing facet dislocation to occur prior to the patient's head striking an object, imparting hyperextension.

Several case reports have been published describing patients who have sustained high-energy hyperextension injuries in motor vehicle accidents presenting with head and facial injuries, posterior ring fractures of C1 (2 of 4 patients), and subaxial fracture-dislocations.[4, 77, 83] Varying degrees of frank dislocation were present, from less than 25% subluxation and perched facets in one report[83] to 100% displacement in another.[4] Interestingly, neurologic injury was not noted in all patients as posterior element fractures at the site of dislocation can contribute to indirect decompression of the cord.[4]

Definitive management consists of a careful reduction and stabilization of the spine. Given the extreme disruption of all three columns, circumferential surgical arthrodesis with instrumentation is likely indicated, though a more conservative instrumented one-column approach has been advocated by some authors.[4, 77] The small numbers of patients with this specific lesion reported may not allow for a meaningful prediction of outcome.

SUMMARY

We have discussed the etiology, pathomechanics, evaluation, and treatment of a wide variety of clinical entities presenting after hyperextension injuries. The wide variation in clinical presentation is presumed to be a function of differences in load magnitudes, vectors, and points of application. More important, the presentation also appears to be age and tissue dependent. Concomitant spinal cord injuries are seen in those with underlying spondylosis, stenosis, and ankylosis, as well as in children with normal-appearing spines. Whiplash remains a challenging condition.

REFERENCES

1. Agha FP, Raji MR: Case reports: Oesophageal perforation with fracture dislocation of cervical spine due to hyperextension injury. Br J Radiol 55:369–372, 1982.
2. Aufdermaur M: Spinal injuries in juveniles. J Bone Joint Surg Br 56:513–519, 1974.
3. Bailes JE, Hadley MN, Quigley MR: Management of athletic injuries of the cervical spine and spinal cord. Neurosurgery 29:491–497, 1991.
4. Baker RP, Grubb RL: Complete fracture-dislocation of cervical spine without permanent neurological sequelae. J Neurosurg 58:760–762, 1983.
5. Ball GV: Ankylosing spondylitis. In McCarty D (ed): Arthritis and Allied Conditions, ed. 11. Philadelphia, Lea & Febiger, 1989, pp 934–941.
6. Barnsley N, Bogduk N, Lord S, et al: Cervical zygapophysial joint pain in whiplash: A double-blind, controlled prevalence study. Presented to 20th Annual Meeting of the Cervical Spine Research Society, Palm Desert, CA, Dec 3–5, 1992, abstr. No. 8.
7. Barnsley L, Chahl J, Lord S, et al: Diagnosis of cervical zygapophyseal pain by double blind differential anaesthetic blocks. Presented to 20th Annual Meeting of the Cervical Spine Research Society, Palm Desert, CA, Dec 3–5, 1992, abstr. No. 7.
8. Benzel EC, Hart BL, Ball PA, et al: The definition of soft tissue injury associated with acute cervical spine trauma by MRI, Presented to 20th Annual Meeting of the Cervical Spine Research Society, Palm Desert, CA, Dec 3–5, 1992, abstr. No. 6.
9. Bohlman HH: Acute fractures and dislocations of the cervical spine. J Bone Joint Surg Am 61:1119–1142, 1979.
10. Boismare F, Boquet J, Morre N, et al: Hemodynamic, behavioral and biochemical disturbances induced by an experimental cranio-cervical injury (whiplash) in rats. J Auton Nerv Syst 13:137–147, 1985.
11. Bracken MB, Shepard MJ, Collins WF, et al: A randomized, controlled trial of methylprednisolone or naloxone in the treatment of acute spinal-cord injury. N Engl J Med, 322:1405–1411, 1990.
12. Brieg A, Turnbull I, Hassler O: Effects of mechanical stresses on the spinal cord in cervical spondylosis. A study of fresh cadaver material. J Neurosurg 25:45–56, 1966.
13. Burke DC: Hyperextension injuries of the spine. J Bone Joint Surg Br 53:3–12, 1971.
14. Capistran TD: Thoracic outlet syndrome in whiplash injury. Ann Surg 185:175–178, 1977.
15. Carter DR, Frankel VH: Biomechanics of hyperextension injuries to the cervical spine in football. Am J Sports Med 8:302–309, 1980.
16. Cattell HS, Filtzer DL: Pseudosubluxation and other normal variations in the cervical spine in children. J Bone Joint Surg Am 47:1295–1309, 1965.
17. Cheng CLY, Wolf AL, Mirvis S, et al: Bodysurfing accidents resulting in cervical spine injuries. Spine 17:257–260, 1992.
18. Chester JB Jr: Whiplash, postural control and the inner ear. Spine 16:716–720, 1991.
19. Colachis SM Jr, Strohm BR: Radiographic studies of cervical

spine motion in normal subjects: Flexion and hyperextension. Arch Phys Med Rehabil, November, pp 753–760, 1965.

20. Darden BV II, Connor PM: Cervical discography. Complications and clinical efficacy. Presented to 20th Annual Meeting of the Cervical Spine Research Society, Palm Desert, CA, Dec 3–5, 1992, abstr. No. 25.

21. Davis SJ, Teresi LM, Bradley WG Jr, et al: Cervical spine hyperextension injuries: MR findings. Radiology 180:245–251, 1991.

22. Dietrich AM, Ginn-Pease ME, Bartkowski HM, et al: Pediatric cervical spine fractures: Predominantly subtle presentation. J Pediatr Surg 268:995–1000, 1991.

23. Epstein JA, Carras R, Hyman RA, et al: Cervical myelopathy caused by developmental stenosis of the spinal canal. J Neurosurg 51:362–367, 1979.

24. Fishman EK, Magid D, Morgan RH: Cervical fracture in ankylosing spondylitis: Value of multidimensional imaging. Clin Imaging 16:31–33, 1992.

25. Fitt G, Hennessy O, Thomas D: Transverse fracture with epidural and small paravertebral hematomata, in a patient with ankylosing spondylitis. Skeletal Radiol 21:61–63, 1992.

26. Foo D, Bignami A, Rossier AB: Two spinal cord lesions in a patient with ankylosing spondylitis and cervical spine injury. Neurology 33:245–249, 1983.

27. Forsyth HF: Extension injuries of the cervical spine. J Bone Joint Surg Am 46:1792–1797, 1964.

28. Gehweiler JA, Clark WM, Schaaf RE, et al: Cervical spine trauma: The common combined conditions. Radiology 130:77–86, 1979.

29. Goldberg AL, Rothfus WE, Deeb ZL, et al: Hyperextension injuries of the cervical spine, Skeletal Radiol 18:283–288, 1989.

30. Grisolia A, Bell RL, Peltier LF: Fractures and dislocations of the spine complicating ankylosing spondylitis. J Bone Joint Surg Am 49:339–344, 1967.

31. Harding JR, McCall IW, Park WM, et al: Fracture of the cervical spine in ankylosing spondylitis. Br J Radiol 58:3–7, 1985.

32. Harris JH, Yeakley JW: Hyperextension-dislocation of the cervical spine. J Bone Joint Surg Br 74:567–570, 1992.

33. Heise AP, Laskin DM, Gervin AS: Incidence of temporomandibular joint symptoms following whiplash injury. J Oral Maxillofac Surg 50:825–28, 1992.

34. Hershman EB, Bercik RJ, Allen SC, et al: Correction of chin-on-chest deformity in ankylosing spondylitis through a fracture site. A case report. Clin Orthop 201:201–204, 1985.

35. Hill SA, Miller CA, Kosnik EJ, et al: Pediatric neck injuries. J Neurosurg 60:700–706, 1984.

36. Hinck VC, Hopkins CE, Clark WM, et al: Sagittal diameter of the cervical spinal canal in children. Radiology 79:97–108, 1962.

37. Ho EK, Chan FL, Leong JC: Postsurgical recurrent stress fracture in the spine affected by ankylosing spondylitis. Clin Orthop 247:87–89, 1989.

38. Hohl M: Soft-tissue injuries of the neck in automobile accidents. J Bone Joint Surg Am 56:1675–1682, 1974.

39. Holdsworth F: Review article—Fractures, dislocations, and fracture-dislocations of the spine. J Bone Joint Surg Am 52:1534–1551, 1970.

40. Howcroft AJ, Jenkins DHR: Potentially fatal asphyxia following a minor injury of the cervical spine. J Bone Joint Surg Br 59:93–94, 1997.

41. Hunter T, Dubo H: Spinal fractures complicating ankylosing spondylitis. Ann Intern Med 88:546–549, 1978.

42. Janecki CJ Jr, Lipke JM: Whiplash syndrome. Am Fam Physician 17:144–151, 1978.

43. Kaplan SL, Tun CG, Sarkarati M: Odontoid fracture complicating ankylosing spondylitis. A case report and review of the literature. Spine 15:607–610, 1990.

44. Kelly JS, Hoover RE, George T: Whiplash maculopathy. Arch Ophthalmol 96:834–835, 1978.

45. Kim KS, Chen HH, Russell EJ, et al: Flexion teardrop fracture of the cervical spine: Radiographic characteristics. AJR 152:319–326, 1989.

46. Kinoshita H, Hirakawa H: Pathological studies and pathological principles on the management of extension injuries of the cervical spine. Paraplegia 27:172–181, 1989.

47. Kischka U, Ettlin T, Heim S, et al: Cerebral symptoms following whiplash injury. Eur Neurol 31:136–140, 1991.

48. Kiwerski J: The influence of the mechanism of cervical spine injury on the degree of the spinal cord lesion. Paraplegia 29:531–536, 1991.

49. Ladd A, Scranton PE: Congenital cervical stenosis presenting as transient quadriplegia in athletes. J Bone Joint Surg Am 68:1371–1374, 1986.

50. La Rocca H: Cervical sprain syndrome-diagnosis, treatment, and long-term outcome. *In* Frymoyer JW (ed): The Adult Spine: Principles and Practice. New York, Raven Press, 1991, pp 31–41.

51. Latimer EA III, Clevenger FW, Osler TM: Tear of the cervical esophagus following hyperextension from manual traction: Case report. J Trauma 31:1448–1449, 1991.

52. Levine AM, Fischgrund J, Edwards CC: Fractures of the C1–2 complex: Concurrent spinal injuries. Presented to 20th Annual Meeting of the Cervical Spine Research Society, Palm Desert, CA, Dec 3–5, 1992, abstr. No. 50.

53. Levine AM, Lutz B: Extension teardrop injuries of the cervical spine. Presented to 20th Annual Meeting of the Cervical Spine Research Society, Palm Desert, CA, Dec 3–5, 1992, abstr. No. 49.

54. Liu YK, Chandran KB, Heath RG, et al: Subcortical EEG changes in rhesus monkeys following experimental hyperextension-hyperflexion (whiplash). Spine 9:329–335, 1984.

55. Macnab I: Acceleration injuries of the cervical spine. J Bone Joint Surg Am 46:1797–1799, 1984.

56. Maimaris C, Barnes MR, Allen MJ: Whiplash injuries of the neck: A retrospective study. Injury 19:393–396, 1988.

57. Marar BC: Hyperextension injuries of the cervical spine. J Bone Joint Surg Am 56:1655–1662, 1974.

58. Maroon JC: "Burning hands" in football spinal cord injuries. JAMA 238:2049–2051, 1977.

59. Matyas JR: The structure and function of tendon and ligament insertions into bone. Thesis, Ithaca, NY, Cornell University, 1985.

60. McLain RF: Innervation of human cervical facets. Presented to 20th Annual Meeting of the Cervical Spine Research Society, Palm Desert, CA, Dec 3–5, 1992, abstr. No. 13.

61. Mealy K, Brennan H, Fenelon GCC: Early mobilization of acute whiplash injuries. Br Med J 292:656–657, 1986.

62. Meyer P Jr: Cervical spine fractures: Changing management concepts. *In* Bridwell KJ, Dewald RL (eds): The Textbook of Spinal Surgery. Philadelphia, JB Lippincott, 1991, p 1004.

63. Mirkovic S, Jain P, Meyer PR, et al: Cervical fractures in DISH: Surgical and clinical evaluation. Presented to 24th Annual Meeting of the Cervical Spine Research Society, Palm Beach, FL, Dec 5–7, 1996, poster No. 20.

64. Mirza S, Chapman J, Anderson P, et al: Assessment of instability in the lower cervical spine: Application of the White and Panjabi criteria and anatomic scoring to cervical spine injuries. Presented to 20th Annual Meeting of the Cervical Spine Research Society, Palm Beach, FL, Dec 5–7, 1996, poster No. 20.

65. Monroe BE, Wagner LK, Harris JH: Hyperextension dislocation of the cervical spine. AJR 146:803–808, 1986.

66. Murray GC, Persellin RH; Cervical fracture complicating ankylosing spondylitis: A report of eight cases and review of the literature. Am J Med 70:1033–1041, 1981.

67. Ohwada T, Tachibana S, Wada K, et al: Cervical myelopathy due to developmental stenosis of the spinal canal. Orthop Trans 2:32, 1978.

68. Olney DB, Marsden AK: The effect of head restraints and seat belts on the incidence of neck injury in car accidents. Injury 17:365–367, 1986.

69. Orenstein JB, Klein BL, Ochsenschlager DW: Delayed diagnosis of pediatric cervical spine injury. Pediatrics 89:1185–1188, 1992.

70. Osgood C, Martin LG, Ackerman E: Fracture-dislocation of the cervical spine with ankylosing spondylitis. Report of two cases. J Neurosurg 39: 764–769, 1973.

71. Pang D, Wilberger JE: Spinal cord injury without radiographic abnormalities in children. J Neurosurg 57:114–129, 1982.

72. Panjabi MM, Lydon C, Vasavada DG, et al: Biomechanical evaluation of diagnostic external fixation. Presented to 20th Annual Meeting of the Cervical Spine Research Society, Palm Desert, CA, Dec 3–5, 1992, abstr. No. 19.

73. Pearce JMS: Whiplash injury: A reappraisal. J Neurol Neurosurg Psychiatry 52:1329–1331, 1989.

74. Pennie BH, Agambar LJ: Whiplash injuries. J Bone Joint Surg Br 72:277–279, 1990.

75. Penning L: Some aspects of plain radiography of the cervical spine in chronic myelopathy. Neurology 12:513–519, 1962.

76. Penning L: Prevertebral hematoma in cervical spine injury: Incidence and etiologic significance. AJR 136:553–561, 1981.

77. Pitman MI, Pitman CA, Greenberg IM: Complete dislocation of the cervical spine without neurological deficit. J Bone Joint Surg Am 59:134–135, 1977.

78. Podolsky SM, Hoffman JR, Pietrafesa CA: Neurologic complications following immobilization of cervical spine fracture in a patient with ankylosing spondylitis. Ann Emerg Med 12:578–580, 1983.

79. Robinson MH, Young JD, Burge PD: Retropharyngeal abscess, airway obstruction and tetraplegia after hyperextension injury of the cervical spine: Case report. J Trauma 32:107–109, 1992.

80. Ruge JR, Sinson GP, McLone DG, et al: Pediatric spinal injury: The very young. J Neurosurg 68:25–30, 1988.

81. Schaefer DM, Flanders AE, Osterholm JL, et al: Prognostic significance of magnetic resonance imaging in the acute phase of cervical spine injury. J Neurosurg 76:218–223, 1992.

82. Scher AT: Cervical spine fusion and the effects of injury. S Afr Med J 56:525–527, 1979.

83. Scher AT: Dislocation of the cervical spine—A rare manifestation of hyperextension injury. S Afr Med J 55:998–999, 1979.

84. Scher AT: Diversity of radiological features in hyperextension injury of the cervical spine. S Afr Med J 58:27–30, 1980.

85. Scher AT: Serious cervical spine injury in the older rugby players. S Afr Med J 64:138–140, 1983.

86. Scher AT: Hyperextension trauma in the elderly: An easily overlooked spinal injury. J Trauma 23:1066–1068, 1983.

87. Schneider RC, Kahn EA: Chronic neurological sequelae of acute trauma to the spine and spinal cord. J Bone Joint Surg Am 38:985–997, 1956.

88. Schuyler-Hacker H, Green R, Wingate L, et al: Acute torticollis secondary to rupture of the sternocleidomastoid. Arch Phys Med Rehabil 70:851–853, 1989.

89. Severy DM, et al: Controlled automobile near-end collisions: An investigation of related engineering and medical phenomena. Car Serv Med J 11:727–759, 1955.

90. Shea M, Wittenberg RH, Edwards WT, et al: In vitro hyperextension in the human cadaveric cervical spine. J Orthop Res 10:911–916, 1992.

91. Sherk H: Cervical Spine Research Society, The Cervical Spine, ed 2. Philadelphia, JB Lippincott, 1989, pp 385, 580.

92. Shono Y, McAfee PC, Cunningham BW: Mechanisms of compression injuries in the cervical spine: Non-destructive and destructive investigative methods. Research award paper. Presented to 20th Annual Meeting of the Cervical Spine Research Society, Palm Desert, CA, Dec 3–5, 1992.

93. Smith JP, Morrissey P, Hemmick RS, et al: Retropharyngeal hematomas. J Trauma 28:553–554, 1988.

94. Speer KP, Bassett FH: The prolonged burner syndrome. Am J Sports Med 18:591–594, 1990.

95. Stanley JH, Schabel SI, Frey GD, et al: Quantitative analysis of the cervical spinal canal by computed tomography. Neuroradiology 28:139–143, 1986.

96. Starshak RJ, Kass GA, Samaraweera RN: Developmental stenosis of the cervical spine in children. Pediatr Radiol 17:291–295, 1987.

97. Stringer WL, Kelly DL: Traumatic dissection of the extracranial internal carotid artery. Neurosurgery 6:123–130, 1980.

98. Stringer WL, Kelly DL, Johnston FR, et al: Hyperextension injury of the cervical spine with esophageal perforation. J Neurosurg 53:541–543, 1980.

99. Taylor AR: The mechanism of injury to the spinal cord in the neck without damage to the vertebral columns. J Bone Joint Surg Br 33:543–547, 1951.

100. Taylor AR, Blackwood W: Paraplegia in hyperextension cervical injuries with normal radiographic appearances. J Bone Joint Surg Br 30:245–248, 1948.

101. Torg JS, Vegso JJ, Sennett B, et al: The National Football Head and Neck Injury Registry: 14-year report on cervical quadriplegia, 1971–1984. JAMA 254:3439–3443, 1985.

102. Torg JS, Pavlov H, Genuario SE: Neuropraxia of the cervical spinal cord with transient quadriplegia. J Bone Joint Surg Am 68:1354–1370, 1986.

103. Torg JS, Pavlov H, O'Neill MJ, et al: The axial load teardrop fracture. Am J Sports Med 19:355–364, 1991.

104. Wang JC, Hatch JD, Delamarter RB, et al: Emergent cervical flexion and extension radiographs in acutely injured patients. Presented to 24th Annual Meeting of the Cervical Spine Research Society, Palm Beach, FL, Dec 5–7, 1996, abstract No. 23.

105. Weinberg S, Lapointe H: Cervical extension-flexion injury (whiplash) and internal derangement of the temporomandibular joint. J Oral Maxillofac Surg 45:653–656, 1987.

106. Weinstein PR, Karpman RR, Gall EP, et al: Spinal cord injury, spinal fracture, and spinal stenosis in ankylosing spondylitis. J Neurosurg 57:609–616, 1982.

107. White AA III, Johnson RM, Panjabi MM, et al: Biomechanical analysis of clinical stability in the cervical spine. Clin Orthop 109:85–96, 1975.

108. Whitehill R: Fractures of the lower cervical spine: Subaxial fractures in the adult. Semin Spine Surg 3:71–86, 1991.

109. Wilkenson M, Bywaters EGL: Clinical feature and course of ankylosing spondylitis. Ann Rheum Dis 17:209–228, 1958.

110. Williams JF: The effect of collision severity on the motion of the head and neck during "whiplash." J Biomech 8:257–259, 1975.

THORACOLUMBAR INJURIES

Thoracolumbar Compression Fractures

Mark S. Cohen ‖ *Benjamin Blair* ‖ *Steven R. Garfin*

Compression wedge fractures account for the vast majority of osseous injuries of the thoracolumbar spine. Although epidemiologic studies are lacking, they represent between 48% and 90% of several large series of thoracolumbar spine injuries.[25, 43, 87, 118, 124] The injury mechanism involves a combination of forward flexion and axial compressive loading, producing a characteristic wedge-shaped vertebral deformity.

Prior to the use of computed axial imaging of the spine, all fractures resulting from spinal compression had been grouped similarly. Little emphasis was placed on the presence or absence of retropulsed bony fragments within the vertebral canal.[10, 11, 34, 79] With improved spinal imaging modalities, newer classification systems have been developed for spinal trauma.[19, 26–28, 34, 79] Pure compression fractures are now frequently defined as isolated failure of the anterior column in compression (see Chapter 4). The middle spinal column around the neurologic elements remains intact and functions as a hinge. The posterior column acts to resist generated tensile forces. The intact middle (and usually posterior) column accounts for the rarity of acute neurologic loss in these injuries.[40] This chapter focuses on this concept of pure compression injury and its etiology, biomechanical principles, treatment, and prognosis.

ETIOLOGY

Violent trauma is the most common cause of compression fractures in young and middle-aged people. Motor vehicle accidents and vertical plunges represent the largest sources,[30, 31, 35, 40, 55, 70, 81, 89, 91] followed by sports and recreational activities.[1, 50, 51, 57, 69, 77, 88] A high incidence of compression fractures (up to 30%) is seen in airplane pilots after use of an ejection seat.[52, 76, 114] Rarely, generalized rigidity or convulsive muscle spasms, as described with tetanus, can cause compression fractures.[109] In the elderly, osteoporosis is the most common cause of simple wedge compression fractures of the spine.[13, 29, 46, 56, 121] With osteoporotic bone, the vertebral bodies are especially vulnerable, and minor trauma, such as acutely flexing forward or lifting, may result in a compression fracture.

While the thoracolumbar junction is the most frequently affected area in spinal compression injuries, certain injury mechanisms have a predilection for specific spinal levels. For example, falling onto the buttocks, as occurs in parachute landings, results most commonly in L1 vertebral body fractures.[21, 42, 92] While flexion-compression injuries from aircraft ejections most commonly involve the midthoracic spinal levels,[52, 76] osteoporotic compression fractures have a predilection for the T12 to L4 region.[8, 13, 37, 102]

BIOMECHANICAL CONSIDERATIONS

The mechanism of injury in all wedge compression fractures involves an axially directed central compressive force in combination with an eccentric compres-

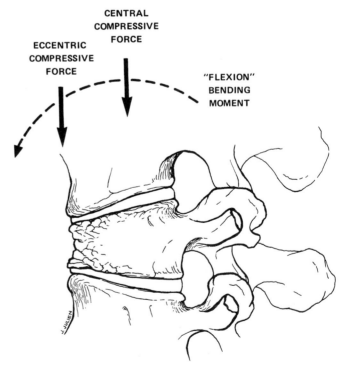

Figure 24–1 ═ Diagram depicting the mechanism of anterior wedge compression fractures of the thoracolumbar spine. An axial centrally directed force works in combination with an eccentric compressive force anteriorly. The latter induces a flexion bending moment. If the forces are great enough to overcome the intrinsic strength of the vertebral body, an anterior wedge compression fracture results.

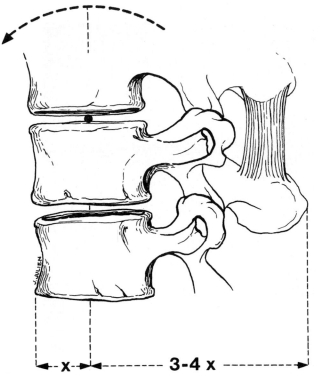

Figure 24–2 = Diagram showing the compressive and tension forces generated during compression injuries in the thoracolumbar spine. The *black dot* at the center of the nucleus pulposus represents the axis of rotation during the injury. The distance from this axis to the posterior border of the spinous process is three to four times as great as the distance to the anterior margin of the vertebral body. Thus, during flexion the anterior vertebral body is subjected to compressive forces three to four times as great as the tensile forces on the posterior ligamentous complex. The integrity of the posterior spinal elements are of great importance in evaluating the stability of wedge compression fractures (see text).

sive force. The latter force falls anterior to the axis of rotation (center of the nucleus pulposus) and results in a "flexion" bending moment (Fig. 24–1). If the forces are great enough to overcome the intrinsic mechanical strength of the vertebral body, an anterior wedge deformity results. The forces lead to progressive vertebral body compression until the energy becomes dissipated and the intrinsic bone strength is equal to or greater than the remaining compressive forces.

The pathologic sequence of vertebral body failure was described by Roaf.[98, 99] With pure flexion-compression forces, failure occurs first in the vertebral body end plate. This is because the intact disc has only limited compressibility and transmits the load to the contiguous bone. Further compression leads to fracture of the vertebral cortical shell. This is followed by compression of the subcortical cancellous vertebral bone.

In pure flexion-compression injuries, the middle column remains intact and acts as a hinge. This is pathognomonic of this injury. The posterior ligaments resist tensile forces, but can fail partially or completely with severe injuries. A simple analysis of the biomechanical moments involved clarifies this point. Anatomic measurements show that during spinal flexion injuries, the distance between the flexion axis (center of the

nucleus pulposus) and the spinous process is three to four times as great as the distance between the axis and the anterior vertebral body[98, 106, 110] (Fig. 24–2). If the compressive load experienced by the anterior vertebral body is force X, the posterior ligamentous complex thus must resist a corresponding tensile load of 1/3 to 1/4 X. As X increases, the load experienced posteriorly eventually exceeds the inherent strength of the ligamentous structures. The integrity of these posterior intervertebral ligaments is of major importance in the determination of mechanical stability (see Clinical Instability).

CLASSIFICATION

Four subtypes of anterior wedge compression fractures have been identified by Denis[26] (Fig. 24–3). The most common, type B, results in failure of the upper end plate with osseous compression of the cancellous bone of the proximal half of the vertebral body. The compression is usually symmetrical bilaterally. Less common patterns of injury involve failure of both end plates (type A), isolated failure of the lower end plate (type C), and a predominantly central failure of the anterior vertebral body (type D).

The lateral wedge compression fracture is a relatively uncommon injury. It accounts for between 8% and 14% of all wedge compression injuries and is most frequently seen in the midlumbar region of the spine.[26, 87, 118] The fracture is believed to be due to the same mechanism as that for anterior compression fractures,

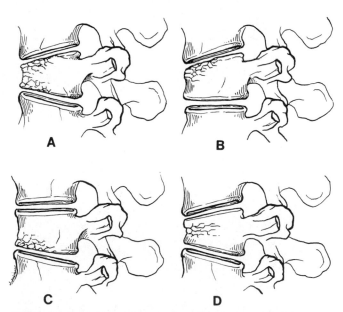

Figure 24–3 = Four subtypes of wedge compression fractures as described by Denis.[27] Type *A* involves a fracture of the superior and inferior end plates. Type *B*, the most common type, involves failure of the superior vertebral end plate with compression of a portion of the superior one half of the anterior vertebral body. Type *C* is an isolated failure of the inferior end plate with involvement of the inferior half of the vertebral body. Type *D* results in failure of the central aspect of the anterior vertebral body with relative preservation of the superior and inferior end plates.

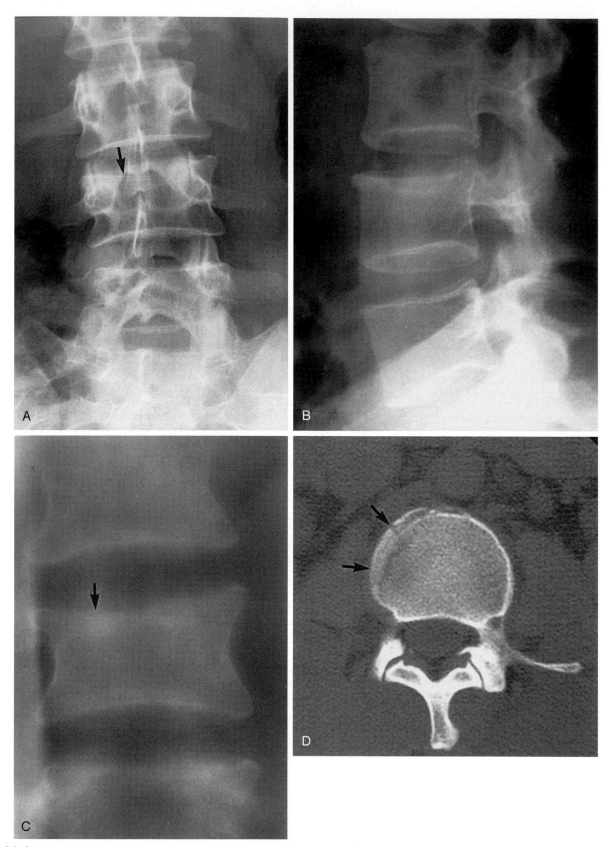

Figure 24–4 = Anteroposterior *(A)* and lateral *(B)* radiographs of a patient with a lateral wedge compression fracture of L4. The AP film shows asymmetrical collapse of the vertebral body *(arrow)*, which can be best appreciated on a plain tomogram in the coronal plane *(C)*. *D,* A CT scan through L4 in the axial plane reveals the asymmetrical fracture of the vertebral body *(arrows)*.

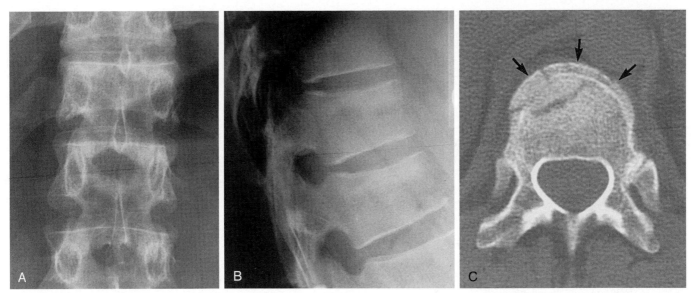

Figure 24–5 ═ Anteroposterior *(A)* and lateral *(B)* radiographs of a patient with adjacent anterior compression fractures of bodies of T12 and L1. Note the anterior wedging of the vertebral bodies with preservation of the posterior vertebral body height and the posterior vertebral body line. C, A CT scan through L1 reveals compression of the superior end plate and anterior vertebral body *(arrows)* with no disruption of the posterior vertebral wall (middle column). The intact posterior vertebral body wall separates the pure anterior wedge fracture from the more unstable burst fracture.

except for asymmetrical collapse of the vertebral body in the sagittal plane (Fig. 24–4).

DIAGNOSIS

The diagnosis of wedge compression fractures depends on a careful review of the anteroposterior (AP) and lateral radiographs, as well as computed tomography (CT) imaging. The AP view shows loss of vertebral height, which is usually symmetrical. The lateral view reveals wedging of the vertebral body with loss of the anterior body height. The posterior vertebral body height is characteristically unchanged (Fig. 24–5A and B).

The plain films must be scrutinized for subtle abnormalities to rule out more severe injuries. For example, if the AP radiograph reveals widening of the interpedicular distance of the fractured vertebral body, a more serious burst fracture has occurred (involvement of the middle column). Similarly, any disruption of the posterior vertebral body cortex on the lateral film denotes a burst injury as opposed to a pure compression injury. Disruption of this line, by definition, implies middle column involvement.[23] McGroy and colleagues have described the use of the posterior vertebral angle to help differentiate compression fractures from minimal burst fractures.[80] This angle is formed by drawing a line parallel with the end plates and a line parallel with the posterior vertebral cortex. An angle greater than 100 degrees suggests a burst fracture. Subluxation of the vertebral bodies on the lateral radiograph indicates a fracture-dislocation injury. Gradations invariably occur between wedge, burst, and fracture-dislocations secondary to forces that are a combination of, or intermediate between, the forces producing the pure

injuries.[27, 62, 99] Ultimately, multiplanar CT (or polytomography) must be utilized to document the intact vertebral ring of the pure wedge compression injury (Fig. 24–5C). This is necessary, as an error rate of up to 25% in differentiating compression fractures from burst fractures based on plain films alone has been reported.[4]

The severity of compression fractures may be defined by the percentage of anterior vertebral body collapse and corresponding kyphotic deformity. The percentage collapse may be calculated by measuring the remaining anterior vertebral body height, divided by the average height of the anterior vertebral bodies above and below the level of injury, as measured on the lateral radiograph.[119] Alternatively, it can be calculated by dividing the remaining anterior vertebral body height by the posterior vertebral body height of the involved vertebra (Fig. 24–6). The angular deformity is measured by the Cobb angle between the first intact end plate on either side of the injured segment.[22]

Upper Thoracic Compression Fractures (T2–10)

The upper thoracic spine, on account of the rib cage, has unique mechanical characteristics and must be discussed separately. The rib cage stiffens the motion segments at each level in the thoracic spine, resisting bending and axial rotation forces. In vitro studies have shown that the load-bearing capacity of the isolated spine can support two to three times greater compressive loads before instability occurs with the addition of the rib cage.[2] Furthermore, the rib cage increases the bending stiffness of the spine in flexion by 27%.[2]

On account of the ribs, considerable force is necessary to produce a compression injury of the upper thoracic spine. These fractures are associated with a

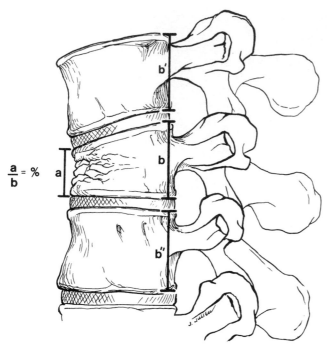

Figure 24–6 = Diagram depicting the calculation of the severity of thoracolumbar wedge compression fractures. The degree of compression is calculated from the measurement of the remaining anterior vertebral body height *a* divided by the posterior height of the involved vertebral body *b*. Alternatively, the remaining anterior vertebral body height *a* can be divided by the average of the anterior vertebral body heights of the adjacent superior and inferior intact vertebral bodies. Note, that in pure anterior compression fractures the posterior vertebral body height remains unchanged (*b* = *b*′ = *b*″).

high degree of concomitant injuries to the chest, head, and cervical spine.[10, 14, 45, 71, 81] Several reports document dislocations of the manubriosternal joint in high thoracic compression fractures due to the large forces accompanying these injuries.[103, 119]

Another important difference between the thoracic spine and the lumbar spine is the presence of the spinal cord. In this region, the spinal canal is narrowed, with less free space between the cord and the osseous ring. The central thoracic spine also has a relatively sparse blood supply.[11, 71, 120] Because of this, spinal cord injury may occur with less percentage of compression or degree of kyphosis than in the lumbar spine. Multiple thoracic wedge compression fractures are the primary exception to the rule that pure flexion-compression injuries do not cause acute neurologic loss.[14, 79, 122]

Thoracolumbar Compression Fractures (T11–L5)

The great majority of compression fractures occur at the thoracolumbar junction (T11–L2), at the fulcrum of motion between the relatively stiff thoracic spine and the mobile lumbar spine.* This region accounts for between 54% and 70% of noncervical wedge compression fractures in reported series.[26, 40, 111, 117, 118, 124] This

---

*References 10, 30, 40, 56, 67, 79, 81, 87, 97, 111, 117, 118, and 124.

is also the most common region for multiple wedge compression injuries, with a lesser peak in the midthoracic region.[111]

The lower lumbar spine (L3–5) accounts for the minority of wedge compression injuries. Normally, very high loads are borne in the lower lumbar region of the spine, and well-developed paraspinal musculature aids in mechanical support of this region. Biomechanical evidence suggests that the lower lumbar vertebrae are mechanically stronger than the upper lumbar vertebrae.[91] Additionally, this area maintains a lordotic posture, which may somewhat shield the vertebral bodies from high direct compressive forces.

CLINICAL INSTABILITY

Mechanical stability reflects the ability of the spine under physiologic loading to limit subsequent deformation and neurologic compromise.[119, 120, 122] Mild wedge compression fractures are generally considered stable injuries. Panjabi et al.[90] have emphasized that biomechanically the middle column is the primary determinant of stability. As compression fractures have, by definition, intact middle columns, they are inherently stable. In more severe wedge compression fractures, stability depends on two factors: the ability of the anteriorly compressed vertebra (anterior column) to withstand further compressive loading and the ability of the interspinous and other posterior ligaments (posterior column) to resist tensile forces. As early as 1949, Nicoll recognized that wedge compression fractures could be unstable if rupture of the posterior ligaments occurred.[87] Failure of these ligaments allows the spine to bend around the hinge of the middle column and, perhaps, collapse further.

Ching and associates[20] assessed the residual stability of thoracolumbar spine fractures as a function of the type of injury. They found increased instability in the sagittal plane in flexion-distraction injuries of 126% compared with only 40% in pure compression fractures. Similarly, flexion-distraction injuries showed an increased torsional instability of 62% compared with the torsional instability for compression fractures, which increased only 3%.

The ability of compressed vertebrae to withstand loading has been studied in vitro. Plaue[93] studied cadaveric specimens and found that compressed vertebral bodies were able to withstand greater than 60% of their original load-bearing capacity. In fact, at 50% compression, the vertebral body began to approach 100% of its original load-bearing ability. This was attributed to impaction of the cancellous vertebral bone, creating "stability." Keaveny and colleagues[65] have also shown that after compression fracture, elasticity of the vertebral body decreases, while overall strength remains unchanged. This remains true until large strain levels occur. The authors attributed this to the fact that for smaller compression fractures the trabeculae are damaged, but the cortical shell remains relatively intact, allowing stress transfer to the cortical bone with strength remaining constant. In vivo, however, untreated severe wedge compression fractures often undergo progressive wedging.[3, 10, 11, 87, 110] Mechanical forces play a major role. The greater the wedging and kyphotic deformity, the greater the moment arm. The greater the moment arm, the greater the tendency toward further progression.[119, 121] A vicious circle can thus ensue.

Another consideration in vertebral body integrity following compression injury involves the occasional occurrence of post-traumatic osteonecrosis (Kümmell's disease).[5–7, 16, 63, 86, 87, 95, 119] In this condition, increased radiodensity of the vertebral body is seen on the radiograph in association with collapse days to years after the injury. Pathologic specimens have supported the concept of osteonecrosis,[63, 73, 104, 105] believed to be secondary to vascular insult at the time of injury. The frequency of this condition is not known, but it is probably more frequent than reported. Patients are generally middle-aged and older. Reported cases principally involve the lower thoracic and upper lumbar spine. Although some think the likelihood of post-traumatic osteonecrosis increases with severity of injury,[87, 119] documented cases describe the process with only minor anterior vertebral wedging after the initial injury[7, 16] (Fig. 24–7). This emphasizes the need for close clinical and radiographic follow-up of all spinal compression injuries. In particular, these patients are at increased risk of delayed neurologic deterioration if further collapse occurs, leading to canal encroachment.[63]

The other major determining factor in the stability of compression injuries is the integrity of the posterior osseoligamentous complex (posterior column). As previously described, anterior vertebral collapse places tensile forces on the posterior ligaments approximately one fourth to one third as great as the anterior compressive forces. A widened interspinous process distance in simple compression fractures is often thought to represent posterior column tension failure.[36, 53, 54] Neumann and co-workers,[85] using a cadaver lumbar spine injury model, found instability exists if a relative increase in interspinous process distance of greater than 33 mm is seen on AP radiographs. However, the posterior spinous ligaments are not taut in neutral position and flexion of the normal spine leads to a physiologic increase in the interspinous process distance. In turn, compression fractures are routinely associated with an increased interspinous process distance geometrically proportional to the deformity of the anterior wedged vertebra.[26–28] The question becomes one of degree, that is, what percentage of compression is necessary to produce posterior ligamentous failure?

White and Panjabi[119] state that wedging of greater than 50% of the vertebral body is suggestive of posterior ligamentous disruption and instability. This figure is cited throughout the literature and is generally accepted as the cutoff for wedge compression fracture stability.* However, this figure is based on "biomechanical theory" as representing greater *likelihood* of posterior ligamentous failure. It is not known exactly how much separation of the posterior elements can reliably be correlated with structural failure of the posterior ligaments. Interestingly, Roaf[98] was unable to cause complete rupture of the posterior ligaments with flexion-compression injuries in cadaveric spines. He found the addition of rotatory forces necessary to produce posterior ligamentous rupture. The integrity of the posterior spinous ligaments may depend on the magnitude, direction, and rate of the applied forces, as well as the patient's age and location of the fracture. Flexion radiographs may be helpful in determining the status of the posterior spinal column soft tissues. Magnetic resonance imaging (MRI) has made it possible to identify injuries to the posterior ligamentous structures as noted by increased signal intensity between spinous processes on T2-weighted images.[15]

At this time, it can only be concluded that the theoretical probability of mechanical instability in wedge compression fractures is (1) increased with increasing severity of vertebral wedging and comminution, (2) affected by the presence or absence of post-traumatic osteonecrosis, and (3) related to the integrity of the posterior ligaments. Finally, although rare, the presence of a neurologic deficit indicates clinical instability.[39, 119] For obvious reasons, wedge compression fractures must never be treated with laminectomy. The isolated surgical removal of the posterior column is associated with progressive spinal instability.[11, 14, 35, 74, 84, 100, 119, 123]

TREATMENT

The classic management of stable thoracolumbar compression fractures consists of postural reduction by hyperextension and immobilization in a plaster jacket.[3, 9, 24, 101, 115, 118] Almost all authors today consider wedge fractures with compression to less than 30% to 40% of the original vertebral height to be stable injuries. Current treatment guidelines include a short term of bed rest, from days to a few weeks, followed by active mobilization. During ambulation the spine can be either unprotected or supported in a brace or appropriately molded orthosis for 3 to 6 months.[10, 60, 79, 119] Almost all patients benefit symptomatically from some type of orthosis, even if not rigid. We generally use a rigid orthosis for symptomatic treatment and molded jackets if correction of a deformity is achievable. Long-term radiographic follow-up is necessary to evaluate healing and document lack of kyphotic progression.

Compression fractures greater than 50% of the original height of the vertebral body in physiologically "young" patients are believed by the majority of authors to be unstable with the potential for further progression and collapse.* This is related to the fact that the force required to fracture healthy vertebrae this much often leads to posterior element disruption. However, few long-term clinical or biomechanical data are available to support this view. Progression may be secondary to anterior bony column failure by a mechanical lever arm, or it may be due to a higher

---

* References 14, 28, 33, 34, 60, 61, 71, 81, 117, and 122.

* References 14, 28, 33, 34, 60, 61, 71, 81, 117, and 119.

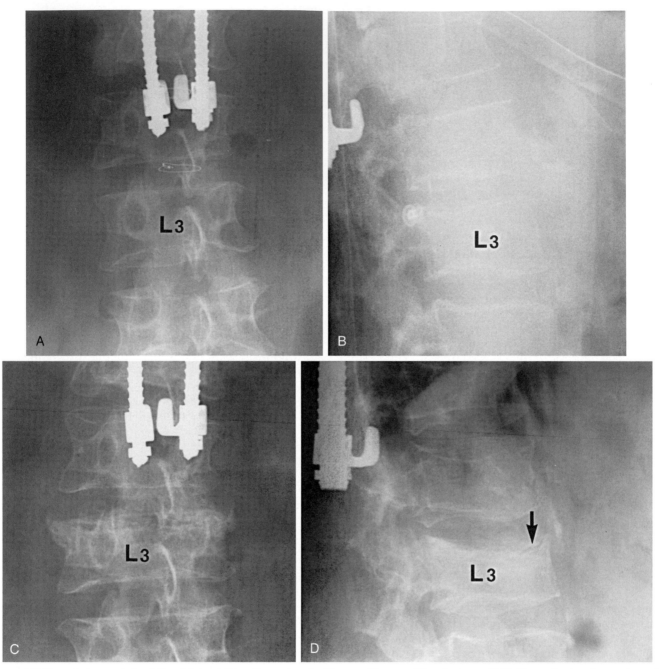

Figure 24–7 = Anteroposterior *(A)* and lateral *(B)* radiographs of a 55-year-old man with a fracture of L12. The patient underwent anterior decompression and posterior instrumentation and fusion from T11 to L1 at the time of injury. Note the preservation of the L3 vertebral body height. He presented at approximately 6 months post injury with progressive low back pain. *C* and *D*, Radiographs revealed collapse of the body of L3. Note the relative radiodensity of the entire vertebral body and intraosseous vacuum within the vertebral body *(D, arrow)* consistent with post-traumatic osteonecrosis (Kümmell's disease).

probability of posterior ligamentous failure. In any regard, there is little disagreement on surgical treatment in severely wedged vertebral compression injuries.

The treatment of wedge fractures with compression to between 30% and 50% of the original vertebral body height is less clearly defined. Bohlman[10] suggests operative reduction and fixation for wedge compression injuries greater than 40%, whereas others think this only results in cosmetic benefit.[110] We frequently treat wedge compression injuries greater than 30% to 40% in young and middle-aged adults operatively, taking

patient age, activity level, medical condition, and associated trauma into consideration. Operative fixation has several advantages in addition to treating potential instability. These include earlier mobilization and rehabilitation; decreased incidence of pulmonary, deep venous thrombotic and decubitus ulcer complications; the avoidance of disuse osteoporosis; and a decrease in the potential for the psychological sequelae of prolonged bed rest. This is especially true in patients suffering from multiple trauma. The more anatomic reduction offered by distraction rodding has the additional advantage of restoring normal posture. Any residual kyphosis secondary to a wedge fracture is often compensated by hyperlordosis of the caudal spinal segments to regain a balanced vertical posture. Compensatory hyperlordosis may be a potential source of chronic low back pain following more severely wedged compression injuries.[31, 56, 61, 122]

High Thoracic Fractures

The treatment of high thoracic compression fractures requires special mention. Fractures between T2 and T10 are believed by some to be stable injuries owing to the rib cage functioning as a stabilizing outrigger.[10, 11] However, because of the rib cage, much higher forces are necessary to cause compression injuries in this area. In addition, the normal kyphosis of the thoracic spine mechanically predisposes to further deformity by the increasing moment arm that accompanies increases in kyphotic angulation.[119, 121] Bohlman[10] believes the major indication for treatment of wedge compression injuries in this area is a thoracic kyphosis of greater than 40 degrees. Edwards and Levine[31] state that late pain is not uncommon with greater than 20 degrees of residual post-traumatic kyphosis. McAfee and co-authors[79] state the only indication for operative fixation is progressive angulation with an associated neurologic deficit. Other authors, including ourselves, treat these fractures under the same guidelines used for other thoracolumbar compression injuries.

Multiple Wedge Compression Fractures

The treatment of multiple adjacent wedge compression fractures (see Fig. 24–5) is currently poorly defined. As previously mentioned, when in the thoracic spine, these injuries may be associated with acute neurologic compromise.[14, 79, 122] In cases without neurologic involvement, several reports document multiple wedge compression injuries leading to progressive deformity and spinal instability.[14, 111, 112] For a given patient, no clear guidelines exist for these injuries. For example, should two adjacent wedge compression injuries, 30% each, be considered a stable injury, or is this equivalent to one 60% vertebral body compression fracture? Theoretically, the probability of posterior ligamentous failure is not additive, as the tensile forces are spread over two adjacent intervertebral segments. However, the magnitude of the acute kyphosis resulting from multiple anterior wedge fractures is additive and must be considered. The greater the angular deformity, the greater the chance for additional angulation due to the increased moment arm related to the deformity. Increased kyphosis also increases the need for compensatory hyperlordosis of the lumbar spine and postural difficulties.

We generally recommend operative reduction and fusion in any case involving neurologic compromise or if any of the following criteria are met: (1) if the compression in any of the multiple adjacent vertebral wedge fractures measures over 35% to 40% in a young or middle-aged adult, (2) if the compression percent-ages for the adjacent vertebral wedge fractures add to greater than 50%, or (3) if an acute kyphosis is present. For borderline cases, the aforementioned advantages of operative fixation apply and should be considered for each patient.

Surgical Instrumentation

Posterior distraction rodding and fusion is the traditional treatment modality for vertebral compression injuries. Posterior distraction instrumentation produces a bending moment that acts to reduce the kyphotic deformity. The intact anterior longitudinal ligament helps maintain the integrity of the vertebral body (ligamentotaxis) and prevents overdistraction. While some authors prefer anterior strut grafting[122] or anterior distraction rodding,[33] most authors agree that compression injuries, if treated early, can be managed by a posterior approach. Standard straight Harrington rod instrumentation for spinal trauma requires long instrumented segments to reduce the fracture, and is associated with fairly high complication rates.[11, 28, 38, 78] Current improvements in instrumentation for spinal trauma include the square-ended rod of Moe and Denis[83] and the rod sleeve system introduced by Edwards and Levine.[31] The sleeves allow for rigid three-point fixation and provide a dynamic corrective force leading to a more anatomic long-term reduction (Fig. 24–8). With this instrumentation, fusion can be limited to one to two interspaces beyond the injured spinal segments in the majority of cases.[31] This can also be achieved by short segment fixation with a pedicle-based fixation system. These, however, do not provide three-point fixation, and collapse or loss of alignment may occur, particularly at the thoracolumbar junction. Compression injuries treated after approximately 14 to 21 days or injuries operated on for late progressive spinal instability require an anterior approach for ligament and disc release, partial vertebrectomy, and strut grafting with or without a concomitant posterior stabilizing procedure. Alternatively, and as preferred by us, anterior instrumentation may be used.

PROGNOSIS

Wedge compression fractures are often complicated by long-term complaints of back pain. Controversy exists regarding the contribution of fracture severity to late symptoms. In 1949, Watson-Jones wrote, "Perfect recovery is possible only if perfect reduction is insisted upon . . . even slight degrees of wedging of the vertebra may cause persistent aching pain."[116] Several long-term follow-up studies on compression fractures have yielded conflicting results regarding this point.

In 1949, Nicoll reported on 88 anterior wedge thoracolumbar compression fractures in coal miners treated symptomatically with and without plaster jackets.[87] At follow-up, approximately 70% of patients complained of residual pain. In nearly three quarters of these, the pain was referred to the lower lumbar spine regardless of the fracture level. Nicoll attributed this pain to soft

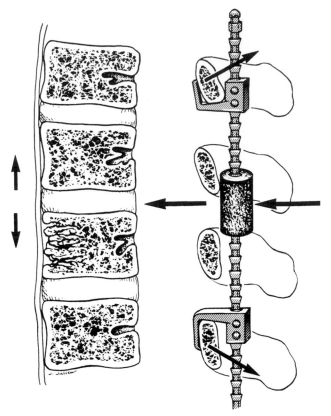

Figure 24–8 = Diagram depicting the biomechanics of the rod sleeve system used to reduce compression fractures. Sleeves added to the posterior distraction rods provide a dynamic corrective force at the fractured vertebral body. Corrective moments are generated through moment arms about the hooks resulting in both distraction and hyperextension of the anteriorly compressed vertebral body.

tissue injury of the spinal muscles and ligaments. Importantly, approximately 40% of his patients were able to return to manual labor irrespective of fracture severity. He concluded that a marked deformity was compatible with a good functional result.

Young[124] and Hazel and associates[48] support this concept. Young evaluated over 600 patients from 3 to 8 years following thoracolumbar spinal injuries, the majority being compression fractures. Although 70% of his patients complained of some degree of back pain (22% incapacitating), he could show no correlation between fracture severity and symptoms at follow-up.[124] Hazel and colleagues[48] reviewed 25 patients an average of 12 years after thoracolumbar compression injuries. While 45% of patients had occasional back pain and 25% complained of frequent pain, these investigators also could demonstrate no correlation between degree of compression and late symptoms.[48]

Several studies challenge this premise. In 1951, Westerborn and Olsson[118] reported on 104 patients with thoracolumbar injuries (83% anterior wedge, 7% lateral wedge) with an average follow-up of over 5 years. Patients were initially treated with hyperextension and plaster immobilization. While 90% of patients were able to return to their preinjury employment and activity, approximately 30% complained of residual symptoms from their injury. Low back pain was again more

common than pain at the site of injury. After reviewing outcomes in their patients, these authors concluded that a marked persistent kyphosis affects the end result.

In 1951, Baab and Howorth[3] reviewed 125 cases of compression fractures treated with a hyperextension jacket with a 5-year average follow-up. Approximately 17% of patients suffered disabling residual pain. Multiple fractures and lateral compression fractures had less satisfactory results, and these authors also concluded that the greater the compression, the more severe the symptoms at the time of follow-up.

Later studies report similar findings. Day and Kokan[25] studied 220 patients (greater than 90% wedge compression) and found half with residual symptoms, 25% disabling. They found lumbar fractures to carry a worse prognosis than thoracic compression injuries, and again the severity of compression correlated with a negative outcome. Soreff[108] reviewed 147 compression injuries and found that objective radiographic abnormalities correlated with symptoms and disability, with lumbar fractures causing greater long-term disability than thoracic injuries. Harkonen and co-workers[43–45] reviewed 242 Finnish patients with thoracic and lumbar fractures and found approximately 75% of patients complaining of late occasional or continuous pain. Kyphotic deformity again correlated with poorer clinical results. Interestingly, they found age greater than 40 years to predispose toward pain and disability. Gertzbein[39] performed a prospective multicenter study on thoracic and lumbar spine fractures, including a subset of 104 compression fractures. He found a positive relationship between the presence of a kyphotic deformity at 1 year post injury and pain. In particular, an increased incidence of moderate to severe pain was noted in kyphotic deformities of greater than 30 degrees.

In sum, it appears that a subset of patients with wedge compression injuries will have residual complaints related to the back. Low back pain appears to be more common than pain at the fracture site, and this may be related to compensatory hyperlordosis. There is evidence suggesting that more severe fractures carry a worse prognosis if treated conservatively and not anatomically corrected. These facts lend support to a more aggressive treatment of compression injuries, particularly with marked compression. For patients with chronic pain, good results with anterior corpectomy and strut fusion have been described.[12]

PEDIATRIC COMPRESSION FRACTURES

Several differences make spinal compression fractures in children different from those in adults. Vertebral bodies in children are well mineralized, and the spinal column in children is more elastic. This makes fractures of the spine in children uncommon. The discs are healthy and have a high turgor pressure. This allows the transmission of force to multiple spinal levels. Finally, the vertebral body epiphyses are open. This allows for a remodeling of the compressed vertebra,

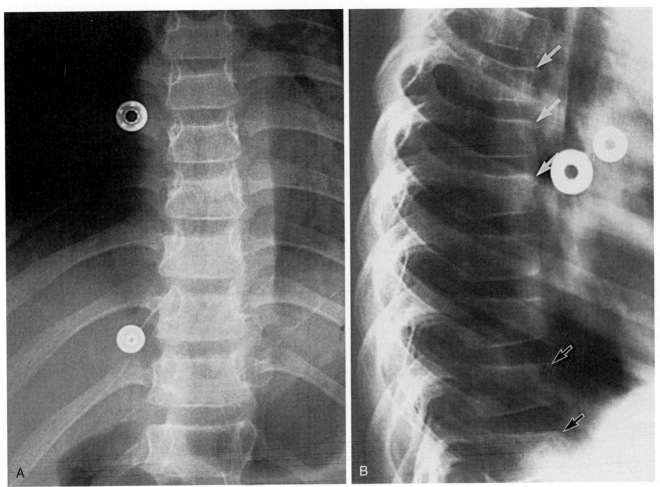

Figure 24–9 = Anteroposterior *(A)* and lateral *(B)* radiographs of a 9-year-old boy with multiple compression fractures of the thoracolumbar spine. The child presented with acute midthoracic as well as thoracolumbar junction pain following a motor vehicle accident. Note the subtle anterior wedging and comminution of T4–6 *(white arrows* in *B)* and the additional compression of the T9 and T10 *(black arrows)* vertebral bodies.

and an infrequent occurrence of late kyphotic deformities.

Several reports on thoracolumbar compression fractures in children between the age of 2 and 15 years exist and document the differences between this age group and adults.[49, 55, 57, 58] Multiple-level compression injuries are the rule, constituting between 66% and 90% of reported series (Fig. 24–9). Of note, some authors have remarked on the relative difficulty in interpretation of radiographic studies, particularly CT scans, in pediatric patients with compression fractures, making the diagnosis at times difficult.[40] The average patient has two to four affected vertebrae, with 11 compressed vertebrae being the highest number reported.[49] The primary location of fractures in this age group is the thoracic spine, especially midthoracic. At follow-up, some restoration of vertebral height is seen in almost all patients. Recovery of vertebral height is proportional to the severity of the compression and the age of the patient. Restoration is generally complete prior to the age of 10. A slight, clinically insignificant scoliosis (less than 10 degrees) is common and is believed to be secondary to uneven compression of the epiphysis. Progression of deformity is uncommon, as are posttraumatic degencrative changes.

Follow-up studies indicate that, even in children, a number of patients report long-term back pain after compression fractures, up to a mean of 16 years post injury.[55] Back pain affects from 38% to 67% of patients and is generally mild and intermittent without functional disability.[55, 57, 58] Treatment of these fractures is generally symptomatic in the younger ages. Short-term bed rest is followed by early mobilization with or without extension supports. By approximately 10 years of age, the thoracolumbar spine approaches the adult spine in biomechanical properties,[50] and by the teens, the indications for operative treatment are similar to those for adults.

OSTEOPOROTIC COMPRESSION FRACTURES

The characteristics of the elderly spine are opposite to those of the child or adolescent. The spine is less flexible, with poorly mineralized vertebral bodies and degenerative intervertebral discs. Recently, a number of studies have shown that the occurrence of compression fractures can be predicted by measuring, with a number of modalities, bone mineral density in the lumbar

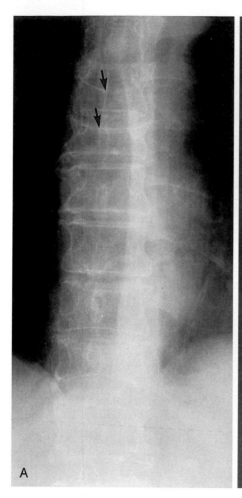
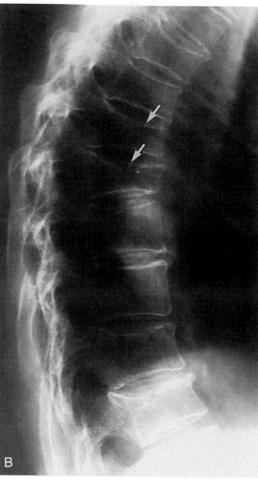

Figure 24–10 = Anteroposterior (A) and lateral (B) radiographs of an elderly patient with multiple osteoporotic thoracolumbar wedge compression fractures. Note the generalized osteopenia and the biconcave profile (codfish) appearance of the fractures (arrows).

spine.[40, 47, 64] Aside from overall decreased bone mass, changes in the geometric properties of the vertebral body increase further the risk of compression fractures in the elderly population.[107] Wedge compression fractures, often multiple, account for the vast majority of vertebral fractures in the elderly. It is estimated that by the eighth decade of life, 50% of women will develop spinal compression fractures.[41, 59, 72] Although common, these fractures are not innocuous, with studies showing decreased physical, functional, and psychosocial performance in elderly patients with osteoporotic compression fractures compared with those without.[75]

As organ transplantation programs multiply, there is also an increasing number of young patients with osteoporotic compression fractures, probably related to immunosuppressive therapy.[66, 96, 113] Another population at risk for osteoporotic compression fractures is patients with ankylosing spondylitis, with some authors attributing the spinal deformities seen with the disease to multiple compression fractures in the thoracic and lumbar spine.[94]

The mechanism for fracture remains a combination of flexion with axial compression. However, as the load-bearing capacity of the vertebral bodies decreases with age, minor events (bending, lifting) can lead to the so-called atraumatic vertebral compression fracture in the elderly.[17, 18, 32, 37] Mizrahi and associates[82] performed finite element stress analysis of osteoporotic

lumbar vertebral bodies and found peak stresses to rise by 250% when the vertebral body is loaded asymmetrically, compared to a normal vertebral body. Because the disc is no longer able to act as a fulcrum, the vertebral body not infrequently compresses uniformly. The characteristic biconcave profile of the vertebral bodies (codfish vertebrae) results[87, 95, 110, 118] (Fig. 24–10). The condition has a predilection for the T12–L4 vertebral area, with the L1 vertebral body being exceptionally susceptible.[8, 13, 37, 102]

The diagnosis of osteoporotic compression fractures is based chiefly on radiographic evidence of significantly decreased bone density. On plain radiographs, this is seen as a decrease in both number and size of trabeculae in the cancellous vertebral body. It requires up to 30% loss of bone mineral, however, before changes become obvious on plain radiographs. Therefore, other, more sensitive methods are required to determine those at risk. Currently, dual-energy x-ray absorptiometry (DEXA) is the modality of choice for determining bone mineral density.

These fractures can be treated symptomatically with a corset or hyperextension brace if tolerated. Early mobilization and avoidance of prolonged bed rest are important. Late collapse is a possibility in these patients, and close clinical and radiographic follow-up is critical. Kaneda and colleagues[63] reported on 22 patients with osteoporotic compression fractures who were initially neurologically intact. Over an interval of 1 to 12 months the patients developed neurologic deficits. These patients underwent anterior corpectomy and placement of a bioactive ceramic vertebral spacer as well as the Kaneda device for anterior fixation. The authors were able to correct kyphosis from an average of 27.8 degrees preoperatively to 13.3 degrees postoperatively, with little deterioration at follow-up. Interestingly, they studied histologically the bone resected from the collapsed vertebrae and found necrosis secondary to ischemia. This supports the concept of late collapse being due to avascular necrosis. All patients in the study had excellent functional return.

PATHOLOGIC COMPRESSION FRACTURES

Compression fractures accompany a variety of systemic disorders involving bone. In the child, spinal compression fractures are associated with lymphoma, eosinophilic granuloma, Gaucher's disease, the mucopolysaccharidoses, osteogenesis imperfecta, and idiopathic juvenile osteoporosis.[50] In older patients, metabolic and metastatic disease may contribute to compression injuries. Less commonly, infection may be a cause of vertebral collapse, especially in high-risk and immunocompromised patients.

REFERENCES

1. Alexander MJ: Biomechanical aspects of lumbar spine injuries in athletes: A review. Can J Appl Physiol 10:1–20, 1985.
2. Andriacchi T, Schultz A, Belytschko T, et al: A model for studies of mechanical interactions between the human spine and rib cage. J Biomech 7:497–507, 1974.
3. Baab OD, Howorth MB: Fractures of the dorsal and lumbar vertebrae. JAMA 146:2, 1951.
4. Ballock RT, Mackersie R, Abitbol J-J, et al: Can burst fractures be predicted from plain radiographs? J Bone Joint Surg Br 74:147–150, 1992.
5. Bedbrook GM: Stability of spinal fractures and fracture-dislocations. Paraplegia 9:23–32, 1971.
6. Benedek TG, Nicholas JJ: Delayed traumatic vertebral body compression fracture; part 2: Pathologic features. Semin Arthritis Rheum 10:271, 1981.
7. Benedek TG, Nicholas JJ, Reece GJ: Kümmell's disease: A rare cause of post-traumatic back pain. Arthritis Rheum 23:653, 1980.
8. Bick EM, Copel JW: Fractures of the vertebrae in the aged. Geriatrics 5:74, 1950.
9. Böhler L: Treatment of Fractures, ed 5, vol 2. New York, Grune & Stratton, 1957.
10. Bohlman HH: Treatment of fractures and dislocations of the thoracic and lumbar spine. J Bone Joint Surg Am 67:165–169, 1985.
11. Bohlman HH, Ducker TB, Lucas JT: Spine and spinal cord injury in the spine. In Rothman RH, Simeone FA (eds): The Spine, ed 2. Philadelphia, WB Saunders, 1982, pp 661–756.
12. Bohlman HH, Kirkpatrick JS, Delmarter RB, et al: Anterior decompression for late pain and paralysis after fracture of the thoracolumbar spine. Clin Orthop 300:24–29, 1994.
13. Boukhris R, Becker KL: The inter-relationship between vertebral fractures and osteoporosis. Clin Orthop 90:209–216, 1973.
14. Bradford DS, Akbarnia BA, Winter RB, et al: Surgical stabilization of fracture and fracture-dislocations of the thoracic spine. Spine 2:185–196, 1977.
15. Brightman RP, Miller CA, Rea GL, et al: Magnetic resonance imaging of trauma to the thoracic and lumbar spine. Spine 17:541–550, 1992.
16. Brower AC, Downey EF Jr: Kümmell disease: Report of a case with serial radiographs. Radiology 141:363, 1981.
17. Buchanan JR, Myers CA, Greer RB: A comparison of the risk of vertebral fracture in menopausal osteopenia and other metabolic disturbances. J Bone Joint Surg Am 70:704–710, 1988.
18. Buchanan JR, Myers CA, Greer RB: Determinants of atraumatic vertebral fracture rates in menopausal women: Biological versus mechanical factors. Metabolism 37:400–404, 1988.
19. Bucholz RW, Gill K: Classification of injuries to the thoracolumbar spine. Orthop Clin North Am 17:67–73, 1986.
20. Ching RP, Tencer AF, Anderson PA, et al: Comparison of residual stability in thoracolumbar spine fractures using neutral zone measurements. J Orthop Res 13:533–541, 1995.
21. Ciccone R, Richman RM: The mechanism of injury and the distribution of three-thousand fractures and dislocations caused by parachute jumping. J Bone Joint Surg Am 30:77–97, 1948.
22. Cobb JR: Outline for the study of scoliosis. Instruct Course Lect 5:261–275, 1948.
23. Daffner RH, Deeb ZL, Rothfus WE: The posterior vertebral body line: Importance in the detection of burst fractures. AJR 148:93–96, 1987.
24. Davis AG: Fractures of spine. J Bone Joint Surg 11:133–156, 1929.
25. Day B, Kokan P: Compression fractures of the thoracic and lumbar spine from compensable injuries. Clin Orthop 124:173–176, 1977.
26. Denis F: The three column spine and its significance in the classification of acute thoracolumbar spinal injuries. Spine 8:817–831, 1983.
27. Denis F: Spinal instability as defined by the three-column spine concept in acute spinal trauma. Clin Orthop 189:65–76, 1984.
28. Denis F: Thoracolumbar injuries. Instruct Course Lect 230, 1988.
29. DeSmet AA, Robinson RG, Johnson BE, et al: Spinal compressive fractures in osteoporotic women: Patterns and relationship to hyperkyphosis. Radiology 166:497–500, 1988.
30. Dickson JH, Harrington PR, Erwin WD: Results of reduction and stabilization of the severely fractured thoracic and lumbar spine. J Bone Joint Surg Am 60:799–805, 1978.
31. Edwards CC, Levine AM: Early rod-sleeve stabilization of the injured thoracic and lumbar spine. Orthop Clin North Am 17:121–145, 1986.
32. Ekin JA, Sinaki M: Vertebral compression fractures sustained during golf: Report of three cases. Mayo Clin Proc 4:4758–5120, 1993.
33. Esses SI: The placement and treatment of thoracolumbar spine fractures: An algorithmic approach. Orthorp Rev 17:571–584, 1988.
34. Ferguson RL, Allen BL Jr: A mechanistic classification of thoracolumbar spine fractures. Clin Orthop 189:77–88, 1984.
35. Flesch JR, Leider LL, Erickson DL, et al: Harrington instrumentation and spine fusion for unstable fractures and fracture/dislocations of the thoracic and lumbar spine. J Bone Joint Surg Am 59:143–153, 1977.
36. Gehweiler JA Jr, Daffner RH, Osborne RL Jr: Relevant signs of stable and unstable thoracolumbar vertebral column trauma. Skeletal Radiol 7:179–183, 1981.
37. Gershon-Cohn J, Rechtman AM, Schraer H, et al: Asymptomatic fractures in osteoporotic spines of the aged. JAMA 153:625, 1953.
38. Gertzbein SD: Harrington instrumentation for fixation in fractures of the spine. J Bone Joint Surg Br 64:526–529, 1982.
39. Gertzbein SD: Scoliosis research society: A multicenter spine fracture study. Spine 17:528–540, 1992.
40. Glass RBJ, Sivit CJ, Sturm PF, et al: Lumbar spine injury in a pediatric population: Difficulties with computed tomographic diagnosis. J Trauma 37:815–819, 1994.
41. Goh JCH, Low SL, Bose K: Vertebral body index and bone mineral density in women with spinal fractures. Acta Orthop Scand 65:522–524, 1994.
42. Grech P: Falls from coconut trees. East Afr Med J 41:64–68, 1964.
43. Harkonen M, Kataja M, Keski-Nisula L, et al: Fractures of the lumbar spine: Clinical and radiological results in 94 patients. Arch Orthop Trauma Surg 94:43–48, 1979.
44. Harkonen M, Kataja M, Keski-Nisula L, et al: Injuries of the

thoracolumbar junction: Clinical and radiological results in 149 patients. Arch Orthop Trauma Surg 94:35–41, 1979.

45. Harkonen M, Kataja M, Lepisto P, et al: Fractures of the thoracic spine: Clinical and radiological results in 98 patients. Arch Orthop Trauma Surg 94:179–184, 1979.

46. Harma M, Heliovaara M, Aromaa A, et al: Thoracic spine compression fractures in Finland. Clin Orthop 205:188–194, 1986.

47. Harrison JE, Patt N, Muller C, et al: Bone mineral mass associated with postmenopausal vertebral deformities. Bone 10:243–251, 1990.

48. Hazel WA, Jones RA, Morrey BF, et al: Vertebral fractures without neurological deficit: A long-term follow-up study. J Bone Joint Surg Am 70:1319–1321, 1988.

49. Hegenbarth R, Ebel KD: Roentgen findings in fractures of the vertebral column in childhood: Examination of 35 patients and its results. Pediatr Radiol 5:34–39, 1976.

50. Hensinger RN: Fractures of the thoracic and lumbar spine. In Rockwood CA Jr, Wilkins KE, King RE (eds): Fractures in Children. Philadelphia, JB Lippincott, 1984, pp 706–731.

51. Herkowitz HN, Samberg LC: Vertebral column injuries associated with tobogganing. J Trauma 18:806–810, 1978.

52. Hirsch C, Nachemson A: Clinical observations on the spines in ejected pilots. Aviat Space Environ Med 34:629, 1963.

53. Holdsworth FW: Fractures, dislocations, and fracture-dislocations of the spine. J Bone Joint Surg Br 45:6–20, 1963.

54. Holdsworth FW, Hardy A: Early treatment of paraplegia from fractures of the thoracolumbar spine. J Bone Joint Surg Br 35:540–550, 1953.

55. Horal J, Nachemson A, Scheller S: Clinical and radiological long-term follow-up of vertebral fractures in children. Acta Orthop Scand 43:491–503, 1972.

56. Howorth MB: Fracture of the spine. Am J Surg 92:573–593, 1956.

57. Hubbard, DD: Injuries of the spine in children and adolescents. Clin Orthop 100:56–65, 1974.

58. Hubbard DD: Fractures of the dorsal and lumbar spine. Orthop Clin North Am 7:605–614, 1976.

59. Iskrant AP: The etiology of hip fractures in females. Am J Public Health 58:485–490, 1968.

60. Jacobs RR, Asher MA, Snider RK: Thoracolumbar spinal injuries: A comparative study of recumbent and operative treatment in 100 patients. Spine 5:463–477, 1980.

61. Jacobs RR, Casey MP: Surgical management of thoracolumbar spinal injuries. Clin Orthop 189:22–35, 1984.

62. Jelsma RK, Kirsch PT, Rice JF, et al: The radiographic description of thoracolumbar fractures. Surg Neurol 18:230–236, 1982.

63. Kaneda K, Asano S, Hashimoto T, Satoh S, et al: The treatment of osteoporotic-posttraumatic vertebral collapse using the Kaneda device and a bioactive ceramic vertebral prosthesis. Spine 17: S295–S303, 1992.

64. Kaplan FS, Dalinka M, Fallon MD, et al: Quantitative computed tomography reflects vertebral fracture morbidity in osteopenic patients. Orthopaedics 12:949–955, 1989.

65. Keaveny TM, Wachtel EF, Guo E, et al: Mechanical behavior of damaged trabecular bone. J Biomech 27:1309–1318, 1994.

66. Kelly PJ, Epstein S: Transplantation bone disease. J Bone Miner Res 7:123–126, 1992.

67. Kelly RP, Whitesides TE Jr: Treatment of lumbodorsal fracture-dislocations. Ann Surg 167:705–716, 1968.

69. Keene JS: Thoracolumbar fractures in winter sports. Clin Orthop 216:39–49, 1987.

70. Kilcoyne RF, Mack LA, King HA, et al: Thoracolumbar spine injuries associated with vertical plunges: Re-appraisal with computed tomography. Radiology 146:137–140, 1983.

71. King AG: Spinal column trauma. Instruct Course Lect 35:40–51, 1986.

72. Lane JM, Healey JH, Bansal M, et al: Overview of geriatric osteopenic syndromes: Definition and pathophysiology. Orthop Rev 17:1131–1139, 1988.

73. Leidholt JD, Young JJ, Hahn HR, et al: Evaluation of late spinal deformities with fracture-dislocations of the dorsal and lumbar spine in paraplegics. Paraplegia 7:16–23, 1969.

74. Lonstein JE: Post-laminectomy kyphosis. Clin Orthop 128:93–100, 1977.

75. Lyles KW, Gold DT, Shipp KM, et al: Association of osteoporotic vertebral compression fractures with impaired functional status. Am J Med 94:595–601, 1993.

76. Lyons TJ, Ficke AJ: Cases from the aerospace medicine residents' teaching file: An aviator with multiple compression fractures of the spine secondary to high speed ejection. Aviat Space Environ Med 58:379–381, 1987.

77. Marcus NA, Sweetser ER, Benson RW: Hot-air ballooning injuries. Am J Sports Med 9:318–321, 1981.

78. McAfee PC, Bohlman HH: Complications following Harrington instrumentation for fractures of the thoracolumbar spine. J Bone Joint Surg Am 67:672–686, 1985.

79. McAfee PC, Yuan HA, Fredrickson BE, et al: The value of computed tomography in thoracolumbar fractures: An analysis of 100 consecutive cases in a new classification. J Bone Joint Surg Am 65:461–473, 1983.

80. McGroy BJ, Vanderwilde RS, Currier BL, et al: Diagnosis of subtle thoracolumbar burst fractures: A new radiographic sign. Spine 19:2282–2285, 1993.

81. Meyer PR Jr: Posterior stabilization of thoracic, lumbar, and sacral injuries. Instruc Course Lect 35:401–419, 1986.

82. Mizrahi J, Silva MJ, Keaveny TM, et al: Finite-element stress analysis of the normal and osteoporotic lumbar vertebral body. Spine 18:2088–2096, 1993.

83. Moe JH, Denis F: The iatrogenic loss of lumbar lordosis. Orthop Trans 1:131, 1977.

84. Morgan TH, Wharton GW, Austin GN: The results of laminectomy in patients with incomplete spinal cord injuries. J Bone Joint Surg Am 52:822, 1970.

85. Neumann P, Nordwall A, Osvalder AL: Traumatic instability of the lumbar spine: A dynamic in vitro study of flexion-distraction injury. Spine 20:1111–1121, 1995.

86. Nicholas JJ, Benedek TG, Reece GJ: Delayed traumatic vertebral body compression fracture, part 1: Clinical features. Semin Arthritis Rheum 10:264, 1981.

87. Nicoll EA: Fractures of the dorso-lumbar spine. J Bone Joint Surg Br 31:376–394, 1949.

88. Odom JA, Brown CW, Messner DG: Tubing injuries. J Bone Joint Surg Am 58:733, 1976.

89. Osebold WR, Weinstein SL, Sprague BL: Thoracolumbar spine fractures: Results of treatment. Spine 6:13–34, 1981.

90. Panjabi MM, Oxland TR, Kifune M, et al: Validity of the three-column theory of thoracolumbar fractures: A biomechanic investigation. Spine 20:1122–1127, 1995.

91. Perey O: Fracture of the vertebral end-plate in the lumbar spine: An experimental biomechanical investigation. Acta Orthop Scand Suppl 25:10–89, 1957.

92. Petras AF, Hoffman EP: Roentgenographic skeletal injury patterns in parachute jumping. Am J Sports Med 11:325–328, 1983.

93. Plaue R: Die Mechanik des Wirbelkompressionsbruchs. Zentralbl Chir 98:761, 1973.

94. Ralston SH, Urquhart GDK, Brzeski M, et al: Prevelence of vertebral compression fractures due to osteoporosis in ankylosing spondylitis. Br Med J 300:563–565, 1990.

95. Resnick D, Niwayama G: Diagnosis of Bone and Joint Disorders, ed 2. Philadelphia, W B Saunders, 1988, pp 3265–3267.

96. Rich GM, Mudge GH, Laffel GL, et al: Cyclosporin A and prednisone associated osteoporosis in heart transplant recipients. J Heart Lung Transplant 11:950–958, 1992.

97. Riggins RS, Kraus JF: The risk of neurologic damage with fractures of the vertebrae. J Trauma 17:126–133, 1977.

98. Roaf R: A study of the mechanics of spinal injuries. J Bone Joint Surg Br 42:810–823, 1960.

99. Roaf R: Biomechanics of injuries of the spinal column. In Vinken PJ, Bruyn GW (eds): Handbook of Clinical Neurology, vol 25, Injuries of the Spine and Spinal Cord. New York, American Elsevier, 1975, pp 123–140.

100. Roberts JB, Curtiss PH: Stability of the thoracic and lumbar spine in traumatic paraplegia following fracture or fracture-dislocation. J Bone Joint Surg Am 52:1115–1130, 1970.

101. Rogers WA: Treatment of fractures of vertebral bodies uncomplicated by lesions of the cord. Arch Surg 30:284–324, 1935.

102. Saville PD: Observations on 80 women with osteoporotic spine fractures. In Barzel US (ed): Osteoporosis. New York, Grune & Stratton, 1970, p 38.

103. Scher AT: Associated sternal and spinal fractures. S Afr Med J 64:98–100, 1983.

104. Schinz HR, Baensch WE, Friedle E: Roentgen Diagnostics, vol 2. New York, Grune & Stratton, 1964, pp 1554–1556.

105. Schmorl G, Junghanns H: The Human Spine in Health and Disease, ed 2. New York, Grune & Stratton, 1971, pp 268–296.

106. Smith WS, Kaufer H: Patterns and mechanisms of lumbar injuries associated with lap seat belts. J Bone Joint Surg Am 51:239–254, 1969.

107. Snyder BD, Piazza, S, Edwards WT, et al: Role of trabecular morphology in the etiology of age-related vertebral fractures. Calcif Tissue Int 53:S14–S22, 1993.

108. Soreff J: Assessment of Late Results of Traumatic Compression Fractures of the Thoracolumbar Vertebral Bodies. Stockholm, Karolinska Hospital, 1977, pp 1–88.

109. Srinivas N, Reddy MSK, Muvagopal S, et al: Dorsal spine compression fractures in tetanus. J Indian Med Assoc 92:57–58, 1994.

110. Stauffer E, S, Kaufer H, Kling TF: Fractures and dislocations of the spine. In Rockwood CA Jr, Green DP (eds): Fractures in Adults, ed 2. Philadelphia, JB Lippincott, 1975, pp 987–1092.

111. Sutherland CJ, Miller F, Wang G-J: Early progressive kyphosis following compression fractures: 2 case reports from a series of "stable" thoracolumbar compression fractures. Clin Orthop 173:216–220, 1983.

112. Tupper JW, Gunn DR, Mullen MP: Double level compression fractures: More unstable than you think. Presented to Ninth Annual Scoliosis Research Society Meeting, San Francisco, September 1974.

113. Van Cleemput J, Daenen W, Nijs J, et al: Timing and quantification of bone loss in cardiac transplant recipients. Transplant Int 8:196–200, 1995.

114. Visuri T, Aho J: Injuries associated with the use of ejection seats in Finnish pilots. Aviat Space Environ Med, 63:727–730, 1992.

115. Watson-Jones R: Treatment of fractures and fracture-dislocations of the spine. J Bone Joint Surg 16:30–45, 1934.

116. Watson-Jones R: Fractures and Joint Injuries, ed 3. Edinburgh: E & S Livingstone, 1943.

117. Weitzman G: Treatment of stable thoracolumbar spine compression fractures by early ambulation. Clin Orthop 176:116–122, 1971.

118. Westerborn A, Olsson O: Mechanics, treatment, and prognosis of fractures of the dorso-lumbar spine. Acta Chir Scand 102:59–83, 1951.

119. White AA III, Panjabi MM: Clinical Biomechanics of the Spine. Philadelphia, JB Lippincott, 1978, pp 115–190, 236–276.

120. White AA III, Panjabi MM, Posner I, et al: The spine: Spinal stability: Evaluation and treatment. Instruct Course Lect 30:457–483, 1981.

121. White AA III, Panjabi MM, Thomas CL: The clinical biomechanics of kyphotic deformities. Clin Orthop 128:8–17, 1977.

122. Whitesides TE Jr: Traumatic kyphosis of the thoracolumbar spine. Clin Orthop 128:78–92, 1977.

123. Whitesides TE Jr, Shaw S, Ghazanfar A.: On the management of unstable fractures of the thoracolumbar spine: Rationale for use of anterior decompression and fusion and posterior stabilization. Spine 1:99–107, 1976.

124. Young MH: Long-term consequences of stable fractures of the thoracic and lumbar vertebral bodies. J Bone Joint Surg Br 55:295–300, 1973.

CHAPTER 25

Flexion-Distraction Injuries of the Thoracic and Lumbar Spine

Frank J. Eismont

Flexion-distraction injuries of the thoracic and lumbar spine were first described by G. Q. Chance in 1948.[3] He did not mention a mechanism of injury in his three cases, but he included an example and a drawing showing the typical posterior distraction and the commonly seen anterior vertebral body wedging. He also noted that hyperextension should achieve an excellent reduction and that bone-to-bone opposition should allow excellent healing and provide an excellent clinical prognosis. Although there have since been significant additions to these concepts concerning mechanism of injury, further classification of the pathology, and alternative treatment options, Chance's astute clinical observations have generally remained true.

It is the purpose of this chapter to facilitate prompt recognition and appropriate treatment of patients with flexion-distraction injuries of the thoracic and lumbar spine. No mention will be made of thoracic and lumbar spine facet dislocations. These are discussed in Chapter 26.

SEAT BELTS

Although any accident providing significant forward flexion combined with distraction can produce this type of injury, it is most commonly the result of a motor vehicle accident (MVA) with the victim wearing a lap seat belt.

The question of whether seat belt use predisposes to any particular injury was first raised in 1962 by Garrett and Braunstein in their article entitled "The Seat Belt Syndrome."[9] They believed that the use of a lap seat belt made injuries to the lumbar spine "somewhat more frequent." This has subsequently been further developed and discussed in many articles.*

In a study of 303 patients admitted to a level I trauma center with spine or abdominal injuries as a result of MVAs over a 5-year period from 1984 to 1988, Anderson and co-authors[1] reviewed the association of various spine injuries with types of restraints used and occupant position in the vehicle. Thirteen (81%) of

the 16 persons with lumbar flexion-distraction injuries were restrained compared with 8 (14%) of 59 patients with cervical spine injuries. Also, none of the 59 cervical injuries or 71 thoracic injuries were using lap belts alone, but 10 (62%) with lumbar flexion-distraction injuries were using lap belts without a shoulder harness. In this series, 26.8% of all those injured in MVAs used some type of restraint, with 13.9% using lap and shoulder restraints and 8.3% using lap belts.

Furthermore, although only 12.9% of all victims in their study were known rear-seat passengers, 67% of those with lumbar flexion-distraction injuries were rear-seat passengers. This association is not surprising considering that most vehicles with lap-only seat restraints have these in the rear seat.

In this same review by Anderson and colleagues,[1] 32% of patients with small bowel injuries and 29% of patients with colon injuries were wearing lap belts alone compared to 10% of patients with liver injuries, 3% of those with spleen injuries, and 8% of patients with pancreas injuries. Those using lap belts alone were 10 times more likely to have a small bowel injury compared to those passengers using no restraints, and those using lap-shoulder harnesses were 4.4 times more likely to have small bowel injuries compared to those using no restraints.

Since the mechanisms of hollow-viscus injury and of lumbar spine flexion-distraction injuries are similar in those using lap seat belts, we would expect many patients to have injuries to both of these areas. In fact, in this same review, 10 of the 16 patients with lumbar flexion-distraction injuries had hollow-viscus injuries—nine had small bowel injuries and seven had colon injuries requiring surgery.

These statistics should warn us that any patient brought to the hospital for evaluation of injuries sustained in an MVA and especially in those patients with a seat belt contusion of the abdomen or a history of being a rear-seat occupant or of lap seat belt use should be thoroughly evaluated for both lumbar spine flexion-distraction injuries and for hollow-viscus injuries.

After emphasizing these injuries and their association with seat belts, it should be emphasized that seat restraints have reduced fatalities 40% to 50%.[7, 8, 29, 31]

---

*References 1, 5, 11–13, 16, 19, 21, 22, 27–30, and 32.

Also, considering nonfatal crash victims, restrained occupants generally have less severe injuries than those not restrained.[17, 26] In a recent study at the Maryland Institute for Emergency Medical Services Systems, unrestrained occupants had a mean injury severity score of 22.9 compared with those restrained occupants with a mean injury severity score of 10.8, which is a significant difference at $P < .0005$.[17] They also found that the medical cost was reduced in those restrained victims with a significance value of $P < .025$. In a review of 1019 spine fracture patients conducted through the Scoliosis Research Society, Gertzbein[10] found that there was a highly significant relationship between wearing a seat belt and neurologic status. Those wearing a belt were much less likely to have a complete paralysis with a significance of $P = .007$.

As of 1990, the use of restraints by vehicle occupants varied from 42% to 82%, depending on the area surveyed.[20, 34] Hopefully, the use of full lap-shoulder restraints will increase and the use of isolated lap belts will be seen less often. Since 1990, rear-seat restraints have included lap-shoulder restraints. The use of air bags should also have significantly reduced the incidence of these injuries, but data concerning their use are not yet available.

BIOMECHANICS OF INJURY

Flexion-distraction injuries should involve a forward flexion with the axis of rotation in the middle column of the spine or more anterior. This would explain the posterior column separations commonly seen and would explain anterior axial load injuries such as wedge compression fractures or burst fractures which are seen in up to 70% of these injuries. Unfortunately, this cannot explain the common lap belt injury because the axis of rotation is the seat belt across the anterior abdominal wall which is anterior even to the anterior column of the spine.

Research by Begeman and co-authors[2] in 1973 helps to explain these associated anterior vertebral body wedge compression and burst fractures. They found that with rapid deceleration using lap belts and using lap-shoulder restraints, the initial loading of the spine was an axial load (Fig. 25–1). This peaked rapidly and slowly decreased throughout the deceleration. There was also a second peak in the axial loading at the termination of the deceleration injury when the torso was thrown back into the seat. Begeman and colleagues also found that greater axial loads were seen in the upright spine supported by a combined lap and shoulder harness. The magnitude of the initial axial loading was proportional to the deceleration gravity force G. Hence, there is more likely to be an associated anterior vertebral wedge compression fracture when the initial deceleration G force is the greatest. Conversely, injury is likely to be limited to the posterior flexion-distraction component when the initial deceleration G force is smaller.

Other basic research concerning flexion-distraction injuries of the lumbar spine has been performed using isolated two-vertebrae segments in mechanical testing.[22–24] It was found that the first point of substantial structural injury occurred at a mean flexion angulation of 16 degrees[22] and a mean flexion angulation of 20 degrees.[23] These are surprisingly close to the angulation cited in clinical reviews beyond which nonoperative treatment failed, that is, 20 degrees by Glassman and co-authors[12] in 1992 and 17 degrees by LeGay and colleagues[19] in 1990.

There are also many potential considerations to explain why this flexion-distraction injury of the spine has occurred so often in young children. They may be limited to riding in the back seat and the back seat more commonly will have had only a lap seat belt, both factors which predispose to this particular injury. Biomechanically, the center of gravity is higher in a child than in an adult[25] and, with the pelvis fixed to the vehicle with a lap seat belt, the flexion-distraction forces may be increased relative to the strength of the bone and ligaments.[28] There is also concern that in children, for various anatomic reasons, the seat belts tend to be worn too high to grab the pelvis (as in adults) and instead compress only the midabdomen and flexible lumbar spine. To minimize this, some have suggested using a bolster on which the child should sit while using the lap belt.

CLINICAL ASSESSMENT

As noted in the discussion concerning seat belts, the clinician should be wary of spine flexion-distraction injury in any patient with a history of involvement in an MVA, especially with documented use of a seat belt. The suspicion should be raised further if the victim is a child, a back-seat occupant, and if only a lap restraint was used.

Physical examination should always be comprehensive for accident victims but special attention should be given to palpation of the spine for tenderness and for any gaping space between adjacent posterior elements. The abdomen should also be inspected looking for any "seat belt sign," that is, any ecchymosis or contusion of the abdomen (see Fig. 25–7). The presence of an ileus would be expected with a flexion-distraction injury of the spine but it should be remembered that the incidence of an associated abdominal injury requiring surgery (Fig. 25–2) is 45% from a combined review of 10 series of patients (Table 25–1). There are also examples in the literature of victims having computed tomography (CT) scans of the abdomen and even mini-laparotomies which do not detect the perforated hollow viscus and hence persistent reevaluation may be necessary in these victims to detect and treat their intra-abdominal problem. Some of the patients have also presented late (at 4 to 6 weeks after their accident)[14] with intestinal obstruction due to narrowed ischemic bowel or obstructing hernias through the mesentery or even hernias through the posterior abdominal fascia.[33]

Neurologically, the majority of patients with lumbar flexion-distraction injuries remain normal. In Denis's

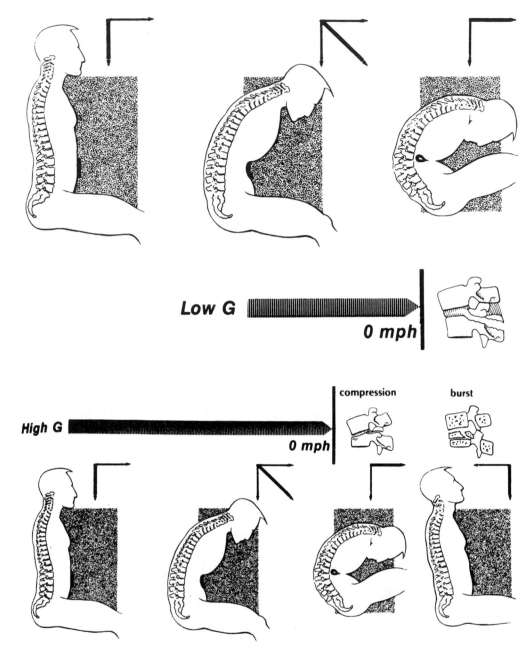

Low G

0 mph

compression   burst

High G

0 mph

Figure 25–1 = *A*, This shows a flexion-distraction injury occurring with low G forces. The axial component of the force is relatively small and hence no wedge compression fracture or burst fracture occurs. A typical distraction injury of the posterior elements of the spine occurs. *B*, In sudden deceleration injuries with high G forces there is an initial significant axial load force which can result in either a wedge compression fracture or burst fracture anteriorly. As the injury progresses the standard posterior distraction injury occurs. At the termination of the motion the body is thrown back into the sitting position and further injury to the vertebral body may occur at this time. (From Gertzbein SD, Court-Brown CM: Flexion distraction injuries of the lumbar spine: Mechanisms of injury and classification. Clin Orthop 227:52–60, 1988.)

review[6] of 19 patients, none had paralysis secondary to their seat belt–type injury. Other series, however, have had up to 30% of patients with paralysis.[28] Adding 10 series of patients (see Table 25–1), the chance of paralysis is 13%. Although it is extremely uncommon, patients may also develop a progressive paraparesis secondary to an associated epidural hematoma at the site of a flexion-distraction injury of the lumbar spine. In most cases, in patients with stable neurologic deficits, immobilization in the supine position on a rotating treatment frame or rigid bed will tend to reduce and

stabilize the injury until definitive treatment with bracing, cast application, or surgery can be performed.

RADIOGRAPHIC ASSESSMENT

Plain x-ray films will usually be adequate to demonstrate flexion-distraction injuries of the lumbar spine. The bony anatomy of the injury is best demonstrated either by anteroposterior (AP) and lateral tomograms or by CT scan with thin cuts and with good sagittal and

Table 25–1 = **PATIENTS REQUIRING ABDOMINAL SURGERY AND PATIENTS WITH PARALYSIS FOLLOWING FLEXION-DISTRACTION INJURY**

SERIES	PATIENTS REQUIRING ABDOMINAL SURGERY	PATIENTS WITH PARALYSIS
Anderson et al.[1]	10/16	—
Dehner[5]	3/7	0/7
Denis[6]	—	0/19
Gertzbein & Court-Brown[11]	9/19	5/19
Glassman et al.[12]	5/12	0/12
Gumley et al.[13]	8/20	2/20
LeGay et al.[19]	7/18	2/18
Newman et al.[21]	4/9	2/9
Reid et al.[27]	3/7	1/7
Rumball & Jarvis[28]	4/10	3/10
Totals	53/118 = 45%	16/121 = 13%

coronal reconstruction (Fig. 25–3). Standard transverse cuts with the CT scanner will tend to minimize or may even miss the injury if the cuts are too wide, especially since the plane of injury is horizontal and parallel to the CT cuts. The CT scan is especially helpful in those victims with anterior vertebral body axial load injuries (up to 85% of cases) to be certain that there is no burst fracture present (up to 15% of cases). This is especially important information if surgery is planned since it will dictate whether or not a compression instrumentation system can be used.

With any patient with a neurologic deficit or any patient scheduled for surgery, it is also important to obtain either a magnetic resonance imaging (MRI) scan or a myelogram followed by a CT scan since these patients may also have disc abnormalities or unsuspected spinal stenosis which might alter the treatment plan.[15]

The injuries are best classified according to Gertzbein and Court-Brown[11] (Fig. 25–4) since their system addresses both the flexion-distraction component as well as any vertebral body axial load injuries which may be present. It is a modification of the classification systems of Gumley and co-authors,[13] and of Denis.[6] Type I is used to categorize the posterior fracture symmetrically, splitting the spinous process, laminae, pedicles, and transverse processes. Type II denotes that the fracture is similar to type I but the fracture line enters at the base of the spinous process. Type III denotes that the fracture posteriorly is asymmetrical, involving more of the posterior elements on one side than the other. Gertzbein and Court-Brown found that 10% of their injuries were type I, 65% were type II, and 25% were type III.[11]

The injury involving the disc or vertebral body is categorized as A when the injury exits through the

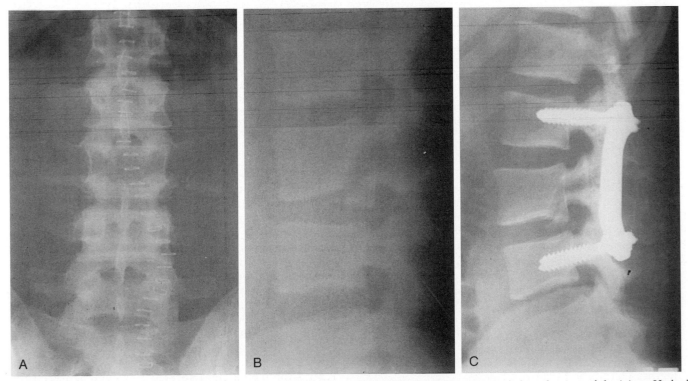

Figure 25–2 = This young man was involved in a motor vehicle accident and was using a lap seat belt at the time of the injury. He had sustained a rupture of his colon which was diagnosed and treated acutely. He was immobilized on a Roto-Rest bed before and after the abdominal surgery until it was certain that his bowel repair was satisfactory. A, This AP radiograph shows anterior abdominal skin clips overlying the lumbar spine. It can be seen quite clearly that the L3 transverse processes, as well as the pedicles are split. B, The lateral film shows that the injury line goes through the inferior end plate of L3 and into the L3–4 disc space. C, This lateral view taken postoperatively shows that the fracture has been well reduced. Considering the pattern of the injury, it was not possible to utilize a shorter construct. This patient was fully mobilized following the spine surgery which facilitated his recovery. This injury would be classified as I, C-2, F after the Gertzbein–Court-Brown classification.

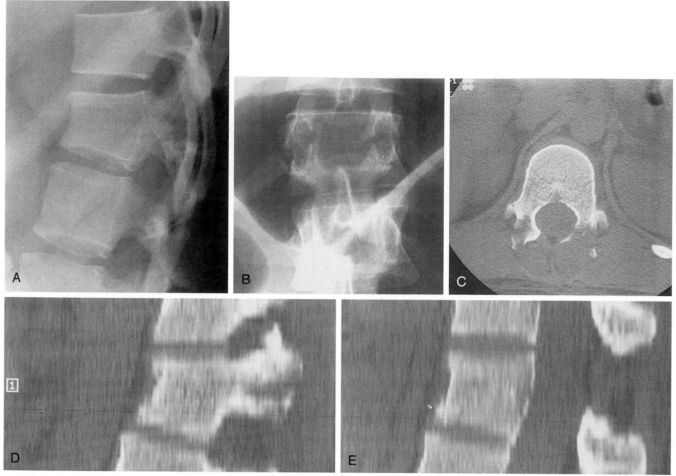

Figure 25–3 = An excellent radiographic example of the flexion-distraction injury as originally described by Chance. *A,* The cone-down lateral radiograph shows the T12 vertebra is slightly compressed anteriorly as with a wedge compression fracture and is distracted posteriorly with the fracture line proceeding through the pedicles. *B,* This cone-down AP film shows that the fracture line divides the pedicles of T12 bilaterally. It can also be appreciated that there is significant spread between the spinous process of T11 and the spinous process of T12. *C,* A typical appearing CT section through the level of injury. The fracture lines are not clearly defined since the cut is exactly parallel to the line of injury. *D,* With reconstruction, it can be seen that the fracture line proceeds directly through the pedicle. *E,* This midsagittal CT reconstruction shows that the fracture line goes into the posterior aspect of the vertebral body. This also very clearly shows the spread of the T11 and T12 spinous processes posteriorly. This would be categorized as a II, B, D injury according to the Gertzbein–Court-Brown classification.

disc, as B when the injury is limited to the body, and as C when the bony injury proceeds through an end plate and into the disc. C-1 denotes an injury through the superior end plate and C-2 denotes an injury through the inferior end plate. Gertzbein and Court-Brown found that 5% of their injuries were type A, 20% were type B, 25% were type C-1, and 50% were type C-2.

Finally, the state of the vertebral body is assessed. If there is a typical wedge compression fracture it is classified type D, if there is an associated vertebral burst fracture it is classified type E, and if the vertebral body is intact it is classified as type F. They found that 70% of their injuries were type D, 15% were type E, and 15% were type F.

TREATMENT

The initial assessment has been discussed above and the emphasis is placed on recognition of the spine injury and adequate evaluation of intra-abdominal injury which is seen in 45% of these patients. The abdominal evaluation may include a peritoneal lavage or minilaparotomy or both.

Associated bowel disruption obviously takes priority over operative treatment of the spine injury. If the bowel surgery involves the colon, spine surgery should be postponed until it is certain that there will be no bouts of septicemia. If the surgery involves the duodenum or jejunum, however, and the general surgeons are pleased with the adequacy of repair, then spine surgery could be performed at any time.

The spine can be initially treated with bed rest on a rigid turning frame such as a Roto-Rest bed. This allows adequate stabilization of the spine injury and lying supine on a rigid surface may even achieve some degree of injury reduction. At this point, decisions are made concerning operative or nonoperative treatment. Surgery is usually recommended under the following circumstances:

1. A progressive neural deficit with proven neural compression.

2. A static neural deficit which occurred at the time of injury with seat belt flexion-distraction injury is usually due to tensile disruption of the neural elements and is not often associated with residual neural compression. Surgery is most helpful in these patients to stabilize the spine to facilitate mobilization and rehabilitation (Fig. 25–5).

3. Many of these patients have multiple trauma and surgery can allow rapid mobilization which may be needed to help with pulmonary function and so forth.

4. There are reviews of flexion-distraction injuries which find poor results with nonoperative treatment if the original deformity is greater than 17 degrees (Le Gay and co-workers[19]) or 20 degrees (Glassman and colleagues[12]). Because of these data we recommend surgical treatment for flexion-distraction injuries with the original deformity 17 degrees or more.

5. Those patients with primarily soft tissue involvement, such as type IIA injuries, will generally heal poorly and will do best with operative treatment.

For those patients who are neurologically intact and have an isolated flexion-distraction injury, the decision between operative and nonoperative treatment is a relatively easy one. In that uniform group of patients (isolated injury in a neurologically intact patient), the decision concerning the type of treatment is based on the (1) presumed outcome for spinal stability and (2) the ability to obtain a reduction. The first issue centers on understanding the nature of the injury. Looking at all classifications of injury, three common generic injury types exist. The first comprises of purely bony injuries with a fracture line through the spinous process, lamina, pedicle, and body. If these heal in a relatively anatomic position, no potential instability can exist. The second group of injuries are combined osseoligamentous with either posterior element disruption through the ligamentous complex combined with a body fracture or posterior element fracture through the bony portion with an anterior disc disruption. The former most commonly results in ligamentous instability even if an anatomic reduction can be obtained. The latter can have a variable outcome. The third type is the purely ligamentous disruptions (facet dislocations), which always result in stability and most often cannot be anatomically reduced.

Figure 25–4 = This shows a useful classification system for discussing flexion-distraction injuries of the spine. *A,* A posterior fracture is characterized as I, where the fracture proceeds through the superior aspect of the spinous process through the pedicle and transverse processes; II, where the fracture line enters at the base of the spinous process, or III, where the fracture lines enter obliquely involving more of the posterior elements on one side than the other. *B,* The anterior fracture is either categorized as A, which shows the plane of injury going through the disc space only; B, which shows the plane of injury is a fracture line through the vertebral body proceeding from posterior to anterior; C-1, which breaks through the superior end plate of the vertebral body and into the disc space; and C-2, which proceeds through the inferior end plate of the vertebral body and into the disc space. *C,* The state of the body is categorized as D, which represents a simple anterior wedge compression fracture; E, which denotes a burst fracture component; or F, which denotes an intact vertebral body (From Gertzbein SD, Court-Brown CM: Flexion-distraction injuries of the lumbar spine: Mechanisms of injury and classification. Clin Orthop 227:52–60, 1988.)

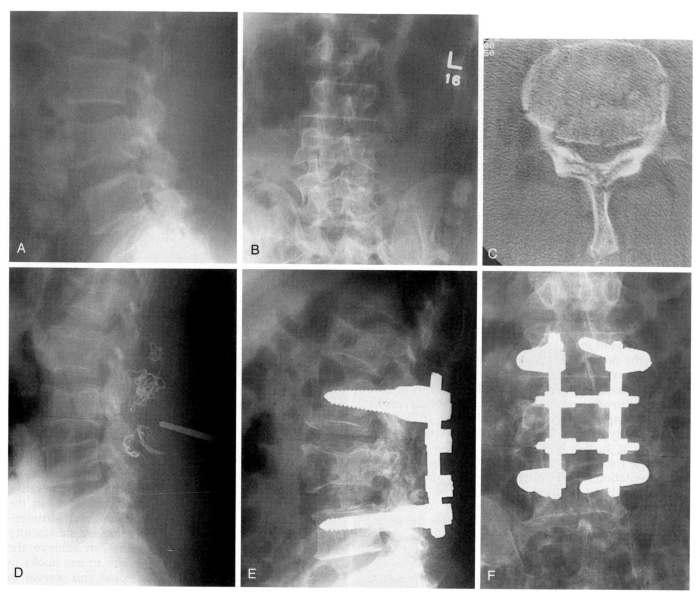

Figure 25–6 = A 56-year-old man sustained this L3 fracture. *A*, The patient has an apparent burst fracture of the L3 vertebra and a partially sacralized L5 vertebra. *B*, This AP radiograph shows significant spread of the pedicles of the L3 vertebra consistent with a significant burst component. *C*, This transverse section on the CT scan reveals that there is a significant burst component to this fracture as was suspected from the plain lateral film. There is also a fracture of the base of the spinous process and lamina. *D*, This lateral intraoperative radiograph is the first picture that clearly shows the fracture of the pars interarticularis of L3. *E*, This lateral radiograph shows that the spine was stabilized at surgery with a neutralization type of construct after a laminectomy had been performed at L3 combined with a bilateral posterolateral decompression to remove the bone from the spinal canal that resulted from the burst fracture. Use of a compression construct under these circumstances would force more bone out into the spinal canal and can be associated with an increased neurologic deficit. *F*, This AP view shows the neutralization construct. Keeping the construct short is important to maintain as many mobile segments as possible.

Figure 25–7 = This 46-year-old woman was involved in a motor vehicle accident and presented with significant thoracolumbar pain and a significant "seat belt sign." *A*, This photograph of the patient's lower abdomen shows the typical ecchymoses consistent with a seat belt injury. This should alert the clinician to possible hollow-viscus injury and to flexion-distraction injuries of the spine. This patient did not have an associated intra-abdominal injury. *B*, This lateral radiograph of the thoracolumbar junction reveals a flexion-distraction injury of T11. This could easily be mistaken for a benign compression fracture of T11. *C*, This AP view of the thoracolumbar and lumbar spine barely shows the T11 vertebra and still does not indicate this to be a flexion-distraction injury. *D*, This AP tomogram shows the fracture lines proceeding through the midpedicles of T11 bilaterally. The fracture through the superior aspect of the lamina of T11 can also be vaguely seen. *E*, The lateral tomogram at the level of the pedicles again shows the fracture line proceeding through the pedicle. *F*, This midsagittal tomogram confirms that the anterior compression of the T11 vertebra is approximately 40% to 50%, but it also reveals a burst component of the fracture. The posterior laminar fracture can also be seen at the top of the T11 spinous process. *G*, This lateral film was taken more than 1 year after operative fixation of the fracture. The Edwards system using sublaminar hooks and rod sleeves to achieve distraction and three point bending was utilized to achieve optimal reduction. The spine alignment has been restored to normal. The length of this construct is not of concern since it only goes down to L1. This leaves many open mobile levels in the lumbar spine. *H*, This AP radiograph shows the position of the rod sleeves over T11. Posterolateral fusion can be seen bilaterally. If a compression system had been utilized to treat this injury, bone could have been further displaced into the spinal canal, causing neurologic deterioration.

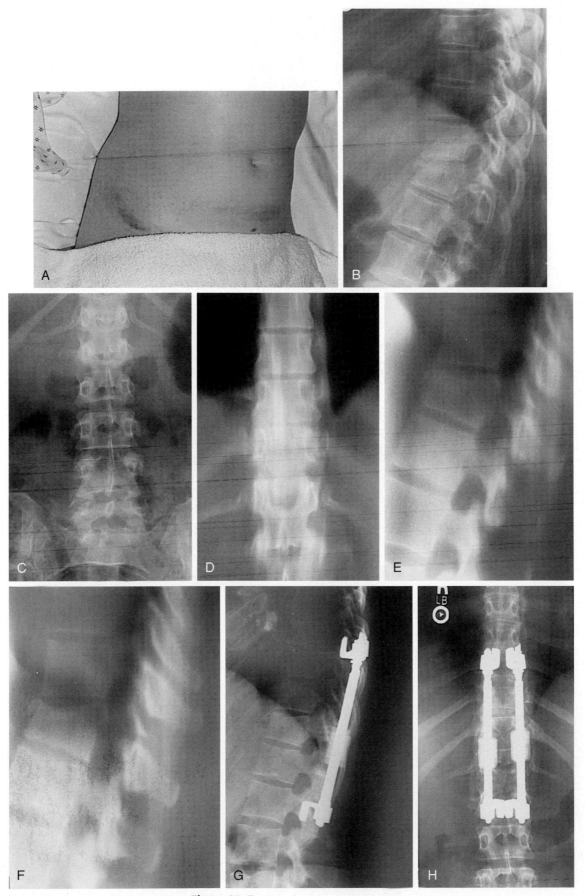

Figure 25–7 = *See legend on opposite page*

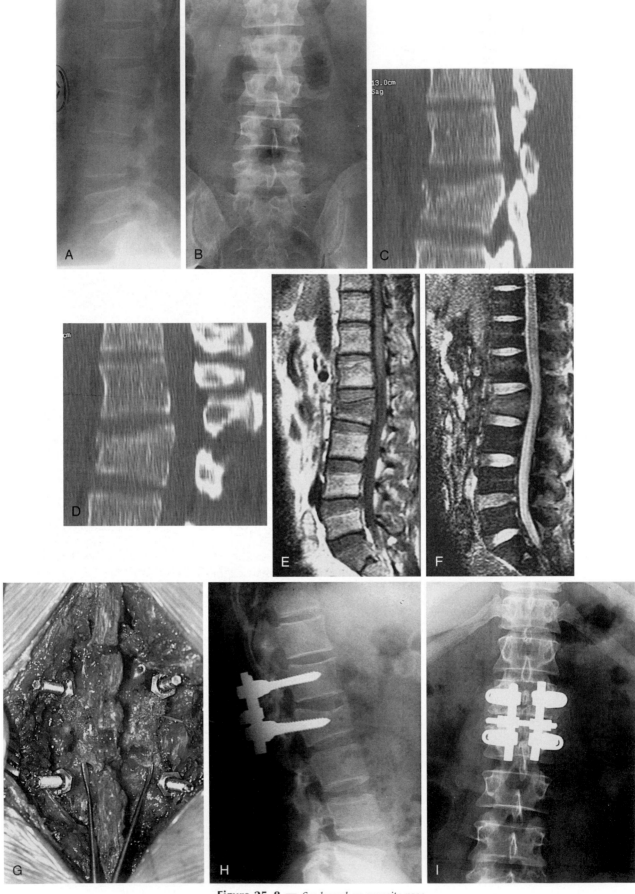

Figure 25–8 = *See legend on opposite page*

option. If this course is taken a custom-made TLSO brace is fitted with the patient lying prone and slightly hyperextended. The fitting is usually done within the first day and it usually takes a few more days to fabricate the brace. Once it is ready, the patient is taught how to roll into the two-piece brace and apply it and tighten it while still lying down. The patient is then taught how to get out of bed safely and ambulate under the direct supervision of a physical therapist. The patient is allowed out of the brace when in bed but instructed to always use it when out of bed. When in bed, the patient is encouraged to lie prone and hyperextend the injury.

After being out of bed and ambulating for 12 to 24 hours, a new standing radiograph is obtained. If there is no loss of position as indicated by an increase in angulation or displacement, then the patient is discharged from the hospital and scheduled for regular follow-up as an outpatient at short initial intervals and longer final intervals. If there is a deterioration in spinal alignment, the patient is readmitted for surgical treatment of the spine injury.

RESULTS

The literature is sparse concerning the clinical results of patients who have been treated for flexion-distraction injuries of the thoracic and lumbar spine. The Scoliosis Research Society's prospective review, including all types of thoracic and lumbar spine fractures, has established some general principles which apply to treating these injuries.[10] A positive relationship was found between the amount of kyphotic deformity present at 1 year after injury and the amount of pain which was present at 1 year for all fracture patients, including those treated operatively as well as nonoperatively ($P < .02$). A kyphosis of greater than 30 degrees was also associated with an increased incidence of more intense back pain but no statistical significance could be determined since the numbers of patients allowed to keep this degree of deformity was very small.

There are three articles dealing specifically with flexion-distraction injuries of the thoracic and lumbar spine which address the patient's pain at follow-up. In the series of Glassman and co-workers[12], 10 of 12 (83%)

had no significant pain at follow-up. Of the two patients with pain, one had been treated operatively and one had been treated conservatively. In the series of LeGay and colleagues,[19] 13 (76%) of 17 patients had no pain or mild pain at follow-up and the majority of patients had been treated nonoperatively (i.e., only three (18%) of those with follow-up had been treated operatively). In the series of operatively treated patients described by Triantafyllou and Gertzbein,[32] 16 patients had been treated with one-level fusions and 14 (87%) had no pain or mild pain at the time of follow-up. The results from each of these reviews show that the majority of patients with these spine fractures do relatively well as regards pain.

The only article specifically addressing function at follow-up was that by LeGay and co-authors.[19] They found that 11 (65%) of their patients reported they were able to participate in all normal activities and four (24%) reported that they had to slightly alter their activities because of their injuries. The remaining two patients had a major change in their activities, but both had sustained multiple injuries which probably contributed to their limitations.

The results concerning paralysis are very vague. We know that approximately 13% of patients with these flexion-distraction injuries have some degree of paralysis, but each series of patients is so small that no comments can be made regarding the outcome of the paralysis and its relationship to the type of treatment given.

SUMMARY

Flexion-distraction injuries of the thoracic and lumbar spine are often seen in young rear-seat passengers using lap seat belt restraints alone. A surprising 45% of these patients have significant bowel injuries which may be occult. Spinal surgery is indicated for those patients with initial kyphotic deformities of greater than 17 to 20 degrees, especially when associated with ligamentous and disc injuries and with pars interarticularis fractures. Short surgical constructs utilizing compression or neutralization are extremely effective in treating these injuries. Special care should be taken with those patients with associated burst fracture or

---

Figure 25–8 = This 36-year-old construction worker was injured in a fall from a height. *A*, The lateral radiograph shows a wedge compression fracture of the L2 vertebra and some separation can be seen between the L1 and L2 posterior elements. *B*, The AP view shows a fracture through the spinous process of L1 and gives a suggestion of a fracture at the level of the L1 pars interarticularis. *C*, This sagittal CT reconstruction shows the fracture in the pars interarticularis of L1. *D*, This midsagittal CT reconstruction shows the fracture through the L1 spinous process as well as the 40% anterior compression fracture of L2. *E*, This midsagittal T1-weighted MRI scan shows that the patient has a relatively narrow spinal canal in both the thoracic and lumbar regions. *F*, This gradient echo image again confirms that the patient has a relatively narrow spinal canal of both the thoracic and lumbar spine. These MRI studies also clearly show that there is no protrusion of either the disc or the vertebral body into the spinal canal at the level of injury. *G*, This intraoperative radiograph shows pedicle screws inserted at the L1 and L2 levels bilaterally. A Penfield elevator has been placed in the fractures of the pars interarticularis bilaterally. *H*, Pedicle screws were especially useful to treat this patient's injury since he has a small spinal canal. Use of laminar hooks could easily produce "steel stenosis" from the instrumentation. The use of pedicle screws allows compression forces to be applied to close the posterior defect without narrowing the spinal canal. At 8 months after surgery, it can be seen that the anterior vertebral body height has been improved at L2, although it has not been improved to normal. *I*, This AP film at 8 months after surgery shows the configuration of the short instrumentation from L1 to L2 and shows a solid posterolateral fusion.

disc disruption in order to avoid neurologic deterioration. Fortunately, the vast majority of patients with this type of spine injury have a successful final outcome regarding pain, function, and stability.

REFERENCES

1. Anderson PA, Rivara FP, Maier R, et al: The epidemiology of seatbelt-associated injuries. J Trauma 31:60–67, 1991.
2. Begeman PC, King AI, Prasad P: Spinal loads resulting from −G acceleration. *In* Proceedings of the 17th Stapp Car Crash Conference, New York, Society of Automotive Engineers, 1973, pp 343–360.
3. Chance GQ: Note on a type of flexion fracture of the spine. Br J Radiol 21:452–453, 1948.
4. Cochran T, Irstam L, Nachemson A: Long-term anatomic and functional changes in patients with adolescent idiopathic scoliosis treated by Harrington rod fusion. Spine 8:576–582, 1988.
5. Dehner JR: Seatbelt injuries of the spine and abdomen. AJR 111:833–843, 1971.
6. Denis F: The three column spine and its significance in the classification of acute thoracolumbar spinal injuries. Spine 8:817–831, 1983.
7. Evans L: The effectiveness of safety belts in preventing fatalities. Accid Anal Prev 18:229–241, 1986.
8. Evans L: Rear seat restraint system effectiveness in preventing fatalities. Accid Anal Prev 20:129–136, 1988.
9. Garrett JW, Braunstein PW: The seat belt syndrome. J Trauma 2:220–238, 1962.
10. Gertzbein SD: Multicenter spine fracture study, Scoliosis Research Society. Spine 17:528–540, 1992.
11. Gertzbein SD, Court-Brown CM: Flexion-distraction injuries of the lumbar spine. Mechanisms of injury and classification. Clin Orthop 227:52–60, 1988.
12. Glassman SD, Johnson JR, Holt RT: Seatbelt injuries in children. J Trauma 33:882–886, 1992.
13. Gumley G, Taylor TKF, Ryan MD: Distraction fractures of the lumbar spine. J Bone Joint Surg Br 6:520–525, 1982.
14. Hardacre J, West K, Rescorla F, et al: Delayed onset of intestinal obstruction in children after unrecognized seat belt injury. J Pediatr Surg 25:967–969, 1990.
15. Heller JG, Garfin S, Abitbol J-J: Disk herniations associated with compression instrumentation of lumbar flexion-distraction injuries. Clin Orthop 284:91–98, 1992.
16. Howland WJ, Curry JL, Buffington C: Fulcrum fractures of the lumbar spine. JAMA 193:140–141, 1965.
17. Kaplan B, Cowley A: Seatbelt effectiveness and cost of noncompliance among drivers admitted to a trauma center. Am J Emerg Med 9:4–10, 1991.
18. Kitchel S, Eismont FJ, Green BA: Closed subarachnoid drainage for management of cerebrospinal fluid leakage after an operation on the spine. J Bone Joint Surg Am 71:984, 1989.
19. LeGay D, Petrie D, Alexander D: Flexion-distraction injuries of the lumbar spine and associated abdominal trauma. J Trauma 30:436–444, 1990.
20. National Highway Traffic Safety Administration: Occupant Protection Facts. Washington, DC, Department of Transportation, June 1989.
21. Newman K, Bowman L, Eichelberger M, et al: The lap belt complex: Intestinal and lumbar spine injury in children. J Trauma 30:1133–1138, 1990.
22. Neumann P, Osvalder A, Nordwall A, et al: The mechanism of initial flexion-distraction injury in the lumbar spine. Spine 17:1083–1090, 1992.
23. Osvalder AL, Neumann P, Lovsund P, et al: Ultimate strength of the lumbar spine in flexion—An in vitro study. J Biomech 23:453–460, 1990.
24. Osvalder AL, Neumann P, Lovsund P, et al: A method for studying the biomechanical load response of the (in vitro) lumbar spine under dynamic flexion-shear loads. J Biomech 26:1227–1236, 1993.
25. Palmer CE: The center of gravity of the human body during growth. Am J Phys Anthropol 11:423–455, 1928.
26. Reath DB, Kirby J, Lynch M, et al: Injury and cost comparison of restrained and unrestrained motor vehicle crash victims. J Trauma 29:1173–1176, 1989.
27. Reid AB, Letts RM, Black GB: Pediatric Chance fractures: Association with intra-abdominal injuries and seatbelt use. J Trauma 30:384–391, 1990.
28. Rumball K, Jarvis J: Seat-belt injuries of the spine in young children. J Bone Joint Surg Br 74:571–574, 1992.
29. Rutledge R, Thomason M, Oller D, et al: The spectrum of abdominal injuries associated with the use of seat belts. J Trauma 31:820–825, 1991.
30. Smith W, Kaufer H: Patterns and mechanisms of lumbar injuries associated with lap seat belts. J Bone Joint Surg Am 51:239–254, 1969.
31. Sullivan P: Number of traffic deaths plummets, experts say MDs can help trend continue. Can Med Assoc J 145:249, 1991.
32. Triantafyllou S, Gertzbein S: Flexion distraction injuries of the thoracolumbar spine: A review. Orthopaedics 15:357–364, 1992.
33. Wang SE, Tiu CM, Chou H, et al: Obstructive intestinal herniation due to improper use of a seatbelt: A case report. Pediatr Radiol 23:200–201, 1993.
34. Williams A, Wells J, Lund A: Seat belt use in cars with air bags. Public Health Brief 80:1514–1516, 1990.

Facet Fractures and Dislocations of the Thoracolumbar Spine

Alan M. Levine

Although all classifications involving flexion-distraction injuries of the thoracolumbar spine recognize the presence of a completely ligamentous form of the injury,[18, 20, 28, 31, 44] few have categorized it as anything other than a variant pattern. However, many reasons exist for considering the purely ligamentous flexion-distraction injury occurring in the thoracolumbar spine as a completely separate entity. As discussed in the previous chapter, the flexion-distraction mechanism produces a wide variation in injuries in the thoracolumbar spine. These have been classified either with great meticulousness, subdividing them into many different categories,[18] or by lumping them into a few categories. Prognostically, it is most effective to consider flexion-distraction injuries in the thoracolumbar spine as being divided into three major categories. The first category includes the pure bony flexion-distraction injuries; these are characterized by a fracture line propagating from posterior to anterior through the spinous process and lamina, into the pedicles, and into the vertebral body (Chance fracture). The second major category has both a bony component and a ligamentous injury. One injury variant occurs through the interspinous ligament and facet capsules in the posterior column, followed by bony injury occurring at the base of the pedicle into the middle and anterior columns of the vertebral body. A related injury is the converse: the fracture line occurs through the posterior bony elements and then proceeds anteriorly into the disc space. This may appear as a variant in children in which the cartilaginous endplate separates from the vertebral body instead of the usual discal injury. The third type of injury is the purely ligamentous injury. Again, the line of injury emanates from posterior through the interspinous ligament into the facet capsule and then across, from a posteroanterior direction into the joint, hinging off the anterior longitudinal ligament. Although this injury bears a great deal of resemblance to the bilateral facet dislocations in the cervical spine, the analogous characteristics of cervical and thoracolumbar injuries have not been discussed frequently. On closer inspection, the similarities between bilateral facet dislocations in the cervical spine and those in the thoracolumbar spine make analysis of components of

diagnosis, treatment, and prognosis more reasonable. This chapter discusses the pure ligamentous variant of the flexion-distraction injury, drawing on similarities to other flexion-distraction injuries in other areas of the spine. The differences between this injury and other flexion-distraction injuries of the thoracolumbar spine are emphasized as well.

ANATOMY

The distribution of these injuries in the thoracic, lumbar, and lumbosacral spine strongly suggests that the variation in the anatomy of the facet complex plays a large role in the genesis of this injury. The majority of these injuries occur at the thoracolumbar junction, with 40% in one series[23] occurring at the T12–L1 interspace and 60% at the thoracolumbar junction. Other authors, including Lewis and McKibbin,[26] showed that 51% of all facet dislocations occurring outside of the cervical spine occurred at the thoracolumbar junction. The possibility of a bilateral facet dislocation occurring in the thoracic region of the spine is more remote,[37] owing to both the orientation of the facet joints and the supporting structures of the ribs. The orientation of the facet joints in the thoracic spine is essentially coronal, with slight orientation toward the anterior portion of the spine. However, the predominant reason for the occurrence of few facet injuries at this level is the large amount of energy required to disrupt the rib cage. Thus, rather than the orientation of the facet joints, the junctional nature of the T12–L1 interspace is the chief reason for the high occurrence of injuries at that location. There is a reasonably rigid segment above, in the thoracic spine, with a transitional level facet joint occurring at T12–L1. The orientation of the facet joints at the thoracolumbar junction has not converted to the sagittal plane, as seen in the lower lumbar spine, thus making a flexion moment more likely to cause dissociation of the superior and inferior facets. With progression more caudally in the spine, the facet joints are oriented almost purely in a sagittal plane, with slight convergence of approximately 10 to 15 degrees toward the midline. The junctional nature of the

T12–L1 facet and, to a lesser extent, the L1–2 facet as a transition between the coronal plane of the thoracic joints and the parasagittal plane of the lumbar joints adds to the overall junctional nature of this level. Thus, the combination of the facet orientation, and the fact that a significant lever arm occurs above the level that is most often disrupted, provides the rationale for the frequent involvement of this level.

Another site of peak occurrence of facet injuries is located at the L5–S1 joint in the spine. As is discussed later, the mechanism of injury is often very different from those that occur at the thoracolumbar junction; but again, this represents a transitional zone. The sacrum forms a rigid kyphotic segment that is connected to the more flexible portion of the lumbar spine. In this area, the anatomic configuration of the facet joint contributes less to the occurrence of injury than does the transitional nature of the L5–S1 articulation.

MECHANISM OF INJURY

It is quite clear that for the majority of bilateral facet dislocations that occur in both the thoracic and the lumbar spine, the predominant mechanism of injury is flexion and distraction. Holdsworth and Hardy[19] originally thought that this injury was the result of severe flexion alone, resulting in failure of the posterior elements. As in the cervical spine, to cause anterior translation of the more superior segment over the inferior segment, it is necessary to distract the posterior ligamentous tissues so that the facet joints can clear one another as flexion occurs. Kelly and Whitesides[21] recognized this bilateral facet dislocation as a rare flexion-distraction injury. Much of the confusion concerning the nature of these injuries is related to this mechanism. A similar-appearing group of injuries with different prognostic significance and stability can easily be confused with this group, however. It is important to differentiate *facet dislocations* from *fracture dislocations* in the thoracolumbar spine. These represent a continuum of injuries ranging from a pure ligamentous bilateral facet dislocation with little or no body disruption, to a dislocation with anterior column comminution, to a dislocation associated with a burst fracture of the inferior level, and, finally, to a fracture-dislocation as the result of shear injury. If a relatively pure mechanism of flexion and distraction occurs, the injury will be reflected predominantly in ligamentous disruption. That is, as the distraction portion of the injury occurs, the interspinous ligament, facet capsules, and ligamentum flavum are disrupted and fail in tension. The inferior facet at the injury segment is distracted to a point at which it clears the tip of the superior facet, and as flexion occurs, disruption of the posterior longitudinal ligament and disc takes place in a posterior-to-anterior direction. The anterior longitudinal ligament is generally spared, as the center of rotation for this injury is approximately located at this juncture. In pure distraction injuries, all ligamentous connections are disrupted.[6] The anterior longitudinal ligament may, depending on the degree of flexion, be stripped off of the superior portion of the more caudal body in the injury segment. What is more important, if the flexion is greater, the probability exists that the anteroinferior portion of the upper vertebral body will be jammed into the superoanterior portion of the inferior body, thus causing some fracturing of the anterior portion of the inferior body. This is a limited anterior column injury with no significance to the ultimate degree of instability. There is, however, in this injury mechanism, no comminution of the middle column or the posterior wall of the vertebral body. The posterior wall is spared and remains intact, as it has been cleared by the initial distraction portion of the mechanism. Thus, depending on the degree of flexion imparted during the injury, the anterior column injury may simply consist of disc disruption up to but not including the anterior longitudinal ligament; or it may result in stripping of the anterior longitudinal ligament from the anterior portion of the body, with the ligament remaining intact; or, finally, a triangular fracture may occur off of the anterior portion of the inferior body, which generally remains in continuity with the intact anterior longitudinal ligament. If, after the dislocation occurs, an axial loading force is imparted to the injured segment, a two-column burst fracture may be associated with the facet dislocation. Treatment of this combined injury needs to take into account both the facet dislocation and the disruption of the anterior and middle columns from the burst fracture component. Occasionally a unilateral facet dislocation can occur as a result of both flexion-distraction and rotation forces.[27]

These injuries must be carefully differentiated from a fracture-dislocation of the thoracolumbar spine. In that type of injury, there is little or no distraction imparted to the posterior elements. Thus, as the translational deformity occurs by application of a shear force, the posterior elements (facets) are fractured, with the remainder of the injury line proceeding either through the disc or the vertebral body. There are many variants of this fracture-dislocation, which may include partial distraction of the posterior elements with either complete or incomplete fracture of one or both of the facets. This may also include a shear-type mechanism combined with axial compression, which causes a bursting injury to accompany the shear component. In this case, comminution of the entire vertebral body occurs, involving not only the anterior but also the posterior columns. A third variant of this shear injury is one in which a rotational moment is imparted. In this case, one facet is generally fractured and the other may be dislocated or may even remain intact, with obliteration of the canal owing to a shearing rotational force. It is important to differentiate the flexion-distraction (bilateral facet dislocation) injury from the shear injuries, as the degree of instability is much more significant in the latter. Recognition of the difference between these two injuries may make a critical difference in the planning and the durability of the instrumentation construct.

True bilateral facet dislocations at the lumbosacral junction are very rare. The reason is, again, related to the mechanism of injury. At the lumbosacral junction, the majority of injuries tend to be related to major trauma involving the pelvis. Thus, the cause of the injury is frequently either a fall from a height, where the direction of impact of the patient's pelvis and sacrum determines the force applied, or ejection from a motorcycle or motor vehicle. This is significantly different than the previously mentioned mechanisms for flexion-distraction–type injuries. Thus, as demonstrated in a variety of case reports and other published material, many of these patients have associated sacral fractures or other disruptions about the pelvis.

Facet dislocations at the thoracolumbar spine, as is the case with other flexion-distraction injuries, are the result of similar types of trauma as cause other types of spinal fractures. In one large series of bilateral facet dislocations,[23] 14 of 30 patients were injured in motor vehicle accidents: however, 1 injury was the result of a motorcycle accident, 9 were the result of falls from heights, 4 were the result of having heavy objects fall onto the back, and 3 were bicycle-related accidents. Any mechanism that pins the pelvis in a fixed location (e.g., a seat belt), or a free fall with resultant motion of the chest cage after the lumbosacral spine and pelvis are pinned at a fixed angle, can result in this type of flexion and distraction. The use of seat belts alone, as opposed to seat belts and shoulder harnesses, has been implicated as a cause of flexion-distraction injuries.

PATIENT EVALUATION

The evaluation of patients with possible facet injuries in the thoracolumbar spine differs little from that described for other types of major trauma. The critical steps, as outlined in the other chapters, begin with a comprehensive evaluation of the patient in an organized and sequential manner. The injury severity score[2] in a large series of these injuries[23] was 33 for thoracic injuries and 25 for lumbar injuries. Approximately half of all patients with this injury will have some other serious trauma as a result of the force of the impact. This reflects the high degree of force necessary to create this particular injury pattern. In addition, there is a known association of intra-abdominal trauma with flexion-distraction injuries in the thoracolumbar spine. Approximately 50% of all of the injuries that result from motor vehicle accidents with the use of lap belts include some degree of intra-abdominal injury,[1, 41] and the hallmarks of abdominal trauma in spinal injury patients have been well described.[39] The only unique distinguishing feature on initial evaluation is the kyphosis that may be associated with facet dislocations in the thoracolumbar spine. This is a more fixed kyphosis than is present with burst fractures, as a result of the locking of the facets. It has significant implication both for diagnosis and for treatment. It is critical to palpate the entire length of the spine in a potentially injured patient. Most patients present in the supine position and will need to be rolled gently into a semi-lateral position for the examiner to be able to palpate any deformity along the thoracolumbar spine. It has been shown that patients with dislocations have a significant kyphotic deformity.[23] This is much more obvi-

ous than bilateral facet dislocations in the cervical spine, especially when it occurs in the area from T11–L4. The implication for treatment, based on this physical examination, is related to the neurologic status of the patient. These are devastating injuries, and it has been shown that as a result of the intact neural arches, which translate one across the other, the incidence of complete and irrevocable paraplegia is higher in this injury than in any other single type of spinal injury. Depending on the series, approximately 90% of the patients with bilateral facet dislocations occurring in the thoracic spine (above T10) will have a complete paraplegia,[17, 22, 23, 37] but only 60% of the patients with bilateral facet dislocations below T10 will have complete paraplegia at the time of presentation.[23] The percentage of patients with significant spinal cord injury is much higher for bilateral facet dislocations in the thoracic and lumbar spine than for any other type of spinal fracture. Even teardrop fractures and bilateral facet dislocations in the cervical spine do not demonstrate a neural injury incidence of 80%. Certainly, even burst fractures of the thoracolumbar spine do not exceed a 40% neural injury rate. Thus, if a patient with a thoracolumbar dislocation is placed in the supine position, the extension of the thoracolumbar spine at the level of the relatively fixed deformity (kyphosis that results from the injury) causes further narrowing of the canal. It is possible to demonstrate that a patient with an incomplete spinal injury from a bilateral facet dislocation who is placed in the lateral position with the knees flexed will regain some function that was lost when the same patient was placed in the supine position. Therefore, in patients with incomplete injury who have a demonstrated facet dislocation, it is preferable to place them in the lateral position with the spine slightly flexed. This minimizes the intrusion of the superior facets into the canal and may preserve some function. It is possible to do a computed tomographic (CT) scan by placing the patient into the scanner in a lateral position, thus allowing the workup to proceed. The patient's position will also be important when attempting to reduce the facet dislocation. Thus, during the physical examination for thoracolumbar spine dislocation, it is important to examine the patient's neurologic status in both the lateral slightly flexed and the supine positions.

RADIOLOGIC EVALUATION

As with other injuries in the thoracolumbar spine, the radiologic evaluation is relatively straightforward, although a number of pathognomonic features can be identified with this injury. Once the patient has been carefully examined for neurologic status as well as deformity, appropriate radiographs are done. Victims of polytrauma should undergo a standard workup that includes, at least, a lateral cervical spine radiograph, anteroposterior (AP) and lateral views of the thoracic spine, AP and lateral views of the lumbar spine, chest x-ray, and AP view of the pelvis. If this injury occurs at the thoracolumbar junction and is not well centered on either the thoracic or lumbar spine, then additional spot radiographs should be taken with the beam centered on the injury to optimally define the injury. This particular injury pattern in the thoracolumbar spine has a very distinctive radiologic appearance that is usually evident on the plain radiographs. The integrity of the posterior walls of the two vertebrae that make up the injury segment should be carefully inspected on the lateral radiograph (Fig. 26–1). In distinction to fracture-dislocations, the height and concave contour of the posterior wall at both levels remains totally intact. There is also significant translation of the superior level over the inferior level. The range of translation is from approximately 10% to 60% (mean, ~40%) based on the width of the intact body. The integrity of the posterior wall is easier to evaluate from T12–L5 than it is in the thoracic spine, and CT reconstructions may be required to make that differentiation. As mentioned previously, the anterior column, or anterior portion of the vertebral body, may in fact be slightly compressed. This does not change the nature of the injury. It is simply a manifestation of the angle of flexion of the superior body at the time of impact, and the anterior column can

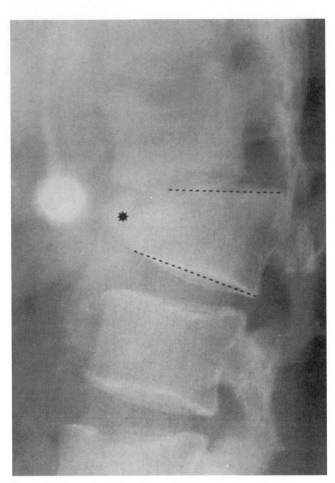

Figure 26–2 = Lateral radiograph demonstrates anterior compression of the lower vertebral segment (*dotted lines*). In addition, a small fragment from the anterosuperior portion of the body (*star*) frequently is fractured off as the anterior longitudinal ligament is stripped from the body. (From Levine AM, Bosse M, Edwards CC: Bilateral facet dislocation in the thoracolumbar spine. Spine 13:632, 1988.)

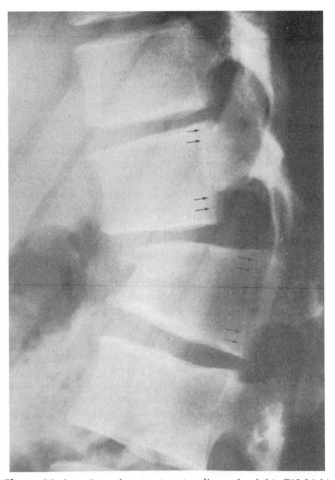

Figure 26–1 = Lateral pretreatment radiograph of this T12-L1 bilateral facet dislocation demonstrates significant translation out of proportion to the degree of body comminution. In addition, the posterior walls of both the superior and inferior vertebral bodies are intact (*arrows*). (From Levine AM, Bosse M, Edwards CC: Bilateral facet dislocation in the thoracolumbar spine. Spine 13:632, 1988.)

vary from having no bony injury to slight compression (approximately 20%) to a small fragmentary avulsion off the anterior superior corner that remains attached to the anterior longitudinal ligament (Fig. 26–2). The dislocation of the facets can sometimes be appreciated on a lateral radiograph of injuries that occur in the lumbar spine, but rarely in the thoracic spine. In only approximately 33% of dislocations that occur in the thoracic spine are facet dislocations clearly demonstrated on the lateral radiograph, whereas in the thoracolumbar junction and the lumbar spine, approximately 75% were clearly demonstrated. However, interpretation of the AP radiograph is important for two reasons. First, it is essential to differentiate a facet dislocation from a fracture dislocation (shear injury), and this can often be done with the AP radiograph. The majority of shear injuries demonstrate bidirectional displacement. By definition, there is anterior translation in a bilateral facet dislocation demonstrated on the lateral film. However, if this is a straight bilateral facet dislocation, the AP film will show relatively satisfactory alignment of the upper and lower portions of the injury segment. However, if this is a shear injury, lateral translation will generally be demonstrated on the AP radiograph. Lateral translation cannot easily occur if the inferior facet of the level above is intact and is wedged firmly within the spinal canal. Additionally, on the AP radiograph, because of the distraction of the posterior column, an increased space is seen between the spinous processes. This can usually be easily identified. In addition, the dislocation of the facets in both the thoracic and the lumbar spine can usually be clearly identified. In more than 50% of the cases, the facet dislocation could be clearly seen on the AP radiograph. Additionally, the fracture patterns may be differentiated from burst fractures in that the interpedicular distance remains constant, as the ring of the neural canal is not disrupted in this flexion-distraction injury.

Preoperative evaluation with a CT scan is routine for these patients. Generally, 3-mm axial sections are used. The empty facet sign as described by O'Callaghan and co-workers[33] and Denis[8] is present in the large majority of patients (Fig. 26–3). Other features noted on the axial sections of the CT scan are marked compromise in the canal diameter and residual area on static analysis.[16, 17, 35, 42, 44] The double-body sign is also present in a majority of cases, as the flexion component of the injury generally brings a portion of the superior body down to the level of the superior portion of the inferior body, with the result that both are visible on a single section of the CT scan (see Fig. 26–3). The CT scan can be used to critically evaluate all of the spinal elements and to better understand the nature of the instability.[29]

Sagittal reconstructions constitute one of the most effective means to demonstrate the degree of canal compromise. As demonstrated by Gellad and associates,[17] the midsagittal reconstruction can be very effective in determining prognosis. Based on a true measurement of the residual midsagittal diameter, it was found that patients who were neurologically intact or who had incomplete lesions at the time of presentation, had a residual midsagittal diameter ranging from 8 to 15 mm (mean, 11.2 mm). The patients who were neurologically complete at the time of presentation had a midsagittal diameter ranging from 5 to 8.5 mm (mean, 6.6 mm). Obviously, location within the spine is critical to those measurements. The canal diameter is larger and the space required for the neural elements is smaller in the lumbar spine; in the thoracic spine, the converse is true.

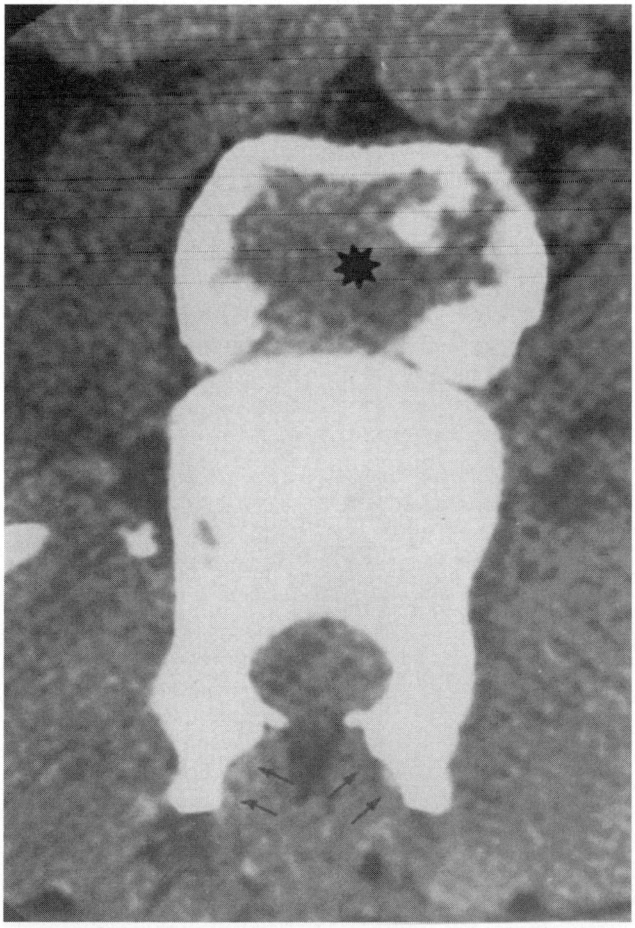

TREATMENT

Treatment of facet dislocations in the thoracolumbar spine has involved little controversy. Postural reduction is ineffective in bilateral facet dislocations,[7] and it may in fact account for the 13% failure rate originally reported by Frankel and colleagues.[15] The nonoperative treatment is a failure for two basic reasons. The first is that despite the significant degree of disruption in all of the ligamentous structures, nonoperative reduction of this injury is essentially impossible. The degree of disruption of the interspinous ligament facet capsules, ligamentum flavum, and disc is very similar to that which occurs in bilateral facet dislocations in the cervical spine. However, it is impossible to apply equivalent amounts of axial traction to disengage the facets and allow postural reduction. This was recognized very early by Bedbrook,[4] who, despite advocacy of postural reduction, thought that bilateral facet dislocation was a cause for immediate surgical reduction. The second reason for the potential failure of nonoperative treatment is that if it were possible to accomplish reduction nonoperatively, with complete disruption of all of the ligamentous structures, with the best result, a kyphotic deformity would exist at the conclusion of treatment, and with the worst result, a redislocation would occur. Disruption of the posterior ligamentous complex and the anulus leads to chronic instability in the majority of cases.[20, 44] Thus, it is the consensus of the majority of authors that the treatment goals for bilateral facet dislocations are reduction of the deformity, adequate decompression of the dural contents, and stabilization, with resultant fusion of the spine. Although it may appear that reduction of the vertebral bodies and stabilization should result in complete clearance of any

Figure 26–3 ＝ Preoperative CT scan demonstrates both the empty facet sign (*arrows*) and the double-body sign (*star*). (From Levine AM, Bosse M, Edwards CC: Bilateral facet dislocation in the thoracolumbar spine. Spine 13:632, 1988.)

canal compromise, this can be a misconception. Recognition of the severity and the significance of the disc disruption at the injury segment between the two dislocated levels is a central concept in the management of thoracolumbar bilateral facet dislocations. There is general agreement that the posterior approach is the most reasonable way to deal with these injuries,[4, 5, 14, 31, 36, 40, 43, 44] although posterior compression fixation had been thought to be the most appropriate method of fixation until recently.[4, 5, 14, 25, 30, 31, 35] Thus, the type of instrumentation must deal appropriately with the ligamentous nature of the injury and the discal disruption.

The initial consideration in operative treatment of facet dislocations in the thoracolumbar spine is positioning. Use of standard techniques of hyperextension positioning to reduce burst fractures is counterproductive in facet dislocations. Because postural reduction cannot occur, and reduction requires distraction of the posterior elements, hyperextension positioning for injuries in both the thoracic and lumbar areas will, in fact, make the reduction more difficult. Generally, reduction can be aided by placement of the patient in the prone position with the table flexed to accommodate the resting position of the spine. This causes relaxation of the posterior elements and makes reduction of the dislocated facets easier. This positioning can be done either on a spinal frame that allows the position to be changed from flexion to extension during the procedure or, preferably, on longitudinal rolls, with the table flexed at the outset. A midline approach is used. The defect between the spinous processes at the level of injury is almost always palpable. On incision of the skin, the massive disruption of the soft tissues is usually evident. In the thoracic spine, this may take the form of a subcutaneous dissection over the posterior aspect of the chest wall on both sides, with a large hematoma. It may, however, simply be evident in either the thoracic or the lumbar spine as a defect that is visible and palpable immediately after incision of the skin. Careful dissection is necessary along intact spinous processes at least one segment distal or proximal to the injury segment. Dissection at the level of the injury should be avoided until more proximal and distal segments are exposed. Subperiosteal dissection of the proximal and distal segments will then place the intermediate soft tissues on stretch, and they can be gradually and gently stripped from their attachments on the spinous processes of the two involved vertebrae. Care must be taken in the midline, however, to avoid dissection, as there are frequently no structures superficial to the dural sac. If the soft tissues are significantly disrupted and devascularized, they can be debrided at the time of exposure. Once exposure is completed down to the level of injury, care is taken to carefully expose the facet joints. The cartilage of the superior facet will be evident in the wound dorsal to the bony elements of the inferior facet. The disrupted ligamentum flavum and interspinous ligament can be very carefully debrided from the injured interspace to allow visualization of the spinal canal elements. In the thoracic spine, in patients with complete injuries, it is not

unusual to encounter complete disruption of the dural tube.[38] When looking into the disrupted segment, no structures may be visible except the posterior wall of the vertebral bodies. It is not recommended that this be probed, as clot, which will prevent subsequent dural leak, is generally evident in the canal. If the dural sac is intact, the disrupted soft tissues are removed sufficient to evaluate it. Before achieving reduction of the dislocation, it is reasonable to denude the cartilage from the exposed superior facets. In some instances, a small chip may be fractured off of the superior aspect of the superior facet, but this is of little consequence. It is not recommended to resect the superior facets to allow ease of reduction, because this will result in increased instability and more difficulty in attaining adequate fixation. Once the level is thoroughly debrided of soft tissues and the anatomy is fully visualized, a laminar spreader (Fig. 26–4) can be placed at the base of the two spinous processes of the involved levels. Generally, neither towel clips nor any other bone-holding clamps allow sufficient gradual pressure necessary to achieve this reduction, and a large amount of distractive force is necessary to disengage the facets at almost any level from T2 down to L5. The laminar spreader is gently distracted, one click at a time, until the tip of the inferior facet just reaches the level of the tip of the dislocated superior facet. If the table or the patient is in extension, this requires an inordinate amount of force, whereas if the patient is in slight flexion, the amount of force required to achieve this degree of distraction is minimal. This will re-create, to some degree, the direction of the injury, but not sufficiently to cause any damage to the dural contents. Once the sufficient amount of distraction has been achieved to disengage the facets, it is recommended that the towel clips, or other bone-holding forceps, be placed on the spinous processes on either side of the injury, and while the surgeon gently rotates the laminar spreader to cause the inferior segment to translate anteriorly, the assistant, with his bone-holding clamps, pushes forward on the inferior segment, and pulls gently back on the superior segment until the facet tips are in proper alignment. At that point, the laminar spreader tension is gently reduced, allowing the facets to seat in normal alignment. It will generally not be possible to effect a complete and symmetrical reduction at this point. However, once the facets are in proper orientation to each other, the table can be gently brought to either a neutral position or to a position of very slight extension. Additionally, an interspinous wire can be placed through the spinous process of the superior level and around the inferior portion of the lower level of the dislocation; this is gently tightened until the reduction appears to be complete with reference to the alignment of the facet joints. This should not be overtightened, as it can cause compression of the disc; in the neurologically incomplete or normal patient, overtightening has the potential to cause neurologic deficit by resultant extrusion of the disc.

The consideration of methods of stabilization can be based both on the biomechanical constraints of the injury and on personal preference. Although it seems

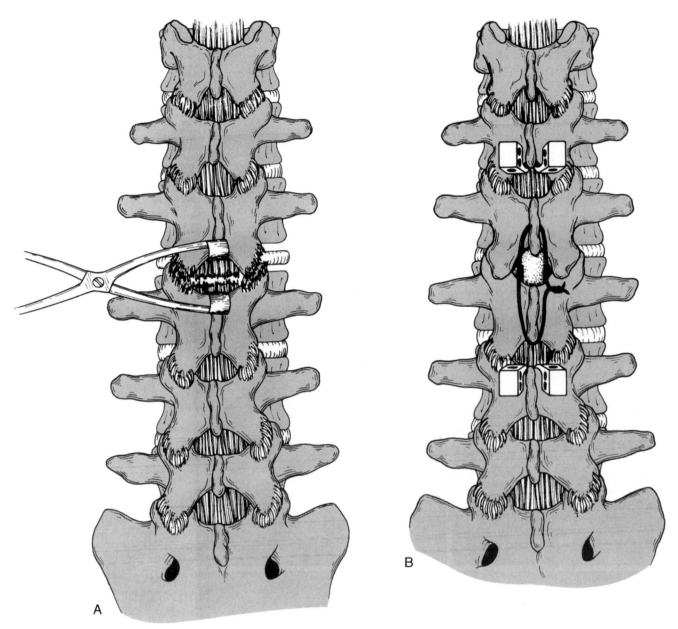

Figure 26–4 = It should be possible to accomplish reduction of bilateral facet dislocation in the lumbar spine in a controlled fashion with preservation of the facets to allow reestablishment of stability. Dissection of the soft tissues is accomplished, and the facet dislocations are identified. Ruptured ligamentum flavum is removed, as are the disrupted facet capsules. Cartilage is removed for the superior facet of the lower level under direct vision. A laminar spreader is then placed between the two spinous processes and is gently manipulated until the facets are distracted. When the tips of the facets are disengaged, the laminar spreader is tipped, pushing the inferior facet anteriorly and pulling the superior facets posteriorly. The distraction on the laminar spreader is then released, allowing the facets to engage in a normal position. *A*, An interspinous wire is placed across the involved level and tightened to complete the reduction and reestablish stability. A short rod-sleeve construct can then be applied. *B*, The slight distraction applied by the rod-sleeve construct does not cause redislocation, as the primary force is lordotic, which counteracts the flexion moment of the original injury. (From Levine AM: Lumbar and sacral spinal trauma. *In* Browner BD, Jupiter JB, Levine AM, et al (eds): Skeletal Trauma: Fractures, Dislocations, Ligamentous Injuries, vol 1. Philadelphia, WB Saunders, 1992, p 844.)

reasonable that a construct that applies extension and compression would counteract the deforming forces of a flexion-distraction mechanism of injury and prevent redislocation, this premise must be examined carefully. If just the bony elements of the injury were being considered, this would be a very reasonable assumption. In addition, the use of compression constructs, because of their intrinsic stability, can generally be shorter in number of segments instrumented than other types of spinal instrumentation. Compression constructs, which are shorter, are less subject to bending moments, which increases their stability. Second, axial loading in a compression construct is borne in part by the facets, rather than by the instrumentation alone. Third, the compressed facets provide some rotational stability. Stauffer and Neil[40] and Pinzur and co-workers[34] showed that stability of compression fixation increased in posterior column injuries caused by tension

Thoracolumbar Burst Fractures

Mark M. Scheffer || *Bradford L. Currier*

The evaluation and management of burst fractures of the thoracolumbar spine have changed dramatically in the past 20 years. Improved imaging techniques such as computed tomography (CT) and magnetic resonance imaging (MRI) have led to a better understanding of fracture patterns, neural compression, and spinal instability. Instrumentation systems have evolved rapidly and have allowed surgeons to decompress and stabilize the spine in various ways.

Surgical management offers distinct advantages over nonoperative management for unstable burst fractures, but the precise indications for operative intervention are still being defined. The purpose of this chapter is to review the historical development and current concepts of the evaluation and treatment of burst fractures.

Our current classification schemes evolved from studies of thoracolumbar spine injuries performed around the time of World War II.[47, 84] In 1943, Watson-Jones[84] noted that 15% of the injuries were comminuted wedge fractures, which would later be known as burst fractures.

In 1949, Nicoll[70] proposed the first widely accepted classification of thoracolumbar injuries. The classification was based on 166 injuries he treated in coal miners; he classified injuries as anterior wedge fractures, lateral wedge fractures, fracture-dislocations, and neural arch fractures. Again, what would later be known as burst fractures were termed anterior wedge fractures with comminution. Unstable burst fractures that displayed facet joint subluxation or posterior element fractures may have been classified as fracture-dislocations. Nicoll observed that anterior wedge fractures with severe comminution almost invariably were associated with damage to the disc, interspinous ligaments, or both.[70] Although he recognized that collapse of comminuted wedge fractures into some degree of kyphosis was inevitable, he classified anterior wedge fractures as stable injuries.

Holdsworth[39, 40] was the first to use the term "burst fracture" to describe the fracture produced by extreme flexion. He recognized that this fracture resulted from the disc rupturing through the vertebral end plate into the vertebral body and causing it to explode or burst. His classification, based on Nicoll's, divided spine injuries into stable and unstable injuries. Stable injuries included compression wedge fractures and compression burst fractures. Unstable injuries included dislocations, extension fracture-dislocations, and rotational fracture-dislocations. He thought that stability after an injury was based on the integrity of the posterior ligamentous complex (PLC), composed of the facet joints, neural arch, interspinous and supraspinous ligaments, and the ligamentum flavum. Holdsworth maintained that direct longitudinal pull along the fibers of the posterior ligaments rarely resulted in rupture and that with the introduction of twisting and pulling, these ligaments were readily torn. He believed that because burst fractures resulted from pure vertical compression, the PLC should remain intact and this injury should be stable.

In 1968, Kelly and Whitesides[47] published an article based on Holdsworth's classification scheme in which they stated that the spine functions as two columns: an anterior column composed of solid bone, disc, anterior longitudinal ligament (ALL), and posterior longitudinal ligament (PLL), and a posterior column composed of the PLC. They slightly modified Holdsworth's classification by placing burst fractures in the unstable category.

McAfee and co-authors[65] added to the understanding of the unstable burst fracture in an article published in 1983 in which they noted that Holdsworth's classification did not include burst fractures with associated PLC disruptions. The authors recognized the potential for these fractures to develop late instability characterized by decreased vertebral height, posterior laxity, and progressive kyphosis. Their criteria for instability were based on neural deficit, PLC disruption, deformity, and canal compromise[65] (Table 27–1).

Their conclusions supported previous observations by Bradford and colleagues[8] that patients with unstable burst fractures who were treated nonoperatively tended to develop post-traumatic spinal stenosis, increased kyphosis with mechanical back pain, and increased neural deficits.

In 1983, Denis[17] proposed the three-column theory of

Table 27–1 == **THE UNSTABLE BURST FRACTURE**

1. Progressive neural deficit
2. Posterior ligamentous complex disruption
3. Kyphosis progressing 20 degrees or more with neural deficit
4. More than 50% loss of vertebral body height with facet joint subluxation
5. Computed tomographic demonstration of free bony fragments within a compromised spinal canal associated with incomplete neural deficit

From McAfee PC, Yuan HA, Lasda NA: The unstable burst fracture. Spine 7:365, 1982.

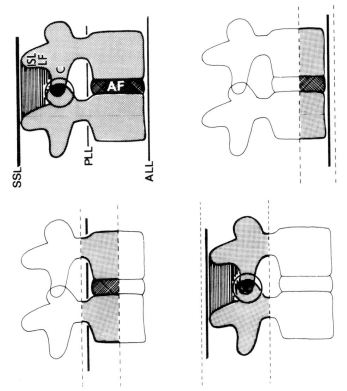

Figure 27–1 = Anterior, middle, and posterior columns, as defined by Denis.[17] *AF*, anulus fibrosus; *ALL*, anterior longitudinal ligament; *C*, facet joint capsule; *ISL*, intraspinous ligament; *LF*, ligamentum flavum; *PLL*, posterior longitudinal ligament; *SSL*, supraspinous ligament. (From Denis F: The three column spine and its significance in the classification of acute thoracolumbar spinal injuries. Spine 8:817, 1983.)

Table 27–2 = **CLASSIFICATION OF THORACOLUMBAR FRACTURES BASED ON THREE-COLUMN CONCEPT**

TYPE OF FRACTURE	COLUMN		
	Anterior	*Middle*	*Posterior*
Compression	Compression	None	None or distraction (severe)
Burst	Compression	Compression	None
Seat belt	None or compression	Distraction	Distraction
Fracture-dislocation	Compression, rotation, or shear	Distraction, rotation, or shear	Distraction, rotation, or shear

From Denis F: The three column spine and its significance in the classification of acute thoracolumbar spinal injuries. Spine 8:817, 1983.

quires decompression. Denis defined three types of instability: mechanical (first-degree), neurologic (second-degree), and combined mechanical and neurologic (third-degree).

Shortly after the Denis three-column theory was published, McAfee and co-workers[64] published their own classification scheme, which was intended to combine into a simplified classification the individual merits of the Denis scheme and the biomechanical scheme proposed by White and Panjabi.[86] This scheme was composed of six injury types: (1) wedge-compression

spinal instability and altered Holdsworth's classification scheme to include flexion-distraction ("seat belt") injuries. Denis divided Holdsworth's anterior column into two parts: the newly described anterior column included the ALL and the anterior half of the vertebral body and anulus fibrosus; the middle column included the PLL and the posterior half of the vertebral body and the anulus fibrosus; and the posterior column was the previously defined PLC (Fig. 27–1). The three-column theory was based on experimental studies that showed that instability occurred only after disruption of the middle column in addition to either the posterior or anterior column. The classification of Denis divided injuries into compression fractures, burst fractures, seat belt injuries, and fracture-dislocations on the basis of the columns involved and the mode of failure (Table 27–2). Burst fractures were defined as injuries involving compression failure of the anterior and middle columns. Burst fractures were further subdivided into five subtypes (Fig. 27–2). Further studies will be necessary to determine whether the subclassification of burst fractures is clinically helpful. One beneficial aspect of the subdivision of burst fractures is that it focuses attention on the area of greatest neurologic compression. Although most burst fractures are associated with canal compromise from fracture of the superior end plate, occasionally the inferior end-plate region re-

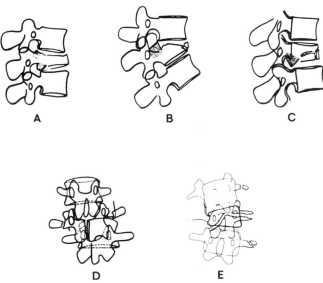

Figure 27–2 = Subclassification of burst fractures. *A*, Fracture of both end plates from a pure axial load. This pattern most commonly occurs in the low lumbar region and does not lead to kyphosis. If operation is indicated, decompression is necessary at two levels. *B*, Fracture of the superior end plate from axial load and flexion. This is the most common pattern of burst fractures and generally occurs at the thoracolumbar junction. When indicated, decompression is necessary only at the upper level. *C*, Fracture of the inferior end plate from axial load and flexion. This is a rare injury. *D*, Burst rotation secondary to axial load and rotation. This may be misdiagnosed as a fracture-dislocation. The lateral radiograph would resemble a type A pattern. *E*, Burst lateral flexion secondary to axial load and lateral flexion. Lateral radiograph may resemble type A, B, or C. (From Denis F: The three column spine and its significance in the classification of acute thoracolumbar spinal injuries. Spine 8:817, 1983.)

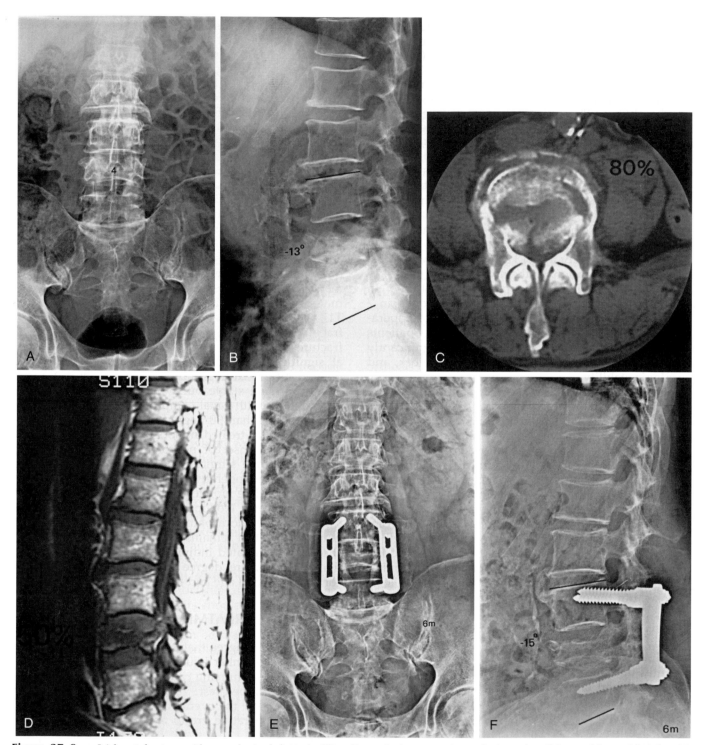

Figure 27–8 = L4 burst fracture with neurologic deficit. *A*, AP radiograph demonstrating splaying of pedicles and loss of height of L4 vertebral body. *B*, Lateral radiograph showing fracture of both end plates of L4, typical of low lumbar fracture (Denis type A pattern). Lordosis of L3–5 is 13 degrees. *C*, CT scan demonstrating canal compromise of 80% at L4. *D*, Sagittal MRI scan showing 50% loss of vertebral body height and bone retropulsed into the canal. *E*, AP radiograph obtained 6 months postoperatively showing laminectomy of L4 and posterolateral fusion of L3–5 with VSP plate instrumentation. VSP plates were chosen because the spinal deformity was not great and reduction was unnecessary. *F*, Lateral radiograph obtained 6 months postoperatively showing fusion in situ with 15 degrees of lordosis at L3–5.

mentation with Harrington rods and other types of rod-hook systems have been popularized for the treatment of burst fractures.

Distraction instrumentation allows reduction of intracanal fragments by ligamentotaxis. Reduction by lig-

amentotaxis has been thought to occur when the intact PLL becomes taut during distraction and pushes the retropulsed fragments anteriorly, away from the canal. Recently, work by Fredrickson and co-workers[31] showed that it may be the anulus and not the PLL that is responsible for reduction by ligamentotaxis. Willén and co-authors[90] showed that indirect canal decompression with Harrington distraction instrumentation increased canal patency from 58.7% preoperatively to 73.6% postoperatively when the operation was performed within 3 days of injury. When the operation was delayed more than 3 days after injury, very little change in canal patency occurred (from 66% to 71%); this result indicates that as the fracture begins to consolidate, indirect reduction becomes less likely.

A disadvantage of this type of instrumentation is that at least two levels above and below the level of injury must be fused. On the basis of a series of 95 patients reported in 1978, Dickson and associates[19] recommended fusing two levels above and two levels below the injured vertebra. Purcell and co-workers[73] performed a biomechanical study on rod fixation of the thoracolumbar spine and concluded that the most stable construct involved rodding three vertebrae above and two vertebrae below the fracture. Adding the additional vertebra above the fracture increased the failure moment by an average of 65% compared with instrumentation of two vertebrae above and below the fracture. The mode of failure changed from slipping out of the upper hooks as a result of vertebral tilt to total laminar failure when longer instrumentation was used. Long rods are necessary because increasing the distance from the fracture site decreases the force on the hooks, reducing the risk of cutout or dislodgment of the hooks.[50] Some authors have recommended the "rod long–fuse short" technique, in which three levels above and below the injury are immobilized with Harrington rods but only one level above and below is

actually fused.[78] The rods are then removed 12 to 24 months postoperatively with the hope that the unfused, immobilized motion segments regain pain-free motion. However, examination of the immobilized but unfused facet joints has shown that the cartilage undergoes degenerative changes that may lead to chronic pain.[43, 44]

The stability of Harrington rods can be enhanced by fixation of the rods to the spine with sublaminar wires.[33, 80] Sullivan[80] recommended fusing three levels above and two levels below the fracture site. The sublaminar wires are passed at two levels below the superior hook and one level above the inferior hook.

High-density polyethylene sleeves placed over the rods can also enhance the stability of Harrington rod instrumentation. According to Edwards and Levine, "the rod-sleeve construct corrects post-traumatic kyphosis by producing an extension 'moment' to directly oppose the flexion 'moment' that caused the deformity"[21] (Fig. 27–9). If the posterior elements are not involved, a single rod-sleeve can be placed on each side of the spinous process directly posterior to the fractured vertebra, but if the posterior elements are fractured, two sets of sleeves are used, one above the fracture and one below, on each side of the spinous processes; this is called a bridging construct.[21] Edwards sleeves provide three-point fixation and allow the construct to store elastic energy. In a series of patients treated with the rod-sleeve construct, kyphosis was reduced from 14 degrees to 0 degrees, and vertebral body height was increased from 68% of normal to 96%. Also, canal patency was increased from 55% to 87% in patients operated on within 3 days.[21]

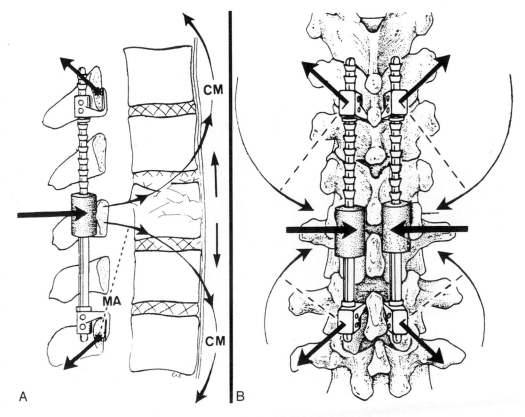

Figure 27–9 = Biomechanics of rod sleeve construct. *A,* Corrective moments *(CM)* are generated by an anterior force from the sleeves acting through the moment arms *(MA),* which pivot about the hooks *(asterisk).* The corrective moments create simultaneous hyperextension and distraction. *B,* Forces are directed medially from the sleeves and laterally from the hooks to enhance rotational stability and correct medial-lateral translation and scoliosis. (From Edwards CC, Levine AM: Early rod-sleeve stabilization of the injured thoracic and lumbar spine. Orthop Clin North Am 17:121, 1986.)

Burst fractures of the relatively immobile thoracic spine can be treated with Harrington rod distraction instrumentation without regard to the long fusion mass required. Fusion of vital motion segments in the lumbar spine, especially L4 and L5, should be avoided, however, and methods of instrumentation that allow a shorter fusion should be used.[53]

Reduction of intracanal fragments with distraction instrumentation may be insufficient to relieve cord or cauda equina compression. Further decompression may be achieved either posterolaterally or anteriorly. Some authors have recommended the use of intraoperative ultrasound to assess canal patency after distraction with reduction (Fig. 27–10).[23, 83] In a prospective study by Eismont and co-workers,[23] intraoperative ultrasonography demonstrated persistent cord or root

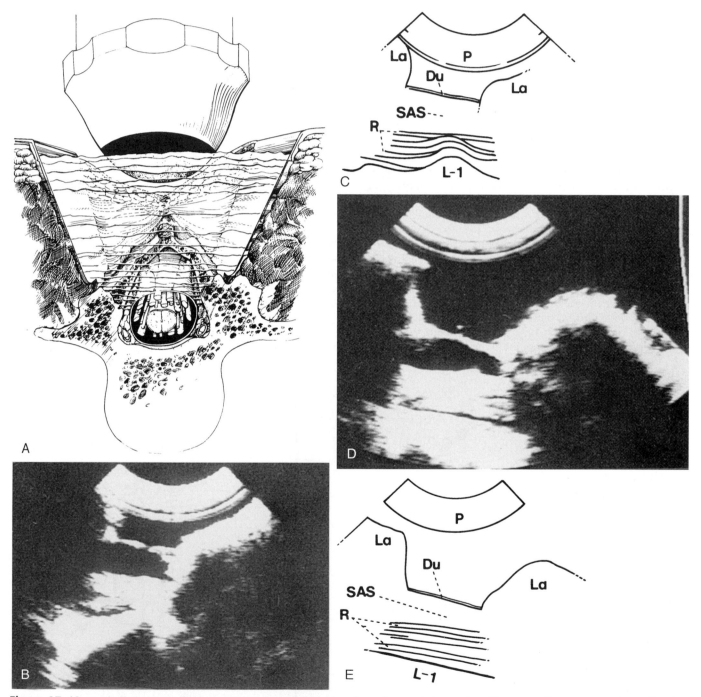

Figure 27–10 = Intraoperative ultrasonography. *A*, Ultrasound probe submersed in sterile saline several centimeters from the dura. Transverse and sagittal sections are obtained by rotating the probe 90 degrees about its longitudinal axis. *B*, Midsagittal plane ultrasound scan of L1 burst fracture demonstrating anterior impingement on the cauda equina. *C*, Sketch of *B*. *Du*, dura mater; *La*, lamina; *L-1*, L1 vertebral body; *P*, ultrasound probe tip; *R*, nerve rootlets; *SAS*, subarachnoid space. *D*, Midsagittal ultrasound scan obtained after posterolateral decompression. Fragment of bone impinging nerve rootlets has been removed and subarachnoid space is now present anterior to the cauda equina. *E*, Sketch of *D*. Abbreviations are the same as those in *C*. (From Eismont FJ, Green BA, Berkowitz BM, et al: The role of intraoperative ultrasonography in the treatment of thoracic and lumbar spine fractures. Spine 9:782, 1984.)

compression in 12 of 16 burst fractures after Harrington rod distraction instrumentation. Patients with incomplete reduction of the canal underwent posterolateral decompression. Eight of the 12 fractures were evaluated postoperatively with CT and all eight showed 100% or near 100% canal patency. Intraoperative myelography may also be used to assess cord compression after distraction instrumentation.

McAfee and colleagues[65] reported a series of 17 patients with neurologic deficits treated with Harrington rod instrumentation and posterolateral decompression: 2 improved two Frankel grades, 7 improved one grade, 3 did not improve, and all 5 patients with conus lesions had complete resolution of their deficits. None of the patients deteriorated neurologically.

Decompression of burst fractures by laminectomy should be condemned.[8] Laminectomy disrupts the posterior column and further destabilizes the spine.[8] The neural elements are compressed anteriorly in a burst fracture and unless the fracture occurs in the lordotic lumbar spine, removing the lamina will not achieve decompression. An exception to this is patients with laminar fractures associated with burst fractures. These patients seem to have an increased incidence of dural laceration with neural element entrapment in the lamina fracture site[11] (see Fig. 27–4). Cammisa and co-workers[11] reviewed 60 thoracolumbar burst fractures and found that 11 of 30 patients with associated lamina fractures had dural tears. Four of the 11 patients had neural elements interposed in the laminar fracture site. From this important study, one can conclude that patients with an associated lamina fracture and a neurologic deficit should have decompression from a posterior approach to exclude the possibility that neural elements are caught in the laminar fracture site and to repair a dural laceration if present.

Anterior decompression and fusion may be performed after posterior distraction instrumentation in patients with incomplete neurologic deficits and persistent neural compression.[63] Many authors believe that the canal can be decompressed most effectively from the anterior approach.[12, 42, 63] Bradford and McBride[9] compared neurologic recovery in patients with thoracolumbar spine fractures treated with either anterior or posterior decompression. They found that neurologic recovery after decompression was 88% in the anterior group and 64% in the posterior group. They thought that the poorer results in the posterior group resulted from the greater amount of postoperative residual canal compromise demonstrated in that group on CT. Anterior decompression is the most direct means of removing the retropulsed bone and disc from the anterior aspect of the thecal sac and does not require any manipulation of the neural elements. After decompression, bone graft can be fashioned from a tricortical iliac crest graft, fibular graft, rib graft, or even femoral allograft. The graft can be fashioned to key into the vertebral body above and below the fractured vertebra. Caution should be used in approaching the spine anteriorly from T8 to L2 because the major medullary feeder vessel, the artery of Adamkiewicz, is located in a variable position in that region.[42] The blood supply to the cord can be protected by avoiding dissection around the collateral vessels located in the neural foramina.

Further decompression is indicated in patients with a neurologic deficit if a significant amount of canal compromise persists after posterior distraction instrumentation. Opinions vary regarding how much canal compromise is considered significant. In a series reported by Edwards and co-workers,[22] 23 patients with thoracolumbar burst fractures treated with early rod-sleeve instrumentation had residual canal compromise of more than 20%. After an average follow-up of 21 months, canal patency increased from an average of 56% to 87%, presumably from resorption and remodeling of the bone fragments. The authors concluded that if "posterior instrumentation restores normal spine alignment and reduces fragments actually compressing the cord, there is no need for further surgery."[22]

Pedicle Screw Fixation

Roy-Camille and co-workers[76] began using a pedicle screw fixation device in 1961. They devised a system in which intrapedicular screws and precontoured plates are used throughout the entire thoracolumbar spine. This construct is semirigid in that there is motion at the screw-plate junction, which necessitates the instrumentation of two levels above and below the fractured vertebra and the use of a hyperextension orthosis or jacket to achieve stabilization.[15, 24]

The use of dynamic compression plates and pedicle screws for the treatment of thoracolumbar burst fractures has been reported. In a series by Sasso and co-workers,[77] dynamic compression plates with pedicle screws were used to treat seven lumbar burst fractures. These fractures were instrumented two vertebrae above and two below the fractured vertebra. Of note is the fact that none of the patients were placed in casts or orthoses postoperatively. All of the patients achieved union at the fusion site, but loss of alignment was common. Although the traumatic kyphosis was corrected at operation, most of the patients had lost correction by 3 months postoperatively. The authors concluded that the recurrence of deformity was due to the plate-screw construct acting as a tension band, and load sharing by the vertebral column is necessary. In the case of burst fractures, the load-sharing capacity of the vertebral bodies is impaired and immobilization in a hyperextension cast or orthosis is necessary.[77]

Other pedicle screw and plate systems have been designed by Steffee and colleagues[79] and Luque and Rapp.[59] The advantage of these systems is that a relatively rigid fixation can be achieved by the instrumentation of only two motion segments, one vertebra above the fracture and one vertebra below the fracture. The disadvantages are that the plate must be contoured before insertion and therefore a good reduction is necessary before instrumentation. The implant itself cannot be used very effectively to help achieve reduction of the kyphotic deformity or decompression of the intracanal fragments. These devices are most useful

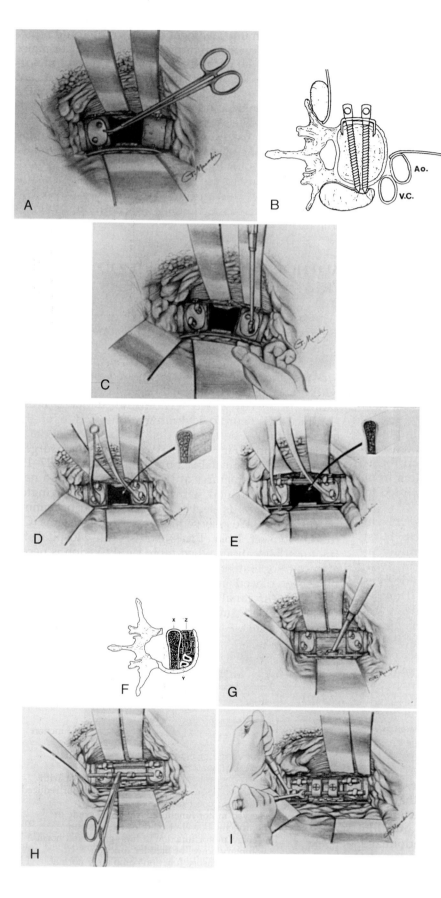

Figure 27–13 = *A*, Application of the vertebral plate. *B*, Direction of screw insertion. *C*, Checking for penetration of the screw chip on the contralateral vertebral cortex. *D*, Correction of kyphosis and insertion of an iliac crest as a strut. *E*, Correction of kyphosis in patients with combined burst fracture and flexion-distraction injury. *F*, Transverse section of bone grafting. *X*, iliac crest; *Y*, rib; *Z*, bone chip from the resected vertebral body. *G*, Bone grafting. *H*, Application of the paraspinal rods. *I*, Application of the transverse fixators and tightening of the nuts. (From Kaneda K: Kaneda anterior spinal instrumentation for the thoracic and lumbar spine. *In* An HS, Cotler JM (eds): Spinal Instrumentation. Baltimore, Williams & Wilkins, 1992, p. 413.)

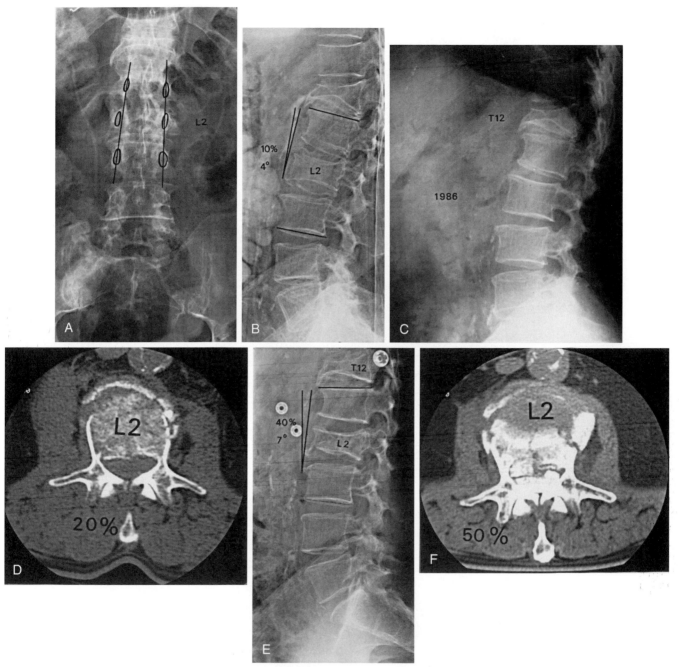

Figure 27–14 = Failure of nonoperative management of L2 burst fracture. Unusual case of a 76-year-old man who sustained an L2 burst fracture with minimal deformity and canal compromise and no neurologic deficit. He was treated with 3 weeks of bedrest and then gradual mobilization in a custom-molded TLSO. On standing in the brace, he had significant lower extremity pain, and 3/5 weakness in multiple muscle groups of both legs. He underwent anterior decompression and fusion in which the Kaneda device was used for fixation. Close follow-up of patients with burst fractures is essential. *A*, AP radiograph demonstrating an L2 burst fracture with splaying of the pedicles. An old T12 fracture is identified. *B*, Lateral radiograph demonstrating a mild L2 burst fracture and an old T12 compression fracture. *C*, Radiograph taken 6 years previously demonstrating the T12 fracture. Patient was asymptomatic in the interval before his L2 fracture. *D*, CT scan of L2 demonstrating 20% canal compromise and no disruption of posterior elements. *E*, Lateral radiograph taken 3 weeks after injury when the neurologic deficit developed. There has been loss of vertebral body height with 3 degrees of increase in the kyphosis. *F*, Postmyelographic CT scan demonstrating that canal compromise has increased to 50%.

Illustration continued on following page

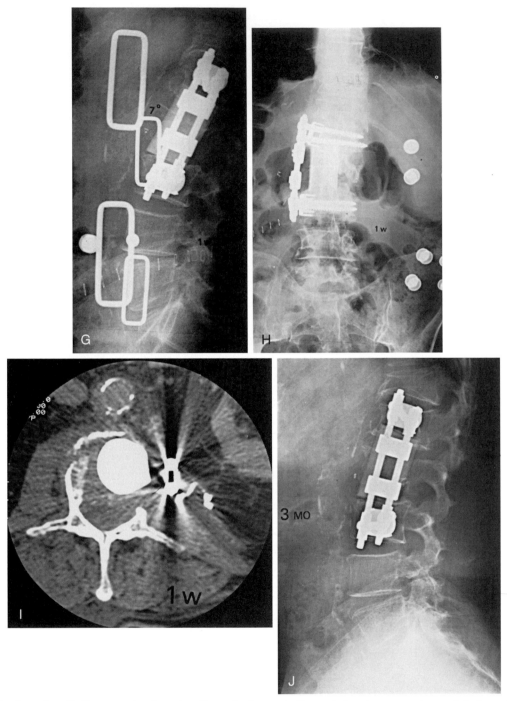

Figure 27–14 *Continued* = G, Postoperative lateral radiograph demonstrating anterior decompression and fusion with Kaneda device instrumentation from L1 to L3. A femoral allograft was packed with autogenous bone and used as a strut graft. *H*, Postoperative AP radiograph 1 week later demonstrating Kaneda device fixation. *I*, Postoperative CT scan demonstrating complete decompression of the spinal canal, lateral position of the Kaneda device, and placement of the femoral allograft. The right side and anterior aspects of the vertebral body were left as a rim to contain additional autogenous graft. *J*, Lateral radiograph obtained 3 months postoperatively demonstrating maintenance of alignment. The patient wore a TLSO for 3 months. He had minimal low back discomfort and no neurologic deficit.

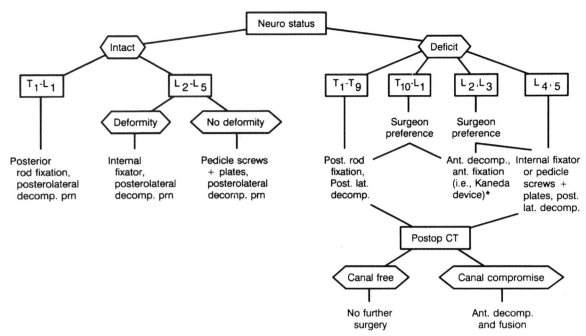

Figure 27–15 = Algorithm for surgical management of unstable thoracic and lumbar burst fractures. *If there is significant posterior instability or a lamina fracture with a possibility of entrapped nerve roots, the spine should be approached posteriorly.

interne or VSP plates to preserve motion segments. If the spinal alignment is satisfactory, we use VSP plates, but if any significant reduction is required, we prefer the internal fixator. A posterolateral decompression is performed if indicated by intraoperative ultrasound.

Unstable burst fractures with an incomplete neural deficit are treated as follows. At T9 and above, a Harrington rod sleeve construct with sublaminar or spinous process wires is used in conjunction with a posterolateral decompression. If significant canal compromise exists after the posterolateral decompression, then an anterior decompression and fusion are performed secondarily. For fractures at T10 to L1, anterior decompression and fusion with the Kaneda device is used, except for fractures with severe posterior column involvement or cases of lamina fracture and suspected dural tears or entrapped nerve roots (in which case we manage the fracture with posterior decompression and instrumentation). If the surgeon prefers to approach the spine posteriorly, it is reasonable to treat fractures from T10 to L1 with a rod sleeve construct or short-segment pedicular fixation even in the absence of a lamina fracture. A rod sleeve construct, however, requires instrumentation of an additional motion segment at the lower end of the fusion. If a pedicle screw system is chosen for the thoracolumbar junction, consideration should be given to transpedicular grafting or an anterior fusion to avoid fatigue fracture of the screws (see Fig. 27–12). Finally, fractures from L2–5 that require operation are treated with the fixateur interne or VSP plates with a posterolateral decompression guided by intraoperative ultrasound (see Fig. 27–8). An anterior decompression is used if the posterolateral decompression is insufficient. Anterior decompression and fusion with Kaneda device instrumentation may also be used for L2 and L3 fractures but

not L4 or L5 fractures because of the lateral position of the iliac vessels in the lower lumbar spine.

For fractures with complete neurologic deficits above the conus medullaris, posterior instrumentation promotes speedier rehabilitation and easier nursing care than nonoperative management. We follow the same guidelines as for patients without a neural deficit. We do not distinguish between complete and incomplete injuries below the conus because the prognosis of cauda equina lesions is better than that of spinal cord injuries.

These recommendations are for fractures that are less than 1 week old. After 1 week, the extent of fracture consolidation is such that correction of kyphosis and decompression through ligamentotaxis is less likely to occur with posterior distraction instrumentation, and consideration must be given to anterior decompression and stabilization or to combined anterior and posterior procedures. Of course, none of these guidelines are absolute and will be modified as new techniques and fixation devices become available.

For burst fractures that present with late kyphotic deformity or neurologic loss or progression, we generally rely on front and back procedures that include anterior decompression and fusion and posterior instrumentation (Fig. 27–16).

SUMMARY

The purpose of this chapter was to describe the historical development of classification schemes of burst fractures. We discussed the anatomy of the thoracolumbar spine and how it relates to spinal stability and the pathogenesis of burst fractures. The clinical and radiographic evaluation of burst fractures were

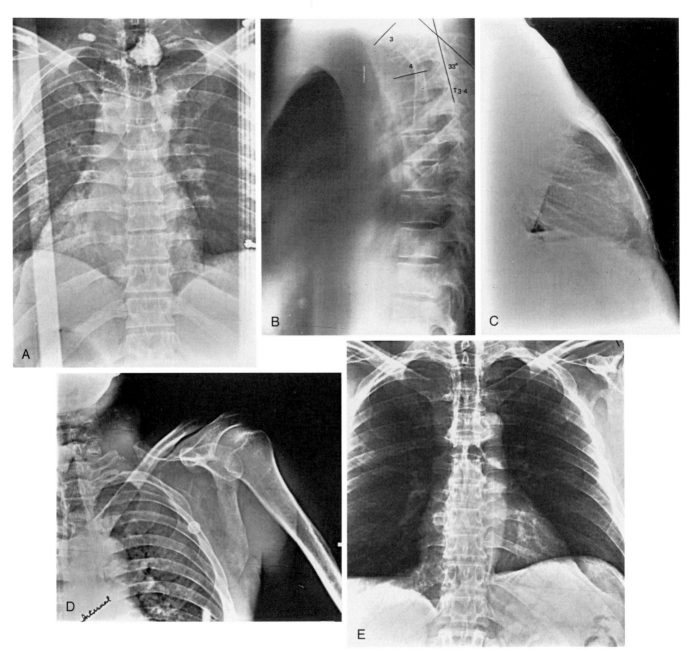

Figure 27–16 = Late PA decompression and stabilization of a T3 burst fracture in 38-year-old man who was involved in a motor vehicle accident. He also sustained a right scapular fracture and a manubrial fracture. Only the scapula fracture was recognized. The burst fracture went untreated. He developed progressive kyphosis associated with loss of height and severe upper back pain with radicular pain around his chest. *A,* AP radiograph obtained at the time of injury. *B,* Lateral radiograph obtained at the time of injury showing 33 degrees of kyphosis of T3–4 from the unrecognized T3 burst fracture. *C,* Unrecognized manubrial fracture. *D,* Scapular fracture for which the patient was treated symptomatically. *E,* AP radiograph obtained at the time of presentation 1 year after injury.

Figure 27–16 *Continued* = *F*, Lateral radiograph demonstrating fracture of the manubrium and kyphotic deformity from the T3 burst fracture. *G*, Lateral tomogram demonstrating 49 degrees of kyphosis of T2–4 and 36 degrees of anterior compression of T3. *H*, Sagittal T1-weighted MRI scan demonstrating T3 burst fracture with impingement on cord, which is draped over the retropulsed posteroinferior aspect of the T3 vertebral body. *I*, Axial MRI scan demonstrating flattening of the cord and loss of anterior subarachnoid space. *J*, One year postoperatively, the PA radiograph demonstrating the fibular strut graft that had been placed after anterior decompression and the posterior CD (Cotrel-Dubousset) rod instrumentation. *K*, One year postoperatively, lateral radiograph demonstrating improvement in overall alignment of the spine.

reviewed, and treatment options based on the location and stability of the injury were discussed.

We have proposed an algorithm for the surgical management of burst fractures. We believe that it is a reasonable approach to these injuries which is based on the current literature. It is not intended to be all-inclusive or to be a rigid protocol because many effective treatment options are available. Each case must be evaluated individually and, if operation is necessary, the approach chosen should be based on the principles discussed and the experience of the surgeon.

REFERENCES

1. Aebi M, Etter C, Kehl T, et al: Stabilization of the lower thoracic and lumbar spine with the internal spinal skeletal fixation system: Indications, techniques, and first results of treatment. Spine 12:544, 1987.
2. Andriacchi T, Schultz A, Belytschko T, et al: A model for studies of mechanical interactions between the human spine and rib cage. J Biomech 7:497, 1974.
3. Angtuaco EJC, Binet EF: Radiology of thoracic and lumbar fractures. Clin Orthop 189:43, 1984.
4. Ballock RT, Mackersie R, Abitbol J-J, et al: Can burst fractures be predicted from plain radiographs? J Bone Joint Surg Br 74:147, 1992.
5. Bayley JC, Yuan HA, Fredrickson BE: The Syracuse I-plate. Spine 16 (suppl):S120, 1991.
6. Been HD: Anterior decompression and stabilization of thoracolumbar burst fractures by the use of the Slot-Zielke device. Spine 16:70, 1991.
7. Berry JL, Moran JM, Berg WS, et al: A morphometric study of human lumbar and selected thoracic vertebrae. Spine 12:362, 1987.
8. Bradford DS, Akbarnia BA, Winter RB, et al: Surgical stabilization of fracture and fracture dislocations of the thoracic spine. Spine 2:185, 1977.
9. Bradford DS, McBride GG: Surgical management of thoracolumbar spine fractures with incomplete neurologic deficits. Clin Orthop 218:201, 1987.
10. Brown LP, Bridwell KH, Holt RT, et al: Aortic erosions and lacerations associated with the Dunn anterior spinal instrumentation. Orthop Trans 10:16, 1986.
11. Cammisa FP, Eismont FJ, Green BA: Dural laceration occurring with burst fractures and associated laminar fractures. J Bone Joint Surg Am 71:1044, 1989.
12. Clark WK: Spinal cord decompression in spinal cord injury. Clin Orthop 154:9, 1981.
13. Court-Brown CM, Gertzbein SD: The management of burst fractures of the fifth lumbar vertebra. Spine 12:308, 1987.
14. Dall BE, Stauffer ES: Neurologic injury and recovery patterns in burst fractures at the T12 or L1 motion segment. Clin Orthop 233:171, 1988.
15. Daniaux H, Seykora P, Genelin A, et al: Application of posterior plating and modifications in thoracolumbar spine injuries: Indication, techniques, and results. Spine 16 (suppl):S125, 1991.
16. Davies WE, Morris JH, Hill V: An analysis of conservative (nonsurgical) management of thoracolumbar fractures and fracture-dislocations with neural damage. J Bone Joint Surg Am 62:1324, 1980.
17. Denis F: The three column spine and its significance in the classification of acute thoracolumbar spinal injuries. Spine 8:817, 1983.
18. Denis F, Armstrong GWD, Searls K, et al: Acute thoracolumbar burst fractures in the absence of neurologic deficit: A comparison between operative and nonoperative treatment. Clin Orthop 189:142, 1984.
19. Dickson JH, Harrington PR, Erwin WD: Results of reduction and stabilization of the severely fractured thoracic and lumbar spine. J Bone Joint Surg Am 60:799, 1978.
20. Dunn HK: Anterior spine stabilization and decompression for thoracolumbar injuries. Orthop Clin North Am 17:113, 1986.
21. Edwards CC, Levine AM: Early rod-sleeve stabilization of the injured thoracic and lumbar spine. Orthop Clin North Am 17:121, 1986.
22. Edwards CC, Rosenthal MS, Gellad F, et al: The fate of retropulsed bone following thoracolumbar burst fractures: Late stenosis or resorption? Orthop Trans 13:32, 1989.
23. Eismont FJ, Green BA, Berkowitz BM, et al: The role of intraoperative ultrasonography in the treatment of thoracic and lumbar spine fractures. Spine 9:782, 1984.
24. Esses SI, Bednar DA: The spinal pedicle screw techniques and systems. Orthop Rev 18:676, 1989.
25. Esses SI, Botsford DJ, Kostuik JP: Evaluation of surgical treatment for burst fractures. Spine 15:667, 1990.
26. Esses SI, Botsford DJ, Wright T, et al: Operative treatment of spinal fractures with the AO internal fixator. Spine 16 (suppl):S146, 1991.
27. Ferguson RL, Allen BL Jr: Mechanistic classification of thoracolumbar spine fractures. Clin Orthop 189:77, 1984.
28. Finn CA, Stauffer ES: Burst fracture of the fifth lumbar vertebra. J Bone Joint Surg Am 74:398, 1992.
29. Flynn JC, Hogue MA: Anterior fusion of the lumbar spine: End result study with long-term follow-up. J Bone Joint Surg Am 61:1143, 1979.
30. Frankel HL, Hancock DO, Hyslop G, et al: The value of postural reduction in the initial management of closed injuries of the spine with paraplegia and tetraplegia. Paraplegia 7:179, 1969.
31. Fredrickson BA, Edwards WT, Rauschning W, et al: Vertebral burst fractures: An experimental morphologic and radiographic analysis. Presented to the meeting of the International Society for Study of the Lumbar Spine, Chicago, 1992.
32. Fredrickson BE, Yuan HA, Miller H: Burst fractures of the fifth lumbar vertebra. J Bone Joint Surg Am 64:1088, 1982.
33. Gaines RW, Munson G, Satterlee C, et al: Harrington distraction rods supplemented with sublaminar wires for thoracolumbar fracture dislocation: Experimental and clinical investigation. Orthop Trans 7:15, 1983.
34. Gertzbein SD, Crowe PJ, Fazl M, et al: Canal clearance in burst fractures using the AO internal fixator. Spine 17:558, 1992.
35. Goldberg AL, Deeb ZL, Rothfus WE, et al: Magnetic resonance imaging in evaluation of acute spinal trauma. Spine 3:339, 1989.
36. Haas N, Blauth M, Tscherne H: Anterior plating in thoracolumbar spine injuries: Indication, technique, and results. Spine 16 (suppl):S100, 1991.
37. Harrington PR: Treatment of scoliosis: Correction and internal fixation by spine instrumentation. J Bone Joint Surg Am 44:591, 1962.
38. Hashimoto T, Kaneda K, Abumi KA: Relationship between traumatic spinal canal stenosis and neurologic deficits in thoracolumbar burst fractures. Spine 13:1268, 1988.
39. Holdsworth FW: Fractures, dislocations, and fracture-dislocations of the spine. J Bone Joint Surg Br 45:6, 1963.
40. Holdsworth F: Fractures, dislocations, and fracture-dislocations of the spine. J Bone Joint Surg Am 52:1534, 1970.
41. Jacobs RR, Asher MA, Snider RK: Thoracolumbar spinal injuries: A comparative study of recumbent and operative treatment in 100 patients. Spine 5:463, 1980.
42. Johnson JR, Leatherman KD, Holt RT: Anterior decompression of the spinal cord for neurological deficit. Spine 8:396, 1983.
43. Kahanovitz N: The effect of internal fixation without arthrodesis on human facet joint cartilage. Orthop Trans 7:14, 1983.
44. Kahanovitz N, Arnoczky SP, Levine DB, et al: The effects of internal fixation on the articular cartilage of unfused facet joints in dogs. Orthop Trans 6:10, 1982.
45. Kaneda K, Abumi K, Fujiya M: Burst fractures with neurologic deficits of the thoracolumbar-lumbar spine: Results of anterior decompression and stabilization with anterior instrumentation. Spine 9:788, 1984.
46. Keene JS: Radiographic evaluation of thoracolumbar fractures. Clin Orthop 189:58, 1984.
47. Kelly RP, Whitesides TE Jr: Treatment of lumbodorsal fracture-dislocations. Ann Surg 167:705, 1968.
48. King AG: Burst compression fractures of the thoracolumbar spine: Pathologic anatomy and surgical management. Orthopedics 10:1711, 1987.
49. Kostuik JP: Anterior fixation for fractures of the thoracic and

lumbar spine with or without neurologic involvement. Clin Orthop 189:103, 1984.

50. Krag MH: Biomechanics of thoracolumbar spinal fixation: A review. Spine 16 (suppl):84, 1991.

51. Krompinger WJ, Fredrickson BE, Mino DE, et al: Conservative treatment of fractures of the thoracic and lumbar spine. Orthop Clin North Am 17:161, 1986.

52. Kulkarni MV, McArdle CB, Kopanicky D, et al: Acute spinal cord injury: MR imaging at the 1.5 T. Radiology 164:837, 1987.

53. Levine AM, Edwards CC: Low lumbar burst fractures: Reduction and stabilization using the modular spine fixation system. Orthopedics 11:1427, 1988.

54. Lindahl S, Willen J, Irstam L: Computed tomography of bone fragments in the spinal canal: An experimental study. Spine 8:181, 1983.

55. Lindsey RW, Dick W: The Fixateur Interne in the reduction and stabilization of thoracolumbar spine fractures in patients with neurologic deficit. Spine 16 (suppl):140, 1991.

56. Louis R: Surgery of the Spine: Surgical Anatomy and Operative Approaches. Berlin, Springer-Verlag, 1983.

57. Louis R: Spinal stability as defined by the three-column concept. Anat Clin 7:33, 1985.

58. Lucas D, Bresler B: Stability of the ligamentous spine. Biomechanics Laboratory Report No. 40, University of California, San Francisco.

59. Luque ER, Rapp GF: A new semirigid method for intrapedicular fixation of the spine. Orthopedics 11:1445, 1988.

60. Magerl F, Harms J, Gertzbein SD, et al: A new classification of spinal fractures. Presented to the Société Internationale Orthopédie et Traumatologie Meeting, Montreal, Sept 9, 1990.

61. Magerl FP: Stabilization of the lower thoracic and lumbar spine with external skeletal fixation. Clin Orthop 189:125, 1984.

62. Malcolm BW, Bradford DS, Winter RB, et al: Post-traumatic kyphosis: A review of 48 surgically treated patients. J Bone Joint Surg Am 63:891, 1981.

63. McAfee PC, Bohlman HH, Yuan HA: Anterior decompression of traumatic thoracolumbar fractures with incomplete neurological deficit using a retroperitoneal approach. J Bone Joint Surg Am 67:89, 1985.

64. McAfee PC, Yuan HA, Fredrickson BE, et al: The value of computed tomography in thoracolumbar fractures: An analysis of one hundred consecutive cases and a new classification. J Bone Joint Surg Am 65:461, 1983.

65. McAfee PC, Yuan HA, Lasda NA: The unstable burst fracture. Spine 7:365, 1982.

66. McEvoy RD, Bradford DS: The management of burst fractures of the thoracic and lumbar spine: Experience in 53 patients. Spine 10:631, 1985.

67. McGrory BJ, VanderWilde RS, Currier BL, et al: Diagnosis of subtle thoracolumbar burst fractures: A new radiographic sign. Presented at the Annual Meeting of the Minnesota Orthopedic Society, Minneapolis, 1992.

68. Meyer PR Jr: Surgery of Spine Trauma. New York, Churchill Livingstone, 1989.

69. Mumford J, Spratt KF, Weinstein JN, et al: Thoracolumbar burst fractures: The clinical efficacy and outcome of non-operative management. Presented to the Meeting of the International Society for Study of the Lumbar Spine. Chicago, 1992.

70. Nicoll EA: Fractures of the dorso-lumbar spine. J Bone Joint Surg Br 31:376, 1949.

71. Panjabi MM, Oxland TR, Lin RM: Thoracolumbar burst fractures:

72. Perey O: Fracture of the vertebral end-plate in the lumbar spine: An experimental biomechanical investigation. Acta Orthop Scand 25 (suppl):5, 1957.

73. Purcell GA, Markolf KL, Dawson EG: Twelfth thoracic–first lumbar vertebral mechanical stability of fractures after Harrington-rod instrumentation. J Bone Joint Surg Am 63:71, 1981.

74. Rissanen PM: The surgical anatomy and pathology of the supraspinous and interspinous ligaments of the lumbar spine with special reference to ligament ruptures. Acta Orthop Scand Suppl 46:5, 1960.

75. Roaf R: A study of the mechanics of spinal injuries. J Bone Joint Surg Br 42:810, 1960.

76. Roy-Camille R, Saillant G, Mazel C: Plating of thoracic, thoracolumbar, and lumbar injuries with pedicle screw plates. Orthop Clin North Am 17:147, 1986.

77. Sasso RC, Cotler HB, Reuben JD: Posterior fixation of thoracic and lumbar spine fractures using DC plates and pedicle screws. Spine 16 (suppl):134, 1991.

78. Stauffer ES: Current concepts review: Internal fixation of fractures of the thoracolumbar spine. J Bone Joint Surg Am 66:1136, 1984.

79. Steffee AD, Biscup RS, Sitkowski DJ: Segmental spine plates with pedicle screw fixation: A new internal fixation device for disorders of the lumbar and thoracolumbar spine. Clin Orthop 203:45, 1986.

80. Sullivan JA: Sublaminar wiring of Harrington distraction rods for unstable thoracolumbar spine fractures. Clin Orthop 189:178, 1984.

81. Trafton PG, Boyd CA Jr: Computed tomography of thoracic and lumbar spine injuries. J Trauma 24:506, 1984.

82. Triantafyllou ST, Gertzbein SD: Management of low lumbar (L4 and L5) burst fractures. Presented to the Meeting of the International Society for Study of the Lumbar Spine, Chicago, 1992.

83. Vincent KA, Benson DR, McGahan JP: Intraoperative ultrasonography for reduction of thoracolumbar burst fractures. Spine 14:387, 1989.

84. Watson-Jones R: Fractures and Joint Injuries, ed 3, vol 2. Edinburgh, E S Livingston, 1943.

85. Weinstein JN, Collalto P, Lehmann TR: Thoracolumbar "burst" fractures treated conservatively: A long-term follow-up. Spine 13:33, 1988.

86. White AA, Panjabi MM: Clinical Biomechanics of the Spine. Philadelphia, JB Lippincott, 1978.

87. White AA, Panjabi MM: Clinical instability of the spine. *In* Evarts CM (ed): Surgery of the Musculoskeletal System, ed 2. New York, Churchill Livingstone, 1990, p 2151.

88. White AA III, Panjabi MM: Clinical Biomechanics of the Spine, ed 2. Philadelphia, JB Lippincott, 1990.

89. Whitesides TE: Traumatic kyphosis of the thoracolumbar spine. Clin Orthop 128:78, 1977.

90. Willén J, Lindahl S, Irstam L, et al: Unstable thoracolumbar fractures: A study by CT and conventional roentgenology of the reduction effect of Harrington instrumentation. Spine 9:214, 1984.

91. Willén J, Lindahl S, Nordwall A: Unstable thoracolumbar fractures: A comparative clinical study of conservative treatment and Harrington instrumentation. Spine 10:111, 1985.

92. Wimmer B, Hofmann E, Jacob A: Trauma of the Spine: CT and MRI. Berlin, Springer-Verlag, 1990.

CHAPTER 28

Low Lumbar Spine Trauma

Alan M. Levine

BASIC CONSIDERATIONS

Treatment of injuries to the lumbar spine requires consideration of a number of additional factors beyond those relevant to injuries of the thoracic and thoracolumbar spine. These are related to the anatomic complexity of the lumbar spine as well as the lordosis and increased normal mobility of the lumbosacral junction. Throughout the 1970s and 1980s, the lack of satisfactory techniques for reduction and stabilization of injuries in the low lumbar spine frequently resulted in less than optimal treatment results leading some authors to espouse nonoperative techniques as a better alternative.[23, 49] Occasional reports surfaced, however, suggesting that an operative approach yielded better anatomic results and perhaps even better functional outcomes.[88, 122] Even with the more widely accepted use of pedicle screw fixation in the lumbar spine in North America, some early poorly conceptualized operative approaches to fractures in this region also led to early failure.[3, 5, 74, 136] This caused some surgeons to accept chronic pain and failure to return to preinjury occupation in this very young group of patients as the norm. Since 1992, a number of studies have appeared suggesting that nonoperative treatment yields satisfactory results in this group of patients but all studies have a very short follow-up (less than 4 years) in a group of predominantly young male patients (mean, 27 years old) more often than not employed in manual labor tasks.[18, 45, 107] In the lumbar spine, anatomic and motion considerations have made instrumentation more difficult than in other regions of the spine. Injuries to the lumbar spine disrupt the normal lordotic alignment of the spine, and restoration of that lordotic alignment is critical to overall vertebral mechanics and spinal alignment in the sagittal plane. Failure to maintain or restore the normal sagittal alignment in the lower lumbar spine, after either elective fusions or fractures, has led to degenerative changes and symptoms in longterm follow-up. The lumbosacral junction in particular must resist a number of large forces, but must also permit a significant amount of motion. It has therefore been difficult to obtain anatomic reduction and reconstruction of the lumbar spine and sacrum until the most recent advances in instrumentation. This has led many authors to suggest limited procedures and goals, or "benign neglect," as methods of treatment of low lumbar injuries. These numerous features and problems separate fractures of the lower lumbar spine from the more numerous and common fractures at the thoracolumbar junction.

More accurate diagnostic imaging studies, as well as advances in instrumentation techniques, should now allow us to treat injuries of the lumbar spine with the same degree of accuracy and competence as more proximal spinal injuries. To do this, however, we must have a clear understanding of the anatomic and functional differences that distinguish the lumbar spine from the more proximal areas of the spine. As described in previous chapters, there are a specific set of technical considerations and fixation methods which are applicable to treatment of spinal trauma in the thoracic region (T2–10) and similarly a set for the thoracolumbar junction (T10–L1). Fractures of L2 form a transitional group, both functionally and technically, between those of the thoracolumbar junction (T10–L1) and the lumbar area (L3 through the sacrum). The major differences in anatomic considerations and techniques apply predominantly to L3 through the sacrum, whereas L2 should be considered as the transitional level, borrowing techniques from above and below.

The treatment goals for spine trauma in general are (1) anatomic reduction of the injury, (2) rigid fixation of the fracture and, when necessary, (3) decompression of the neural elements. For treatment of the lumbar and sacral spine we must add the considerations of (4) maintenance of sagittal alignment, (5) conservation of motion segments, and (6) prevention of frequent complications (e.g., hook dislodgment, loss of sacral fixation, pseudarthrosis, and so forth). As we review the characteristics of the lumbar spine, it will become evident that techniques that were discussed previously for the treatment of cervical, thoracic, and thoracolumbar spine injuries are not applicable to the treatment of lumbar spine injuries.

ANATOMIC FEATURES

The first critical anatomic consideration is the sagittal alignment of the lumbar spine. Normal kyphosis of the thoracic spine falls within a range of 15 to 49 degrees,[148] whereas normal lumbar lordosis is generally thought to be less than 60 degrees. This is in part determined by the slope of the sacral base, which averages approximately 45 degrees from the horizontal. This angle is critical in determining the amount of shear force[132] to which the lumbosacral junction is subjected (Fig. 28–1). Anatomic differences in the structure of the lumbar

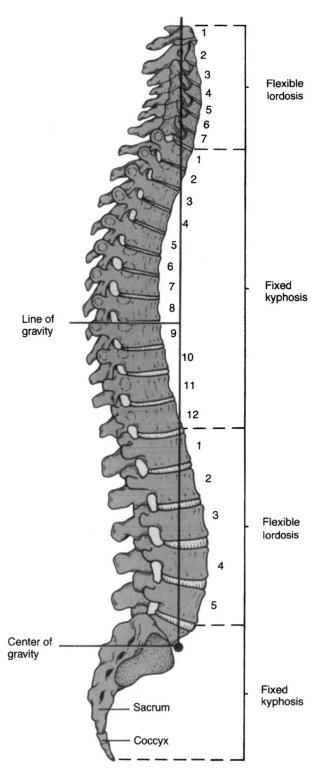

Figure 28–1 = The spine is divided into four segments, two with relatively fixed kyphosis (the sacral and thoracic spine) and two with relatively flexible lordosis (the cervical and lumbar spine). The weight-bearing axis is anterior to the thoracic spine and thoracolumbar junction. It falls posterior to the vertebral bodies of the lumbar spine, making the pattern of fracture with axial-loading injuries significantly different in the lumbar spine compared with the thoracic and thoracolumbar spine. (From Levine AM: Lumbar and sacral spine trauma. *In* Browner BD, Jupiter JB, Levine AM, et al (eds): Skeletal Trauma: Fractures, Dislocations, Ligamentous Injuries, vol 1. Philadelphia, WB Saunders, 1992.)

vertebrae influence therapeutic decisions and affect attachment of fixation devices differently than for proximal levels in the thoracic and lumbar spine.

With caudal descent in the lumbar spine, the overall dimensions of the canal enlarge, whereas the area occupied by the neural elements decreases. The cord in the thoracic region measures approximately 86.5 mm² and is housed within a canal that is generally 17.2 × 16.8 mm². Thus, in the thoracic region, the cord occupies about 50% of the canal area. In the thoracolumbar region the conus broadens, as does the canal. The spinal cord usually terminates at approximately L1. In the lumbar region the canal is typically large (23.4 × 17.4 mm).[39, 118] Here the roots of the cauda equina are the only contents. In addition, the size and shape of the laminae change configuration at the various levels of

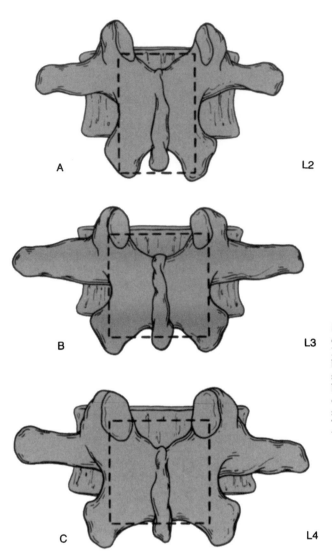

A L2

B L3

C L4

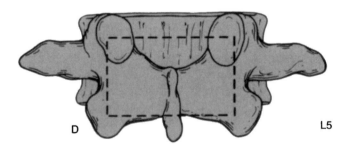

D L5

Figure 28–2 = *A–D*, The shape of the lumbar laminae and relative size of the pedicles dramatically influence our ability to position hardware. From L2 to L5 the length of the laminae becomes less and the width becomes greater. Therefore, hook placement proximally is easier in the spine but may cause impingement when placed over the lamina of L5 because of its relatively short length. However, pedicle fixation is easier distally with the larger pedicle size. (From Levine AM: Lumbar and sacral spine trauma. *In* Browner BD, Jupiter JB, Levine AM, et al (eds): Skeletal Trauma: Fractures, Dislocations, Ligamentous Injuries, vol 1. Philadelphia, WB Saunders, 1992.)

the spine. The laminae in the thoracic and thoracolumbar region are rectangular in shape, being somewhat longer than wide. In the midlumbar spine the width and length of the laminae equalize. At L5 the lamina is considerably wider than long (Fig. 28–2). The sacral laminae are extremely thin, and might be absent in some areas. Similarly, it has been shown that in the lumbar spine the minimum and maximum pedicle diameters increase to a mean minimum diameter of approximately 10 mm at L5 and 8.5 mm at L3.[126]

With the increasing emphasis on innovative methods of fixation for injuries in the low lumbar spine, an understanding of the pertinent anatomic dimensions takes on new significance, whereas previously, with hook fixation or sublaminar wiring to the posterior elements, the only important consideration was posterior topographic anatomy. However, the dimensions, position, and orientation of the pedicles, as well as the shape of the vertebral body, are likewise critical. The initial anatomic description of pedicle morphology referable to pedicle screw fixation was done by Saillant in 1976[123] and was confirmed by two later studies from

North America.[78, 150] The critical features are the sagittal and transverse width of the pedicles, pedicle length, pedicle angle, and chord length (depth to the anterior cortex along a fixed orientation). These dimensions vary widely within regions of the spine (thoracic vs. lumbar) but also vary in the lumbar spine with progression from L1 to L5. The mean transverse diameter measured either on computed tomograph (CT) scan or anatomic specimen was approximately 9 mm at L1, increasing to as much as 18 mm at L5 (Fig. 28–3A). The sagittal width in the lumbar spine is relatively constant with a mean of between 14 to 15 mm at all levels (Fig. 28–3B). The angle of the pedicle axis generally increases in the lumbar spine with a mean of about 11 degrees at L1, 15 degrees at L3, and over 20 degrees at L5 (see Fig. 28–3A). Finally, the angle of insertion of the screw is critically important since the shapes of the lumbar vertebrae change dramatically from L1 to L5. Since the distance between the pedicles is greater at L5 and the anteroposterior (AP) diameter of the vertebral body is

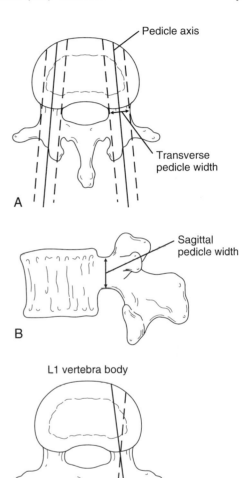

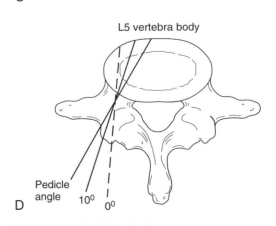

Figure 28–3 ═ *A*, This axial view of a lumbar vertebral body shows the transverse pedicle width which increases from L1 to L5. It also demonstrates the pedicle axis which likewise increases from L1 to L5. *B*, The sagittal view of the vertebral body shows the sagittal pedicle which is relatively constant in the lumbar spine. *C*, This diagram shows an L1 axial view with the axis of the pedicle demonstrating the larger cortex-to-cortex distance. *D*, The axial view of L5 demonstrates how the AP length can increase with increasing angle. (Redrawn from Levine AM: Lumbar and sacral spine trauma. *In* Browner BD, Jupiter JB, Levine AM, et al (eds): Skeletal Trauma: Fractures, Dislocations, and Ligamentous Injuries, ed 2, vol 1. Philadelphia, WB Saunders, 1998.)

effectively less at that location, the chord length or distance from posterior cortex to anterior cortex can vary dramatically with the angle of insertion. If screws are inserted perpendicular to the posterior cortex along a 0-degree axis, as originally described by Roy-Camille and colleagues,[122] the mean depth at L1 is about 4 mm, whereas at L5 it is only 35 mm. Increasing the angle of insertion to 10 or 15 degrees, or increasing the angle of the axis of the pedicle can increase the cortex-cortex distance by as much as 5 mm at L1 (to 50 mm) and 15 mm at L5 (to about 50 mm).

The next significant anatomic feature is the extreme flexion-extension mobility of the lumbar spine compared with the mobility of other areas. The thoracic spine is relatively stiff as a result of the orientation of the facet joints. Flexion-extension in the thoracic spine is limited and, in fact, rotation exceeds flexion-extension at each level. At the thoracolumbar junction flexion-extension increases, whereas lateral bending and rotation decrease. The facet joint orientation in the lumbar spine becomes sagittal and the facet joints quite large.[144] Therefore, from L1 to L5 there is a progressive increase in the degree of freedom of motion in flexion-extension and a decrease in rotation. Flexion-extension increases from approximately 12 degrees at the L1–2 level to 20 degrees at the L5–S1 level, with lateral bending remaining similar at about 6 degrees.[143] This extreme flexion-extension mobility needs to be taken into account in considering injuries of the lumbar spine, because the relative position and orientation of one vertebra to another can change according to the position of the victim at impact. The extreme lumbar lordosis and lumbosacral angle can be flattened dramatically by sitting and the spine oriented in a vertical rather than lordotic position. This contributes to the differing relative incidence of specific types of injuries in the lumbar spine, compared with those in more proximal regions.

LUMBAR SPINE INJURY PATTERNS

Most operatively treated fractures of the thoracic, thoracolumbar, and lumbar spine occur at the thoracolumbar junction. As a result of the anatomic differences previously discussed, the relative incidence pattern of injuries is different in the lumbar spine than in the thoracic or thoracolumbar spine. The thoracic spine is additionally stabilized by the rib cage while the thoracolumbar junction is a transitional zone at the end of a relatively stiffer segment. The lumbar spine is protected only by the abdominal and paraspinous musculature and is more subject to forces such as distraction and shear. Additionally, factors extrinsic to the spine such as the type of accident (motor vehicle accident [MVA] vs. fall) and the use of restraints such as lap belt vs. shoulder harness also influence the number and types of injuries. For instance, the use of a lap belt alone as a passenger in an MVA predisposes to flexion-distraction injuries of the lumbar spine.[6, 113] Since the lower lumbar spine and lumbosacral junction normally are quite lordotic, severe flexion injuries are less com-

mon than in the thoracic or thoracolumbar spine. The extreme flexion-extension range of motion frequently tends to negate the flexion moment of an injury. Therefore, more low lumbar injuries are axial loading injuries as the spine is brought to a straight neutral position at the moment of impact and is then axially loaded. Some flexion-distraction injuries occur as the pelvis or low lumbar spine becomes fixed in a given position and the remainder of the body is flexed and distracted over it.

A variety of different injury patterns can occur in the lumbar spine. The purpose of dividing them into subgroups and classifying the injuries is to be able to predict their natural history and behavior. Easy recognition of these subgroups is important for determining optimal treatment. Additionally, the classification should help the treating physician understand the nature of the instability and thus construct a treatment regimen based on counteracting that instability.[145] Although many classification systems exist, none have been totally successful in achieving those goals.[103] Therefore, as in the other sections describing spinal injuries, these injuries are grouped and described by both radiologic criteria as well as their major deforming forces. The major forces contributing to injuries are flexion and extension, compression, lateral bending, rotation, distraction, and shear. Most injuries are not caused by a single force, but by a major force with minor components from other, different types of forces.

Soft Tissue Injuries, Avulsion Fractures, and Ligamentous Injuries

Although conceptually this group of injuries may appear to be quite simple to understand and treat, they may be the most challenging since they constitute a large and highly variable group. Until the last 5 years, they were very poorly imaged, since we were reliant on plain films and CT scan findings which were merely indirect evidence of the soft tissue and ligamentous injury. In some cases these findings reflect poorly the force imparted to the spine or the subsequent severity of the injury. The improved use of magnetic resonance imaging (MRI) has at least allowed the physician to directly visualize the location of the injury. The direct correlation between the visualized soft tissue or ligamentous injury and its effect on spinal stability has still not been clarified. The significant force needed to overcome the muscular and ligamentous restraints of the lumbar spine should be considered in evaluating these problems. For example, fractures of the transverse processes of the lumbar spine may represent several different injuries depending on the mechanism. The significance of an L5 transverse process fracture associated with a vertical shearing injury to the pelvis is different from that of multiple transverse process fractures. The force of the injury to the lumbar spine is greater in a pedestrian being struck by a motor vehicle with resultant transverse process fractures than in indirect muscle forces causing avulsion fractures. Significant muscular forces produced by the paraspinous musculature at the time of impact can result in an avulsion fracture of the transverse process (Fig. 28–4). In the more severe form they can be accompanied by nerve root avulsion at the same level. Prior to any treatment, and especially in combination with other significant bony injuries, avulsion fractures should be thoroughly investigated to ascertain that the nerve root exiting at the level of the transverse process is intact. Preoperatively, myelography often does not demonstrate dye leakage at the level of the avulsion, but preoperative MRI or intraoperative exploration at the time of surgery for an associated injury might confirm the diagnosis (see Fig. 28–4).

End-plate avulsions[106] are a recognized phenomenon in the adolescent patient. Disc herniation can occur in the adult who sustains significant trauma, whereas in the child the ligamentous attachments are somewhat stronger than the bony attachment of the end plate (Fig. 28–5). Therefore, end-plate avulsion with displacement and neurologic findings might be present. This can be visualized by a combination of CT scan and MRI, and should be treated by excision of the end-

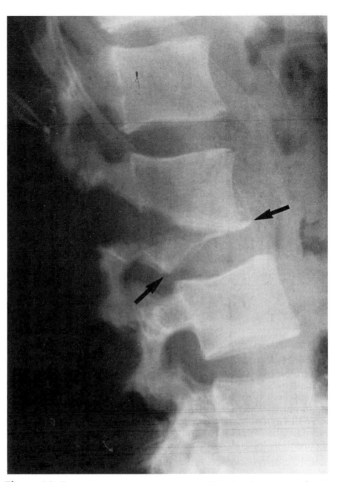

Figure 28–5 = This lateral radiograph of the lumbar spine of a 16-year-old girl demonstrates an end-plate avulsion. She was involved in a motor vehicle accident and sustained complete paraplegia from the flexion-distraction injury several levels above the area of bony injury. Note the avulsion of the end plate of the vertebral body *(arrows)* with translation of the end plate anteriorly in addition to the flexion and distraction of the posterior portion of the end plate. (From Levine AM: Lumbar and sacral spine trauma. *In* Browner BD, Jupiter JB, Levine AM, et al (eds): Skeletal Trauma: Fractures, Dislocations, Ligamentous Injuries, vol 1. Philadelphia, WB Saunders, 1992.)

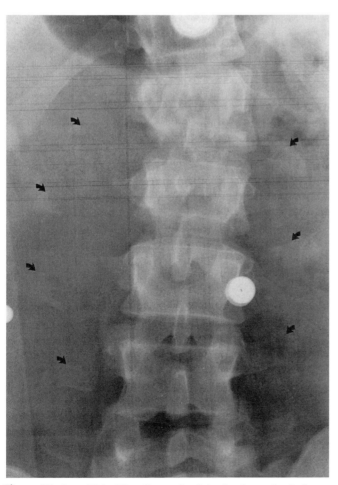

Figure 28–4 = This AP radiograph of the lumbar spine is from a 24-year-old man involved in a motorcycle accident. The patient had a burst fracture of L1 and multiple avulsion fractures of the transverse processes at L1–4 *(arrows)*. (From Levine AM: Lumbar and sacral spine trauma. *In* Browner BD, Jupiter JB, Levine AM, et al (eds): Skeletal Trauma: Fractures, Dislocations, Ligamentous Injuries, vol 1. Philadelphia, WB Saunders, 1992.)

plate fragment, which usually resolves the neurologic symptoms completely. These are most frequently seen in the adolescent and young adult at the L4–5 and L5–S1 level.[40] In the younger child it might occur only with avulsion of the cartilaginous ring apophysis. In adolescents and young adults an isolated portion of the limbus or the entire bony end plate can fracture off.[40] The neural impingement is the result of both the bony fragment and the disc herniation.[40, 60, 138]

Disruption of the posterior ligamentous complex (i.e., supraspinous ligament, intraspinous ligament, facet capsules, ligamentum flavum) constitutes a continuum of injuries usually occurring in concert with other bony flexion injuries.[54, 57] If a significant ligamentous injury occurs alone or in combination with a very innocent-appearing bony injury, an insignificant anterior compression of the vertebral body (Fig. 28–6), they may be easily overlooked initially. If the patient has considerable spasm from the soft tissue injury, the full

equina syndrome. This is often seen with severe burst fractures with canal retropulsion and large amounts of bone within the neural canal. The second type of injury is the isolated root injury or combinations of root injuries. These may be nonrecoverable root avulsions, which can occur in combination with transverse process avulsions. Lesser degrees of root injury occur with canal impingement. Isolated root injury is common with a retropulsed fragment of bone that catches the exiting root between it and the undersurface of the lamina. Root deficits are also common in patients with low lumbar fractures that have sagittal splits in the lamina associated with dural tears. Posterior dural tears allow herniation of the roots outside the dural sac or entrapment within the spinous process or laminar fracture.[22, 30, 84] Canal narrowing by translational deformity, as in bilateral facet dislocation, is less likely to cause severe neurologic deficit in the low lumbar spine than at the thoracolumbar junction. Burst fractures of the lumbar spine are associated with neurologic deficit in about 50% of patients.

MANAGEMENT

Indications

Various systems have been devised in an attempt to classify spinal injuries, according to both mechanism and degree of instability. In addition, a number of definitions have been proposed—for example, stable vs. unstable. A generic definition of spinal stability includes those fracture patterns that are not likely to change position with physiologic loads and therefore will not cause additional neurologic deficit or increasing deformity. Although many systems have been proposed that are applicable to lumbar spine injuries, no pragmatic system has been devised that clearly groups the injuries so as to differentiate treatment approaches. Most systems of thoracolumbar trauma classification have either an anatomic reference[13, 65] or a mechanistic reference,[42] but all clearly fail to achieve the desired goal of classifying injuries according to subsequent treatment categories. Therefore, other criteria must be used to aid in making decisions about the treatment of lumbar fractures.

In general terms, the indications for surgery in lumbar injuries are the following: (1) the presence of detectable motion at the fracture site that cannot be controlled by nonoperative methods (instability); (2) neurologic deficit; or (3) severe disruption of axial or sagittal spinal alignment. In lumbar and sacral fractures the presence of neurologic deficit can indicate gross instability. With a large canal-to-neural element ratio, significant translation or angulation must take place in order to have neural injury. This is not a universal rule, however, since transverse process fractures and avulsions can have accompanying nerve root avulsions. Also, in children, the neurologic injury can occur at a level above that of the actual bony injury because of the differential elasticity of the cord and spinal elements.

Instability

In lumbar fractures certain patterns of injury can be defined as unstable, even in the absence of neurologic deficit. Those patients with severe posterior ligamentous complex disruption from a flexion or flexion-distraction injury are considered to have unstable injuries. Treatment is clearly indicated, and there is little controversy as to the appropriate treatment. Most authors believe that nonoperative treatment of ligamentous injuries does not restore stability, and prefer limited operative stabilization. Similarly, flexion-distraction injuries, such as bilateral facet dislocations with complete disruption of the posterior ligamentous complex and the disc, are considered to have gross ligamentous instability which will result in continued loss of sagittal alignment. Shear injuries with circumferential disruption are also known to be grossly unstable and in fact require operative stabilization. Burst fractures present a much more complex problem as they represent a spectrum of injuries. Patients who are neurologically intact with minimal deformity require less aggressive treatment than those with more severe injuries. The problem is predicting behavior of the injury based on static radiographic studies. Burst injuries that demonstrate significant canal compromise, disruption of the anterior and posterior portions of the vertebral body, and laminar fractures are commonly considered to be unstable and require aggressive treatment. Mixed instabilities with gross displacement and shear injuries demonstrate markedly unstable clinical behavior.

Neurologic Deficit

The second criterion that constitutes an indication for treatment is neurologic deficit. There is considerable controversy about the benefits of operative treatment for spinal injury as related to neurologic recovery for cord level injuries,[20, 21, 24, 61, 82, 110, 129] but there is general agreement about surgery in the lumbar spine since the majority involve root injuries.[22, 68, 82] Because the canal-to-neural element ratio is very large, a small degree of canal compromise (30%) in the absence of severe deformity (kyphosis) tends not to be significant in regard to neural recovery. A larger degree of canal compromise (50%), accompanied by high-grade neurologic compromise (cauda equina syndrome), can often be treated successfully by direct neural decompression.[85, 101] In addition, specific root involvement with localized compression of the root can be improved by direct exploration of the root and decompression. Finally, those patients with sagittal spinous process fractures, neurologic deficit, and dural tears with roots outside the dural sac also benefit from direct decompression and dural repair.[22, 30, 84]

Disruption of Axial or Sagittal Spinal Alignment

The next indication for treatment is severe sagittal or coronal plane deformity. Most fractures of the lumbar spine result in kyphotic deformities, and may be accompanied by translational and rotational deformities. Because maintenance of normal lumbar sagittal alignment (i.e., lordosis) is critical for the normal weight-bearing axis of the body, and therefore for optimal function of the paraspinous musculature, restoration to normal is an indicated criterion for treatment to obtain long-term pain-free functional results. However, the validity of this statement has not been fully verified since most of these injuries occur in relatively young persons and the follow-up in most operative and non-operative series is still relatively short.[3, 5, 18, 45, 71, 74, 107, 136] Clinically stable fractures that do not have significant kyphosis or scoliosis associated with them can be optimally treated with external immobilization. Those fractures, however, that have significant kyphosis or other deformities that cannot be reduced and maintained in external immobilization need operative intervention for reestablishment of normal spinal alignment. Less emphasis was given to operative intervention previously because of the lack of appropriate methods to restore spinal alignment in a predictable manner. In fact, the use of spinal instrumentation for fractures of the lumbar spine resulted not in restoration of spinal alignment, but in iatrogenic flat back and other significant alignment deformities with secondary symptoms. If the aim of treatment is accurate restoration of alignment, the surgeon must be certain that the method selected can achieve that goal.

Treatment Options

A number of treatment options exist for the management of low lumbar fractures, generally consisting of either nonoperative or operative treatment. Two major points of controversy obviously exist when deciding on treatment of these injuries. The first is the role of operative treatment and how often it should be applied. As previously mentioned, 10 years ago operative treatment was rarely utilized, not because there was not a role for it but rather that the fixation techniques and instrumentation were not capable of yielding consistently satisfactory results in this area of the spine. Now that more satisfactory methods exist for operative treatment, its role must be reassessed in relation to realistic outcome goals. Secondly, nonoperative treatment consists mainly of bed rest and postural reduction in combination with external immobilization by cast or orthosis. With the possible exception of pelvic and sacral fractures, the role of traction or external fixation is limited. Operative intervention can involve various procedures, including the following: (1) reduction, stabilization, and fusion of spinal fractures from a posterior approach; (2) indirect or direct decompression of neural elements from a posterior or posterolateral (transpedicular) approach; and (3)anterior decompression or reduction, stabilization, fusion, and fixation from an anterior approach.

Nonoperative Treatment

Nonoperative treatment can be used for both stable and unstable injuries of the lumbar region.[66] However, considerable debate and variation are present when trying to decide on the optimal type of nonoperative treatment. Thus treatment may range from application of a lumbosacral corset and immediate mobilization to as much as 3 months at bed rest in a cast. Two major elements are open to debate in nonoperative treatment. The first is the role of recumbency and the duration of that recumbency. The second is the type of external immobilization to be used to treat low lumbar fractures. Clearly, part of this debate can be obviated by considering the type of low lumbar injury to be treated and the relative degree of instability that is present. It is most often indicated for minor fractures such as spinous process fractures and transverse process fractures where a lumbosacral corset with immediate mobilization gives sufficient support to decrease discomfort in fractures without any true degree of instability. Compression fractures with less than 50% anterior compression can generally be treated with immediate mobilization in a total contact orthosis (TCO) for levels above L5 but with thigh extension for level L5 fractures. The use of the proper orthosis to achieve the treatment goal is often a problem with treatment of lumbar fractures. There is a misconception that orthoses that provide satisfactory immobilization in the thoracolumbar spine are also useful for the lumbar spine. Although the studies are relatively few in number, it has been well shown that improper selection of an orthosis for the desired level can lead to increased motion at the injured level by immobilizing the levels above it. On the other hand, Chance fractures may in fact require application of an extension cast to achieve any degree of reduction of the deformity, which most often cannot be reduced with the use of an extension brace or TCO. Some burst fractures[18, 65] can be regarded as stable and therefore appropriate for nonoperative treatment. The major consideration in making that decision, however, is that there be minimal disruption of the posterior wall of the vertebral body and minimal disruption of alignment. The debate here becomes more complex as there have been no well-designed studies documenting the outcome in low lumbar burst fractures with reference to maintenance of alignment. In the neurologically intact patient with any degree of body comminution and retropulsion, the goals of treatment are to maintain optimal reduction of alignment and allow the fracture to go on to union. In the low lumbar spine extension casting is usually of little value in improving the reduction and thus a TCO is just as satisfactory for immobilization. For fractures of L2–4 a standard TCO is acceptable, but certainly for the L5 burst fracture a thoracolumbosacral orthosis (TLSO) (leg included) is mandatory to immobilize the pelvis and prevent flexion at the fracture site. Optimal nonoperative treatment of lumbar burst fractures should probably involve prolonged bed rest (3 to 6 weeks) prior to mobilization in an appropriate orthotic device. This issue of the role of recumbency and its duration is unclear as most studies fail to adequately analyze alignment parameters for low lumbar fractures and in addition have treated a "mixed bag" rather than a uniform group of injuries. Failure to provide sufficient protection from axial loading forces with the use of bed rest can result in further deformity and neurologic deficit. Advocates of postural reduction have indicated that certain fracture patterns, such as bilateral facet dislocations, are not amenable to postural reduction and must be treated surgically without regard to the neurologic status.

It should be reemphasized that most fractures of the low lumbar spine require immobilization of the pelvis by a single-leg spica cast or a TLSO to fix the relation of the low lumbar spine. Immobilization by standard lumbar orthoses could actually accentuate the motion at L4–5 and L5–S1.[44, 114] For upper lumbar fractures, a molded TCO provides optimal immobilization. Care should be taken not to use a thoracolumbar extension orthosis (e.g., a Jewett brace) in the lumbar spine, because it might increase motion at the index level by rigidly immobilizing more proximal levels. Thus pain and deformity might increase in the low lumbar spine.

Some authors have advocated the use of nonoperative treatment for unstable injuries. This treatment consisted mainly of using bed rest to reduce gross malalignment and allow the fracture to begin to consolidate in the supine position before mobilization. Although this was once an accepted method of treatment,[10, 47] the current demands to reduce the length and cost of hospitalization combined with the effectiveness of operative methods render nonoperative treatment less desirable for unstable fractures.

Operative Treatment Goals and Instrumentation

Once the decision has been made to consider surgery for a patient with spinal injury, the goals must be clearly defined to aid in selecting the appropriate procedure to achieve optimal results. With specific reference to the lumbar spine and sacrum, the goals of operative treatment are reviewed here and the various surgical methods by which those goals can be achieved are discussed. Details of the operative methods for specific injuries and their treatment patterns are described subsequently.

The major goals of treatment of lumbar spine and sacral injuries are anatomic reduction of the injury deformity, rigid fixation, neural decompression (when indicated), maintenance of sagittal alignment, minimization of fixation length, and reduction of the incidence of complications. The time from injury must also be considered, because the efficacy of various methods changes with the time course.

The controversy concerning the relative benefits and risks of operative vs. nonoperative treatment of fractures of the lumber spine continues to rage. Over the last 5 years with the advent of patient satisfaction scales, outcome of the treatment has become more objective and is now to be considered as important as the objective neurologic and radiologic criteria. A major problem still exists when attempting to decide on the optimal treatment for lumbar burst fractures. The average age of patients sustaining these injuries is around 27 years and many of the patients are employed at the time of injury doing manual labor. Although short-term studies have suggested that the fractures go on to healing relatively reliably, it is unclear as to the long-term outcome. If we are able to technically restore the anatomic alignment of the spine, do those patients do better with less pain and return to previous employment in both short- and long-term evaluation? Part of the problem in decision making is that some surgical techniques were used that did not either restore or maintain an anatomic alignment.[3, 135] Thus the appropriate comparison is restoration of alignment with nonoperative treatment. With relatively short follow-up (less than 4 years) trends in current studies suggest that those patients with neurologic deficit appear to recover more quickly and more completely with surgical intervention.[68, 107] Some authors believe that nonoperative treatment of low lumbar burst fractures gives satisfactory short-term results but when the data are critically analyzed most patients have a significant degree of residual back pain and disability, even in the short term.[3, 5, 19, 45] More accurate reduction and longer-term follow-up will yield different conclusions. In a yet unpublished series of 29 patients with a range of follow-up of 5 to 11 years (mean 8.2 years) with anatomic restoration of alignment in the majority of patients, the incidence of back pain was less than 20% and the norm was return to preinjury employment.[85] Thus the current trend is nonoperative treatment for those patients who are neurologically intact with minimal to moderate deformity. For those with significant deformity or neurologic deficit, operative treatment should give better long-term results.

Anatomic Fracture Reduction

The first goal of operative intervention is anatomic reduction of the fracture. A general principle of achieving anatomic reduction is that the deforming forces that have caused the injury must be directly counteracted by the instrumentation system used to achieve the reduction. In addition, in the lumbar spine, the deforming influence of normal physiologic forces must also be counteracted, specifically the shear force acting at the lumbosacral junction. For the lumbar spine, selection of an instrumentation system should be determined by the ability of that system to achieve a reduction of the deformity and by the relative length of the instrumentation required to do so. If a shorter construct can achieve the same degree of reduction and rigid fixation, it should be used preferentially to maintain as many mobile levels as possible in the lumbar spine. Flexion and axial loading contribute in varying degrees to most deformities in the lumbar spine, and counteracting those forces should be carefully considered. The fixation procedure used should have an element of distraction and lordosis to restore the normal alignment. Experimental data have demonstrated that devices offering variable and independent application of distraction and lordosis are better able to achieve anatomic reduction.[14, 152]

Not all instrumentation systems can achieve optimal results in all portions of the spine. In the following paragraphs some general types of instrumentation and their feasibility for use with different types of injury in the lumbar spine are considered.

Rod Systems. Straight Harrington distraction rods impart distraction, but fail to produce or restore lordosis. Although operative position can restore lumbar lordosis in a lumbar fracture at surgery, the use of a distraction system alone placed posterior to the center of rotation of the vertebra cannot maintain it. Either continued distraction removes all the lumbar lordosis or incomplete tightening of the system leaves a gap between the instrumentation and the posterior portion of the spine. This results in either continued fracture kyphosis and collapse as the patient is mobilized or an iatrogenic flat back syndrome. Segmental spinal instrumentation can achieve extension and some rotational stability, but offers no axial control.[5] Although restoration of height might be achieved during reduction, the spine then collapses with ambulation. Contoured rod systems with segmental fixation, by either wires or hooks (e.g., Moe rods, Harri-Luque, Cotrel-Dubousset,[104] Synthesis, Texas Scottish Rite Hospital, or TSRH), allow correction of deformity and restoration of sagittal alignment for many patients with midlumbar fractures. A relative disadvantage is the length of the instrumentation necessary to achieve that result. Most require two or three levels of fixation above and below the fracture for adequate lever arms and fixation, and this could involve fixation of the entire lumbar spine. For upper and midlumbar fractures the rod sleeve method allows anatomic reduction with distraction and lordosis and maintenance of alignment with rigid fixation.[36]

Pedicle Screw Systems. Although still not yet approved by the Food and Drug Administration (FDA) pedicle screw systems have a major advantage in the reduction and fixation of lumbar injuries because they reduce the number of levels that need instrumentation to achieve adequate reduction or rigid fixation. Although there is no appreciable improvement in outcome for treatment of thoracolumbar fracture,[149] the differences are more pronounced in the low lumbar spine. In addition, most pedicle screw systems can achieve rigid fixation and maintenance of sagittal contours. The length of instrumentation does not need to be increased when removing portions of the posterior elements for monitoring by intraoperative ultrasonography or when laminectomy is necessary for repair of dural lacerations or for direct root decompressions.

Pedicle screw systems are of three basic types: (1) plate-based systems; (2) rod-based systems; and (3) external and internal fixators. Most plate-based systems have no significant capability for achieving reduction other than by postural reduction on the operating table.[34, 94, 122, 135] Rod-based pedicle fixation devices such as the modular system or internal and external spinal fixators[32, 77, 95, 96, 116] allow progressive reduction of deformities after screw fixation with maintenance of correction. However, fixator-type systems relying on one pair of screws proximally and one pair distally have a higher failure rate than systems using three or more pairs of screws.

Anterior Procedures. Anterior procedures for decompression, reduction of deformity, and stabilization have been used in the acute setting. In the absence of instrumentation, the long-term results of anterior correction of deformity with the use of the strut graft have been poor in terms of maintenance of anatomic alignment.[101] A tricortical bone graft cannot provide progressive correction. Results with more recent types of anterior instrumentation such as the Kostuik-Harrington,[75] Kaneda devices,[72, 73] and several different types of plate systems have indicated an ability to achieve and maintain reduction. The ability to slightly compress and distract is now built into the slotted holes and instrumentation of several different plate designs. This is an improvement over previous plates which simply functioned as neutralization devices. These plate systems now allow decompression and reasonable stabilization to be accomplished from an anterior approach for upper lumbar spine fractures. However, most anterior plate systems are not designed for fixation to the L5 or S1 segments as a result of the position of the lumbosacral plexus and the iliac artery and vein. This distinctly limits the ability to achieve adequate stabilization for either L4 or L5 fractures from an anterior approach.

For the correction of deformity from spinal fractures that are more than 6 weeks old, the mechanics of correction are different because secondary changes have occurred that complicate the fracture deformity. Primary healing of the cancellous fractures has begun, along with scarring of the soft tissues. At this stage an anterior procedure for release of tissues becomes important for achieving and maintaining correction as the complexity and stiffness of the deformity increase. When a reduction is attempted with posterior instrumentation alone more than 6 weeks after injury, it is difficult to overcome the kyphosis that has resulted from the shortening of anterior structures and the formation of anterior bony bridges. There is now some preliminary evidence that an anatomic reduction can be achieved and maintained using a posterior approach with appropriate application of forces if no synostosis has formed anteriorly. Total reduction from an anterior approach alone can be difficult in these late cases, because posterior scarring or healing of posterior element fractures might have occurred. In addition, most anterior spinal devices lack sufficient lever arms and rigidity of fixation points to be able to apply forces adequate for achieving total reduction.

Maintenance of Correction

The second goal of surgical treatment, maintenance of correction, is related to the rigidity of fixation and to the ability of the selected instrumentation to counteract both the deforming forces and the normal physiologic forces of the lumbar spine. Long-term results in terms of the rigidity of fixation have been poor for devices that do not counteract all the deforming forces, such as straight distraction rods and segmental spinal instrumentation. In addition, in the lumbar spine where construct length is important, shorter constructs impart more load bearing to the hardware and therefore may have a higher failure rate. The concept of load sharing either with intact posterior elements or with a supplemental anterior graft should be considered. Experimental data on short constructs for the lumbar spine often lead to the conclusion that restoration of the anterior column using a strut graft is important,[34, 58, 76, 97, 130] although load sharing with the intact posterior elements, when properly applied, seems be sufficient. In addition, in areas of the spine where construct stability is compromised by inadequate terminal fixation (i.e., the sacrum), maintenance of long-term anatomic restoration of alignment has been unsatisfactory. Posterior devices that achieve rigid fixation and counteract deforming forces can achieve satisfactory results with hook or pedicle screw fixation. The use of anterior grafts as the sole stabilizer after anterior decompression and correction of deformity has had disappointing results. More rigid anterior devices have been effective in maintaining satisfactory long-term results.[98]

Decompression of Neural Elements

The third goal, decompression of neural elements, is not always a critical goal of surgical treatment of lumbar burst fractures. Although originally it was thought that the patient who was neurologically intact with significant canal compromise might benefit from neural decompression, it has been shown that the assumption was false. Late spinal stenosis does not occur in patients either operated on or not operated on in whom a reasonably anatomic reduction occurs. It has been demonstrated that resorption of residual bone within the canal predictably occurs both with and without surgery.[17, 80, 129] Thus the sole indication for neural decompression is the patient with neural deficit. Neural decompression can be achieved in several different ways both directly and indirectly and the optimal method is dependent on the specific clinical situation. Laminectomy alone plays no role in neural decompression. In upper lumbar spine injuries there is significant experimental[48, 62] and clinical evidence[24, 33, 89, 128, 140, 147] that immediate indirect decompression by ligamentotaxis and complete correction of the deformity can provide adequate decompression of the neural elements. This technique has been shown to be most effective in the first 48 hours after injury. Transpedicular decompression is a direct posterior technique,[61, 139] but with limited visibility of the anterior portion of the dural sac and results which do not differ from indirect decompression. In the low lumbar spine and sacrum, however, indirect decompression is not as successful because the technique depends on distraction and tension of the posterior longitudinal ligament. It is therefore less effective in an area of extreme lordosis or kyphosis. Thus at L4 and L5 direct decompression using a laminectomy or laminotomy can be effective in revealing the area of compression and allowing decompression by removal of the bone fragments that are compressing the dural sac or nerve roots. This is possible because limited retraction of the dural sac to achieve exposure is possible at this level. This technique is only recommended for those areas of the spine involving the cauda equina or roots of the sacrum. For transverse fractures of the sacrum, laminectomy and direct removal of fragments impinging on the roots or

dural sac can be effective. Direct decompression is most easily done when the compression is one-sided so that bilateral exposure is not necessary. It is technically easier when carried out within the first 2 weeks of injury, because the fragments are more mobile and more easily removed. In the upper lumbar spine, a transpedicular posterolateral approach for direct decompression might be indicated. In this case, removal of a portion of the lamina and the pedicle exposes the dural sac adequately on one side and allows direct decompression. Performing a laminectomy or laminotomy at the same time allows direct monitoring of the decompression by ultrasonography.[38]

For patients who have had an inadequate indirect decompression with posterior instrumentation or who present late (more than 2 weeks after injury) and require decompression of the dural sac, anterior corpectomy and direct decompression are the most effective. Some authors have advocated direct anterior decompression and stabilization in the immediate acute setting for the treatment of lumbar trauma, but the increased morbidity and decreased stabilization potential of the anterior approach makes this a somewhat less attractive alternative. In addition, the use of pedicle fixation for the stabilization of especially low lumbar fractures allows laminectomy and posterior decompression along with very short construct length, without compromising the quality of the reduction and stabilization.

Maintenance of Sagittal Alignment

The next important goal in the treatment of lumbar fractures is the maintenance of sagittal alignment. Any instrumentation system used for these fractures should be able to impart and maintain the lordosis of the lumbar spine and lumbosacral junction. Thus, distraction instrumentation with augmentation by sublaminar wires is rarely indicated for low lumbar fractures. When crossing the lumbosacral junction, as is the case with many low lumbar fractures, adequate fixation to the pelvis needs to be obtained to maintain lordosis. This is not obtained with any type of hook fixation. The use of Luque-Galveston fixation might augment fixation to the pelvis, but its complexity and the failure of Luque instrumentation to provide axial control makes this an unsatisfactory alternative. Most fixation constructs crossing the lumbosacral junction require screw fixation. This is especially critical in maintaining the lumbosacral angle, lumbosacral lordosis, and overall sagittal alignment of the spine.

Minimizing Fixation Length

Minimizing fixation length to maintain the maximal number of mobile lumbar segments is the next important treatment goal and consideration in instrumentation of fractures of the lumbar spine. However, there must be a satisfactory balance between the number of levels requiring instrumentation to achieve satisfactory reduction and stabilization and the preservation of important lumbar motion segments. Fixation rigidity should not be compromised to shorten levels, as with the use of Luque rectangles in fractures of the lumbar spine. Similarly, plate fixation requires adequate numbers of screws above and below the fracture. Even the Cotrel-Dubousset system has been found to be inadequate with the use of short constructs (less than four levels) in maintaining alignment[2, 7, 8] and requires augmentation with an anterior strut graft to achieve an anatomic reduction. Thus, with selection of the construct, the surgeon should keep in mind both the rigidity of fixation and the length so as not to compromise other treatment goals.

Minimizing Complication Rate

The final treatment goal for lumbar and sacral fractures is to minimize the extremely high complication rate associated with instrumentation of these injuries. The major complications are pseudarthrosis, hook dislodgment,[37] failure of sacral fixation, and iatrogenic flat back.[81] Care must be taken in achieving the other treatment goals so that the instrumentation system used will not jeopardize the results with an unacceptably high complication rate.

Standard Techniques for Specific Types of Injuries

Minor Bony, Disc, and Ligamentous Injuries

Most minor bony injuries, such as avulsion fractures, spinous process fractures, and ligamentous strains, are satisfactorily treated by external immobilization for symptomatic relief. A major consideration in this group of patients concerns those with posterior ligamentous instability without significant fracture. These patients might not be initially recognized but once the spasm of the acute injury has subsided, flexion-extension radiographs can define any significant instability related to profound disruption of the intraspinous and supraspinous ligaments and facet capsules. With a minor degree of disruption (sprain), external immobilization for 6 weeks to 2 months can allow sufficient healing to achieve symptomatic relief and stability. If the disruption is complete, with tearing of the ligamentum flavum and anulus and anterior wedging of the disc space on flexion-extension radiographs, an arthrodesis might be necessary to restore sagittal alignment and control the ligamentous instability (Fig. 28–20). Avulsion fractures of the transverse processes can be treated symptomatically by external immobilization to support the severe muscular trauma associated with the more minor bony injury. Transverse process fractures associated with more severe bony injury can be treated secondarily by immobilization of the primary injury. Endplate avulsions in children simulating disc herniation in the acute injury setting require surgical intervention for direct decompression after appropriate diagnostic studies.[36, 40, 138] A laminotomy as used for a discectomy is generally sufficient to allow excision of the protruding portion of the end plate. The remaining portion of the end plate generally heals without further intervention.

Anterior Wedge Compression Fractures

Compression fractures of the lumbar spine are relatively frequent either as single or multiple injuries. Their outcome is usually favorable except in the osteopenic patient. The most frequent problems are either failure to recognize accompanying severe ligamentous disruption or mistakenly identifying a burst fracture as merely a compression fracture. In evaluating these

Figure 28–20 ═ A 44-year-old woman whose initial radiographs are shown in Figure 28–6 presented 5 months postinjury with severe kyphosis and ligamentous instability. Unfortunately, her maximal hyperextension radiograph (A) shows only minimal correction of the kyphosis. The patient underwent posterior correction, stabilization, and fusion of the kyphosis. She went on to solid arthrodesis and is pain-free with no evidence of instability (B). (From Levine AM: Lumbar and sacral spine trauma. In Browner DB, Jupiter JB, Levine AM, et al (eds): Skeletal Trauma: Fractures, Dislocations, Ligamentous Injuries, vol 1. Philadelphia, WB Saunders, 1992.)

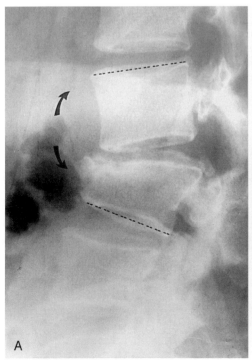
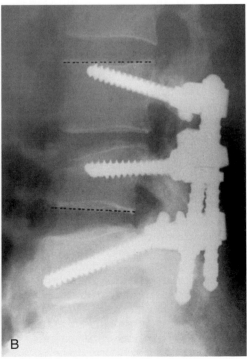

A B

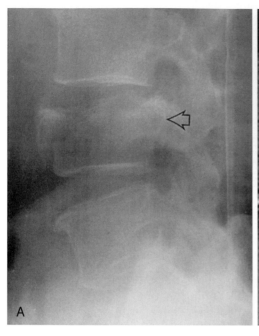 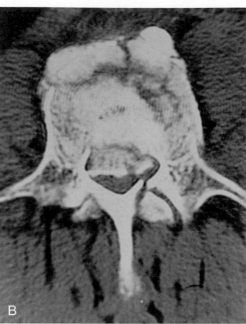

Figure 28–21 = *A*, This lateral radiograph of an L4 burst fracture might be mistaken for a simple compression fracture of L4. The key to the diagnosis is the posterosuperior corner of the affected vertebral body (L4). The posterosuperior corner is retropulsed into the canal as confirmed on CT scans (*B*). Although the comminution of the vertebral body and the loss of height is unimpressive, the degree of canal occlusion and the overall structural disruption of the vertebral body is not fully appreciated except on CT scan. (From Levine AM: Lumbar and sacral spine trauma. *In* Browner BD, Jupiter JB, Levine AM, et al (eds): Skeletal Trauma: Fractures, Dislocations, Ligamentous Injuries, vol 1. Philadelphia, WB Saunders, 1992.)

injuries care must be taken to confirm that the posterior wall of the vertebral body remains intact.

A common pitfall in the treatment of these injuries is the failure to recognize the extent of the injury. Although the degree of sagittal plane deformity might not be severe, CT scanning is indicated to confirm the integrity of the posterior wall of the vertebral body. Careful examination of well-centered AP and lateral plain films will differentiate the two injuries in most cases. Often, a clue is available on the lateral view showing displacement of the posterosuperior corner (Fig. 28–21). Comminution of the posterior wall converts the injury to the more significant burst pattern, which alters the prognosis and treatment program. In addition, the surgeon must be certain that the compression fracture is not accompanied by ligamentous disruption (see Fig. 28–20).

For those wedge compression fractures with loss of less than 50% of the height of the vertebral body, no ligamentous instability generally exists. The goal of treatment is to prevent further anterior compression and residual kyphosis. Nonoperative treatment, even in hyperextension, cannot restore vertebral height, but such patients are still best treated nonoperatively. Careful attention needs to be paid to the ability of the orthosis chosen to immobilize that segment of the spine. Compression fractures of L2–4 are not hyperextended by a Jewett brace and might in fact be made worse. These require a lumbar orthosis, such as a chair back, Norton-Brown brace, or TCO. Compression fractures of L5 are not well immobilized by the standard lumbar orthoses, and, in fact, motion at the L5 level is accentuated by the use of a lumbar orthosis, which blocks movement at the other levels.[44, 114] Immobilization of L5 fractures requires a single leg included in the orthosis to immobilize the lumbosacral junction. Immobilization needs to be extended for a period of 3 months, until the vertebral body has consolidated. Post

immobilization, the patient should be checked with flexion-extension radiographs to determine if any residual instability is present. Increasing compression during the course of treatment interfering with the normal lordotic sagittal alignment of the spine might require a change in treatment, surgical restoration of alignment, and single-level arthrodesis.

Burst Fractures of the Lumbar Spine

The majority of the patients sustaining injuries of the lumbar spine requiring operative stabilization have burst fractures. The key to selecting the most appropriate treatment for these patients is recognition of the components of the fracture pattern. As previously described all burst injuries have comminution of the anterior portion of the body and significant involvement of the posterior wall (middle column), with retropulsion of bone into the canal. The two most common types of burst fractures seen in the lumbar spine are Denis A (comminution of the entire body and the body-pedicle junction with or without posterior element involvement) and Denis B (comminution of only the upper end plate with an intact body-pedicle junction usually sparing the posterior elements). These two fracture types have reasonably equal distribution at L2 and L3, but the Denis B fracture predominates at L4 and L5. Lateral burst fractures (Denis E) are also occasionally seen. Review of the care of these injuries illustrates most of the techniques required for the surgical treatment of lumbar injuries. Differentiation of treatment of upper and lower lumbar fractures is necessary for optimal results.

Flexion-compression (Denis B) injuries represent a subset of burst fractures that have a fracture of the posterior wall of the vertebral body with retropulsion of the posterosuperior corner into the spinal canal, causing compression. The critical feature on the AP view and on the CT scan is that the pedicles are not splayed apart. On the CT scan it is evident that they are still attached to the lateral sides of the vertebral body, although there is a large central fragment that can cause canal compression. This is usually accompanied by a significant degree of kyphosis. Recognition of this particular pattern of injury in the lumbar spine is critical to treatment. It allows use of a very short rod construct with the application of a three-point bending force applied through the pedicles of the fractured body to achieve anatomic reduction and rigid fixation (Fig. 28–22). In the upper lumbar spine (L2 and L3

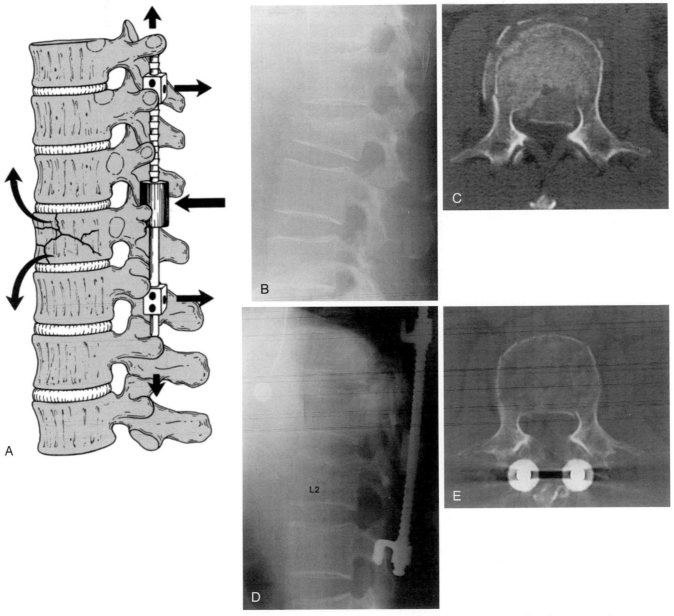

Figure 28–22 = *A,* The use of a rod sleeve technique allows correction of both the flexion component as well as the compression component of the deformity. The use of a rod sleeve directly over the apical portion of the kyphosis (which is at the level of the pedicle of the injured body) will create a three-point bending moment to correct a flexion deformity. After complete correction of the flexion deformity, residual compression may then be corrected by ratcheting the rod for distraction. The use of the rod sleeve and the three-point bending will prevent kyphosis with the use of distraction applied posterior to the axis rotation of the spine. The rod sleeve technique requires a minimum of 3 cm from the center of the sleeve to the hook for maximal lever arm. Therefore, for upper lumbar fractures, based on the length of the lamina, this will encompass one level below the injury and two levels above for a total of three fused interspaces and four segments. This 43-year-old man was riding his bicycle and was struck by a motor vehicle; he sustained this L2 burst fracture. *B,* On the initial lateral radiograph he had comminution of the upper 60% of the vertebral body and 29 degrees of kyphosis and was neurologically intact with the exception of inability to void. *C,* Preoperative CT scan showed 60% canal compromise. This fracture was thought to be a Denis type B burst fracture with intact body pedicle junction and posterior elements. Thus, a single sleeve construct could be utilized with the point of lordosis centered directly over the L2 pedicle with the distal extent of the instrumentation only going to L3. *D,* On the postoperative lateral view restoration of vertebral height and sagittal alignment were achieved. *E,* The postoperative CT scan at exactly the same level as the preoperative scan shows restoration of the canal area as well as the placement of the sleeves. (From Levine AM: Lumbar and sacral spine trauma. *In* Browner BD, Jupiter JB, Levine AM, et al (eds): Skeletal Trauma: Fractures, Dislocations, Ligamentous Injuries, ed 2, vol 1. Philadelphia, WB Saunders, 1998.)

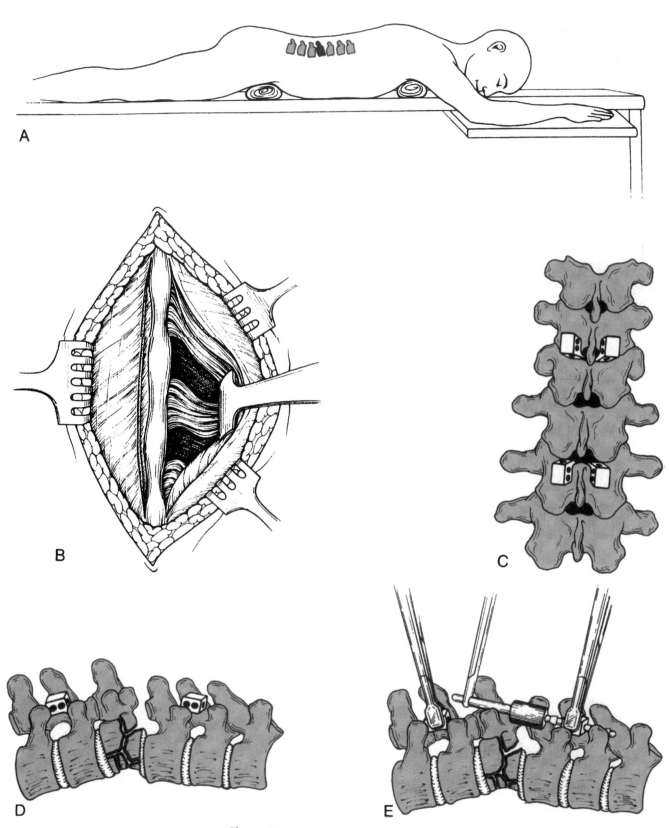

Figure 28–23 == *See legend on opposite page*

fractures) this immobilizes and fuses only four verte-bral segments and three interspaces. The predominant advantage is that the construct is shortened on the distal end minimizing intrusion into the critical motion segments of the lumbar spine. Thus for an L2 fracture, the distal end of the construct is at L3, which is no different from a pedicle screw or anterior plate con-struct. However, sufficient lever arms are maintained to achieve an anatomic reduction (Fig. 28–22A–E). Al-though this short rod technique has been attempted with several different instrumentation systems, it has not been uniformly successful because of differing bio-mechanical characteristics of the systems. Early experi-ence with the Cotrel-Dubousset instrumentation for four-level constructs has resulted in a high incidence of laminar fracture, loss of correction, and infection.[1, 7, 9]

Rod-Sleeve Technique. The rod-sleeve technique has been effective in achieving satisfactory application of this short rod technique.[90] Thus, for an L2 fracture, the sleeves are placed over the L1–2 facets and centered over the L2 pedicle, with distal hooks placed over the superior edge of the L3 lamina and superior hooks at the inferior edge of the T12 lamina. If, however, the patient is relatively small or great difficulty is encoun-tered in assembling the instrumentation, the proximal hooks can be moved up one level to T11, making assembly easier and decreasing the risk of hook failure at the proximal end while maintaining the advantage of limited involvement of the lumbar spine. Similarly, at L3, the distal hooks can be placed at L4 and the proximal hooks at L1 or T12. This does not extend any further distally in the lumbar spine than a pedicle screw system, carries a lower overall risk to the patient, and interferes minimally with the important distal mo-tion segments in the lumbar spine. This technique can achieve excellent control of the fracture and stabiliza-tion, with an acceptably high fusion rate.[90]

Preoperative evaluation of the spinal injury should consist of a minimum of high-quality AP and lateral views of the spine, centered at the fracture. A CT scan of the injury must include at least a level above and below the fracture. The patient is placed on a Stryker frame for minimal movement. After induction of anes-thesia, the patient is rolled into the prone position on the Stryker frame, with transverse rolls placed at the level of the clavicles and at the level of the pubic symphysis (Fig. 28–23). This aids in the postural reduc-tion of the fracture and allows adequate room for ve-nous return.

A routine posterior approach to the spine is taken. Care is taken in incising the lumbodorsal fascia. Two longitudinal incisions are made in the fascia along the lateral edge of the spinous processes of T12, L1, L2, and L3. Throughout this procedure the construct can be seated at the T11 level in a very small patient. This leaves the intraspinous ligament intact (Fig. 28–23). Using a cautery, the paraspinous musculature is stripped subperiosteally from the lamina, facet joints, and transverse processes without undue motion of the spine and minimal bleeding. Exposure is carried out to the tips of the transverse processes at T12–L3. A lateral localization radiograph is taken with a marker placed on a spinous process. All facet capsules are then re-moved.

Care is taken to size the spine for placement of the sleeve. The appropriate rod sleeve is placed at the level of the facet joint at L1–2 directly over the L2 pedicle. In a small man or woman a medium-sized rod sleeve is usually long enough and, in a larger person, a large rod sleeve is appropriate. The distance from the center of the rod sleeve to the hook is measured; it should be at least 3 to 4 cm to provide an optimal lever arm for maximal reduction.

At this point, using a small curette, the ligamentum flavum is removed from the undersurface of the T12 lamina. A medium-profile anatomic hook can then be advanced into position beneath the lamina. The hook is not placed in the facet but is situated medially be-tween the facet and the spinous process beneath the lamina. It should seat easily. If the lamina of T12 is excessively thick, a hook with a higher profile can be

---

Figure 28–23 = Surgical technique for the rod sleeve procedure. For treatment of lumbar injuries with the rod sleeve technique, the patient is placed on a Stryker frame with transverse rolls placed at the level of the clavicle and at the level of the pubis. This serves two purposes. It allows the lumbar spine to fall into lordosis, thus posturally reducing a significant portion of the spinal deformity (A). In addition, it suspends the abdomen off of the Stryker frame, thus reducing resistance to venous return and decreasing blood loss in the field. A longitudinal incision is then made through the skin and subcutaneous tissue, and the tips of the spinous processes are exposed. An effort is made to leave the interspinous and supraspinous ligaments intact if they have not been disrupted by the injury (B). This allows reconstruction of the lumbodorsal fascia at closure. To preserve the supraspinous and interspinous ligaments, longitudinal incisions through the lumbodorsal fascia are made parallel to the edge of the spinous processes using a cutting cautery. The line of incision is not curved into the area of the supraspinous and interspinous ligaments. To keep from moving the spine and potentially causing neural damage, the cautery is used to strip the muscle from the spinous processes and lamina. Exposure is carried out to the tips of the transverse processes. Once exposure is complete, the number of levels to be instrumented is decided on based on the preoperative evaluation of the plain films and CT scans. For a flexion-compression injury where the pedicles and the neural arch are intact but there is a large central portion of retropulsed bone and kyphosis, a four-segment–three-interspace construct is selected. Therefore, for an L2 fracture, hooks would be placed over the top of the L3 lamina and on the undersurface of the T12 lamina (C and D). Care is taken in hook placement not to damage the surface of the lamina on which the hook is placed. Notching the lamina can create a stress riser sufficient to cause failure of the hook purchase site. At the lower hook site, care should be taken that both hooks can be placed in the canal without overlap. An appropriately sized rod and sleeve are selected. The rod is advanced up through the upper hook at T12 so that the end clears the hook over the top of the L3 lamina. The operating surgeon then places a hook holder on the L3 hook and a rod holder on the tip of the rod with the sleeve placed over the L2 pedicle. Direct downward pressure is applied progressively until the tip of the rod can be articulated with the hole in the hook (E). At this point the surgeon's assistant uses a spreader to distract the rod down into the distal hook and engage the hook. The process is repeated on the opposite side. Prior to applying distraction to the construct, the sleeves are placed in appropriate position over the L1–2 facet and the L2 pedicle.

Illustration continued on following page

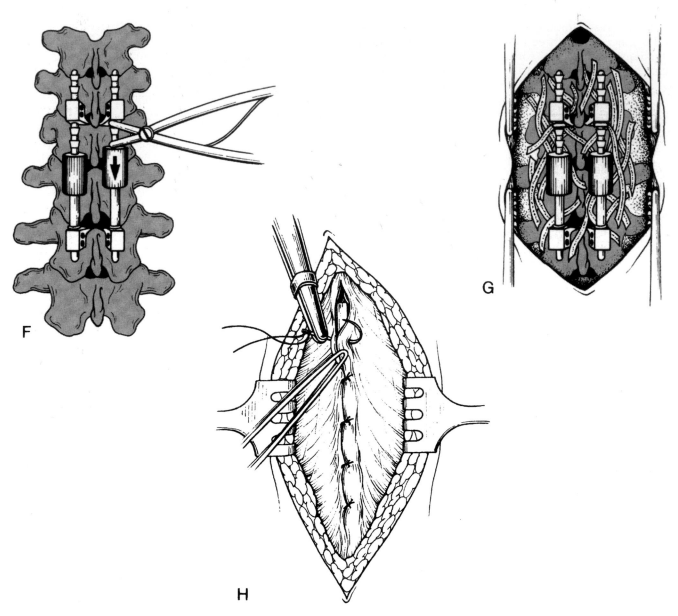

Figure 28–23 *Continued* ▭ The sleeve can be moved by using a rod spreader *(F)*. The pressure on the sleeve should be sufficient to prevent it from being moved by hand. Distraction is then progressively applied to the system until all components are tight. With the use of stress relaxation during the harvesting of the bone graft, the system will allow an additional bit of distraction after approximately 10 to 15 minutes. On the lateral radiograph a slight bow should be apparent in the rods. C washers are then placed and the harvested cortical cancellous graft is placed on decorticated transverse processes from T12 down to L3 *(G)*. The lumbodorsal fascia is then closed back to the supraspinous ligament to recreate the appropriate tension *(H)*. (From Levine AM: Lumbar and sacral spine trauma. *In* Browner BD, Jupiter JB, Levine AM, et al (eds): Skeletal Trauma: Fractures, Dislocations, Ligamentous Injuries, vol 1. Philadelphia, WB Saunders, 1992.)

used instead. Hook sizes can be changed, depending on the size of the patient.

Attention is then turned to the L2–3 interspace. The ligamentum flavum is excised from the interspace, exposing the epidural fat. A small portion of the inferior portion of the L2 lamina is removed so that a high-profile hook can be easily placed over the superior portion of the L3 lamina. Under no circumstances should a portion of the L3 lamina be removed, thus recessing the hook distally on the lamina to accommodate seating. This simply thins the pars interarticularis, recesses the hook, and potentially allows a secondary fracture.[43] The laminotomy, however, should be widened laterally and might require excision of the medial portion of the facet so that the two hooks at the L3 level can be placed in the canal without any overlap (Fig. 28–23C and D).

Once both laminotomies are made, the reduction maneuver is begun. The rod sleeve is placed over the rod, and the rod sleeve combination is advanced up through the proximal hook. When the rod has cleared the distal hook, the operating surgeon places the high-profile lower hook over the top of the L3 lamina (Fig. 28–23E). A rod holder is placed on the end of the rod and the surgeon's assistant takes a rod spreader in preparation for advancing the rod down into the distal hook. The surgeon applies pressure directly downward using the rod sleeve to reduce the kyphosis by centering it over the apex of the kyphosis. When the end of the rod is at the level of the hole in the distal hook, the assistant gently distracts the rod until the rod engages the distal hook. Downward pressure should be maintained on the rod until the end of the rod is fully engaged in the hook.

If difficulty is encountered in engaging the rod into the distal hook, several alternatives are available. First, the sleeve should be pushed distally on the rod off the apical facet, which allows easier engagement. Second, the next smaller sleeve can be substituted if the initial choice is too large. If, after the reduction with a smaller sleeve, the sleeves are not snug, they can again be substituted one at a time for the next larger size, which should now be easier because the reduction has been partially achieved. Third, the construct can be extended one level more proximally. Before any tension is placed on the rod using a spreader, the rod sleeve is advanced to its proper position (Fig. 28–23F). The rod is then gently distracted to two-finger snugness.

At this point the rod sleeve should be wedged tightly between the spinous process and the facet in a mediolateral direction, and wedged tightly against the posterior aspect of the lamina. The same procedure is repeated on the opposite side and the two rods are distracted equally to achieve full reduction. The position is checked by lateral radiographs. A slight bow in the rod can be noted on the intraoperative radiographs if proper tension is achieved.

Intraoperative reduction of intraspinal fragments is optimal within the first 48 hours. It can be checked by intraoperative ultrasonography,[38] which might be difficult because of sleeve position and the importance of maintaining the spinous process, or by intraoperative myelography. At this point a bone graft is harvested from the iliac crest, usually by an extension of the midline incision in subcutaneous dissection to the appropriate iliac crest. Generally, it is suggested that the right iliac crest be used so that the left is preserved if an anterior approach and stabilization are necessary. After obtaining the bone graft, some stress relaxation will have occurred in the spine and additional tension can be added to the rod by distracting one or two more ratchets. The lordotic force on the rods should be such that slight bowing of the rods occurs within their elastic range. C washers are then placed inferior to the upper hooks. Two ratchets should be visible above the tops of the hooks to prevent dislodgment. The transverse processes are thoroughly decorticated and the fusion should extend from the tips of the T12 transverse processes to the tips of the L3 transverse processes (Fig. 28–23G). Care should be taken so that the transverse processes and the lamina of T12 are fully decorticated, because they lie proximal to the hook placement site and are sometimes neglected.

In closure the surgeon should take care to suture the lumbodorsal fascia back to the remaining interspinous ligament to restore normal function to this musculoligamentous complex (Fig. 28–23A). The incision is closed over a closed suction drain system. On the sec-

ond to third postoperative day, a mold is made for a TCO jacket and the patient is generally mobilized on the sixth to seventh postoperative day in the TCO. Radiographs are taken postoperatively and after all transfers to ascertain that reduction remains stable. In patients with neurologic deficit, postoperative CT scans are obtained on the fifth postoperative day to confirm that indirect decompression of the neural canal has been achieved.

This technique works satisfactorily for Denis B–type burst fractures at the L1, L2, and L3 levels. With fractures of this type at L3, the hooks only extend to L4. It is not recommended that the technique be used for L4 fractures, because hook placement on the lamina of L5 can entail the risk of compression of the neural canal, depending on the extent of lordosis at that level.

As the predominant force across the spinal segments changes from flexion to a more axial load, the nature of the injury changes to that of a Denis A burst fracture. This is characterized on the AP view by spreading of the pedicles and on the lateral view by severe comminution of the body, usually with less kyphotic deformity than the previously described flexion-compression injuries. CT scans generally show retropulsion of significant central bony fragments as well as comminution of the pedicles, or at least of the pedicle-body junction (Fig. 28–24). If there is a lateral bending force applied, the compression might be asymmetrical to one side or the other, with resulting scoliosis. This injury in the upper lumbar spine can be treated adequately by the use of posterior distraction rod techniques, such as the Harri-Luque, multiple hook and rod, or rod sleeve. Since the pedicles at the apical level are comminuted, however, direct lordotic pressure over that area might tend to narrow the canal rather than produce lordosis. The fragmented pedicles could simply be driven into the comminuted vertebral body and not achieve the lordosis and ligamentotaxis necessary (Fig. 28–25). Therefore, a modified technique is necessary.

A "bridging" technique is used, in which rod sleeves are placed at the intact pedicles above and below the level of injury (Fig. 28–26). This necessarily increases the length of the construct. For an L2 burst fracture, sleeves are placed over the L1 and L3 pedicles. This necessitates hook placement at T11 and L4. The length of the construct is increased by two interspaces and two segments. This achieves the desired goal of anatomic reduction and rigid fixation, but sacrifices additional lumbar motion segments. This length of instrumentation is similar to that required in burst fractures of this type fixed with any of the multiple hook-rod systems.[104, 133] In order to maintain adequate stability and fixation on the distal end, that technique mandates a bilaminar placement (indirect distal claw) to prevent early laminar failure. Because of this, some authors have recommended pedicle fixation for these fractures to preserve more distal intact segments. The risks of pedicle instrumentation must be balanced against the benefits, and the long-term results are not yet available.

The use of the rod sleeve technique for a bridging construct is the same as described previously for short rod sleeve fixation, with two exceptions. First, the con-

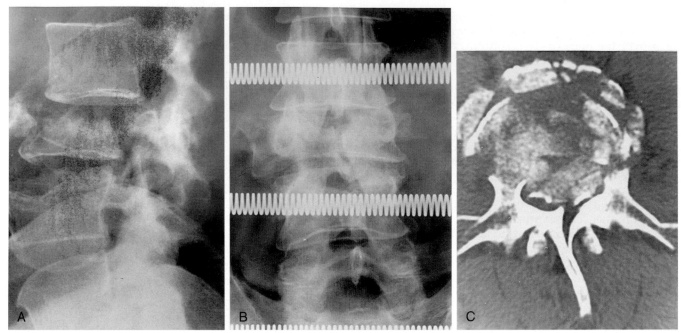

Figure 28–24 = This 63-year-old man sustained a burst fracture of L3. *A,* The lateral preoperative radiograph demonstrates severe destruction and axial compression of the L3 body. There is slight posterior translation but little angulation associated with the fracture. *B,* The AP radiograph demonstrates severe comminution of the vertebral body with spreading of the pedicles and posterior element fractures. *C,* The CT scan of the affected level demonstrates the critical radiographic features. There is complete comminution of the entire vertebral body and significant retropulsion of bone into the canal with nearly complete occlusion of the canal and comminution of the pedicles. Pressure applied to these pedicles would only drive the pedicles into the severely comminuted body and would not cause resultant lordosis and ligamentotaxis. (From Levine AM: Lumbar and sacral spine trauma. *In* Browner BD, Jupiter JB, Levine AM, et al (eds): Skeletal Trauma: Fractures, Dislocations, Ligamentous Injuries, vol 1. Philadelphia, WB Saunders, 1992.)

struct is longer and the hooks are placed one more level proximally and one more level distally. Second, the hook and rod sizes might need to be varied to achieve a tight construct. Because the upper sleeves are placed at the L1 level, it might be necessary to place medium-sized sleeves at the L1 level and larger sleeves at the L3 level. In addition, a high-profile hook is placed over the top of the L4 lamina. It might be

necessary to vary the hook size or sleeve placement at the proximal end to obtain tight contact between the sleeves and posterior bony elements. This can be done by using combinations of medium-sized proximal hooks and medium sleeves or, if that does not achieve tight contact, by changing to high-profile hooks proximally and using larger sleeves to allow for optimal fixation.

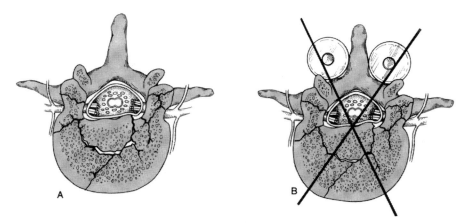

Figure 28–25 = The use of a standard rod sleeve technique with application of three-point bending applied at the comminuted pedicles of a true burst fracture does not result in the desired indirect decompression of the neural canal and ligamentotaxis. The differentiation on CT scan of intact pedicles and neural arch vs. comminuted pedicles and neural arch is critically important. *A,* The pedicles are severely comminuted, as is the vertebral body. There is a retropulsed fragment causing compression of the neural canal. A single rod sleeve placed over the comminuted pedicles would only drive them into the comminuted vertebral body *(B)* and would not achieve a reduction. A bridging technique is necessary to achieve ligamentotaxis and indirect decompression for this type of fracture. (From Levine AM: Lumbar and sacral spine trauma. *In* Browner BD, Jupiter JB, Levine AM, et al (eds): Skeletal Trauma: Fractures, Dislocations, Ligamentous Injuries, vol 1. Philadelphia, WB Saunders, 1992.)

Figure 28–26 = The same principles of three-point bending used for a flexion-compression fracture with an intact neural arch are applicable to the burst fracture with a comminuted neural arch. However, the sleeves *(A)* are placed at the first intact neural arch above and below the level of the injury. This extends the length of fixation but will effectively achieve three-point fixation and lordosis of the fracture and allow subsequent distraction to regain height without causing a recurrent flexion deformity. *B*, Note the bow of the rod in the reduced position demonstrating the significant three-point bending moment induced by the bridging sleeve construct. (From Levine AM: Lumbar and sacral spine injuries. *In* Browner BD, Jupiter JB, Levine AM, et al (eds): Skeletal Trauma: Fractures, Dislocations, Ligamentous Injuries, vol 1. Philadelphia, WB Saunders, 1992.)

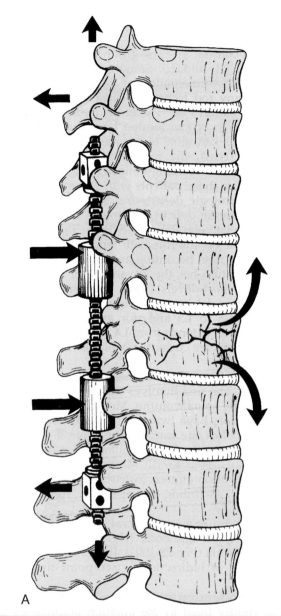

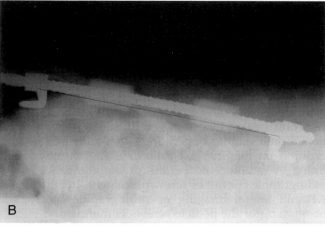

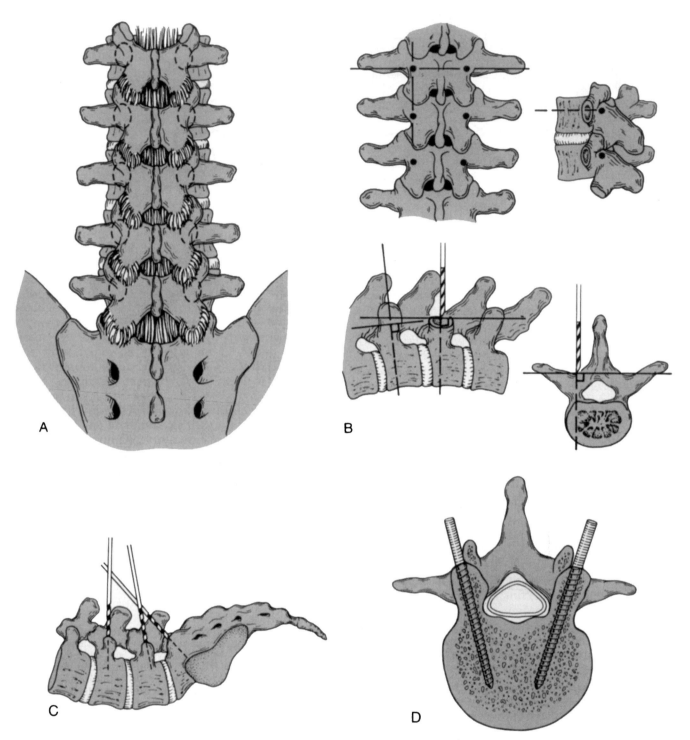

Figure 28–28 = The operative technique for pedicular fixation of low lumbar burst fractures has many similarities from one system to the next. The technique shown emphasizes the critical features. When exposing the spine, care must be taken not to disrupt the interspinous ligament or the facet capsules proximal to the level of instrumentation. In exposing the transverse process opposite the superior pedicle, it is critical that the facet capsule not be disrupted. In view of the location of the pedicle and its proximity to the capsule (A), great care should be taken in this dissection. Screw position can be determined by a number of different techniques. The technique of Roy-Camille (B) positions the entry point at the intersection of a line through the transverse processes and a line through the inferolateral edge of the facet joint. Entry into the pedicle can be facilitated by using a high-speed burr to remove the cortical bone at the location of the suggested entry point. A small probe, sound, or curette can be used to easily traverse the cancellous bone of the pedicle. This technique prevents inadvertent perforation of the pedicle walls. Drill bits can then be placed into pedicles so that the use of intraoperative image intensification or radiographs will allow identification of the position of the drill bits within the pedicles (C). The orientation of the drill bits within the vertebral bodies changes with the level. In view of the angle of the side wall of L5, the screws should be oriented approximately 10 degrees medial and 15 degrees caudal to accommodate the lordosis of L5. D, Orientation within the sacrum, as previously described, can be either medial into the body or lateral out into the sacral ala.

tion and aligned against the inferior edge of the L5 spinous process (if it exists). This should orient the drill with 35 degrees of lateral tilt and 25 degrees of inferior tilt (Fig. 28–28E). The posterior cortex of the sacrum is then drilled in that orientation. The bit is advanced to the anterior cortex of the sacrum simply by pushing it through the soft cancellous bone until the anterior, dense, cortical bone of the sacrum is encountered. The anterior cortex is not drilled at this point, but drill bits are placed as described previously, with one inverted, and their position is checked radiographically. On a true lateral view the drill bit should be oriented parallel to or should slightly converge toward the superior end plate of the sacrum, approximately 1 cm inferior to it. After checking the position, the hole is overdrilled with the appropriate size for the screw.

When drilling the anterior cortex, a hand drill should be used and the drill steadied with both hands to prevent plunging. Once the anterior cortex is felt to be engaged by the drill bit, three quarters of an additional twist is necessary to penetrate the anterior cortex fully. A depth gauge is used to measure screw length and care should be taken that the foot of the depth gauge is oriented medially, so that the shortest possible length is used to engage the cortex (the ala slopes laterally,

and therefore lateral measurements are always longer). If medial screw orientation into the vertebral body of S1 is necessary for the fixation device, the S1 pedicle must be located. An entrance hole is made at the base of the superior facet of S1 and the pedicle is probed and located in the standard fashion. Because of the severe medial slope of the sacrum, 20 to 30 degrees of medial and 25 degrees of inferior orientation of the screw are necessary to attain adequate fixation in the sacral body.

If an internal fixator[41, 93] is being used, fixation in the fractured body is not necessary. At this point the appropriate screws can be placed, the fixator inserted, and the reduction accomplished by application of lordosis (Fig. 28–28F) and distraction ((Fig 28–28G) to the system. Care should be taken after screw insertion and before application of the device to decorticate the transverse processes and sacral ala adequately, because the bulk of the devices could preclude adequate preparation for fusion after application.

If the pedicle screw system being used can accommodate fixation or requires fixation in the apical or fractured level, certain other factors must be considered. First, the configuration of the fractured body must be clearly delineated on the CT scan before attempting screw placement. The most common pattern for L4 and

Figure 28–28 *Continued* = *E*, Lateral orientation requires a 35-degree lateral tilt and a 25-degree inferior tilt. For internal or external fixators, application of two points of fixation are applied, and reduction is achieved using the device.

Illustration continued on following page

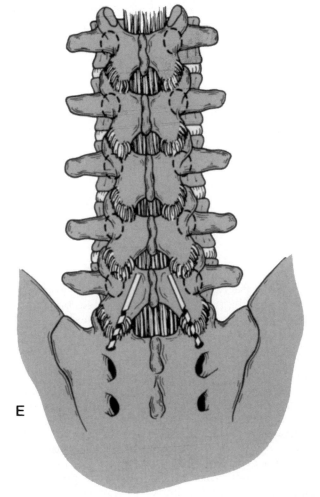

E

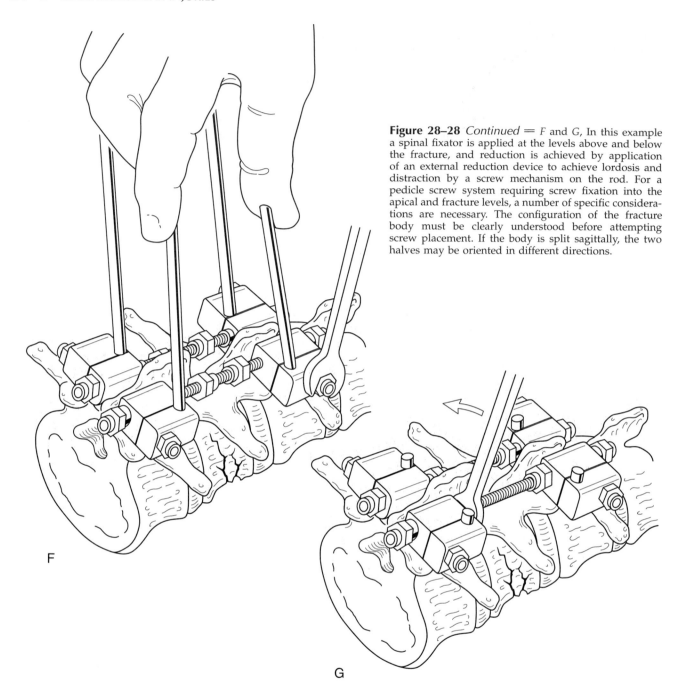

Figure 28–28 *Continued* = F and G, In this example a spinal fixator is applied at the levels above and below the fracture, and reduction is achieved by application of an external reduction device to achieve lordosis and distraction by a screw mechanism on the rod. For a pedicle screw system requiring screw fixation into the apical and fracture levels, a number of specific considerations are necessary. The configuration of the fracture body must be clearly understood before attempting screw placement. If the body is split sagittally, the two halves may be oriented in different directions.

L5 burst fractures is that the superior portion of the body and the pedicle are comminuted, but the inferior portion of the pedicle remains attached to the inferior portion of the vertebral body. This can be accompanied by a sagittal split in the body, so that the two halves of the vertebra are not attached. Most frequently, however, the area of best screw purchase is in the inferior portion of the body. Therefore, placement requires orientation of the drill bit in a much more inferiorly directed position than normally. In addition, if the two halves are split, a more directly anterior position (rather than medial orientation) might also be necessary for good purchase (see Fig. 28–28G).

A common variation is when one pedicle and the lateral cortex of the body on that side are displaced significantly. It might not be possible to reduce this or place the final screw in that pedicle until vertebral height has been restored.

Finally, in placing the screws, other cracks and fissures in the body might be palpable as the vertebral body is probed. The surgeon should always be aware of the exact dimensions of that vertebral body and the depth of insertion of any instrument, so that the anterior cortex of the body is not penetrated through a fracture line. Screw placement at the fracture level is accomplished similar to that at other vertebral levels by opening the posterior cortex over the center of the pedicle using a high-speed burr. This usually requires removal of the inferior portion of the superior facet and probing with a 3-0 curette prior to placement of a

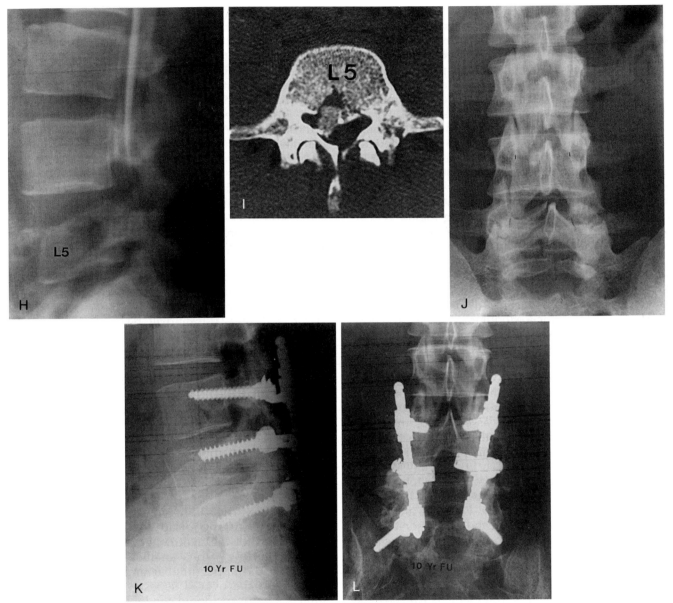

Figure 28–28 *Continued = H,* Therefore, one side may require vertical placement of the screw, whereas the other side, because of orientation, may require slight angulation medially. In addition the screw may traverse a fracture within the body. The surgeon should feel the fracture site as the screws are placed. A transverse connector is recommended to increase the rigidity of the construct. (*A–E* from Levine AM: Lumbar and sacral spine trauma. *In* Browner RB, Jupiter JB, Levine AM, et al (eds): Skeletal Trauma: Fractures, Dislocations, Ligamentous Injuries, ed 2, vol 1. Philadelphia, WB Saunders, 1998.) A 22-year-old man sustained an L5 burst fracture with incomplete neurologic deficit and root involvement at L5 and S1 as a result of canal compromise. *H,* This preoperative lateral view shows minimal distortion of sagittal alignment with anterior compression of L5, but a high-grade block on the myelogram. This is typical of a low lumbar burst fracture with minimal disruption of alignment (i.e., vertebral height and sagittal alignment) but significant canal retropulsion as demonstrated by the patient's CT scan *(I).* The AP radiograph *(J)* shows the split in the lamina with severe posterior element involvement. Follow-up at 10 years *(K)* shows the short construct from L4 to S1 with excellent maintenance of sagittal alignment and restoration of body height. The AP view at 10 years *(L)* shows the results of laminectomy performed to locally remove the retropulsed fragment of bone and decompress L5 and S1 roots, followed by lateral bilateral fusion. The patient had complete neurologic recovery. *(H–J* from Levine AM: The surgical treatment of low lumbar fractures. Semin Spine Surg 2:41–53, 1990.)

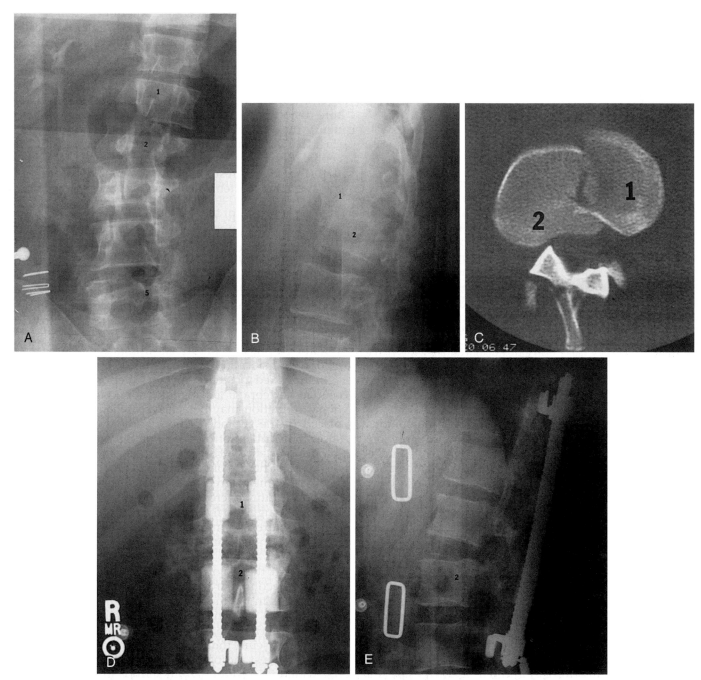

Figure 29–2 = This 25-year-old man was crushed between two whales. Multiple injuries were sustained including a flexion-rotation–type fracture-dislocation at L1–2. The patient suffered a Frankel D neurologic injury as graded for the lower extremities. AP *(A)* and lateral *(B)* radiographs demonstrate lateral dislocation and rotation of L1 on L2. *C,* CT scan. Note the rotational malalignment of L1 on L2 and that the two vertebral bodies are seen on the same axial image as the result of overlap from the dislocation. *D,* Postoperative AP radiograph. Edwards rods with bridging sleeves were used to distract, derotate, and reduce the kyphosis. *E,* Postoperative lateral radiograph. Note excellent reduction with maintenance of normal sagittal alignment. Also note slight overdistraction of the L1–2 disc space attesting to the unstable nature of this injury, including a probable partial disruption of the anterior longitudinal ligament (ALL). If a complete ALL rupture occurs, there may be no end point "felt" during distraction instrumentation. If this is discovered, instrumentation with more rigidity than that shown here should be used.

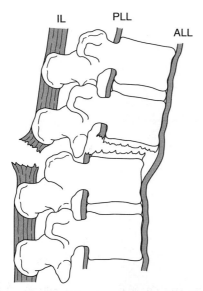

Figure 29–3 = Flexion-distraction–type fracture-dislocation. The injury may occur through soft tissue (as demonstrated here) or bone. The anterior longitudinal ligament may be stretched and stripped off the vertebral body rather than torn. *IL,* interspinous ligament; *PLL,* posterior longitudinal ligament; *ALL,* anterior longitudinal ligament. (Modified from Denis F: The three column spine and its significance in the classification of acute thoracolumbar spinal injuries. Spine 8:817–831, 1983.)

tion may be contraindicated if significant facet fractures, as opposed to facet dislocations, are present.

NEUROLOGIC INJURY

Holdsworth[17] stated that fracture-dislocations invariably result in paraplegia or quadriplegia. Holdsworth's classifications were, however, based on 1000 patients all with neurologic injuries treated at the Spinal Injuries Centre in Sheffield, England. In other series, where spine fractures with and without neurologic compromise are evaluated, neurologic injuries related to fracture-dislocations vary from none to complete neurologic deficit.[6, 7, 11, 13, 19] This is true in the thoracic, as well as the lumbar, spine.

As might be expected, injuries in the thoracic spine and at the thoracolumbar junction have an increased incidence and severity of neurologic injury compared with injuries in the lumbar region.[12, 19] Unfortunately, the thoracolumbar junction is also the most common area in the thoracic or lumbar spine to suffer these injuries.[6, 19] In Kaufer and Hayes's series,[19] there was a 62% incidence of neurologic injury in fracture-dislocations at the thoracolumbar junction, as compared to a 38% incidence in the lumbar region. Two thirds of the lumbar injuries had complete neurologic recovery, but only one quarter of the injuries across the thoracolumbar junction showed any significant neurologic improvement.[19] In Denis's series[6] there was a 75% overall incidence of neurologic injury in fracture-dislocations. Approximately 40% had a complete deficit. No breakdown according to thoracic vs. lumbar levels was presented.[6]

Surprisingly, considering the pathoanatomic changes that occur and the forces applied, there have been multiple case reports of "complete" fracture-dislocations of the thoracic and lumbar spine presenting without evident neurologic injury. In these cases the dislocation is usually associated with bilateral pedicle fractures resulting in anterior or anterolateral dislocation of one vertebral body on the subjacent one, while leaving the posterior elements in a reduced position.[4, 15, 18, 21, 23] This pattern may be considered similar to that seen in traumatic spondylolisthesis of the axis in which the neurologic structures are spared as the space available for the cord increases due to separation of the posterior bony ring from the anterior vertebral body.

TREATMENT

Spine fractures and dislocations with complex, multiplanar instability have been treated in a variety of ways. Postural reduction with subsequent prolonged immobilization,[12, 14, 17, 23] halo-femoral traction followed by immobilization,[18, 21, 23, 24] and surgical reduction with[5, 7, 10, 11, 13, 18, 19, 22] and without[17] instrumentation have all been employed. When examining the literature and comparing recommendations, one must keep in mind the era in which the studies were conducted. Although the healing process has not changed over the years, surgical techniques and instrumentation have advanced. Imaging studies, pedicle and segmental fixation techniques, anterior instrumentation, and improved anesthetic and intraoperative spinal cord monitoring are just some of the advances which make surgical treatment more attractive today than it might have been previously. However, despite continuing controversy which may exist regarding the treatment of other "unstable" patterns, even fairly rigid proponents of nonoperative therapy for most spinal column injuries agree that surgical reduction and stabilization are indicated in those patients with gross, complex displacements.[7, 12]

If reduction can be obtained and there is a significant bony (fracture) component, fracture-dislocations can heal and obtain stability through prolonged immobilization with bed rest.[7, 17] However, this requires weeks to months of hospitalization with intensive attention to nursing care. Risks of immobilization, including deep venous thrombosis, pulmonary emboli, pressure ulcers, deconditioning, increased costs of hospitalization, and a delay in rehabilitation are some of the objections to nonoperative care. Increased deformity (early and late) with resultant pain or neurologic deterioration is also a very real concern when treating highly unstable injuries nonoperatively. Additionally, since the majority of these injuries include significant ligamentous disruption, stability with healing cannot be predicted.

Balancing risks against benefits, surgical stabilization and fusion are indicated in most cases with complex instability. This is true despite the difficulties encountered in safely reducing and rigidly maintaining the dislocated vertebrae, particularly in a patient with multiple spinal fractures and preservation of, at least, some

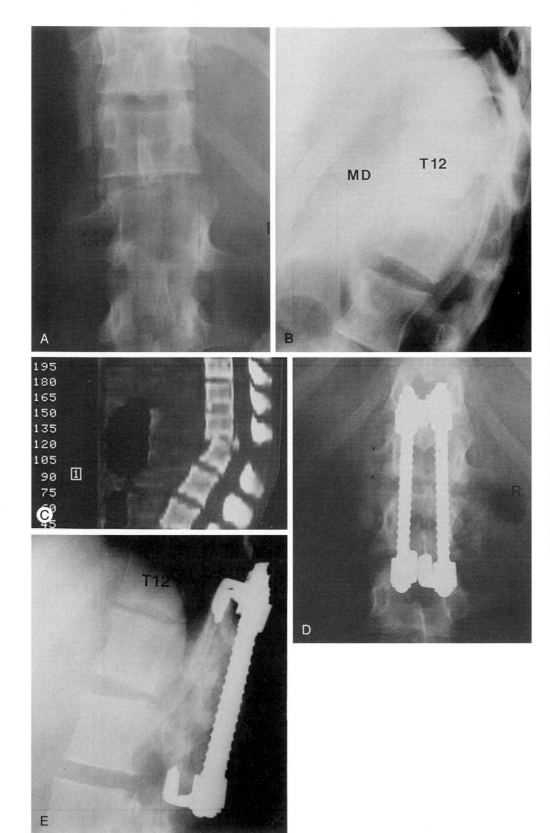

Figure 29–4 = This 32-year-old man was injured in a motor vehicle accident. The patient was wearing his safety belt when he sustained an unstable flexion-distraction–type injury at T12–L1. The patient was neurologically intact. AP *(A)* and lateral *(B)* radiographs demonstrate characteristics of a flexion-distraction–type injury. Note the fracture through the left transverse process and widening between the spinous processes of the injured level. *C,* Subluxation and kyphosis is demonstrated on sagittal CT reconstruction. AP *(D)* and lateral *(E)* postoperative radiographs. Edwards hooks and rods were used in compression to reduce and stabilize this injury *(arrowheads).*

Figure 29–5 = *A*, Posterior-to-anterior fracture-dislocation. Note facet and posterior element fractures. Also note complete disruption of anterior longitudinal ligament *(ALL)*. *B*, Anterior-to-posterior fracture-dislocation. A locked dislocation without bony injury may occur (as demonstrated here). Note complete disruption of all ligamentous restraints. *IL*, interspinous ligament; *PLL*, posterior longitudinal ligament. (Modified from Denis F: The three column spine and its significance in the classification of acute thoracolumbar spinal injuries. Spine 8:817–831, 1983.)

neurologic function. With modern techniques of stabilization and anesthetic care, the risks of neurologic deterioration, as well as late deformity and pain, are decreased with surgical stabilization. The risks of prolonged bed rest are avoided and early rehabilitation is achieved markedly sooner than when a nonsurgical approach is selected. Although major neurologic improvement cannot be counted upon, surgery allows early rehabilitation, which is extremely important psychologically, as well as physically, in the spinal cord–injured patient. Additionally, hospitalization costs have been shown to decrease by approximately 50% in those that have early surgical stabilization followed by rehabilitation, as compared to a nonoperative approach.[5]

In the neurologically incomplete and complete patient, attempts to improve neurologic outcome and decrease the risk of further neurologic damage and deformity must begin immediately. Frequently, on the initial examination, it is impossible to distinguish between a complete and an incomplete neurologic injury as the patient may be obtunded or in spinal shock. These patients should initially be assumed to be "incomplete," treated with emergency spine precautions, and followed closely with serial neurologic examinations to monitor for changes. Patients should be placed at strict bed rest with logrolling only, or preferably, on a Roto-Rest–type bed which continually "turns" the patient while he or she is strapped securely in the bed. This eliminates the need for manual turning of the patient, yet decreases the risks of pressure sores and pulmonary complications.

Although it has not been shown that early decompression is better than late decompression in improving neurologic outcome, attempts should be made to reduce the dislocation in order to obtain a more anatomic and stable position as well as to decompress the neural elements. This is done, initially, with simple positioning in the supine position without attempts at manipulation. An incomplete cord injury may have significant potential for recovery with appropriate, adequate decompression.[2, 20] Imaging studies are extremely important in evaluating the possible need for decompression of the spinal cord or cauda equina in the neurologically incomplete patient. Laminectomy, without instrumentation and fusion, is contraindicated as it may result in greater instability, resulting in increased deformity and pain, as well as new or increasing neurologic injury in these highly unstable injuries.[20]

In spinal injuries with multiplanar instability, the posterior ligamentous complex and posterior elements are severely disrupted. Realignment and stabilization are required. This can be achieved through a posterior approach using instrumentation and posterolateral bone grafting. Anterior surgery with decompression and strut grafting may also be required in the neurologically incomplete patient with significant canal compromise, although with this approach the ability to accurately reduce and realign the deformity may be limited, depending on the pattern of injury, the instrumentation available, and the surgeon's experience.

Techniques of stabilization are changing rapidly. Newer anterior instrumentation, such as the Kostuik-Harrington and Kostuik-Edwards systems and the Kaneda device, is useful if anterior decompression of the thoracic or lumbar spine is indicated. Posteriorly, pedicle for rigid segmental fixation techniques, or both, are beneficial as excellent stability can be obtained. Many of the newer instrumentation systems allow combinations of hooks and screws to be used together as necessary. Additionally, because of the multiple forces involved in creating the injuries, multiple forces (distraction, compression, lateral translation, and rotation) may be required to obtain a reduction and then maintain it in a stable, safe, and rigid position. Because of this, no single system can be recommended, but

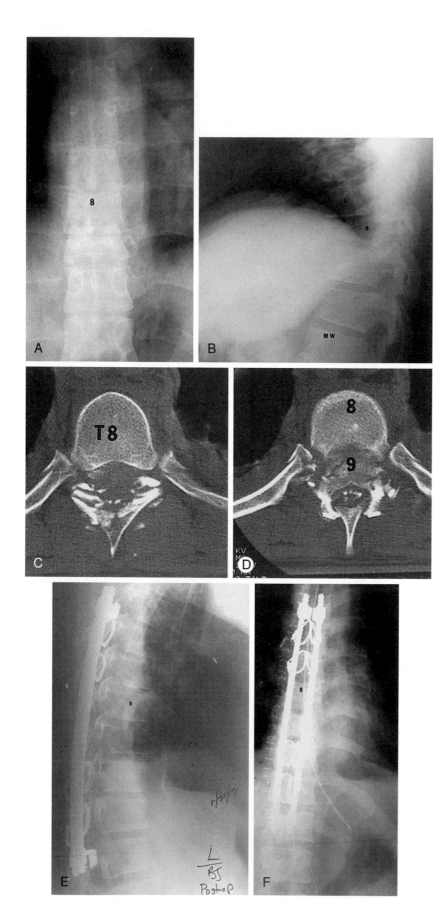

Figure 29–6 = This 31-year-old man was involved in an off-road recreational vehicle accident. There is complete neurologic deficit below T9. *A,* AP radiograph. Note overlap of inferior body of T8 over superior body of T9. *B,* Lateral radiograph demonstrates subluxation of T8 on T9 consistent with a posterior-to-anterior shear injury. *C,* Comminution of inferior T8 and superior T9 facets can be seen on the CT scan, as well as fractures of the eighth ribs bilaterally. *D,* Subluxation of T8 on T9 is demonstrated on the CT scan. Note the bone fragments in the spinal canal. Lateral *(E)* and AP *(F)* views of postoperative alignment. As this patient had a complete neurologic deficit, sublaminar wires were used with Edwards rods and hooks to stabilize the spine and allow rapid mobilization without bracing. Note the reduction of T8 on T9 as well as the restoration of the height of T8.

familiarity with and availability of multiple instrumentation systems are required.

Often, distraction or lateral and posterior translation through the instrumentation is required to gain a reduction. After reduction is obtained, conversion to a rigid mode in compression (through the same instrumentation if possible) is then necessary. At this time, few systems provide this. Pedicle screws fixed to rods or plates through adaptors (e.g., Cotrel-Dubousset [CD] Texas Scottish Rite Hospital [TSRH], Steffee, Edwards, Fixateur Interne systems) are best suited for the lumbar spine while hook, rod, and sleeve (which control lateral motion and rotation) combinations are more often used in the thoracic spine (e.g., CD, TSRH, Edwards systems). In the patient with complete neurologic injury, more conventional rigid fixation over multiple levels (e.g., sublaminar wires to rods) is useful as this can be installed rapidly while providing very rigid fixation without excessive hardware implantation. In patients with complete neurologic injury, the neurologic risk of passing sublaminar wires is not of consequence. The main advantage and perhaps goal of this last technique is to reduce the need for postoperative external immobilization and thereby speed and enhance the rehabilitation effort.

In highly unstable injuries with damaged posterior and anterior longitudinal ligaments, overdistraction is a concern when a distraction device is used to reduce or instrument the spine. Segmental fixation, as discussed later, can decrease the risk of overdistraction while providing rigid fixation. If this is not available, overdistraction in thoracic and lumbar fracture-dislocations may be avoided using traditional (Harrington-type) distraction instrumentation by placing an interspinous wire or small compression rod centrally across the unstable segment, followed by distraction rodding. The interspinous wire prevents overdistraction and creates a fulcrum for reduction when distraction is applied through the rods. This technique helps reduce kyphosis while restoring alignment and height.[11]

In complete dislocations, distraction with outriggers may be helpful. Anterior, three-point pressure and leverage from the rods is, therefore, not possible, so height of the spinal column can only be obtained with the outriggers. AP and vertebral body alignment is then achieved with contoured rods. Sublaminar wiring or spinous process wiring may then be used to segmentally instrument and stabilize the spine. This decreases any dependency on the anterior longitudinal ligament for the maintenance of correction and is essential if the anterior longitudinal ligament is disrupted. Passing sublaminar wires, however, is potentially dangerous in the neurologically intact or incomplete patient. In this setting, the spinous process, button-wire technique of Drummond may be preferred. It has been our preference, when using posterior instrumentation, to use a segmental fixation system that can accommodate hooks as well as screws, which allows distraction as well as compression and provides rigid end-point fixation. CD-type instrumentation (e.g., CD and TSRH) and the Edwards modular system provide this ability in the severely unstable spine. The CD system offers the ability to use multiple points of fixation with hooks and screws. Compression and distraction forces can be applied at different points along the same rod (Fig. 29–7A–E). By contouring the rods and then further rotating or bending them into position, reduction can be achieved without significant distraction.

The Edwards modular system also allows laminar hooks and pedicle screws to be used with the same rod. Using screws and pedicle connectors, anterior, posterior, and lateral subluxations can be reduced without overdistraction. Round and elliptical polyethylene rod sleeves can be placed along the rods to assist with reduction. These sleeves act as a fulcrum creating an extension moment which restores alignment in the sagittal plane. This also helps restore vertebral height. As these sleeves wedge between the spinous processes and facets, they act to increase mediolateral stability. The increased stability of the system related to the sleeves and pedicle screws often allows shorter instrumented segments, as compared to other hook-rod constructs.[8] Edwards Universal rods can be used in compression or distraction. When the distraction system is used, however, the anterior longitudinal ligament must be competent to prevent overdistraction.

In fracture-dislocations resulting from flexion-distraction–type forces, or in pure facet dislocations with disc and ligamentous disruption of the middle and anterior columns, a compression construct should be employed to stabilize the spine. The facets and cortex of the posterior aspect of the vertebral body must, however, be essentially intact if compression is to be used.[8] Additionally, attention should be paid to the possibility of a disc herniation resulting from compression.[16] In a neurologically intact or incomplete patient, a wake-up test or spinal cord monitoring should be performed after the instrumentation is complete in order to evaluate and document neurologic function. In a flexion-rotation–type injury, or unstable three-column burst fracture of the vertebral body, a distraction rod may be employed using minimal distraction while using rod sleeves or screws to help reduce and stabilize the dislocation. Overdistraction should be avoided while reducing the fracture in all planes. Intraoperative radiographs should be closely examined to look for evidence of overdistraction. If instability is so great that overdistraction is still a problem, a more rigid system or anterior stabilization may be required (see Fig. 29–7A–E).

CONCLUSIONS

Unstable, multiplanar spinal injuries are relatively rare. These injuries are best treated surgically regardless of the neurologic status. The surgeon should be familiar with the evaluation of these injuries as well as the potential difficulties encountered in their reduction and stabilization. The treating surgeon should be competent in both anterior and posterior approaches. Familiarity with different instrumentation systems is necessary. No single instrumentation system is optimal, as the patterns of injury vary greatly. Some patterns are

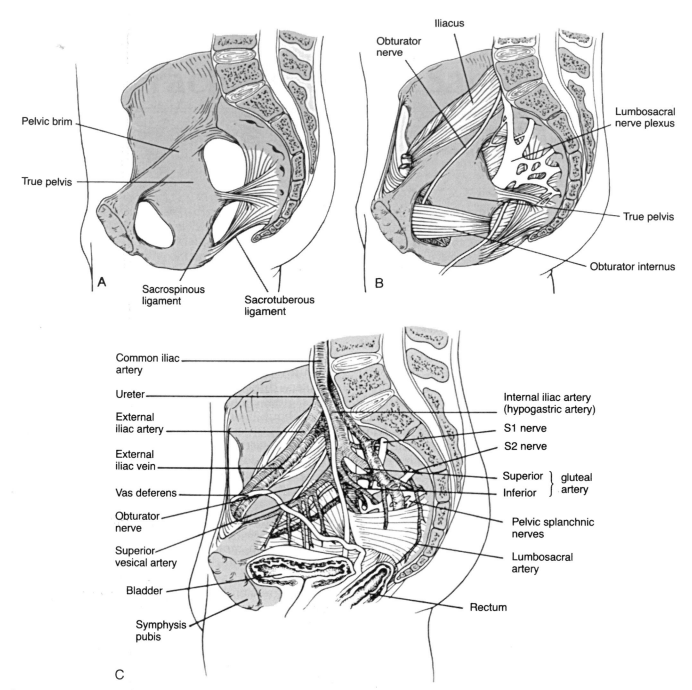

Figure 30–2 = The anatomic relationship of the sacrum to the pelvis and sacral spine determines the nature of the fracture. *A,* The sacrum is secured to the pelvis by the sacrospinous and sacrotuberous ligaments. *B,* The major structures in the inner aspect of the pelvis are the lumbosacral plexus (as it originates from the L5 root and the sacral roots and leaves the pelvis through the greater sciatic notch at the sciatic nerve) and the superior gluteal artery. The internal obturator originates from the obturator membrane and loops out through the lesser sciatic notch. *C,* Anatomy of the internal aspect of the pelvis showing the relationship of the iliac vessels and lumbosacral plexus to the anterior surface of the sacral body and ala. (From Kellam JS, Browner BD: Fractures of the pelvic ring. *In* Browner BD, Jupiter JB, Levine AM, et al (eds): Skeletal Trauma: Fractures, Dislocations, Ligamentous Injuries, vol 1. Philadelphia, WB Saunders, 1992, pp 852–853.)

screws directed from medial to lateral. The entry point is on a line bisecting sequential dorsal foramina. The screws pass obliquely through the vestigial pedicle, traversing as much bone as possible without entering the sacroiliac joint. Pullout strength can be increased by placing successive screws in a convergent superoinferior direction. These anatomic considerations are of

the most significance in transverse and oblique fractures.

The anatomic considerations are somewhat different for vertical fractures that require iliosacral fixation. The sacral ala slopes anteriorly; thus, the borders of the ala on the inlet view can be misleading. The superior border of the ala on the outlet view is actually the posterior portion of the ala. As a result of the concavity of the sacral ala, it is easier to misdirect screws anterior to the ala, where they can potentially jeopardize the neurovascular bundle. A critical feature is the relationship of the starting point of the iliosacral screws to landmarks on the lateral side of the ilium. The inlet and outlet views provide less accurate visualization than does a CT scan with three-dimensional (3-D) reconstruction.[43] With the use of image intensification, careful identification of both the superior and anterior aspects of the sacrum must be identified to establish the safe zone for screw passage. This avoid exiting the ala anteriorly and then reentering it more medially.[49, 50] At the S2 level, the body is usually identifiable, but it lies more posterior in the concavity of the sacrum. Passage of screws at that level is much more dangerous than at S1, and their use should be reserved for instances in which S1 is severely comminuted.

EVALUATION

Following appropriate evaluation and stabilization of cardiovascular and pulmonary systems, the victim and the rescue personnel should be questioned about the details of the accident. Attention should be focused on high-energy deceleration mechanisms, such as jumps or falls from a height, motorcycle accidents, and rollover motor vehicle accidents. These injury mechanisms should serve as a warning sign to the evaluating physician to thoroughly evaluate the pelvic ring for injury. Physical examination should include palpation over the entire spinal column including the sacrum. Commonly, areas of localized tenderness and/or hematoma indicate the presence of a sacral fracture. Manual compression over the iliac crests, both anteroposteriorly (AP) and laterally, can also aid in identifying a pelvic ring injury. As part of the routine examination, the external genitourinary system and the anus and rectum must be assessed for sensory, motor, and reflex function. Perforations through the rectum and disruption of the bladder and ureters must be ruled out, as they are not uncommon with high-energy injuries to the pelvic ring. The patient with a sacral fracture associated with pelvic ring injury may require massive resuscitation efforts and very close monitoring as a result of disruption of sacral vasculature and associated catastrophic bleeding.[29] Mortality rates may be high despite optimal treatment[25, 29] and may require measures such as military antishock trousers (MAST) or a pelvic external fixator[21] to attain initial stability. Embolization may even be necessary to attain hemodynamic stability.[2] Although it is beyond the scope of this discussion, with sacral fractures and/or pelvic disruptions, the surgeon should also be cognizant of and assess for associated injuries such as vaginal, rectal, and genitourinary disruptions.[15, 26, 55] Particularly in the case of a sacral fracture associated with a lumbar spine fracture,[1] careful discrimination in the neurologic examination is critical to proper correlation of neurologic deficit with the appropriate level of injury

After general radiologic assessment appropriate for a polytrauma victim is completed (lateral cervical spine, AP, and lateral radiographic views of the thoracic and lumbar spine as well as AP radiographic views of the pelvis), a more specialized evaluation of the sacrum and pelvis can be undertaken. Injuries to the sacrum may not be obvious on an AP pelvis radiograph because of the 45 degree posterior inclination of the sacrum due to the lumbosacral lordosis. On both the AP and lateral views of the sacrum, detail is often obscured by overlying soft tissue and gas shadows (Fig. 30–3A and B). In addition, the overlying iliac wing makes precise definition of the injury more difficult.[19, 63, 64] The exception to this rule is a vertical fracture of the sacrum, in which unilateral proximal migration of the hemipelvis and/or a transverse process fracture at L5 is usually apparent. A Ferguson AP view using a 30 degree cranial projection makes visualization of the upper sacrum easier, but it does not improve the view of the lower sacrum.[13] Coned-down sacral lateral, inlet, and outlet views should be obtained in every case of suspected sacral injury. Recognizing that these fractures are easily missed on plain radiographs, the films should be closely scrutinized with attention to the bony anatomy as described by Bonnin.[3] The thoracolumbar spine should be assessed carefully for evidence of burst fractures, L5 transverse process fracture, or lumbosacral facet dislocation.[3, 13, 31, 51]

Denis and co-workers noted that 50% of patients with intact neurologic function had inappropriate delays in diagnosis of sacral fracture. Therefore, if the injury mechanism, clinical examination, or plain films raise the suspicion of sacral fracture, ancillary studies should be obtained without hesitation. The computed tomographic (CT) scan has become the standard of care for the evaluation of both pelvic and sacral fractures[13, 24, 31, 32] (Fig. 30–3C). Axial CT scans may pass through the fracture plane and miss the injury completely. However, CT scans with narrow sections (2-mm maximum sections) and appropriate orientation of the gantry, with sagittal and coronal reconstruction, can provide detailed information about the fracture.[48] Attention to gantry orientation is necessary, because even if the plane of the axial section is perpendicular to the proximal two segments of the sacrum, the orientation of the distal portion of the sacrum changes by 20 to 30 degrees. Thus as the images are taken through the area of the fracture, the gantry may not be appropriately aligned, resulting in distortion of the clarity of the fracture lines[53] (Fig. 30–3D).

If neurologic deficit is present, then myelogram and CT scan or magnetic resonance imaging (MRI) would be indicated (Fig. 30–3E). The combination of myelography and CT scan is of less value in this region, because flow of dye into the root sleeves in this area is limited.[15, 17, 26, 48, 55] MRI is now the study of choice, and we have found it to be extremely helpful in the diagnosis and treatment planning of these injuries. The advantages of MRI include the ability to routinely obtain clear sagittal and axial views of the entire sacrum and neural elements (Fig. 30–4). Neural element compression by displaced fracture fragments or hematoma

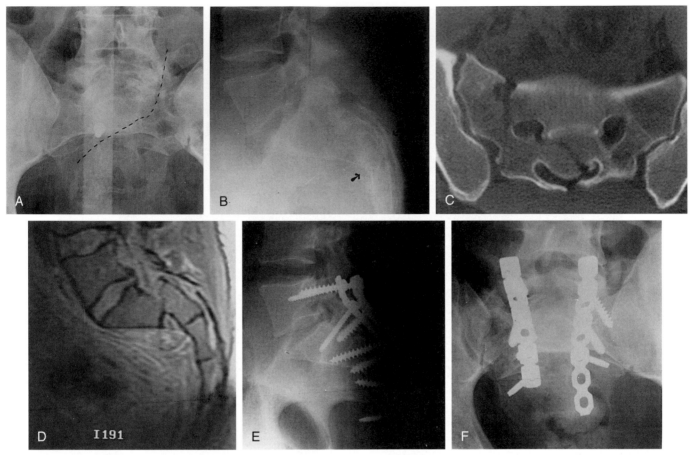

Figure 30–4 = The patient, a 30-year-old-man, fell from a height of 35 ft, landing on both feet and falling backward onto his buttocks; he sustained multiple injuries to both feet and an oblique sacral fracture with a complete neural injury at the S2 level. *A*, The AP radiograph did not clearly demonstrate the oblique nature of the fracture line *(dashed line)* with extension into the L5–S1 articulation on one side. *B*, The lateral view shows the increase in kyphosis apparent at the fracture site *(arrow)*. *C*, The axial CT scan clearly shows the oblique nature of the fracture line as it courses through the floor of the canal into the neuroforamen and into the ventral surface of the sacrum. *D*, The nature of the displacement is better seen on MRI, with the proximal fragment displaced anteriorly and the distal fragment posteriorly. The fracture traversed the base of the S1 facet on the right and therefore required plating to the L5 pedicle (*E* and *F*) to achieve reduction and stabilization.

indirect traumatic mechanisms. Based on this frame-work, nine fractures are described (Fig. 30–5). Low transverse fractures and penetrating injuries (e.g., gunshot wounds) are classified as direct trauma mechanisms. Indirect traumatic mechanisms often resulted in vertical fractures (lateral mass, juxta-articular, cleaving, or avulsion) or a high transverse pattern. Subsequently, Sabiston and Wing reviewed 35 sacral fractures and proposed a similar, but much simpler, classification[52] (Fig. 30–6).

The most comprehensive analysis of sacral fractures has been reported by Denis and associates, consisting of 235 sacral fractures in a series of 776 patients with pelvic injuries.[13] To assist in the analysis of their data, these authors also performed anatomic cadaveric studies of the sacral roots and foramina. Their classification system is based on identifying three vertical zones through the sacrum (Fig. 30–7). Zone 1 is in the region of the sacral ala and ends immediately lateral to the sacral foramina. Zone 2 encompasses the region of the foramina and zone 3 encompasses the region of the central sacral canal. Injuries are assigned to the highest

zone that the fracture line transgresses. Therefore, a fracture that passes through all three zones would be classified as a zone 3 injury (see Fig. 30–7).

Zone 1 injuries ranged from minor avulsion fractures to unstable vertical shear mechanisms with fractures lateral to the sacral foramina. These injuries rarely presented with neurologic deficit (6%) and were limited to either sciatic nerve or L5 root involvement.[13] Zone 2 fractures passed through one or more foramina and carried a 28% incidence of neurologic injury. Because these fractures were usually unilateral and did not involve the central canal, bowel and bladder deficits were not expected. The L5 root may, however, be involved by entrapment in the alar fracture, leading to a "traumatic far out syndrome." Zone 3 fractures, by definition, transgressed the central canal and carried an overall 57% incidence of neurologic injury; 76% of patients presented with bowel, bladder, and sexual function deficit.

Transverse fractures were initially classified as a separate group by Roy-Camille and co-workers[51] and then modified by others.[59] Roy-Camille and colleagues re-

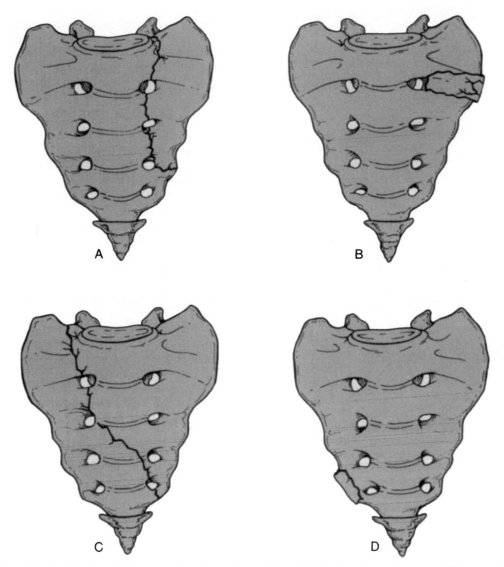

Figure 30–5 = Schmidek classified vertical fractures into four patterns. These include lateral mass fractures *(A)*, juxta-articular fractures *(B)*, cleaving fractures *(C)*, and avulsion fractures *(D)*. (Redrawn from Schmidek HH, Smith DA, Kristiansen TK: Sacral fractures. Neurology 15:735, 1984.)

viewed 13 cases of transverse sacral fractures and also conducted cadaveric experiments to study the fracture mechanism. They noted that 11 of the 13 cases resulted from suicide jumps, implicating axial loading as the predominant force of injury. From their clinical and biomechanical data, three distinct fracture types were described. The type I injury is a flexion injury without significant displacement or deformity. The type II fracture is a flexion injury with posterior displacement of the cephalad fragment. Type III fractures are caused by an extension moment with anterior displacement of the cephalad fragment. Kaehr and co-workers[32] classified 140 fractures with the aid of CT scanning and emphasized the importance of that radiographic tool for complete understanding of the injury. Six types of injuries were visualized. Type I consisted of avulsion injuries, and type II (which were the most common type—45%) were through the ala. Type III injuries were transforam-

inal (23.6%) and type IV were medial to the foramina. Type V were transverse (5%) and type VI were complex variations. Some of the fractures that are considered transverse are in fact oblique, a fact emphasized by Isler[31] but noted previously by Roy-Camille. The L5–S1 articulation can be disrupted by an oblique fracture of the sacrum. Extra-articular fracture of the base of the superior S1 facet may cause instability and listhesis at that level, or alternatively the fracture may disrupt the joint integrity directly. However, for most sacral fractures, treatment decisions are based on three facets of the classification schema. First, it is important to know whether the sacral injury is isolated or is accompanied by a pelvic injury. Second, the fracture line must be identified as either vertical or transverse. Finally, if the fracture is oblique, it is important to ascertain whether it involves the L5–S1 articulation (Fig. 30–8).

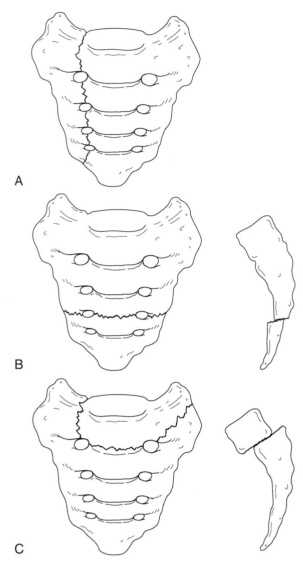

Figure 30–6 ═ Sabiston's classification of sacral fractures had three main types. Type A were vertical fractures. Type B were transverse below the level of the sacroiliac joint and type C were transverse at the level of the sacroiliac joints with vertical components. (Redrawn from Sabiston CP, Wing PC: Sacral fractures: Classification and neurologic implications. J Trauma 26:1114, 1986.)

TREATMENT

The three principal goals in managing sacral fractures are as follows:

1. Reestablishment of stability of the pelvic ring and lumbosacral junction
2. Correction and prevention of angular (kyphotic) and translational (shear) deformities of both the pelvic ring–sacrum and lumbosacral junction
3. Prevention of further neural deficit and treatment of existing neurologic injury with appropriate decompressive and stabilizing procedures

Maintaining pelvic ring stability is important in both the acute and long-term management phases. In the immediate posttraumatic period, unstable pelvic injuries may be associated with significant and sometimes life-threatening hemorrhage, and application of external fixators can help to bring such hemorrhage under control.[33] Likewise, acute stabilization of the pelvic ring may also prevent further neurologic injury. For long-term management, reestablishing pelvic ring stability should ultimately prevent chronic pain and deformity and enhance patient care by allowing earlier mobilization.

The angular (kyphotic) and translational (shear) deformities associated with sacral fractures may be factors in both instability and neurologic injury. The presence of major angular or translational deformity often heralds an unstable injury, and correction of the deformity should accompany stabilization. Furthermore, correction of such deformities may relieve some of the compression of neural elements. Angular and translational deformities should also be corrected to prevent chronic skin problems (e.g., over a sacral gibbus) or difficulty with sitting balance and lumbosacral biomechanics.

Neurologic injury can be caused directly as a result of compression of the sacral roots by fracture fragments, by nerve entrapment at the level of the foramina or ala (L5 root), or by avulsion or laceration of the roots, or it can be caused indirectly by traction on the cauda equina. Depending on the fracture pattern, the

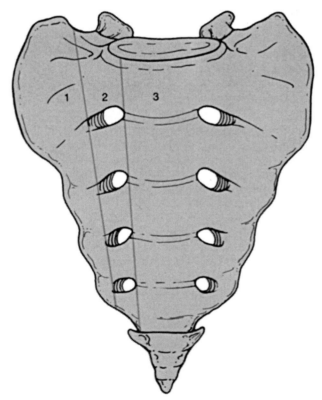

Figure 30–7 ═ Denis and co-workers classified 238 fractures of the sacrum according to zones. Zone 1 was the sacral ala and comprised 118 patients, with only 5.9% having neural deficit. Zone 2 was through the neural foramina and comprised 81 patients, of whom 28.4% had neural deficits. Zone 3 was through the central canal and was seen in only 21 patients, of whom 56.7% had deficits. (Redrawn from Denis F, Davis S, Comfort T: Sacral fractures: An important problem. Clin Orthop 227:67, 1988.)

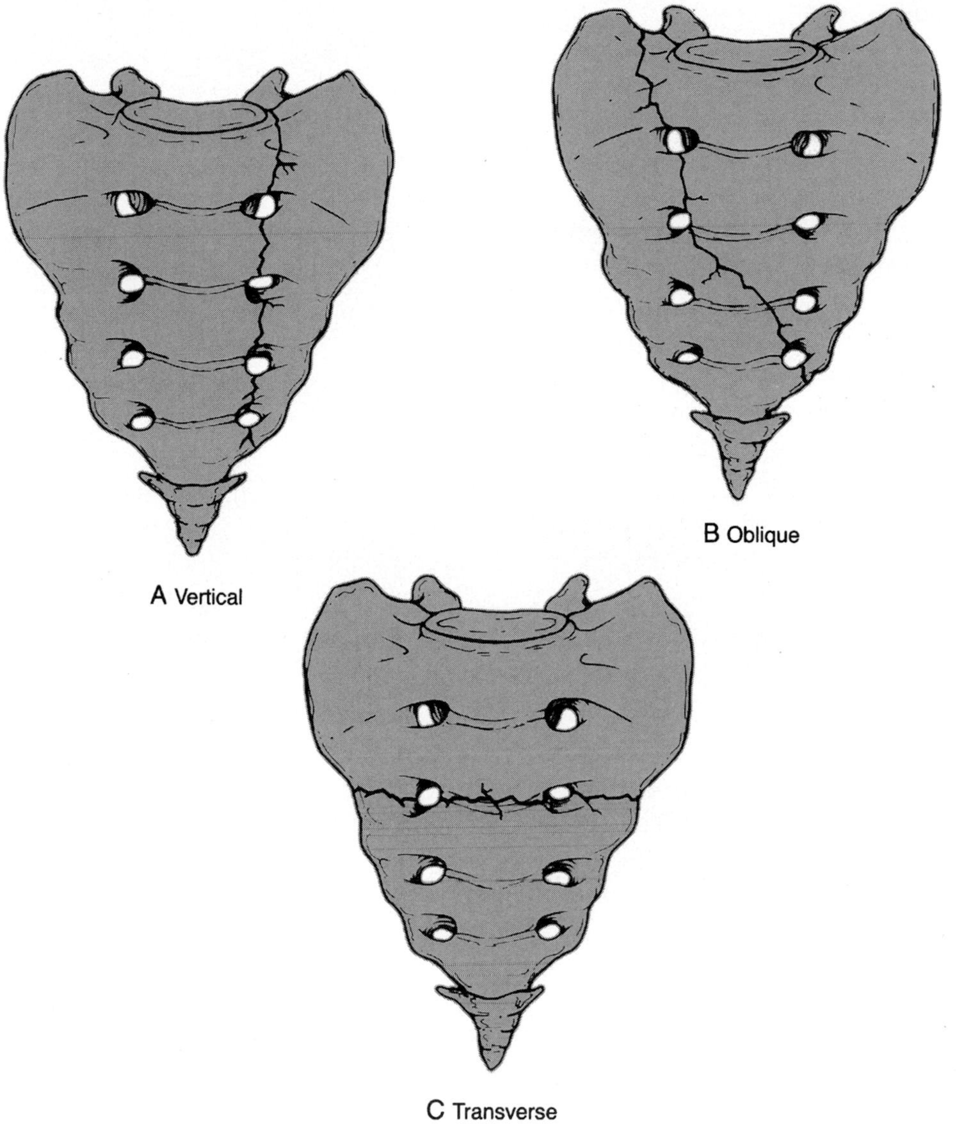

Figure 30–8 = Classification of sacral fractures. *A*, Fractures of the sacrum can be classified in a number of different ways. One of the most common is according to the direction of the fracture line within the sacrum. Therefore, fractures can either be vertical *(A)*, oblique *(B)*, or transverse *(C)*. These fractures can occur at any level in the sacrum. Vertical fractures may occur in the ala or through the foramina. Similarly, oblique fractures can occur at any location. Transverse fractures are less common and more frequently occur at the apex of the sacral kyphosis between S2 and S3, but they may occur as a high transverse fracture at S1 or S2. (From Levine AM: Lumbar and sacral tramua. *In* Browner BD, Jupiter JB, Levine AM, et al (eds): Skeletal Trauma: Fractures, Dislocations, Ligamentous Injuries, vol 1. Philadelphia, WB Saunders, 1992, p 818.)

A Vertical

B Oblique

C Transverse

neurologic deficit can present as an isolated root deficit, sciatica, multiple root deficits, or complete cauda equina syndrome. Reestablishing pelvic ring stability and correction of deformity may alleviate compression of the neural elements and prevent further deterioration. However, if the neural elements remain entrapped despite reduction and stabilization, direct decompression is required as well.

Treatment Protocol

Although some authors have recommended conservative treatment of these injuries,[3, 44, 52] a growing consensus supports surgical management.[13, 18, 45, 51, 54] On the basis of our personal experience, as well as review of the literature, we recommend the following algorithm for the treatment of these injuries.

Because of the unique anatomic relationship of the spine and pelvis to the sacrum, treatment methods need to be tailored to three clinical situations. The first is a sacral fracture in conjunction with a pelvic injury,

the second is an isolated sacral fracture, and the third is a sacral fracture in conjunction with a lumbosacral disruption. For the first group (with a pelvic ring disruption), in addition to preserving neural function the goal is a stable, pain-free pelvic ring. Patients with intact neurologic function and minimally displaced or angulated fractures (e.g., stable zone I and II injuries) may only require a short period of bed rest followed by progressive mobilization in a cast or brace (Fig. 30–9*A*–*C*) and then ambulatory status as tolerated.[1, 3, 10, 35, 38, 46] During this period the patient's neurologic function is carefully monitored and the fracture is assessed with serial radiographs. Given the typically well-vascularized fracture site, these injuries should be fully united by 3 months.

Unstable pelvic injuries should be treated with emergent application of an external fixator as has been described.[30, 33] If vertical displacement is present, then skeletal traction should be added. A number of methods have been described for operative management of pelvic injuries with sacral components including indi-

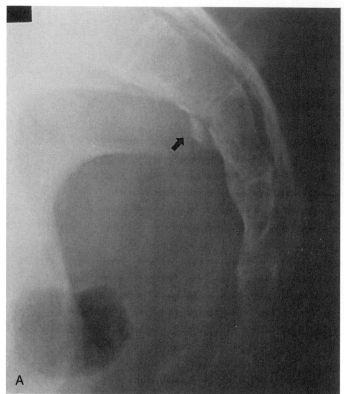

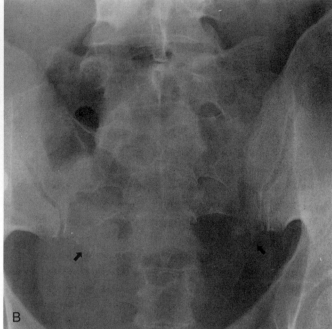

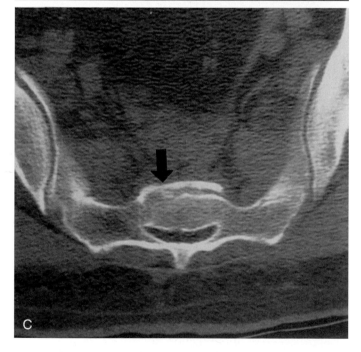

Figure 30–9 = This patient fell from a height and landed on his buttocks. *A,* The lateral radiograph shows an increase in kyphosis and comminution of the anterior cortex *(arrow). B,* On the AP view the fracture line occurred at the level of the termination of the sacroiliac joint and its attachment to the sacrum *(arrows). C,* The CT scan shows minimal comminution with only fracturing of the anterior cortex *(arrow).*

rect reduction with either anterior external fixation or anterior operative stabilization.* Finally, direct reduction and stabilization of vertical sacral fractures has been described[16, 39, 41, 49, 57, 58, 62] using both anterior and posterior sacroiliac plating, sacral bar techniques, and tension band plates across the ilium.[14, 16] Most recently, the percutaneous stabilization technique has been described.[1, 33, 49, 50]

*References 4, 8, 11, 13, 14, 16, 20, 25, 28, 34, 36, 39, 41, 49, 57, 58, and 62.

For vertical fractures, especially in zones 1 and 2, with or without other pelvic involvement, fixation with horizontal compression across the posterior aspect of the ilium and sacrum seems to provide adequate fixation. Although this can be done using sacral bars, the point of compression is posterior to the fracture line, and the potential exists for an opening on the anterior portion of the sacrum unless anterior fixation is also used. In addition, for zone 2 injuries through the region of the foramen, compression is not desirable. The sacral bar technique depends on compression for fixation and thus may compress the comminuted bone in the region of the foramen. Direct screw fixation can be done with little or no compression. Recent biomechanical studies[30, 57] evaluating fixation for transforaminal fractures has shown little difference between one or two iliosacral screws in combination with posterior tension bands or posterior transiliac bar devices. Sacral bars have also been compared with a new plate devised for fixation of these fractures.[30] The technique of iliosacral screw placement, in both prone and supine operative positions, has been well described (Fig. 30–10). Likewise, the verification of reduction and screw placement can either be done with image intensification[49, 50] or CT scan guidance.[43] Whether the patient is in a prone or supine position, the operation must be done on a radiolucent table. With a supine position, a support is placed under the lumbosacral spine to allow sufficient access. The image intensifier is placed on the opposite side from the surgeon. Initial calibration of the angles is performed, which is necessary to obtain simulated inlet and outlet views for monitoring the screw insertion. Next, care is taken that an anatomic reduction is achieved either by positioning or traction, and the reduction is verified by image intensification. The position of the starting hole is the most critical feature in obtaining adequate screw position. A number of different techniques exist for determining the starting hole, but most are based on the intersection of a line from the sciatic notch and one from the posterior superior iliac crest (Fig. 30–11*A* and *B*). Ideally, the screw should be perpendicular to the ilium and should cross the sacroiliac joint and remain within the sacral ala, proximal to the S1 foramen and distal to the L5–S1 disc, entering the vertebral body of S1. For unilateral

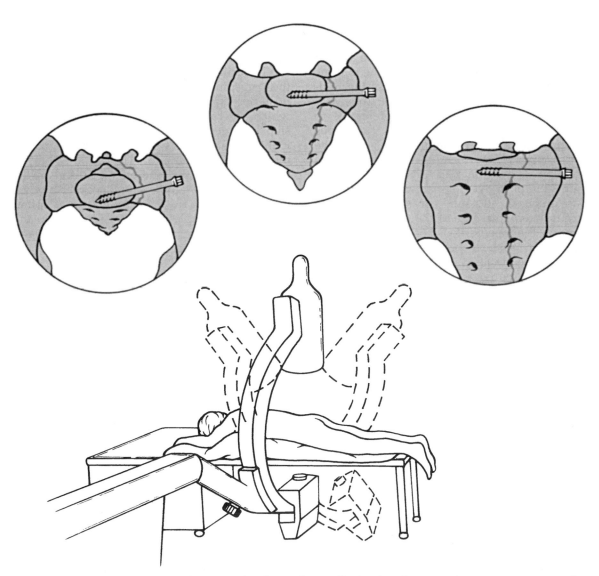

Figure 30–10 ═ Iliosacral screw fixation. To be certain that iliosacral screw fixation into the sacrum is accurate, some type of monitoring is necessary, which in most cases is image intensification. The image must be placed so that 40-degree caudal and 40-degree cephalad views can be obtained. A partially threaded screw can be used for fractures in zone 1, although a fully threaded screw should be used in zone 2 (transforaminal) fractures so that compression is not applied to the comminuted bone, causing further impingement on the exiting roots. (From Kellam JS, Browner BD: Fractures of the pelvic ring. *In* Browner BD, Jupiter JB, Levine AM, et al (eds): Skeletal Trauma: Fractures, Dislocations, Ligamentous Injuries, vol 1. Philadelphia, WB Saunders, 1992, p 888.)

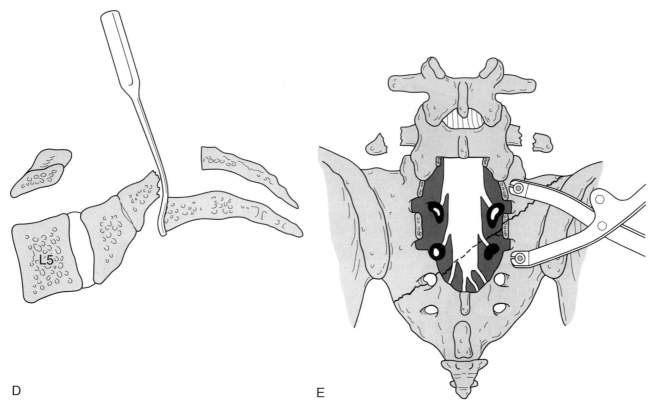

D
E

Figure 30–12 *Continued* = If the proximal fragment is posteriorly displaced (*D*), then the instrument should be placed under the ventral surface of the distal fragment. Separation of the fracture fragments and at least partial reduction are critical before plate fixation is begun. A 3.5- or 4.5-mm pelvic reconstruction plate is selected on the basis of hole spacing and the size of the sacrum. If the anatomic position is achieved manually, then the plate is contoured to directly match the contour of the posterior aspect of the sacrum; if the position is less than anatomic, then the plate is slightly undercontoured. If the fracture is more oblique and shortened, then a temporary screw can be placed in both the proximal and distal fragments and a distraction tool can be applied to achieve length while the final plate is being positioned. *E*, With the exception of the S1 segment, plate placement and screw starting points lie on a line along the dorsal foramen with the screw directed laterally into the residual pedicle. At S1, two screws are placed, the more proximal screw directed laterally from the dimple at the base of the S1 facet.

a pelvic reduction clamp to slightly distract the screws to disimpact the fracture line and achieve length for correction of angulatory deformity. If a large fragment of the floor of the sacral canal continues to compress the dural sac, even after initial temporary reduction, consideration is given to excavation of the sacral ala just lateral to the canal, so that the fragments that are impinging the canal can be removed through an oblique lateral exposure. This may require bilateral excavations at the level of the fracture or simply unilateral excavation. No attempt should be made to tamp the fragments into place. Rather, the fragments should be removed using a pituitary rongeur. Care is taken not to damage the roots during removal of the fragments. Fragments should be put aside for subsequent bone grafting. At this point, internal fixation can be accomplished. Commonly pelvic reconstruction plates are used to achieve stabilization. This may require either a 3.5- or 4.5-mm plate. The characteristics on which the choice of this hardware is based are its malleability over the posterior contours of the sacrum and the correlation of hole spacing with the proper fixation points on the sacrum. For transverse or transverse/ oblique fractures within the body of the sacrum that do not involve the L5–S1 articulation, a minimum of

two sets of screws proximal and distal to the fracture line is preferable. Since bone stock and screw fixation points are limited in the sacrum, reduction should never be attempted using the instrumentation to avoid screw pullout while levering on the plate. If the fracture configuration permits, we prefer to insert both medial and lateral screws into the sacrum at S1, thereby achieving optimum fixation into the superior fragment. The most proximal screw, at the lateral border of the S1 superior facet, is directed approximately 30 degrees medially into the S1 body through the pedicle, aiming at the sacral promontory. The next screw, at the inferior edge of the S1 facet, is directed 35 degrees laterally into the sacral ala and parallel to the sacral end plate. In the remainder of the levels, a single or double screw traversing the pedicle laterally and parallel to the sacroiliac joint is preferred. The average proximal screw inserted at the level of the medial border of the S1 facet is usually directed about 30 degrees medially, entering into the S1 body; screw length generally averages 35 to 45 mm. The next screw is inserted below the inferior edge of the S1 facet and is directed laterally approximately 35 degrees into the sacral ala and parallel into the plane of the sacroiliac joint. The proximal screws average approximately 30 to 45 mm in length. The

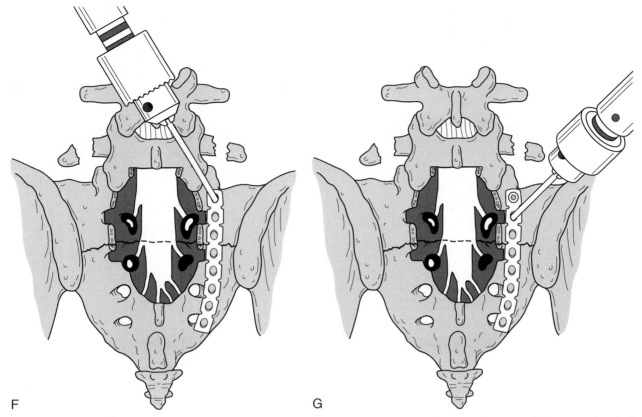

Figure 30–12 *Continued* = *F*, It is drilled bicortically and tapped and then inserted. *G*, The second screw in S1 is inserted and directed medially into the body. It likewise is tapped and inserted either to the full depth of the body or bicortically.

Illustration continued on following page

screws at S2, S3, and S4 are shorter (approximately 20 mm at the most distal point). Trajectory is between 20 and 35 degrees laterally.

If the fracture line is more oblique than transverse and involves the L5–S1 articulation, the most proximal end of the construct needs to be extended to the L5 pedicle (see Fig. 30–4). This is sufficient if there is minimal translation (less than 20% of the body width); however, the construct may need to be extended even more proximally to L4 to achieve adequate purchase on the distal portion of the spine if 50% or more displacement is present at the L5–S1 level. Extending the fixation to L4 is rarely required. After fixation is complete, the canal is reassessed. If the reduction is incomplete and some translational deformity still exists, but the fracture is in a stable position, additional excavation of the floor of the canal will be undertaken to remove any bone that may be pressing on the ventral surface of the sacral roots. Cancellous grafting is usually not necessary for fractures contained totally within the sacrum, although any residual graft can be used to fill in the defects. However, for those that traverse the L5–S1 articulation, standard transverse process sacral alar grafting should be done with autologous cancellous bone. Reapproximation of the paraspinous musculature over the hardware and fracture is critical. Postoperatively, the patients is placed into a custom-molded total-contact orthosis, with one thigh incorporated into the brace. Once in the brace, the patient progresses to

ambulation as tolerated. Bracing is typically continued on a full-time basis for 10 to 12 weeks. We do not advocate routine removal of the plates unless they are causing soft tissue irritation.

For more comminuted fractures of the upper portion of the sacrum (S1 and S2) or for the type with vertical bilateral fractures in the ala (zone 1) and a transverse fracture connecting the two, a different approach must be taken. When minimal comminution is present in the two vertical fractures, and they are extraforaminal, iliosacral screws can be placed bilaterally to stabilize that component followed by plating for the transverse component. Alternatively, a technique using bilateral rod and screw fixation has been described.[59] The fracture is exposed through a posterior approach and reduced using the techniques described previously. Iliac fixation is then done using a combination of the Galveston technique and screws proximally. Fixation of the proximal sacrum is established by screws directed medially into the body of S1 and also into the pedicles of L5. Fixation potential more distally in the sacrum is limited. Rods are connected to the screws, and crosslocking is suggested.[59]

RESULTS

The majority of the literature about sacral fractures consists of case reports and other anecdotal reports*

---

*References 3, 12, 15, 20, 22, 28, 35, 42, 46, 51, 59, 63, and 64.

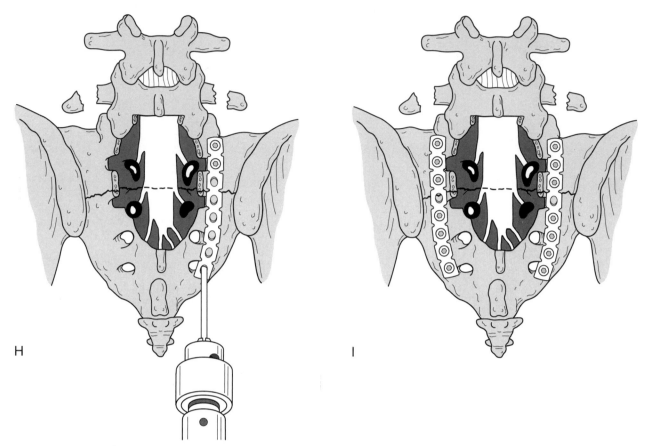

H

I

Figure 30–12 *Continued* = *H,* The starting site for the most distal screw is selected. A minimum of two and preferably three points of fixation need to be present distal to the fracture line. These screws are angled obliquely parallel to the sacroiliac joint for maximal length and fixation. An attempt should be made to place pairs of adjacent screws to converge in the caudocephalad direction for maximal pullout strength. The distalmost screws will rarely exceed 20 mm, whereas the more proximal screws will average between 35 and 45 mm. The screw is tightened into position but is not used to achieve fracture reduction. If the reduction is not complete and the plate is completely in contact with the posterior aspect of the sacrum, further manual reduction is done prior to final tightening of all screws. Screws are then placed in every hole that does not fall directly over a dorsal foramen. *I,* The contralateral side is plated in a similar fashion.

and very few substantial and well-documented series. Denis and co-workers[13] published the most extensive series and found that zone 1 stable injuries were well treated by bed rest and early mobilization. The incidence of neurologic injury and recovery seems to be highly dependent on fracture pattern and severity of neural tissue damage. Zone 1 and 2 fractures typically present with unilateral L5 or S1 root deficit in approximately 6% to 30% of patients.[13, 23] Recovery from deficits caused by root avulsion or transection, which have been found to occur in as many as 40% of autopsy specimens studied,[30] cannot be expected. Recovery from deficits caused by root compression at the level of the sacral foramen, or traumatic "far out" lesions of L5, occurs reliably after either closed reduction or decompression accompanied by open reduction and internal fixation.

Zone 3 injuries result in a greater than 50% incidence of neurologic injury.[13, 23] Transverse zone 3 fractures above the S4 foramen are almost invariably accompanied by severe sacral root deficit, including bowel, bladder, and sexual dysfunction.[13, 19] Recovery from such a deficit is enhanced by direct decompression and stabilization and ranges from 50% to 100%.[13, 19, 23] Root

avulsions are common in transverse fracture patterns, which often occur in the region of the dorsal root ganglion.[30] As shown by Gunterberg, patients with unilateral sacral root disruption retain the potential for voluntary sphincter control, although recovery may take 6 months or longer.[27] To assess and monitor the extent of neural deficit, early and periodic cystometrograms and/or somatosensory evoked potential studies are recommended.[13] In the series of Denis and colleagues,[13] five patients had loss of bowel and bladder function, were treated operatively, and had return of function in all cases, whereas in the three treated nonoperatively, two of three had partial return of function and one a had no return. Denis and co-workers[13] also noted neural fibrosis forming around the roots in cases of decompression following fracture healing. This observation further strengthens the argument for early surgical intervention. Additionally, Gibbons and co-workers[23] found either partial or complete recovery in 7 of 8 patients treated surgically and in only 3 of 15 treated nonoperatively. Additionally, in the series of Albert and colleagues,[1] operatively treated cases showed more consistent return of function than did nonoperatively treated cases. Because these are all root

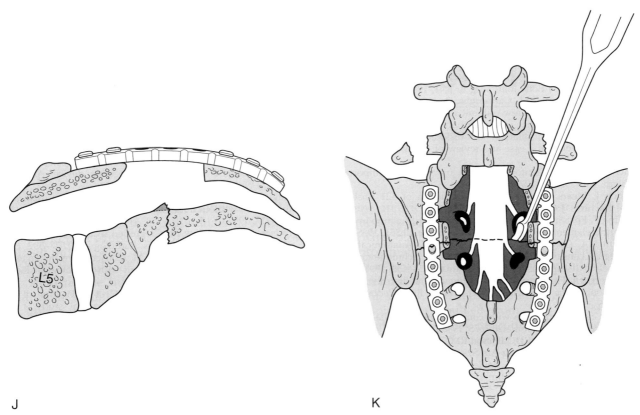

J   K

Figure 30–12 *Continued* = *J* and *K*, Decompression of the sacral roots is checked by gently retracting the roots toward the midline, and any residual impinging bone is removed with a curette or pituitary rongeur. Tamping the fragments down into the sacrum is much less effective. The contralateral side is also checked and if reduction was incomplete, decompression is still possible by resecting the residual bone of the displaced portion of the floor of the canal. Decompression should not be attempted without stabilization, as shifting of the fracture alignment can easily cause compression to recur. (Modified from Levine AM: Lumbar and sacral trauma. *In* Browner BD, Jupiter JB, Levine AM, et al (eds): Skeletal Trauma: Fractures, Dislocations, Ligamentous Injuries, vol 1. Philadelphia, WB Saunders, 1992, p 845.)

injuries, residual compression due to the kyphotic nature of the injury deformity is at least partially responsible for the failure of recovery seen with nonoperative treatment. However, Sabiston and Wing[52] had nine patients with neural deficits, all of whom were treated conservatively with bed rest and traction. All but one showed some improvement.

CONCLUSIONS

Sacral fractures are potentially devastating injuries, they occur most frequently in conjunction with pelvic ring trauma. A high index of suspicion is required when evaluating trauma patients to identify the injuries, as they are difficult to recognize and are frequently overlooked. However, a detailed clinical examination and careful scrutiny of the radiographs often uncover a sacral fracture. In many cases, with unstable injuries and dense neural deficit, aggressive decompression and stabilization can lead to early mobilization and good functional results. Surgical techniques vary on the basis of the constellation of injuries and the direction of the fracture line. Although they have been classified as zone 1 to 3 injuries, considering the direction of the fracture line is most helpful in deciding on the surgical treatment. Vertical fracture lines are

best treated with iliosacral screw fixation. However, for purely transverse and oblique fractures through zone 3, with or without neurologic deficit, fixation techniques have dramatically evolved since the late 1980s. These are best treated with bilateral posterior plating with extension to L5 for oblique injuries involving the L5–S1 articulation. In patients with neural deficit, early recognition, accurate imaging, and surgical stabilization and decompression are essential for optimal recovery of bowel and bladder function in cases of severely displaced fractures.

REFERENCES

1. Albert TJ, Levine AM, An HS, et al: Concomitant noncontiguous thoracolumbar and sacral fractures. Spine 18:1285–1291, 1993.
2. Ben-Menachem Y, Handel SF, Ray R, et al: Embolization procedures in trauma: The pelvis. Semin Intervent Radiol 2:158–181, 1985.
3. Bonnin JG: Sacral fractures and injuries to the cauda equina. J Bone Joint Surg 27:113, 1945.
4. Browner BD, Cole JD, Graham JM, et al: Delayed posterior internal fixation of unstable pelvic fractures. J Trauma 27:998–1106, 1987.
5. Bucknill TM, Blackburne JS: Fracture-dislocations of the sacrum: Report of three cases. J Bone Joint Surg Br 58:467–470, 1976.
6. Carl A, Blair B: Unilateral lumbosacral facet fracture-dislocation. Spine 16:218–221, 1991.

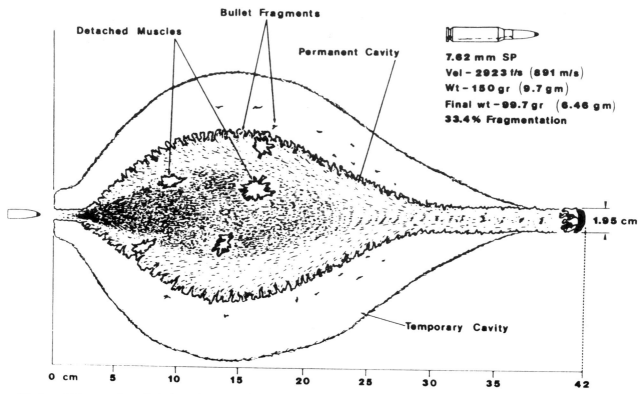

Figure 31–3 ═ This wound profile is from the same rifle represented by the lower graph in Figure 31–2. The permanent cavity is significantly larger in this case, and this is entirely due to the use of a soft-point bullet, which leads to significant bullet fragmentation. (From Fackler ML, Bellamy RF, Malinowski JA: The wound profile: Illustration of the missile-tissue interaction. J Trauma 28(suppl):S21–S29, 1988.)

the spinal canal relative to the size of the spinal cord. In subjects with extremely small canals, the incidence of spinal cord injury was extremely high. The pathologic sections of the spinal cord varied, as would be expected, but it was interesting that significant pathologic changes often were noted within the spinal cord even in some animals that had not sustained any paralysis.

PATIENT EVALUATION

The evaluation of patients with gunshot wounds of the spine should include the same detailed history and physical examination and x-ray evaluation as would be performed for patients with other suspected spine injuries. Attention is first given to the ABCs of emergency treatment protocols.

The history should include a general description of the weapon (e.g., handgun, rifle, assault weapon). Very often this information is not available, but it can be helpful if known. The patient should also be questioned as to whether any paralysis or paresthesias occurred immediately following the injury. If the patient did indeed have an episode of transient paralysis, a more detailed neurologic follow-up would be indicated.

The importance of the physical examination cannot be overemphasized. This should include examination of the entrance and exit wounds, and the tissue should be palpated to assess the presence of crepitance and the general turgor of the tissue. The presence of a very large exit wound and the presence of crepitance and increased tissue turgor are consistent with wounds that have a large permanent cavity and may very well have significant tissue necrosis.[11]

The physical examination should also include a good, detailed neurologic examination, as outlined in Chapter 3. The presence of paralysis or abnormal reflexes should be documented.

The x-ray evaluation of the patient is also extremely important. Attention should be paid to the fracture type and the degree of bone comminution. The radiograph should also be scrutinized to see if the bullet has remained in the torso and to assess the extent of bullet fragmentation. Increased bone comminution and bullet fragmentation should alert the treating physician to a possible association with a significant permanent cavity. Such a case may be one of the few instances in which significant wound debridement is required.[11]

A computed tomographic (CT) scan may help to further assess the extent of the spine injury and the extent of spinal canal encroachment by bone or bullet fragments. The stability of the spine can also be better assessed with the help of a CT scan; this is addressed in the discussion of spine stability. The general surgical team who is helping to assess the patient may recommend other studies to evaluate the extent of soft tissue injuries to structures adjacent to the spine.[2] These might include a barium swallow, arteriography, and intravenous pyelogram.

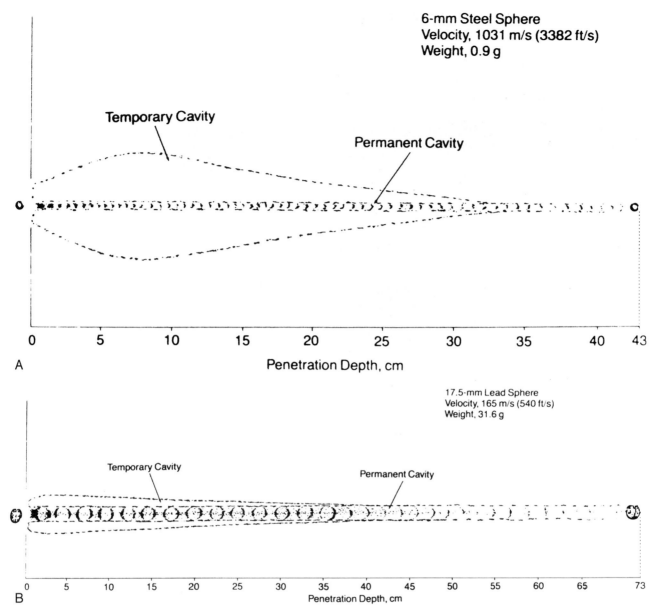

6-mm Steel Sphere
Velocity, 1031 m/s (3382 ft/s)
Weight, 0.9 g

Temporary Cavity

Permanent Cavity

| 0 | 5 | 10 | 15 | 20 | 25 | 30 | 35 | 40 | 43 |

A

Penetration Depth, cm

17.5-mm Lead Sphere
Velocity, 165 m/s (540 ft/s)
Weight, 31.6 g

Temporary Cavity

Permanent Cavity

| 0 | 5 | 10 | 15 | 20 | 25 | 30 | 35 | 40 | 45 | 50 | 55 | 60 | 65 | 73 |

B

Penetration Depth, cm

Figure 31–4 = *A* and *B,* These wound profiles were obtained using a small sphere at a high velocity to compare the injury with a large sphere at a slower velocity. The kinetic energy ($E = mv^2$) is the same in each of the two examples. However, the larger sphere penetrates 30 cm deeper and produces a permanent cavity more than 50 times the volume of that produced by the smaller sphere. (From Fackler ML: Wound ballistics: A review of common misconceptions. JAMA 259:2730–2736, 1988.)

TREATMENT OF GUNSHOT WOUNDS OF THE SPINE

Wound Care

In some cases, performing local wound care is more appropriate in the emergency room and in some cases it is more appropriate in the operating room. The operating room would be more appropriate for large exit wounds and when physical and radiographic findings, discussed previously, suggest the presence of large permanent cavities. Although this type of wound is uncommon in civilian practice, it is important to recognize that such cases may exist.

Because of the proximity of the esophagus, the major blood vessels, and the larynx and trachea in wounds of the neck, general surgeons in the past were extremely aggressive with recommending operative exploration. The traditional recommendation had been to explore all penetrating neck wounds.[40] Now it is more often advocated to explore only those neck wounds with signs of serious injury and to observe those without specific warning signs of major injury.[33, 43] The same is true for penetrating injuries of the chest and abdomen.[2] The availability of emergency arteriography coupled with the use of intravascular hemostatic coils has also changed the indications for emergency exploratory surgery. Many cases previously requiring surgery to achieve hemostasis can now be managed with minimally invasive techniques (Fig. 31–6).

Bullet in the Disc Space

Three factors must be considered in deciding whether surgery is indicated when the bullet is located in the disc space.

The first consideration is whether lead poisoning will develop. Reports in the literature suggest that the lead is leached out of a bullet that is bathed in synovial fluid, and lead poisoning can subsequently occur.[29, 49, 52] One article in the literature has suggested that this may also be the case with a lead bullet located within the disc space.[16] At our institution I have also had a similar encounter with one patient. A review of the literature does not indicate what percentage of patients with bullets in the disc space will develop lead poisoning in the future; hence, it is not possible to make a sound scientific decision about whether surgery should be recommended routinely. An alternative to routine surgical removal would be to obtain a baseline serum lead level, which is followed up first at 6-month intervals and then at yearly intervals. Removal of the bullet should be undertaken if a rise to an abnormal serum lead level is noted.

The second consideration includes the mechanical disruption of the motion segment by the presence of a bullet within the disc space. Medical experience for this problem is also anecdotal. This problem can also be followed on a clinical basis. If mechanical-type symptoms develop (e.g., worsening of local pain with upright posture and activity and decrease in local pain with recumbency), and if the symptoms were not present prior the gunshot wound's being inflicted, then consideration could be given to removal of the bullet with or without local fusion.

The third consideration regarding surgery is whether there has been a disc extrusion as a result of a gunshot wound of the spine. If this has occurred, and if the disc extrusion is causing significant symptomatic neural compression, then surgery would be indicated for removal of the disc fragments to achieve neural decompression. This occurrence is extremely uncommon, but it has been reported in the literature.[37]

Bullet in the Spinal Canal

Many articles have been written concerning removal of bullets from the spinal canal[8, 18, 20, 26, 35, 46, 47, 48, 53]; however, until recently, this problem had not been reviewed in a scientific fashion. For conclusions to be valid, there must be two groups with equivalent pathology, with one group having bullets removed and the other group having bullets left in place. It is also important that this study be done on a prospective basis, recording adequate neurologic information as well as quantitative assessment of complaints of pain, for example. Such a review was performed by Waters and Adkins.[50] They reviewed cases of 90 patients in which 32 had bullet removals and 58 had bullets left in place. They were able to conclude that at the T12–L5 levels, statistically significant neurologic motor improvement occurred with removal of the bullet from the spinal canal (Fig. 31–7). There was no difference,

however, in sensation or in pain experienced by the patients. In thoracic spine injuries, from T1 to T11, no statistical difference was seen for either complete or incomplete injuries, whether or not the bullet was removed. Similarly, no difference was seen with bullet removal in the cervical spine; however, the authors suggest that the patient numbers were too small to be able to draw statistical conclusions about the cervical spine.

Adding my own subjective opinion to these data, I would recommend that patients with cervical injuries undergo bullet removal, as this significantly decreases the degree of spinal cord compression.[5] I even recommend this in cervical complete injuries, not for cord function return, but rather for nerve root improvement at the adjacent level over a period of time. The rationale for doing this would be the same as that for closed spinal cord injuries of the cervical spine accompanied by significant residual neural compression by bone or disc fragments, which can improve following elective decompression.[1, 3]

Everyone would also agree that surgery is indicated in patients with bullets in the spinal canal who are experiencing neurologic deterioration. I would emphasize, however, that surgery should only be performed in patients in whom compression of the neural elements by bone, disc, bullet, or hematoma has been documented. Such deterioration is extremely uncommon but will occasionally be seen (Fig. 31–8). I emphasize that surgery is only indicated with demonstrated compression as it is also known that neurologic deterioration can occur on the basis of ascending spinal cord necrosis with no residual neural compression, and that this particular pathology is not helped by surgery, and in fact, it may be worsened.

Once the decision has been made to surgically remove the bullet from the spinal canal, it is essential that a scout x-ray be taken in the operating room before the incision is made. The reason for this is that the bullet can occasionally migrate within the spinal canal, depending on the position of the patient.[21, 28, 54] This is especially true for patients with large spinal canals and relatively small bullets.

Regarding the timing of surgery for removal of bullets from the spinal canal, we normally recommend that this surgery be performed at 7 to 10 days following the injury, because at this time such problems as cerebrospinal fluid leakage and dural repair will be simplified considerably (Fig. 31–9). (This obviously would not apply in cases of significant neurologic deterioration, which, as stated previously, require immediate surgery.)

Rate of Neurologic Recovery

We know from the established literature that most spinal cord injuries improve to some extent over time. Complete spinal cord injuries usually demonstrate root improvement at one or two levels over time. Incomplete spinal cord injuries have a chance for dramatic improvement over time. For incomplete injuries, this includes both improved spinal cord function as well as

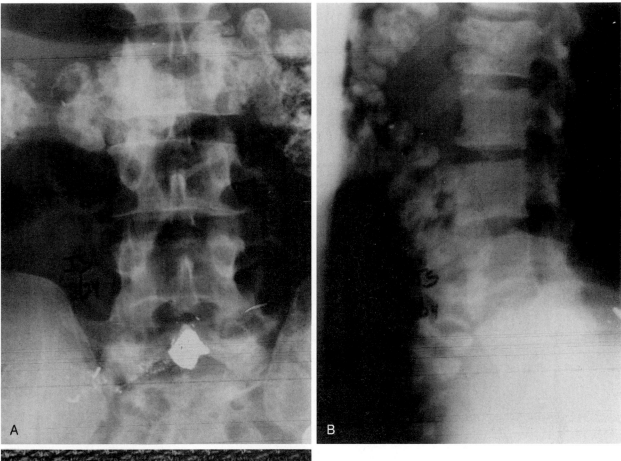

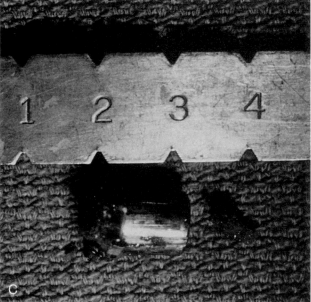

Figure 31–7 = *A–C*, This young man was shot through the flank, and the bullet lodged within the spinal canal at the L5–S1 level. He had normal motor function in his legs but some dysesthesia in the S1 nerve root distribution, and he had some urinary dysfunction with elevated post-void residual volumes. He was taken to surgery 8 days after the injury was inflicted, and the bullet was easily removed. A small dural laceration was easily repaired. The patient had return of normal urologic function. (From Eismont F, Lattuga S: Gunshot wounds of the spine. *In* Browner BD, Jupiter JB, Levine AM, et al (eds): Skeletal Trauma, ed 2. Philadelphia, WB Saunders, 1997, p 1104.)

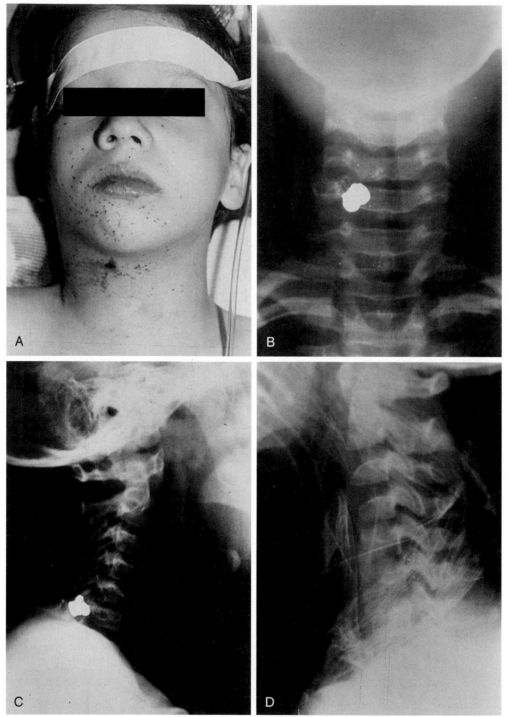

Figure 31–8 = *A–D,* This young boy was accidentally shot in the neck and had progressive quadriparesis. At 24 hours after injury he had lost all motor function in his legs. The plain films revealed that the bullet was filling the right side of the spinal canal. He was taken to surgery emergently and an anterior cervical procedure was performed. The trachea and esophagus were found to be intact. A corpectomy of C5 and C6 was performed to remove the bullet. An anterior cervical fusion was then performed using autologous iliac crest bone graft. The patient regained ambulation, and the only residual weakness involved the arms. (From Eismont F, Lattuga S: Gunshot wounds of the spine. *In* Browner BD, Jupiter JB, Levine AM, et al (eds): Skeletal Trauma, ed 2. Philadelphia, WB Saunders, 1997, p 1106.)

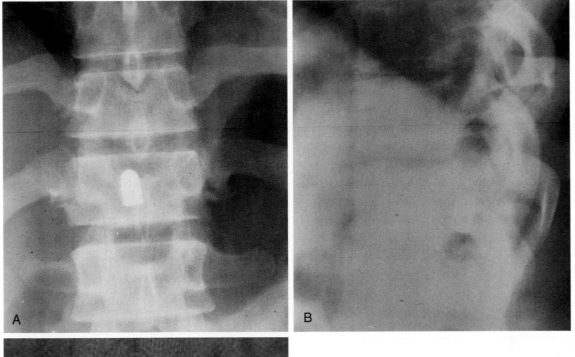

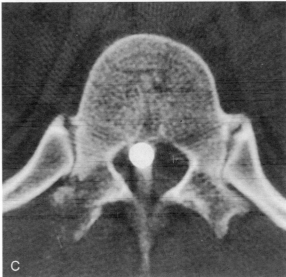

Figure 31–9 = *A–C,* This patient, who had been shot, presented to the emergency room with complete paraplegia, no bowel or bladder function, and no motor or sensory function below L1. His neurologic condition was unchanged for 1 week. He was taken to surgery for removal of the bullet, which was located within the dura. The goal of surgery was not to improve the function of the conus medullaris, but rather to maximize the chance for improvement of the L1–4 nerve rootlets that traveled past the level of injury. (From Eismont F, Lattuga S: Gunshot wounds of the spine. *In* Browner BD, Jupiter JB, Levine AM, et al (eds): Skeletal Trauma, ed 2. Philadelphia, WB Saunders, 1997, p 1107.)

local root function. An early review of closed and open spinal cord injuries at the University of Miami in the early 1980s showed that patients with open spinal cord injuries (the majority of these were due to gunshot wounds) still showed statistically significant neurologic improvement at 6 months follow-up, but the improvements started slightly later than in those with closed injuries. This was true for both incomplete and complete open spinal cord injuries.[15] This is illustrated in Figure 31–10.

COMPLICATIONS OF GUNSHOT WOUNDS OF THE SPINE

Cerebrospinal Fluid–Cutaneous Fistulas

Cerebrospinal fluid (CSF)–cutaneous fistulas have been described after gunshot wounds of the spine.

These can sometimes be seen as a direct result of a gunshot wound of the spine[50]; however, they are seen most commonly following acute surgical treatment with laminectomy (Fig. 31–11). Stauffer and co-workers[48] described their experience with 185 patients and noted that of those not having laminectomies, the incidence of CSF-cutaneous fistulas was 0%. In those treated with laminectomy, "spinal debridement," and bullet removal, the incidence was 6%.

Considering that most of the CSF-cutaneous fistulas are seen following acute surgical treatment, I would emphasize delaying the removal of the bullet for 7 to 10 days, as mentioned in the preceding section. When surgery is performed to remove the bullet, meticulous dural repair and meticulous closure of the paraspinous muscles and deep fascia and skin are necessary to minimize the chance of a postoperative CSF-cutaneous fistula.[10] At the time of repair of the dura, it should be

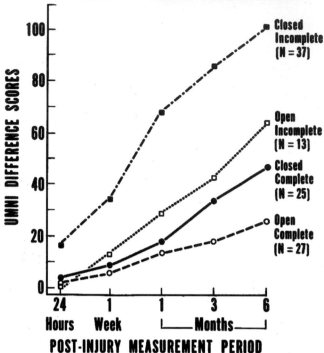

GAIN IN NEUROLOGICAL FUNCTION BY
INJURY ETIOLOGY & INJURY COMPLETENESS

Figure 31–10 = This graph shows that the prognosis for recovery in penetrating injuries of the spine is worse than that for closed injuries. This is true for both complete and incomplete injuries. (From Green BA, Eismont FJ, Klose KJ, et al: A Comparison of Open Versus Closed Spinal Cord Injuries During the First Year Post Injury. Presented at the Annual Meeting of the American Spinal Injury Association, New Orleans, 1981.)

checked with Valsalva maneuvers to make certain that it is indeed water-tight. If a water-tight closure cannot be achieved, then a lumbar subarachnoid cutaneous drain (Fig. 31–12) should be placed to adequately decompress the dural sac to promote proper healing and to prevent such problems as CSF-cutaneous fistulas and subsequent meningitis.[24]

Spine Infections Following Gunshot Wounds

Spine infections occur infrequently following gunshot wounds of the spine. Most follow injuries to the pharynx,[41, 42] esophagus, or colon[38]; they very seldom occur after injury to any other organs, including the stomach or small bowel. Preceding sections have discussed methods of treatment to minimize this complication, including the routine use of prophylactic antibiotics for 72 hours after injury and for 7 to 14 days after injury of a contaminated viscus.[38, 41, 42] The choice of antibiotic is discussed earlier in the chapter.

The other common cause of infection following gunshot wounds of the spine is iatrogenic infection following surgery. Stauffer and co-workers,[48] in their review of patients treated with laminectomy for bullet removal, found that 4% of patients developed a postoperative wound infection,[48] which is treatable like any other postoperative infection of the spine.[14]

In patients without spine infections, significant fistula formation may be seen (Fig. 31–13). In patients with a contaminated viscus injury, a fistula may occur from the viscus to the spine. In these cases, it is not possible to effect resolution of the infection without adequate correction of the pharyngeal, esophageal, or bowel fistula. This may require such tactics as diversionary drainage and prolonged hyperalimentation. Occasionally, patients are seen with cutaneous fistulas leading to vertebral osteomyelitis–disc space infection, but it is much more common for this to occur in patients with a viscus fistula, as described earlier.

The reasons for surgical treatment of patients with spine infections following gunshot wounds are the same as for patients with spine infection from other causes: this would include progressive paralysis associated with the infection, progressive deformity, lack of a known organism, suspected foreign body associated with the infection, and failure of conservative treatment. In most cases, the spine infections are not noted until several weeks following the injury; at that time I would normally recommend a CT-guided needle biopsy of the spine followed by a 6-week course with maximum-dose parenteral antibiotics. Open surgery would be reserved for the cases previously described.

Pain Following Gunshot Wounds of the Spine with Associated Spinal Cord Injury

It is common for patients with spinal cord injuries secondary to gunshot wounds of the spine to have problems with severe deafferent pain. Most commonly this is described as a searing, burning type of pain, which normally radiates into the paralyzed extremities. A local pain may also be present, which is described

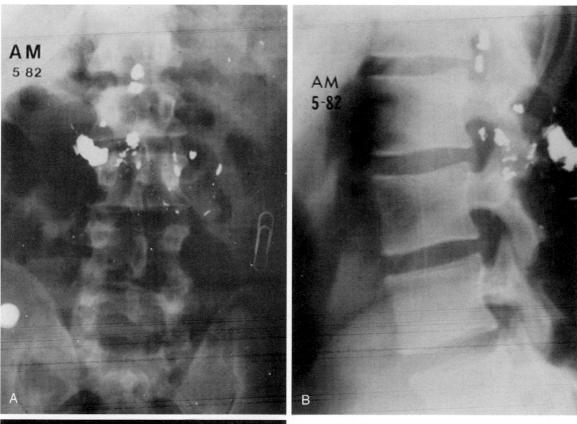

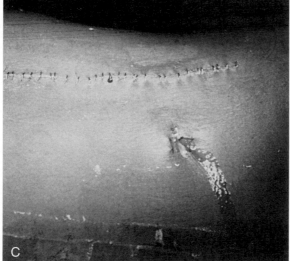

Figure 31–11 ═ *A–C,* This patient was shot in the back and presented with complete paraplegia at the L1 level. He was taken to surgery emergently where a laminectomy was performed. Postoperatively the patient developed a cerebrospinal fluid (CSF)–cutaneous fistula through the site of the bullet wound. It is now appreciated that this type of surgery is ineffectual, because no major bullet fragment is present within the spinal canal. The chance of developing the CSF-cutaneous fistula was also heightened by performing the surgery immediately. Treatment now requires placement of a subarachnoid CSF shunt and revision surgery to treat the CSF-cutaneous fistula, the postoperative infection, and the secondary meningitis. (From Eismont F, Lattuga S: Gunshot wounds of the spine. *In* Browner BD, Jupiter JB, Levine AM, et al (eds): Skeletal Trauma, ed 2. Philadelphia, WB Saunders, 1997, p 1109.)

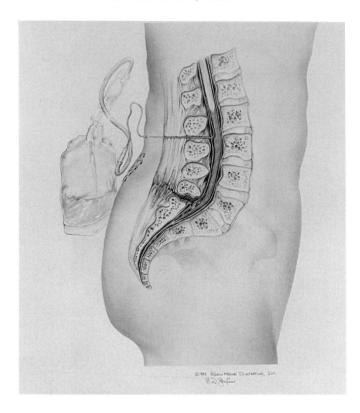

Figure 31–12 = This drawing shows the use of a CSF subarachnoid cutaneous shunt, which allows decompression of the dura and healing of the original CSF-cutaneous fistula. (From Kitchell S, Eismont FJ, Green BA: Closed subarachnoid drainage for management of cerebrospinal fluid leakage after an operation on the spine. J Bone Joint Surg Am 71:984–989, 1989.)

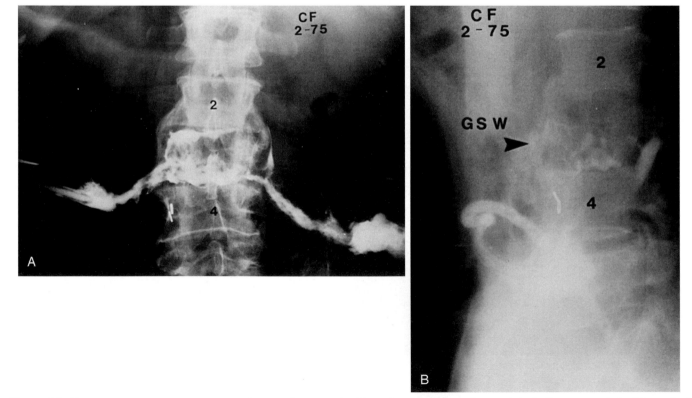

Figure 31–13 = *A* and *B*, This patient sustained a gunshot wound with perforation of the colon, and the bullet traversed the L3 vertebral body. Chronic vertebral osteomyelitis developed, with a sinus draining through each flank. The sinogram reveals the significant vertebral destruction. Treatment for this problem requires assessment of the gastrointestinal tract to rule out any remaining bowel fistula. This should be followed by vigorous spine debridement and packing of the cavity with cancellous bone or viable soft tissue, followed by a protracted course of antibiotics. (From Eismont F, Lattuga S: Gunshot wounds of the spine. *In* Browner BD, Jupiter JB, Levine AM, et al (eds): Skeletal Trauma, ed 2. Philadelphia, WB Saunders, 1997, p 1111.)

more commonly as an ache. These pains usually improve with the passage of time and the use of conservative measures, such as an aggressive course of nonsteroidal anti-inflammatory drugs in combination with amitriptyline (Elavil).[27, 36, 51] Although amitriptyline has not, to my knowledge, been tested in patients with penetrating injuries of the spine, it has been proved to help with burning diabetic neuropathic pain[27] and with postherpetic neuralgia.[51] In my anecdotal experience, it seems helpful in patients with gunshot wounds of the spine. If the amitriptyline is not successful, a course of carbamazepine (Tegretol) would normally be utilized.

If the deafferent type of pain is still present and disabling, decompressive procedures will most likely not make a significant difference in the symptoms (Fig. 31–14). The series by Waters and Adkins,[50] in which bullets were removed from the spinal canal of patients with gunshot spinal cord injury, has shown that although paralysis can be improved with bullet removal in the T12 to L5 region, no difference in pain is noted.[50] If surgery is contemplated for this type of deafferent pain, then use of a DREZ (dorsal root entry zone) procedure, using intraoperative computer assessment, can offer significant pain relief in some patients.[32] This is best utilized in patients without useful distal motor function, because of the risk of increasing distal neurologic deficit with this procedure.

In patients with persistent severe local pain and aching that seems out of proportion to what would normally be expected, evaluation should be undertaken to rule out underlying infection. This would include obtaining a sedimentation rate and a CT scan. Interpretation of the CT scan under these circumstances is always difficult, because the affected vertebra most commonly has sustained a fracture, and only signs of progressive bone destruction allow diagnosis of the infection.

OTHER PENETRATING INJURIES OF THE SPINE

Impalement Injuries

Impalement injuries of the spine are uncommon. Trauma is usually massive and gross wound contamination is more likely to be present than in other injuries to the spine.[19] Patients should be taken to surgery for spine debridement. Cultures for aerobes, anaerobes, and fungus should be carefully obtained. Unlike the relatively clean gunshot wounds described earlier, these injuries require a minimum of 3 weeks of parenteral therapy with broad-spectrum antibiotics specific to the organisms found at the original debridement. It is not uncommon to find a combination of bacteria and fungi. With such injuries it is also extremely important to rule out significant presence of foreign bodies, such as pieces of clothing, which may have been driven into the spine at the time of the impalement injury (Fig. 31–15).

Patients who have had impalement injuries of the spine often have recurrent spine infections and spontaneous drainage from sinus tracts. Successful treatment usually requires sinography to define the course of the sinus, tomograms or CT scans immediately after sinography to define the bone or disc pathologic characteristics, and surgery to debride the spinal source of infection as well as to excise the chronic sinus tract.

Figure 31–14 = *A* and *B*, This patient had incomplete paraplegia following a gunshot wound to the spine. He had some function in almost every muscle group below the level of injury, but the main problem was severe pain radiating into the extremities. Passage of time and medical treatment with amitriptyline were unsuccessful. Following removal of the bullet, the patient had significant improvement of pain. Unfortunately, this type of positive response cannot be predicted with bullet removal. (From Eismont F, Lattuga S: Gunshot wounds of the spine. *In* Browner BD, Jupiter JB, Levine AM, et al (eds): Skeletal Trauma, ed 2. Philadelphia, WB Saunders, 1997, p 1108.)

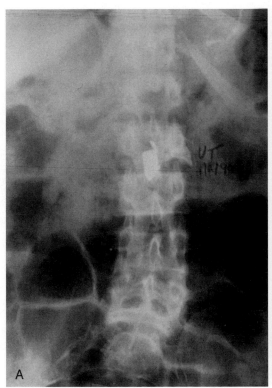
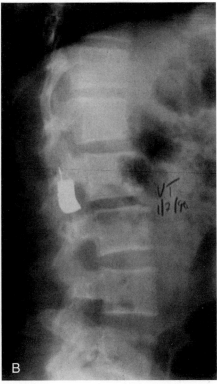

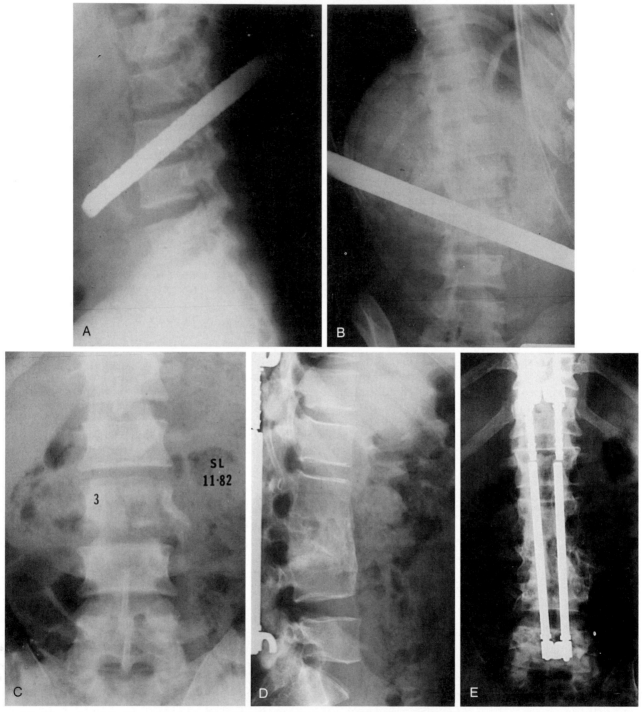

Figure 31–15 $=$ *A* and *B*, This patient was impaled on a reinforcing rod following a motorcycle accident. The rod was removed in the operating room with both anterior and posterior exposure of the spine provided. The spine was cultured and vigorously debrided at the time of initial emergency surgery. Despite 3 weeks' administration of broad-spectrum antibiotics, persistent vertebral osteomyelitis and pain developed and vertebral destruction continued (*C*). At 6 weeks after injury, the patient was returned to surgery for simultaneous anterior and posterior debridement, fusion, and stabilization. *D* and *E*, Pieces of clothing were found within the vertebral body, and cultures at surgery revealed standard pyogenic organisms as well as a fungus infection. Radiographs taken 10 years after injury reveal complete resolution of the infection. Broken rods and a flat-back deformity are now appreciated, but the patient is asymptomatic and is able to participate in full wheelchair activities with no pain. (From Eismont F, Lattuga S: Gunshot wounds of the spine. *In* Browner BD, Jupiter JB, Levine AM, et al (eds): Skeletal Trauma, ed 2. Philadelphia, WB Saunders, 1997, p 1112.)

The injection of methylene blue into the sinus tract helps to identify the tissue that requires excision (Fig. 31–16). Methylene blue should never be used if the possibility of a dural-cutaneous fistula exists; intrathecal injection of methylene blue is fatal.

Stabbing Injuries

Stabbing injuries of the spine are seen much less commonly than gunshot wounds of the spine. In some countries, these are the most common type of penetrating injury of the spine. Radiographs should be taken immediately to make certain that no foreign bodies remain. Any remaining foreign bodies (Fig. 31–17) should be surgically removed. Unlike gunshot wounds

of the spine, which are normally sterile, foreign bodies are not sterile and can be the source of persistent late infections. Stab wounds are very often associated with Brown-Séquard–type paralysis; hence, they have the best prognosis for incomplete spinal injuries. The general prognosis for patients with stab injuries to the spine and incomplete paralysis is significantly better than that for patients with gunshot wounds of the spine and a similar extent of paralysis.

CONCLUSION

Unfortunately, the incidence of spinal cord injuries due to gunshot wounds is rising. Because of this, it is

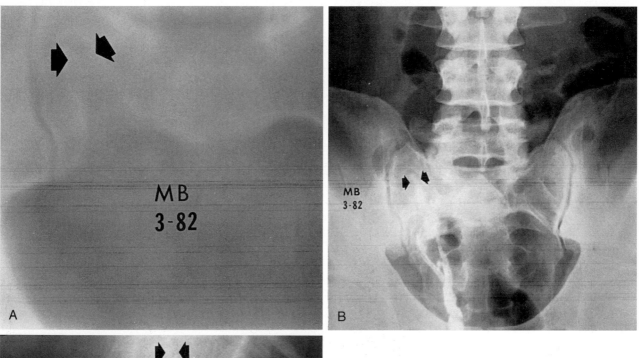

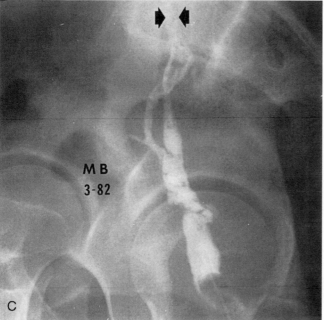

Figure 31–16 ═ This man fell at a construction site and landed on a reinforcing rod, which pierced the perineum and transverse colon and penetrated the sacral ala. He presented to us many months after injury with a persistent perineal fistula, after several courses of antibiotics and anterior abdominal operations failed. *A*, The AP tomogram of the sacrum shows the lytic tract in the ala caused by the penetrating rod and persistent infection (*arrows*). *B*, The AP view of the pelvis immediately after the sinogram shows that the fistulous tract ends in the right ala (*arrows*). *C*, The lateral sinogram also confirms the source of the infection in the sacral ala. This patient was successfully treated with a posterior lateral muscle splitting approach and wide debridement of the sacral ala followed by a 6-week course of antibiotics for all organisms cultured from the alar bone debris. (From Eismont F, Lattuga S: Gunshot wounds of the spine. *In* Browner BD, Jupiter JB, Levine AM, et al (eds): Skeletal Trauma, ed 2. Philadelphia, WB Saunders, 1997, p 1113.)

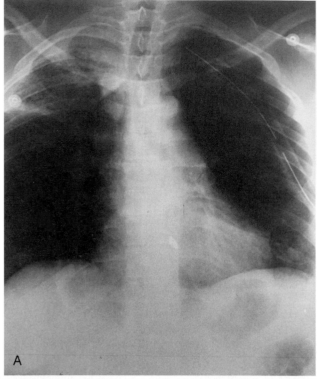

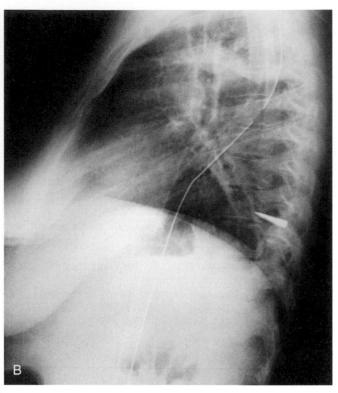

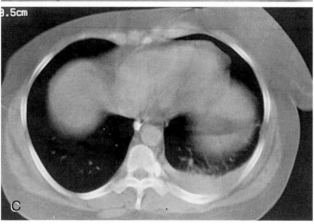

Figure 31–17 = This patient presented to the emergency room after being stabbed with a pair of scissors. After emergency treatment for a pneumothorax, AP *(A)* and lateral *(B)* chest films reveal a metallic foreign body adjacent to the thoracic spine. *C,* A CT scan verifies the location of the foreign body. This patient was taken to surgery for removal of the foreign body to minimize the chance of development of a persistent infection. (From Eismont F, Lattuga S: Gunshot wounds of the spine. *In* Browner BD, Jupiter JB, Levine AM, et al (eds): Skeletal Trauma, ed 2. Philadelphia, WB Saunders, 1997, p 1114.)

necessary for each of us to be familiar with the evaluation and treatment of these injuries. The importance of a good history, physical examination, and radiographic evaluation is emphasized. The reader understands that most gunshot wounds of the spine can be treated nonoperatively, but this does not apply to all cases. It is important not to miss the very rare injury that clinically resembles a typical war injury.

REFERENCES

1. Anderson P, Bohlman HH: Anterior decompression and arthrodesis of the cervical spine: Long-term motor improvement: II. Improvement in complete traumatic quadriplegia. J Bone Joint Surg Am 74:683–692, 1992.
2. Bishop M, Shoemaker WC, Avakian S, et al: Evaluation of a Comprehensive algorithm for blunt and penetrating thoracic and abdominal trauma. Am Surg 57:737-746, 1991.
3. Bohlman HH, Anderson P: Anterior decompression and arthrodesis of the cervical spine: Long-term motor improvement:
I. Improvement in incomplete traumatic quadriparesis. J Bone Joint Surg Am 74:671–682, 1992.
4. Breitenecker R: Shotgun wound patterns. Am J Clin Pathol 52:250–269, 1969.
5. Cammisa FP, Eismont FJ, Tolli T: Penetrating injuries of the cervical spine. *In* Camins MB, O'Leary PF (eds): Disorders of the Cervical Spine. Baltimore, Williams & Wilkins, 1992, pp 317–322.
6. Capen D: Etiology of Spinal Cord Injuries: Significant Changes Over 10 Years. Presented at the Annual Meeting of the American Academy of Orthopaedic Surgeons, San Francisco, February 1993.
7. Cushid JG, Kopeloff LM: Epileptogenic effects of metal powder implants in the motor cortex in monkeys. Int J Neuropsychiatr 3:24–28, 1968.
8. Cybulski GR, Stone JL, Kant R: Outcome of laminectomy for civilian gunshot injuries of the terminal spinal cord and cauda equina: Review of 88 cases. Neurosurgery 24:392–397, 1989.
9. Denis F: The three column spine and its significance in the classification of acute thoracolumbar spinal injuries. Spine 8:817–831, 1983.
10. Eismont FJ, Wiesel SW, Rothman RH: Treatment of dural tears associated with spinal surgery. J Bone Joint Surg Am 63:1132–1136, 1981.

11. Fackler ML: Wound ballistics: A review of common misconceptions. JAMA 259:2730–2736, 1988.
12. Fackler ML, Bellamy RF, Malinowski JA: The wound profile: Illustration of the missile-tissue interaction. J Trauma 28(suppl):S21–S29, 1988.
13. Fackler ML, Malinowski JA: The wound profile: A visual method for quantifying gunshot wound components. J Trauma 25:522–529, 1985.
14. Gepstein R, Eismont FJ: Postoperative spine infections. In Garfin SR (ed): Complications of Spine Surgery. Baltimore, Williams & Wilkins, 1989, pp 302–322.
15. Green BA, Eismont FJ, Klose KJ, et al: A Comparison of Open Versus Closed Spinal Cord Injuries During the First Year Post Injury. Presented at the Annual Meeting of the American Spinal Injury Association, New Orleans, 1981.
16. Grogan DP, Bucholz RW: Acute lead intoxication from a bullet in an intervertebral disc space. J Bone Joint Surg Am 63:1180–1182, 1981.
17. Hales DD, Duffy K, Dawson EG, et al: Lumbar osteomyelitis and epidural and paraspinous abscesses. Spine 16:380–383, 1991.
18. Heiden JS, Weiss MH, Rosenberg AW, et al: Penetrating gunshot wounds of the cervical spine in civilians: Review of 38 cases. J Neurosurg 42:575–579, 1975.
19. Horowitz MD, Dove DB, Eismont FJ, et al: Impalement injuries. J Trauma 25:1–3, 1985.
20. Jacobson SA, Bors E: Spinal cord injury in Vietnamese combat. Paraplegia 7:263–281, 1969.
21. Karim NO, Nabors MW, Golocovsky M, et al: Spontaneous migration of a bullet in the spinal subarachnoid space causing delayed radicular symptoms. Neurosurgery 18:97–100, 1986.
22. Keith A, Hall ME: Specimens of gunshot injuries of the face and spine, contained in the army medical collection now on exhibition in the Museum of Royal College of Surgeons of England. Br J Surg 7:55–71, 1919–1920.
23. Kihtir T, Ivatury RR, Simon R, et al: Management of transperitoneal gunshot wounds of the spine. J Trauma 31:1579–1583, 1991.
24. Kitchell S, Eismont FJ, Green BA: Closed subarachnoid drainage for management of cerebrospinal fluid leakage after an operation on the spine. J Bone Joint Surg Am 71:984–989, 1989.
25. Klemperer WW, Fulton JF, Lamport H, et al: Indirect spinal cord injuries due to gunshot wounds of the spinal column in animal and man. Mil Surg 114:263–265, 1954.
26. Kupcha PC, An HS, Cotler JM: Gunshot wounds to the cervical spine. Spine 15:1058–1063, 1990.
27. Kvinesdal B, Molin J, Frolund A, et al: Imipramine treatment of painful diabetic neuropathy. JAMA 251:1727–1730, 1984.
28. Ledgerwood AM: The wandering bullet. Surg Clin North Am 57:97–109, 1977.
29. Leonard MH: The solution of lead by synovial fluid. Clin Orthop 64:255–261, 1969.
30. Magnuson E, Leviton J, Riley M: Seven deadly days. Time, July 17, 1989, pp 30–61.
31. May M, West JW, Heeneman H, et al: Shotgun wounds to the head and neck. Arch Otolaryngol 98:373–376, 1973.
32. Nashold BS, Ostdahl RH: Dorsal root entry zone lesions for pain relief. J Neurosurg 51:59–69, 1979.
33. Ordog GJ, Albin D, Wasserberger J, et al: 110 Bullet wounds to the neck. J Trauma 25:238–246, 1985.
34. Pal GP, Sherk HH: The vertical stability of the cervical spine. Spine 13:447–449, 1988.
35. Pool JL: Gunshot wounds of the spine: Observations from an evacuation hospital. Surg Gynecol Obstet 81:617–622, 1945.
36. Richards JS: Pain secondary to gunshot wounds during the initial rehabilitation process in spinal cord injury patients. J Rehabil Res Dev 25(suppl):75, 1989.
37. Robertson DP, Simpson RK, Narayan RK: Lumbar disc herniation from a gunshot wound to the spine. Spine 16:994–995, 1991.
38. Roffi RP, Waters RL, Adkins RH: Gunshot wounds to the spine associated with a perforated viscus. Spine 14:808–811, 1989.
39. Romanick PC, Smith TK, Kopaniky DR, et al: Infection about the spine associated with low-velocity-missile injury to the abdomen. J Bone Joint Surg Am 67:1195–1201, 1985.
40. Saletta JD, Lowe RJ, Lim LT, et al: Penetrating trauma of the neck. J Trauma 16:579–587, 1976.
41. Schaeffer SD, Bucholz RW, Jones RE, et al: Treatment of transpharyngeal missile wounds to the cervical spine. Laryngoscope 19:146–148, 1981.
42. Schaeffer SE, Bucholz RW, Jones RE, et al: The management of transpharyngeal gunshot wounds to the cervical spine. Surg Gynecol Obstet 152:27–29, 1981.
43. Sheely CH, Mattox KL, Reul GJ, et al: Current concepts in the management of penetrating neck trauma. J Trauma 15:895–900, 1975.
44. Sherman IJ: Brass foreign body in the brain stem. J Neurosurg 17:483–485, 1960.
45. Sights WP, Bye RJ: The fate of retained intracerebral shotgun pellets. J Neurosurg 33:646–653, 1970.
46. Simpson RL, Venger BH, Narayan RK: Penetrating spinal cord injury in a civilian population: A retrospective analysis. Surg Forum 37:494–496, 1986.
47. Simpson RK, Venger BH, Narayan RK: Treatment of acute penetrating injuries to the spine: A retrospective analysis. J Trauma 29:42–45, 1989.
48. Stauffer ES, Wood W, Kelly EG: Gunshot wounds of the spine: The effects of laminectomy. J Bone Joint Surg Am 61:389–392, 1979.
49. Switz DM, Deyarle WM: Bullets, joints, and lead intoxication. Arch Intern Med 136:939–941, 1976.
50. Waters RL, Adkins RH: The effects of removal of bullet fragment retained in the spinal canal. Spine 16:934–939, 1991.
51. Watson CP, Evans RJ, Reed K, et al: Amitriptyline versus placebo in postherpetic neuralgia. Neurology 32:671–673, 1982.
52. Windler EF, Smith RB, Bryan WJ, et al: Lead intoxication and traumatic arthritis of the hip secondary to retained bullet fragment. J Bone Joint Surg Am 60:254–255, 1978.
53. Yashon D, Jane JA, White RJ: Prognosis and management of spinal cord and cauda equina bullet injuries in 65 civilians. J Neurosurg 32:163–170, 1970.
54. Yip L, Sweeny PJ, McCarroll KA: Spontaneous migration of an intraspinal bullet following a gunshot wound. Am J Emerg Med 8:569–570, 1990.
55. Young JA, Burns PE, et al: Spinal Cord Injury Statistics: Experience of the Regional Spinal Cord Injury Systems. Phoenix, Good Samaritan Medical Center, 1982, pp 1–152.

CHAPTER 32

Management of Pediatric Spinal Cord Injury Patients

Alexander R. Vaccaro ‖ *Peter D. Pizzutillo*

A clear understanding of the anatomic, biomechanical, and physiologic differences between the pediatric and adult spine is essential to the provision of care to the pediatric spine patient. The specific characteristics of the immature spine have a direct impact on the decision-making process in the treatment of acute spinal cord injury in the child. Alterations in normal growth and development of the injured spine require a high degree of vigilance to avoid the complications of chronic, progressive instability and post-traumatic spinal deformity. This chapter presents established principles regarding the acute and chronic surgical management of pediatric spinal cord injury and discusses controversies about management. The management of specific pediatric spinal column lesions is discussed elsewhere in this book.

INCIDENCE

Spinal injury in the pediatric age group is rare. Of the 11,200 spinal injuries reported each year, 1065 occur in the pediatric age range with half requiring hospitalization. Eighty percent of those hospitalized suffer from varying degrees of neurologic impairment.[79, 112] Only 5% of spinal cord injury patients of all age groups with complete neurologic injury occur in patients in the childhood years.[103] The reported incidence of pediatric spinal cord injury ranges from 0.65% to 10% of all reported spinal injuries[9, 38, 69, 71, 79, 93, 108, 111, 117] with two notable age peaks: patients less than 5 years old and those older than 10 years of age.[9, 38] The incidence of osseous injury to the spine increases between the ages of 6 and 15[103] as the spinal column develops adult morphology and decreasing flexibility.[42] Under the age of 12, the incidence of spinal column injury has an equal sex distribution, but a dramatic increase in male incidence is noted after the age of 12.[42]

CAUSES OF INJURY

The causes of pediatric spinal cord injury vary according to the age of the patient.

Birth Trauma

Spinal cord injury secondary to obstetric complications has been reported as the result of difficult cephalic or breech delivery with distraction and hyperextension of the head and neck resulting in injury to the spine.* Hachen[63] reported an infant born with quadriplegia who was delivered by cesarean section and was found on predelivery radiographs to be in extreme cervical hyperextension. Spinal injury may be an unrecognized cause of death in the newborn.[4, 93] Underdevelopment of paracervical musculature and a relatively large head in the neonate potentially increase the risk of cervical injury. Autopsy studies of stillborn infants have documented evidence of cord damage (30% to 50%), including extradural and intradural hemorrhage, nerve root avulsion, and cord transection.[2, 3, 28, 31, 128] Such cord injury can be extensive and suggests the imposition of severe longitudinal forces on the spine. Severe cord injury has been documented in the absence of radiographic evidence of bone or ligament injury.[1, 71, 79, 82]

Child Abuse

Infants and young children who present with avulsion fractures of the spinous process, pedicle fractures of the axis, or multiple compression fractures in the cervical, thoracic, or lumbar spine, should be carefully evaluated to rule out the battered baby syndrome.[38, 108] Associated stigmas of child abuse include skull fractures, rib fractures, associated long bone fractures, and skin lesions in various stages of healing.[38, 93, 108]

General Pediatric Population

The causes of spinal cord injury in the child differ from those in the adult in that injury in children less than 10 years of age is primarily a result of motor vehicle–pedestrian accidents, falls, and firearm injuries. Children older than 10 years tend to be injured in circumstances similar to adults, for example, passenger-related motor vehicle accidents, sporting activities, and falls.[2, 5, 25, 39, 64, 93, 108, 117]

---

*References 3, 26, 43, 63, 69, 76, 108, 122, and 134.

DEVELOPMENTAL PHYSIOLOGY OF THE IMMATURE SPINAL COLUMN

In order to fully appreciate the unique nature of the child's response to injury, developmental stages in the maturation of the spinal cord and vertebral column must be understood.

Nervous System

Spinal cord development begins in the second gestational week with the formation of the notochord through cell migration and invagination within the primitive streak.[102] Ectoderm overlying the notochord subsequently develops into the neuroplate which invaginates to form the neurotube which establishes the primitive central nervous system.

The cells of the neurotube differentiate into three layers: (1) the ependymal lining of the central canal of the spinal cord; (2) the intermediate mantle, which becomes the gray matter; and (3) the peripheral marginal layer, which becomes the white matter. Spinal cord and spinal column growth are disproportionate with the spinal cord terminating at the L1–2 vertebral level at 2 months of age.

During the third week of gestation[104] the paraxial mesoderm forms somites in a cephalocaudad direction. During the fourth week of gestation, the somites differentiate into three colonies of cells giving rise to dermis and subcutaneous tissues (dermatome), the muscles (myotome), and vertebral bodies (sclerotome).

Axial Skeleton

Each sclerotome consists of a cranial half of loosely packed cells and a caudal half of densely packed cells with the developing fissure ultimately forming the perichordal ring, a precursor of the intervertebral disc. Sclerotomal maturation is influenced by the adjacent neurotube, the notochord, and the surrounding neural crest cells.

During the sixth gestational week the mesenchymal vertebral anlagen develop primary centers of chondrification in the body (centrum) and in each neural arch. Concomitantly, the anulus fibrosus evolves from condensing perichordal tissue with a degenerating notochord contributing to the gelatinous core of the nucleus pulposus.[108]

Primary centers of ossification first appear in lower thoracic and upper lumbar vertebral bodies with further development occurring in rostral and caudad directions. The ossification centers of the neural arches appear first in the lower cervical spine.[108] Each vertebral body develops three centers of primary ossification, one in the body and one in each neural arch. The atlas and axis are the only vertebrae with different development. The atlas has two ossification centers in each neural arch and the axis develops from five primary centers of ossification, two in the dens, one in the body, and two in the neural arches.[2, 108]

The ossification centers of the body and neural arches fuse at the neurocentral synchondrosis at 3 to 6 years of age for vertebrae C3–7. This juncture is anterior to the anatomic pedicle and is often confused as a fracture site in the immature trauma patient.[22] The posterior vertebral arches are closed by 2 to 4 years of age. The thoracic and lumbar spine lags behind the development of the cervical spine which is mature at approximately 8 years of age. Continued growth of vertebral bodies occurs through perichondral and periosteal appositional growth and longitudinally through enchondral ossification.[103] The cervical vertebrae achieve one-half adult size by age 2 years[108] with little longitudinal growth occurring beyond the age of 10 years. The longitudinal growth rate of the vertebral column decelerates after 3 years of age and experiences a second growth spurt at the time of puberty.[103] The thoracic vertebral body grows 0.7 mm per year while the lumbar vertebral body grows 1.2 mm per year.[44, 103]

The atlas appears initially as two primary centers of ossification in each lateral mass or neural arch. The primary center of ossification of the body, the centrum, does not appear until 1 year of age and may be singular or multifocal in appearance.[102, 103] The posterior neural arches of the atlas fuse between 3 and 7 years of age. Occasionally closure is incomplete, forming a clinically insignificant posterior spondyloschisis resembling a potential fracture.[108] The atlas reaches adult dimensions by age 4 years with no further enlargement of its spinal canal.[103] The canal diameter for the remainder of the vertebral column remains static from the time of closure of the posterior synchondroses at 3 to 6 years of age.

The axis is formed by five primary ossification centers which appear at the fifth to seventh month of fetal life[108] (Fig. 32–1). The bipartite ossification centers of the dens are usually fused by 3 months of age. Earlier radiographs of the unfused centers from the time of birth may spuriously suggest fracture.[103] The apical cartilaginous dens or chondrum terminale develops a secondary center of ossification at 3 to 6 years.[103] The junction of the chondrum terminale with the body of the dens resembles a transverse or V-shaped cleft. Fusion of this ossification center with the remainder of the dens occurs by age 12. The term *ossiculum terminale* is appropriate when this secondary center of ossification fails to fuse with the body of the dens. This is a normal variant of ossification that is clinically insignificant but may be confused as a fracture.[108]

The junction of the body of the dens with the body of the axis is known as the basilar subdental synchondrosis. Fusion occurs by 6 years of age, but complete fusion may not occur until 11 years of age in 50% of patients.[34, 92] The synchondrosis should not be confused with a fracture.

The vertebral ring apophysis, first appearing at a small recess along the superior and inferior rim of the vertebral bodies at 5 years of age, develops secondary centers of ossification at 6 to 8 years in females and at 7 to 9 years in males. These centers contribute little to longitudinal growth and serve as attachment sites for ligaments and periosteum. Fusion begins at 14 years of age with completion at the age of 24.[104, 108] Trauma may also be suggested by secondary centers of ossification

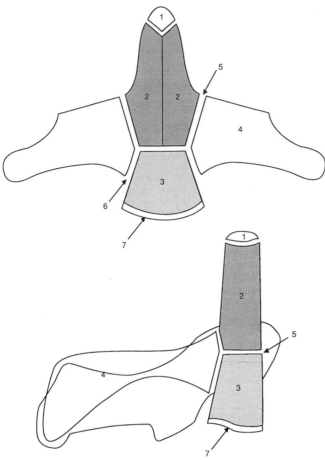

Figure 32–1 ═ Anteroposterior and lateral views of immature axis revealing five centers of primary ossification prior to fusion. *1*, Apical cartilaginous dens or chondrum terminale; *2*, bipartite ossification centers of the dens; *3*, body; *4*, neural arch; *5*, neurocentral synchondrosis; *6*, subdental synchondrosis; *7*, inferior body end plate.

in the transverse and spinous processes, as well as by the normal anterior wedge-shaped vertebral bodies of the immature spine which are squared off by age 7.[108]

Vascular Supply to the Spine

The distribution of the arterial and venous vascular supply to the spine is well established at birth and changes little with development.[104] The anterior spinal artery, a branch of the two vertebral arteries, supplies most of the anterior spinal cord lying along the anterior median fissure. The posterior cord is supplied by two posterior spinal arteries, branches of either the vertebral or inferior cerebellar arteries lying along the posterior lateral sulcus.[37] At birth, the vertebral body is surrounded by an extensive network of arterial branches which extend to the vertebral end plates. The cartilaginous end plate is also supplied by a circumferential network of fine arteries ending in sinusoidal terminals. As ossification proceeds, the majority of the blood supply to the articular surface is terminated with only a subarticular and subchondral horizontal plexus of vessels remaining. The anatomic distribution of the blood supply to the adult cervical spine may be an

important factor in the high incidence of nonunion in Anderson type 2 odontoid fractures. This is not an important factor in the healing process of pediatric odontoid fractures since the basilar subdental synchondrosis, which is the most common point of fracture of the odontoid in the child, is supplied by vessels entering medial to the facet joints (Fig. 32–2). The tip of the dens receives the majority of its blood supply from the surrounding tissues and ligaments (Fig. 32–3).

ANATOMIC, BIOMECHANICAL, AND PHYSIOLOGIC DIFFERENCES IN THE PEDIATRIC AND ADULT SPINAL CORD INJURY PATIENT

There are inherent differences in the anatomy, biomechanics, and physiology of the adult and pediatric spinal column. These differences are extremely important regarding management and prognosis after spinal cord trauma. The cervical and upper thoracic spine are the most frequently injured regions in the pediatric age group.[5, 38, 99, 103, 112] The upper cervical spine is more frequently injured in the child younger than 7 years of age compared with those older than 7 years.[8, 54, 69, 71, 105, 116] Due to the disproportionately large head in the child less than 8 years of age, the fulcrum of flexion and extension is high at the C2–3 or C3–4 level compared with the older child in whom the fulcrum is more caudad at C5–6.[38, 117] This exposes the upper cervical spine to greater inertial loads. Laxity of the interspinous ligaments and joint capsules,[108] the horizontal orientation of the facet joints,[103] the anterior wedging of the vertebral bodies, the poorly developed uncinate processes, and the underdeveloped cervical musculature[38, 121] all contribute to the increased flexibility and hypermobility of the upper cervical spine of young children.[69] These anatomic and biomechanical characteristics may explain the increased pediatric suscepti-

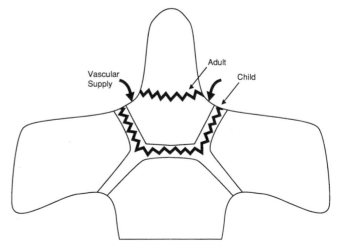

Figure 32–2 ═ The entry of the vascular supply of the immature axis allows continued circulation to the dens after fracture through the subdental synchondrosis. Note how the fracture line in a typical adult dens fracture is above the entry point of the vascular supply to the dens, which results in a high incidence of nonunion.

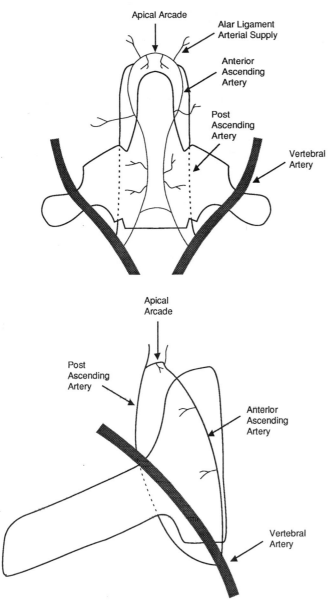

Figure 32–3 = Anteroposterior and lateral views of the mature axis illustrating its extensive blood supply from branches of the surrounding vertebral arteries. Note the apical arcade supplying the tip of the dens.

bility to spinal cord injury[2, 38] without radiographic evidence of abnormality (SCIWORA) in patients younger than 10 years. The high cartilage-to-bone ratio of vertebral bodies, the larger and more resilient intervertebral discs,[84, 92] the strong vertebral end-plate complex,[16] and strong ligamentous structures increase the risk of fracture at the relatively weaker growth plate and apophyseal regions which may be difficult to demonstrate by routine radiography.[11, 117]

Owing to the large amount of force necessary to disrupt the flexible spinal column in children, there is often a greater degree of neurologic compromise at the time of injury.[7, 29, 105, 114, 117, 119] After spinal cord injury, a child less than 10 years of age is twice as likely to be quadriplegic than paraplegic[59] whereas this ratio is

reversed in children older than 10 years,[108] when anatomic and biomechanical differences become much less important.[137]

The most obvious distinguishing factor in the immature spine is the presence of a functioning growth plate. Injury of the growth plates of the vertebral body due to fracture or alteration in applied stress as a result of paralysis results in progressive deformities with possible neurologic deterioration.

INITIAL EVALUATION OF THE PEDIATRIC SPINAL CORD PATIENT

When a child presents with multiple organ system trauma, a high index of suspicion should exist in regard to potential injury of the spinal column.[109] After careful assessment of the patient's cardiopulmonary system, strict immobilization of the spinal column should be initiated at the scene of the accident. In children younger than 8 years of age, because of the relatively large size of the child's head in relation to body size, avoid the use of standard adult spine boards, which would create forced flexion of the cervical spine.[108] Use of shoulder rolls or a spinal board that is recessed in the area of the head is necessary to prevent flexion of the cervical spine (Fig. 32–4). Following a complete physical examination, anteroposterior

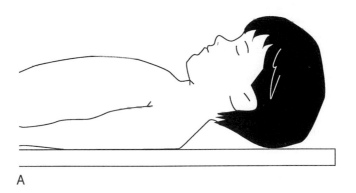

A

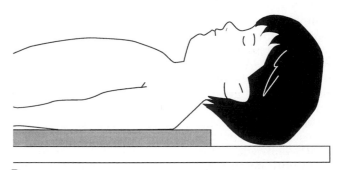

B

Figure 32–4 = *A*, Owing to the disproportionately large head-to-chest ratio in children less than 8 years of age, standard spine boards result in flexion of the cervical spine. *B*, Simple modifications to accommodate the large head size allow neutral positioning of the cervical spine.

and cross-table lateral radiographs of the entire spine are required when spinal injury is suspected.[103] Significant forces are necessary to cause significant spinal injury in this age group, and the evaluating physician should be aware of the high incidence of associated system injuries.[71] It is important to perform a meticulous neurologic examination and in patients with head trauma all attempts must be made to rule out injury of the upper cervical spine. It is easy to miss significant spinal injury in a comatose patient, especially in the absence of radiographic evidence of injury.[63] Sneed and Stover[125] reviewed four children admitted with the diagnosis of brain injury who had delayed diagnosis of spinal cord injury. On the basis of this experience, the authors recommended a detailed search for clues to spinal cord injury. These include flaccidity, diaphragmatic breathing without use of accessory muscles of inspiration, dermatomal pattern sensory loss, the absence of sacral reflexes, bradycardia with hypotension, autonomic hyperreflexia, poikilothermia, priapism, unexplained urinary retention, and the presence of clonus in an unconscious patient without decerebrate rigidity. Bohn and associates[22] identified 19 children who were brought to the emergency department without vital signs. They exhibited severe hypotension that was not explained by blood loss. Upon radiographic evaluation and postmortem evaluation in 16 of these patients, the author determined the cause of injury to be damage to the high cervical spinal column and cord. Patients presenting with hypoxic encephalopathy[125] should be evaluated to differentiate injury to the high cervical cord from head trauma.

The management of spinal cord injury in the pediatric patient requires a multidisciplinary effort involving not only the neurosurgeon and orthopaedist but also the pediatrician, pediatric surgeon, urologist, psychiatrist, psychologist, physical therapist, occupational therapist, social worker, orthotist, and a dedicated nursing staff.[42]

SPINAL CORD INJURY WITHOUT RADIOGRAPHIC ABNORMALITY (SCIWORA)

The capacity for stretch of the immature spinal column is greatest for the bony cartilaginous ligamentous complex, intermediate for the surrounding dura and arachnoid layers, and least for the spinal cord and pia mater.[9, 38, 96] The spinal cord is further restricted in movement by the horizontally departing cervical spinal roots, the attachment of the dura to the foramen magnum, and the lower cervical brachial plexus.[79] Under experimental conditions, the spinal osteochondral elements have been found experimentally to be able to stretch 2 in. without disruption, while the spinal cord could only be stretched 0.25 in.[38, 70, 85, 108] Breig[25] documented elongation of the spinal cord during flexion and shortening during extension. In light of the aforementioned characteristics of the pediatric spinal column, SCIWORA can be explained. One possible mechanism of injury for a child who suffers an impact to

the frontal region of the skull is a temporary hyperextension of the cervical spine with compression of the spinal cord by the ligamentum flavum.[97, 133] A decrease in the anteroposterior diameter of the cord may also have effects on the anterior spinal artery.[79] Cervical hyperflexion may follow and lead to longitudinal traction on the spinal cord with stretching, transection, vascular insufficiency of the spinal cord, herniation of an intervertebral disc, or displacement of a vertebral end plate.[1, 9, 15, 35, 108]

Autopsy findings in patients with SCIWORA reveal segmental atrophy of the spinal cord[59, 82] secondary to probable ischemic infarction[1, 71] with resultant necrosis of the central cord and anterior gray matter. Thus, SCIWORA may be the result of a complex of factors including interference with the intrinsic blood supply of the cord, spinal cord traction, buckling of the ligamentum flavum, acute disc herniation, or disruption of the end plate,[11] without radiographic evidence.

The incidence of SCIWORA is greatest in the pediatric age population (1% to 67%; average, 20%),* with younger patients affected more often than older patients.[64, 105, 136] There is usually a greater degree of neurologic deficit in the patient with SCIWORA, with an incidence of complete cord injury between 40% and 55%.[22] Patients who initially presented with incomplete neurologic deficits have demonstrated a delayed onset of increasing neurologic deficiency as late as 4 days after the original injury.[105]

The evaluation of patients with SCIWORA has been significantly improved by magnetic resonance imaging (MRI) which directly demonstrates cord edema, hemorrhage, or disruption, as well as vertebral end-plate or disc injury.

It is interesting to note that in many of these patients spinal instability cannot be demonstrated by dynamic radiographic testing using lateral flexion and extension radiographs of the cervical spine.[105] When no evidence of instability is found,[9] the treatment of patients with this disorder is supportive.

While the prognosis for neurologic improvement in patients with incomplete cord injury without radiographic abnormality is favorable, only minimal improvement can be expected in patients with complete spinal cord injury.[9, 18]

FRACTURE TYPES

There are five categories of fractures that occur in the pediatric spinal cord injury patient.[38, 42] These include (1) compression fractures with disruption of the anterior column alone or in conjunction with posterior column disruption when more than 50% of the vertebral body height is compressed; (2) burst fractures with disruption of both anterior and middle columns and preservation of the posterior column; (3) Chance fractures that result in compression of the anterior column with distraction of the middle and posterior columns; (4) growth plate and apophyseal fractures; and (5) frac-

---

*References 5, 7, 35, 63, 76, 79, 98, 103, 105, 108, 117, and 144.

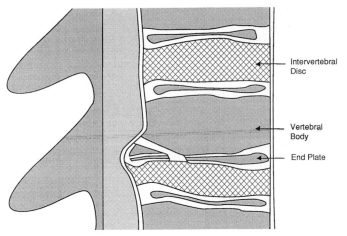

Figure 32–5 ═ An osteochondral end-plate avulsion fracture with an intact posterior longitudinal ligament results in spinal canal occlusion.

ture-dislocations resulting in compression, rotation, and shear of the anterior column with distraction, rotation, and shear of the middle and posterior columns. Fracture dislocations are the result of tremendous force with a concomitant high incidence of neurologic deficit after injury.[69]

Growth plate fractures are the most common type of fracture in the pediatric spine,[61] with injury to the basilar subdental synchondrosis of the odontoid the most common injury.[71] In autopsy studies performed in children under 12 years of age, injuries to the vertebral bodies consist primarily of end-plate disruptions[11, 38] (Fig. 32–5). The growth plate of the developing spine is the weakest component of the osteochondral complex, and is susceptible to tension, rotation, and shear forces.[108] These fractures may only demonstrate isolated widening of the spinous processes on radiographic evaluation and require rigorous evaluation to prove spinal stability.

Nerve root compression is common in cases of osteochondral or apophyseal fractures with the lesion usually identified by MRI, computed tomography (CT), or CT-myelography.[66] If symptomatic spinal stenosis exists with nerve root deficit, surgical removal of the fragment is the procedure of choice.[38] Fractures of the ring of the apophysis, classified into three groups by Takata and co-workers,[132] can mimic a herniated disc in the young adolescent patient. Treatment of persistently symptomatic lesions is surgical excision of the segment of apophysis protruding into the spinal canal.[132]

The goals of treatment of spinal fractures include restoration of spinal column alignment and stability, preservation of neurologic function, prevention of neurologic deterioration, and improvement of existing neurologic function.

The problem in management occurs with end-plate disruption and neurologic impairment (incomplete or complete). It is these patients who are at high risk for progressive post-traumatic deformity.

Instability of the spine has been defined by Denis[41] as disruption of the middle column and by White as the potential for irritation or damage to the spinal cord or nerve roots when the spine is subjected to normal physiologic loads.[60] The difficulty in accurately determining the presence of instability of the bony cartilaginous immature spine makes management of these patients extremely difficult.[97, 103]

CONSERVATIVE TREATMENT

Nonoperative treatment of spine fractures has been shown to be effective as surgery in terms of healing and neurologic outcome in the acute stage of spinal cord injury in patients of all ages.[38, 117, 121] Burke and Murray[30] reported a series of patients with spine injury who were treated with recumbency alone and found that only 2.5% of patients required surgical spinal fusion for late instability. Davies and colleagues[40] noted that neurologic recovery of spinal cord injury patients was the same for patients treated either nonoperatively or by surgery, but patients treated nonoperatively required a longer hospital stay. Jacobs and co-workers[74] performed a clinical review of patients who were treated operatively vs. those treated nonoperatively for spinal cord trauma in terms of functional return to society. The authors found that ambulatory patients who were surgically treated were able to walk 4.6 weeks earlier than those treated nonoperatively, while patients with lower extremity paralysis who were treated surgically were able to use their wheelchair 5.2 weeks earlier than those treated nonoperatively. They also noted an increased incidence of complications in those treated nonoperatively that was due to long-term recumbency, but found no difference in neurologic recovery between the two groups. Therefore, from a functional standpoint, patients treated surgically avoid the adverse consequences of recumbency are able to obtain the upright position sooner, and participate earlier in activities of daily living. Activity is important in paralyzed patients with poor pulmonary reserves, osteopenic bone, and insensate skin.[9] Furthermore, persistent instability of the spine will deter the functional return of adjacent cord segments and nerve roots and may result in ascending cystic degeneration of the spinal cord.[23]

Fortunately, only around 20% of children with significant spinal column disruption will require surgical intervention owing to the child's rapid healing potential of the ligamentous column, bony elements, and osteochondral growth plates.[38, 50, 69] An important problem in the pediatric patient with spinal cord injury is the predictable sequelae of post-traumatic deformity, a complication not seen in the adult patient.[23]

SURGERY IN THE SPINAL CORD INJURY PATIENT

The indications for surgical treatment of acute spinal cord injury are similar in both the adult and pediatric populations. Operative intervention is appropriate in (1) nonreducible or markedly unstable injuries, (2) doc-

and is documented by dynamic testing, then surgical stabilization is indicated.[108]

The surgical approach to the pediatric cervical spine requires meticulous dissection with exposure of only those posterior elements to be included in the fusion area. Unnecessary exposure of other spinal levels may result in the extension of fusion with increased alteration in the growth and mechanics of the child's cervical spine.[55] The use of allograft is not as effective as autograft in attaining a solid fusion mass of the cervical spine in the pediatric patient.[126]

Neonates

The management of cervical spine injury in the infant differs from injury in the older child on the basis of poorly developed paracervical musculature, increased ligamentous laxity, thin cranium, underdevelopment of the osseoscartilaginous structures, and frailty of skin.[56, 95] Fractures such as C2 burst injuries, which are managed easily in the young child by immobilization, may need to be fused in the neonate because of the lack of normal muscular splinting from the hypoplastic surrounding muscular sleeve. The delicate and sensitive skin in these patients lowers a surgeon's threshold for surgical stabilization compared to that in the older child, in whom bracing is less difficult.[90]

Occipitoatlantal Junction

Occipitoatlantal dislocation is frequently a lethal injury in any age group. Instability at this level is exacerbated in the infant and young child by the characteristic anatomic presence of small occipital condyles, the large surface area of the atlanto-occipital joint, and horizontal facet joints.[103, 108] The primary treatment of this injury is an occipital-to-C1[57] or -C2[36] fusion. In pediatric patients, care must be taken during surgical exposure of the posterior elements of the atlas. The tortuous course of the vertebral arteries along the posterior superior arch of the atlas is only 1 cm from the midline.[108]

Fractures at C2

Fractures of the odontoid in children usually involve the basilar subdental synchondrosis with rapid healing occurring following positional reduction and immobilization (Fig. 32–9).[17, 20, 24, 78, 103, 117, 118] The most common type of odontoid fracture in the adult is the Anderson-D'Alonzo type II fracture which occurs at the waist of the odontoid above the facet joints. This fracture site is devoid of an adequate blood supply. While their type II fracture demonstrated a high incidence of nonunion in the adult, Anderson and D'Alonzo reported complete healing of odontoid fractures in four pediatric patients treated by immobilization.[6] The study of Sherk and co-workers[120] of 11 pediatric patients with odontoid fractures supports the expectation of good results with complete healing of fractures in all patients treated by immobilization.

Os odontoideum refers to the round or oval-shaped

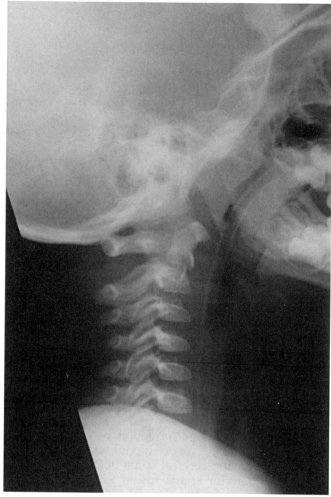

Figure 32–9 = A lateral radiograph in a 6-year-old boy reveals a displaced odontoid fracture through the basilar subdental synchondrosis.

ossicle with smooth cortical borders that is found cephalad to the remainder of the hypoplastic dens.[108] The etiology of os odontoideum is controversial, but there is good evidence to indicate that some of the observed lesions are the result of previous trauma[47, 51] subsequent to nonunion.[103] Alternative etiologies include vascular insufficiency[53] with retraction of the proximal fragment of the odontoid by the alar ligaments and hypertrophy of a remnant of the proatlas that is associated with a hypoplastic dens.[103, 108]

When a patient with an os odontoideum presents with symptoms of upper cervical cord compromise and demonstrates instability at C1–2 on dynamic flexion-extension lateral radiographs, then surgical stabilization of C1 and C2 is indicated. Care must be exercised in applying posterior wire reduction and fixation of C1 and C2 to prevent cord compression by the anterior arch of the atlas and the attached ossicle.

Atlantoaxial Instability

Traumatic atlantoaxial instability may vary from unilateral or bilateral anterior subluxation of the lateral masses of C1 on C2, to fixed rotatory subluxation of C1 on C2, to posterior displacement of one or both lateral masses of the atlas on the axis[49] (Figs. 32–10 and 32–11). Treatment for each disorder must be individualized and may differ from the similar adult condition for which surgical fusion is the usual standard of care.[48, 108] Pediatric patients are frequently treated by closed reduction with traction and immobilized by a halo vest or Minerva cast until stability can be determined. The presence of neurologic impairment, significant anterior displacement of C1 on C2, chronic deformity present longer than 3 months, or recurrent deformity is a factor that may require surgical intervention. The treatment objective in patients with atlantoaxial instability is restoration of anatomic alignment and stability. If nonoperative management is unsuccessful with persistent instability, then surgical arthrodesis is warranted.

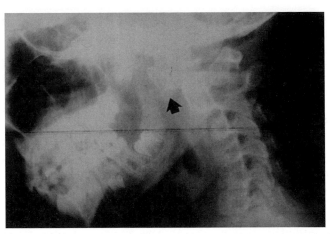

Figure 32–11 = The lateral flexion radiograph illustrates marked widening of the atlantoaxial interval (*arrow*) in a 7-year-old boy after a motor vehicle–pedestrian accident.

Lower Cervical Spine Injuries

Fractures of the subaxial cervical spine are more common in the older adolescent, but may occur in the younger child. While the nature of these fractures may permit successful treatment by traction and immobilization, long-term clinical and radiographic evaluation is required to detect the development of latent instability.

When performing a posterior cervical fusion in a child, single-level arthrodesis is preferred, if possible, to avoid the development of cervical stiffness and reduced range of motion. Birney and Hanley[18] reviewed 61 pediatric cervical spine injuries at 5½ years after surgical arthrodesis. Eight of 13 patients with excessive posterior fusion masses for C1 and C2 bony injuries complained of limitation of cervical motion, a stiff neck, and easy fatigability. A 25% loss of cervical motion was documented. Patients with posterior fusions of the lower cervical spine in the authors' series had similar but milder complaints. Roy and Gibson[116] re-

ported 18 patients who underwent meticulous one-level posterior cervical fusion with no loss of motion at follow-up. Care should be exercised in exposing only those posterior elements necessary for adequate stabilization to avoid the potential of creeping fusion to other uninvolved vertebral levels. Rarely is anterior fusion necessary in the acute treatment of fracture dislocations of the pediatric cervical spine. Poor results had been reported after primary anterior cervical fusion due to damage to the superior and inferior vertebral growth plates.[127]

Thoracolumbar Spine

Compression Fractures

The majority of fractures involving the thoracic and lumbar spine in the child and adolescent are compression injuries which are stable and heal well with nonoperative treatment.[72] When compression of the anterior vertebral body is greater than 50%, the possibility of posterior instability exists and may necessitate surgical stabilization.[38] When surgical arthrodesis of the unstable thoracic spine is required, avoid placing instrumentation into the relatively small spinal canal of the neurointact pediatric patient for fear of spinal cord impingement. Interspinous wiring is a viable alternative if segmental fixation is needed.[38] Unstable anterior compression lesions with posterior ligamentous disruption above the level of L1 often require fusion levels three levels above and two levels below the site of instability.[9]

Fracture Dislocations of the Thoracolumbar Spine

Fracture dislocations of the thoracolumbar spine are extremely difficult to reduce with closed method and are associated with neurologic deficit in 75% to 90% of patients.[42] Treatment frequently involves open reduction and internal fixation with rapid healing owing to

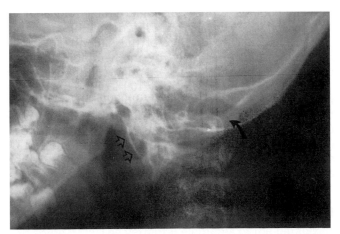

Figure 32–10 = A lateral radiograph reveals atlantoaxial rotatory subluxation in a 5-year-old girl. Note the obliquity of the ring of C1 (*open* and *closed arrows*) in relationship to the standard lateral alignment of the lower cervical vertebrae.

rounding bony elements,[87] by local vascular insufficiency of the spinal cord, or by extradural and intradural fibrosis secondary to local instability.[91] Malcolm and others reviewed 48 patients with post-traumatic kyphosis of whom 13 demonstrated increasing neurologic deficit 3 months to 20 years after the original injury.[90, 91, 97] The work of Malcolm[91] and co-workers[92] and that of Bohlman[21] suggested that late decompression was of benefit in adults with continued or progressive neurologic deficit from post-traumatic deformity.

Treatment of Paralytic Spinal Deformity

Primary immobilization and nonoperative stabilization of the injured pediatric spinal column must be closely observed for development of post-traumatic deformity.[103] Bracing may be used when deformity is of a mild degree of severity and may be continued to allow maximum spinal growth prior to surgical fusion.[27] Bracing within 6 months of injury in certain studies has been shown to decrease the incidence, extent, and progression of post-traumatic deformity in a paralyzed child.[14, 96] Ultimately, 68% of these children will require surgery for their deformity.[94] Surgical fusion should be electively scheduled and performed while the patient's spine is still supple.

Certain principles have evolved regarding the surgical management of paralytic spinal deformity. The surgeon should use the strongest available means of internal fixation to allow early mobilization of the patient.[112] Appropriate anterior release and fusion should be performed in severe degrees of rigid kyphosis or lordosis to reduce the stress on the posterior fusion mass and improve truncal realignment. A large amount of autogenous and allogeneic bone graft[112] should be used to increase the potential of a large bone fusion mass. Only those vertebral areas to be fused should be surgically exposed to prevent spreading fusion. Finally, the younger the patient at the time of surgery, the more extensive the fusion. Fusion to the sacrum in paralytic spinal deformities is recommended to decrease the risk of pseudarthrosis, instrument failure, and the adding on of vertebral bodies to the primary deformity. Soft tissues that impede spinal realignment, such as the lumbodorsal fascia, iliotibial band, or hip joint contractures, should be released.[42]

Scoliosis

Scoliotic curvatures of 40 degrees or more in the pediatric spinal cord injury patient are progressive, resistant to brace interventions, and require surgical intervention.[10, 14, 103] Surgical correction and fusion are difficult in this patient population and have a high complication rate.[96] Campbell and Bonnett[32] reviewed 64 juvenile spinal cord injury patients with fixed spinal deformity. Fifty percent of this group required surgery, with the majority undergoing successful posterior spinal fusions to the sacrum. The authors recommended halo-femoral traction when the preoperative bending films demonstrated little improvement in deformity.

Preoperative halo-femoral traction is dangerous with a fixed spinal deformity or with a previous fusion mass with the potential for excessive traction on a tethered cord. Anterior and posterior approaches to the deformed spine or osteotomy of the spine may be needed.

Kyphosis

The management of post-traumatic kyphosis has been controversial. Kilfoyle and associates,[80] in a review of 104 cases with congenital or acquired paraplegia with kyphosis, recommended in patients with curves greater than 60 degrees of anterior spinal fusion at the apex of the deformity followed by a posterior fusion. The addition of anterior fusion was recommended to remedy the high rate of pseudarthrosis and loss of correction experienced with posterior spinal fusion alone.

Malcolm[90] and colleagues reported a 50% failure rate in 48 patients with post-traumatic kyphosis who were treated solely with anterior spinal fusion. The authors recommended both an anterior and posterior fusion in a patient with post-traumatic kyphosis.

Lordosis

Progressive lordosis is usually seen in patients with complete lower thoracic spinal lesions who have lost abdominal flexor function but have active posterior spinal extensors.[81] Posterior spinal fusion is appropriate for deformities up to 100 degrees, while anterior and posterior spinal fusion are indicated when the deformity exceeds 100 degrees.[103, 112]

EFFECTS OF EARLY FUSION ON THE DEVELOPING SPINE

A major concern when surgical fusion is performed in the young child is the loss of longitudinal trunk growth. An estimate of remaining spinal growth may be obtained by multiplying 0.7 mm times the number of segments fused times the number of years of remaining growth.[100, 139] Winter[138] reviewed 75 patients who had spinal fusion performed prior to the age of 10 and who were followed for 9½ years. He noted cessation of longitudinal growth with an average growth of 1 mm following surgery and also noted bending of the fusion mass at follow-up that averaged between 10 and 15 degrees. If possible, fusion should be delayed until after the age of 10.[83, 138] Letts and Bobechko[83] reported the results of early fusion on 57 patients whose average age at surgery was 4.3 years. The average increase in longitudinal growth was 2 mm and 26% of patients required additional surgery because of progressive curvature of the spine. Dubousset and associates[44] noted a 33% incidence of curve progression in 81 patients fused early for congenital scoliosis. Curve progression and vertebral rotation after fusion of the child's spine have been recognized as a problem.[44, 58, 81, 138, 141]

Hefti and McMaster[68] illustrated the cessation of posterior spinal growth in 24 patients who underwent a posterior spinal fusion, but had continued growth of the unfused anterior spinal column. Dubousset and co-authors[44] termed the continued anterior vertebral growth after posterior spinal fusion in a young child with rotation of the apical vertebrae the "crankshaft phenomenon." The more immature the patient, the greater the resultant rotation regardless of the thickness of the fusion mass or use of instrumentation. The authors recommend anterior spinal fusion when such a deformity occurs.

INSTRUMENTATION WITHOUT FUSION

One method suggested to allow longitudinal vertebral growth while correcting lateral curvature is through vertebral instrumentation without fusion.[58, 89, 100] Internal fixation without fusion was first introduced by Harrington[67] in 1967 but was unsuccessful owing to aggressive subperiosteal stripping with resultant complete fusion of the instrumented spine. Harrington's technique was modified by Marchetti and Faldini in 1977 through their "end fusion technique" in which they fused two vertebral bodies at each end of the curve with application of instrumentation 6 months later.[58] Moe and colleagues[100] further modified their technique by exposing only the posterior elements of the vertebral body at each end of the curve with insertion of hooks and distraction by a subcutaneous rod. The authors reported their results in 20 patients, each of whom underwent two to eight surgical procedures (average 4.5) during their lengthening cycles and had adequate control of scoliosis. While an average 3.8 cm of longitudinal growth was realized prior to fusion, a high number of complications ranging from hook and rod displacement to posterior element fracture were recorded.

CONCLUSION

Understanding the normal variations in the growth and development of the immature spinal column serves as a foundation for appropriate diagnosis and management of the acute pediatric spinal cord injury patient. The goal of medical treatment of any spinal cord injury patient, young or old, is to protect the central nervous system from further injury by appropriate support and stabilization while facilitating, through aggressive rehabilitation, the introduction of the patient into society as a productive, functioning member. Through appreciation of the various anatomic, biomechanical, and physiologic differences between adult and pediatric spinal injury patients, the surgeon can anticipate the potential problems of altered vertebral growth plate development and occult spinal instability, and prevent the complication of severe progressive spinal deformities or neurologic deficit. With careful follow-up and meticulous attention to detail, both in conservative management and in the operative approach to these patients, a surgeon can expect good to excellent results in the majority of these difficult patients.[142]

REFERENCES

1. Ahmann PA, Smith SA, Schwartz JF, et al: Spinal cord infarction due to minor trauma in children. Neurology 25:301–307, 1975.
2. Allen B, Ferguson RL: Cervical spinal trauma in children. In Bradford DS, Hensinger RN (eds). The Pediatric Spine. New York, Thieme, 1985, pp 89–104.
3. Allen JP: Birth injury to the spinal cord. Northwest Med 69:323–326, 1970.
4. Allen JP, Meyers GG, Condon VR: Laceration of the spinal cord related to breech delivery. JAMA 208:1019–1022, 1969.
5. Anderson JM, Schutt AH: Spinal injury in children. A review of 156 cases seen from 1950 through 1978. Mayo Clin Proc 55:499–504, 1980.
6. Anderson LD, D'Alonzo RT: Fractures of the odontoid process of the axis. J Bone Joint Surg Am 56:1663–1674, 1974.
7. Andrews LG, Jung SK: Spinal cord injuries in children in British Columbia. Paraplegia 17:442–451, 1979.
8. Apple J, Kirks DR, Merten DF, et al: Cervical spine fractures and dislocations in children. Pediatr Radiol 17:45–49, 1987.
9. Asher MA, Jacobs RR: Pediatric thoracolumbar spine trauma. In Bradford DS, Hensinger RN (eds): The Pediatric Spine. New York, Thieme, 1985, pp 105–117.
10. Audic B, Maury J: Secondary vertebral deformities in children and adolescents. Paraplegia 7:11–16, 1969.
11. Aufdermaur M: Spinal injuries in juveniles. Necropsy findings in 12 cases. J Bone Joint Surg Br 56:513–519, 1974.
12. Bailey DK: The normal cervical spine in infants and children. Radiology 59:712–719, 1952.
13. Banniza von Bazan VK, Paeslack V: Scoliotic growth in children and acquired paraplegia. Paraplegia 15:65–73, 1977–1978.
14. Bedbrook GM: Correction of scoliosis due to paraplegia sustained in pediatric age group. Paraplegia 15:90–96, 1977.
15. Bedbrook GM: Spinal injuries with tetraplegia and paraplegia. J Bone Joint Surg Br 61:267–284, 1979.
16. Benner B, Molel R, Dickson J, et al: Instrumentation of the spine for fracture dislocations in children. Childs Nerv Syst 3:249–255, 1977.
17. Bhattacharvya SK: Fracture and displacement of the odontoid process in a child. J Bone Joint Surg Am 56:1071–1072, 1974.
18. Birney TJ, Hanley EN: Traumatic cervical spine injuries in childhood and adolescence. Spine 14:1277–1282, 1988.
19. Blasier RD, La Mont RL: Chance fracture in a child: A case report with nonoperative treatment. J Pediatr Orthop 5:92–93, 1985.
20. Blockey NJ, Purser DW: Fractures of the odontoid process of the axis. J Bone Joint Surg Br 38:794–817, 1956.
21. Bohlman HH: Late pain and paralysis following fracture of the thoracolumbar spine. The long term results of anterior decompression and fusion in T1 patients. Orthop Trans 12:60, 1988.
22. Bohn D, Armstrong D, Becker L, et al: Cervical spine injuries in children. J Trauma 30:463–469, 1990.
23. Bonnett CA, Mitani M, Guess V: Spinal cord injury. In Lowell WW, Winter RB (eds): Pediatric Orthopaedics. Philadelphia, JB Lippincott, 1978, pp 495–591.
24. Braakman R, Penning L: Injuries of the Cervical Spine. Amsterdam, Excerpta Medica, 1971, pp 53–76.
25. Breig A: Biomechanics of Central Nervous System. Stockholm, Almguist & Wiksell, 1960.
26. Bresnan MJ, Abroms IF: Neonatal spinal cord transection secondary to intrauterine hyperextension of the neck in breech presentation. J Pediatr 84:734–737, 1974.
27. Brown JC, Swank SM, Matta J, et al: Late spinal deformity in quadriplegic children and adolescents. J Pediatr Orthop 4:456–461, 1984.
28. Burke DC: Spinal cord trauma in children. Paraplegia 8:1–4, 1970.
29. Burke DC: Traumatic spinal paralysis in children. Paraplegia 11:268–276, 1974.

POSTOPERATIVE CARE AND REHABILITATION

antimicrobial concentrations in the blood, muscles, and hematoma of postoperative patients has demonstrated that first-generation cephalosporins reached levels twice that of any second- or third-generation cephalosporin.[6] There is a 10% to 20% incidence of cross-reactivity in patients with penicillin allergies who are administered cephalosporins. Manifestations of the allergic reaction include rash, urticaria, fever, eosinophilia, and anaphylaxis. A test dose of oral cephradine (Velosef) 250 mg is given to screen these patients prior to the first intravenous dose.

POSTOPERATIVE IMMOBILIZATION

The need for postoperative external immobilization depends on the method of stabilization utilized. Our series of 112 patients who underwent posterior stabilization for thoracolumbar (T11–L2) injuries has shown that a 17% incidence of hardware-related complications (failure, pseudarthrosis) accompany the use of Harrington distraction rods alone.[9] An 8% incidence is associated with the use of Drummond wires.[9] Most of these consisted of failures at the bone-hook interface. Supplemental body jacket immobilization is recommended for these patients for a period of 3 months postoperatively to reduce the risk of hardware-related complications. The use of more rigid constraints such as Luque rods with sublaminar wires, Cotrel-Dubousset instrumentation, and pedicle screw constructs which stabilize at least two normal levels above and below the traumatized motion segment may not require postoperative external mobilization. Thus far, there are no satisfactory long-term studies to determine if instrument-related complications are less frequent with these newer types of stabilization methods.

Body jackets (total contact orthoses, TCOs) should be manufactured from a negative plaster mold. These can be molded as early as the second postoperative day, if there is no abdominal distention, and applied to the patient by the fourth postoperative day. Off-the-shelf orthoses may apply abnormally high pressure on the skin, increasing the risk of breakdown. We recommend polypropylene jackets because they are durable and lightweight, thereby facilitating the early rehabilitation period. Jackets should consist of either anterior and posterior shells or one-piece shells for thoracolumbar fracture (T9–L3) with Velcro fasteners which will allow rapid application and removal. This is extremely important in patients with associated chest injuries who may require institution of cardiopulmonary resuscitation. A large anterior thoracic window is important to allow maximum chest expansion and optimize respiratory function. Jackets should be worn 24 hours per day as repeated removal and reapplication may precipitate hardware dislodgment. An undergarment should be worn to cover all exposed skin and changed daily using meticulous hygiene. Daily changing and hygiene allow careful skin inspection.

One must bear in mind that body jacket immobilization in patients with sensory deficits carries a risk of skin-related complications. Our series showed a 4%

Table 33–1 = **REHABILITATION TIME VS. POSTOPERATIVE IMMOBILIZATION**

Body jacket (42 patients)	113 days
No body jacket (18 patients)	69 days

incidence of sacral decubitus ulcers requiring myocutaneous flap reconstruction.[9] Also, patients who require body jackets in the acute postoperative period require a longer time to achieve completion of their initial rehabilitation time (Table 33–1). This is due in part to a significant decrease in the initial hip range of motion (Table 33–2).

Jackets utilized in patients with intact upper lumbar dermatomes may experience numbness over the anterior thigh caused by pressure on the lateral femoral cutaneous nerve. This should not be confused with neurologic progression secondary to the spinal cord injury. It is treated by providing anteroinferior relief to the orthosis or restricting hip flexion when jacket immobilization is required.

Another rare complication of jacket immobilization is due to compression of the superior mesenteric artery and the third part of the duodenum.[2, 4, 5, 10, 11] Patients will exhibit nausea and vomiting. Abdominal distention is not a hallmark feature because the obstruction is in the proximal portion of the gastrointestinal tract. Bowel sounds are normal and flatus and stool are still passed. Postoperative analgesics that also cause nausea and vomiting may delay the diagnosis. Prolonged delay can lead to hypovolemia and hypokalemic alkalosis. Treatment consists of nasogastric suction and intravenous fluid replacement. Electrolytes should be closely monitored as potassium replacement is often necessary. Positional changes such as foot elevation in the supine position may relieve the symptoms. Abdominal windows are usually not successful in alleviating the condition. Symptoms should improve in 48 to 72 hours, and if they do not, jacket removal is necessary.

Since its first description by Perry and Nickel in 1959,[8] halo immobilization has been an important adjunct in the care of the patient with cervical spine trauma. It may be occasionally used with surgical stabilization or applied in the surgical suite for nonoperative treatment. The circumference of the skull is measured above the ears, and the appropriate-size ring is selected. Povidone-iodine preparation is used, and four halo pins are applied to fix the ring to the skull,

Table 33–2 = **HIP RANGE OF MOTION RELATED TO THE USE OF POSTOPERATIVE IMMOBILIZATION**

	DEGREES OF FLEXION
Body jacket	
Hip ROM—initial	93
Hip ROM—final	115
No body jacket	
Hip ROM—initial	117
Hip ROM—final	118

ROM, range of motion.

allowing 1 cm of clearance between the skull and ring circumferentially. Pins are placed in opposite fashion (left posterior and right anterior, then right posterior and left anterior). The posterior pins are placed above the tragus of the ear taking care to avoid the more anterior temporal arteries. Correct anterior pin placement is over the lateral orbit to avoid the more medial supraorbital and supratrochlear nerves as well as the frontal sinus. All pins are tightened 1 in.-lb at a time in opposite fashion using a torque screwdriver. The vest is applied and reduction is checked with a lateral radiograph. Halo pins may be tightened 2 days after initial application to 8 in.-lb. It is critical to readjust the vest after mobility of the patient. We do not recommend further tightening to avoid penetration of the inner table of the skull if the pins are extremely loose. The pins may be retorqued at 7 and 30 days if less than two turns are necessary to achieve tightness. Twenty percent of patients will exhibit pin tract infection. Pin care utilizing povidone-iodine scrub is important to reduce the incidence of infection. Vests should be well padded to avoid skin breakdown. Use of a circumferential halo cast is discouraged because if the need for cardiopulmonary resuscitation arises, the patient's life may depend on the expeditious removal of the vest. The use of a vest with articulated anterior struts is suggested. Intubation of the patient with a halo vest may be difficult otherwise. A tracheostomy tray should be located on the ward where patients with halo casts are located to assure prompt airway access in emergent situations.

COMPLICATIONS

Complications that occur in the acute postoperative period are listed in Table 33–3. The surgeon must be especially aware of progressive neurologic deterioration. This unfortunate complication and uncontrollable bleeding are the only two indications requiring emergent return to the surgical suite. Neurologic deterioration may be due to postoperative hematoma (which must be evacuated), or malposition of hardware or the bone graft, which must be removed or repositioned. Postoperative hematomas in patients who underwent anterior cervical exposure can cause life-threatening airway obstruction. For this reason, anterior cervical procedures require drainage postoperatively. We recommend a tracheostomy tray at the bedside to allow rapid evacuation of the hematoma if this should occur in the early postoperative period.

Esophageal perforation may occur rarely during anterior cervical surgery but is not usually recognized until the early postoperative period. Persistent dysphagia that does not improve by the fourth postoperative day should alert the surgeon to possible esophageal perforation. Patients should be studied with esophagoscopy or an esophagogram. Patients with perforations should be treated with nasogastric suction and intravenous fluids. Small perforations should resolve in 2 to 3 weeks. Patients should be restudied prior to resuming oral intake. Perforations that are refractory to conservative treatment may require sternocleidomastoid flap coverage.[3]

Anterior decompression of the thoracic spine or thoracolumbar junction involves exposure of the chest cavity. A chest tube is placed in the eighth intercostal space postoperatively. Initial management consists of suction through a column of approximately 20 cm H_2O. Chest radiographs are checked daily. Forty-eight hours postoperatively the suction is turned off and the patient is left to water-seal. Air leaks are observed, and if present, suction is continued. Chest tubes should never be discontinued if an air leak is present. This could lead to a tension pneumothorax, requiring reinsertion. Chest tubes are discontinued 24 hours after water seal, if no air leak is present. Removal is performed during maximum inspiration. A pressure dressing is applied and a chest radiograph is immediately taken to rule out pneumothorax. It is important to encourage aggressive respiratory therapy in the early postoperative period. Intercostal nerve blocks are occasionally utilized to assist respiration by preventing splinting of the chest wall secondary to postoperative incisional pain.

Inadvertent dural tears rarely go unrecognized until the postoperative period. However, some may be discovered by clear drainage exuding from the wound on the third to fourth postoperative day. These usually occur after late anterior decompression for a healed vertebral fracture. Recumbency and closed gravity drainage of 200 to 300 mL of cerebrospinal fluid per 24-hour period through an intradural puncture at the third lumbar motion segment for 3 days will usually stop the fluid leak.[7] If drainage does not cease, then reexploration with meticulous dural repair or a dural patch graft is indicated.[1]

Infections are usually due to *Staphylococcus aureus.* Prolonged antibiotics may be appropriate if the infection is recognized within the first 2 weeks after surgery. Late infection requires meticulous debridement of all nonviable tissue to remove the organism's protective environment, and prolonged use of culture-directed antibiotics. Many bacteria secrete a glycocalyx slime that adheres to foreign bodies and nonviable osseous tissue and protects them from systemic antibiotics. Superficial infections involving only soft tissue require a 2-week course, while deep infections involving graft or hardware require 4 to 6 weeks of intravenous antibiotics. In trauma patients postoperative infections are more common in those who have risk factors such as obesity, diabetes, and debilitation, and in those who are immunocompromised.

The long-term mechanical result of the unstable low thoracic or lumbar fracture with neurologic compromise has not been altered by operative intervention. However, surgical stabilization and the current stan-

Table 33–3 = **ACUTE POSTOPERATIVE COMPLICATIONS**

Hematoma	Infection
Hardware failure	Injury to viscera
Hardware malposition	Dural tears
Displaced bone graft	

predominant defense mechanism operating at this juncture to protect the individual from the extent of physical damage and limitations. The patient may strive to seem more like his or her "old" self. There is a determination to work harder, be more hopeful, and think more clearly. Anger easily appears if the individual perceives that his or her reality is being challenged. Forcing acceptance could cause rejection of what is being offered. The consistency of the team approach is crucial at this time. It is important to give consistent information about the injury, including limitations, and to provide it in a supportive manner. If denial is not creating any problems in the treatment program, it is best to leave it alone. It should be pointed out that hope need not represent denial and is often an important mechanism for maintaining the patient's motivation.

As the patient begins to acquire a realistic view of the disability, he or she is said to be in the acknowledgment stage. Depression is the main response as reality imposes itself. The patient may feel sad, helpless, hopeless, and may express suicidal ideation. The expression of suicidal thoughts may represent a level of the person's despair, a symptom of depression, or an intended solution to a dramatic problem. It must always be considered serious and evaluated for its potentiality.

It is also important that the rehabilitation team not confuse depression with "lack of motivation," or feel that the individual is willfully responsible for the depression. The type and level of depression need to be accurately assessed so that all treatments can be considered, including psychiatric evaluation for psychotropic medication, if appropriate. Support and reassurance with a focus on short-term goals is often most helpful.

Adaptation is the final stage, often seen after a period of community reentry, though sometimes seen in the rehabilitation setting. It is a time when the patient has developed a renewed sense of self-worth, having worked through major emotional reactions. The patient is generally more realistic about his or her limitations, focusing on what can be done rather than what cannot be done. This is a time when a sense of well-being and positive self-regard are maintained by the patient.

During the course of rehabilitation it is important for the team to be provided with a forum in which to address patient behaviors which may interfere with progress in the treatment program. Increased levels of depression, decreased frustration tolerance, a premorbid drug and alcohol abuse history, control issues, and so forth, may all produce behaviors which prevent the patient from maximum participation in the program. The team must be able to meet and openly discuss patient behaviors. They must determine what the problems are, where they are occurring, who is having the problems, how they are being addressed, what is working and what isn't, and how they can best be managed in the best interest of patient participation. At some point in the process the patient needs to be involved. Behavior management strategies may need to be developed which require a contract with the patient to set appropriate limits. It may also be appropriate at some point to involve the family.

The patient's family may experience similar reactions. It is important that they be involved in the total rehabilitation process to the limits of their readiness and willingness to do so. They are critical to the adjustment process and need much ongoing support and education.

The area of sexual function or dysfunction is of prime concern to this patient population. The psychologist plays an important role in addressing the area of sexuality. Sexual function is managed in the same fashion as other areas of functioning in an attempt to establish a pattern of life as close to that of premorbid functioning as possible. A formal sexual function program has two components: an educational group series designed to address the issues at a general level, and an individual sexual function evaluation designed to address individual specific sexual function issues with a physician and the psychologist present. The program provides an opportunity to address the areas of sexual dysfunction, alternative behaviors, precautions, and other areas related to sexual counseling.

Surgical Considerations in the Rehabilitative Program

Proper management directed toward stabilizing the spine, preventing further injury, and facilitating mobilization allows the newly injured patient to begin the rehabilitation program soon after injury. Delayed rehabilitation can result from a single poor decision regarding patient management, be it in the field by an emergency medical technician, by an emergency room physician, or in planning and performing surgery by an orthopaedic or neurologic surgeon. Inappropriate decision making in the early postinjury period can lead to disastrous complications, or to multiple surgeries.[54]

Once care of the patient is assumed, the treating physician must initially provide spinal immobilization and assessment. Cervical injuries may be stabilized by use of a cervical collar, sandbags, or traction. Thoracic and thoracolumbar injuries may be stabilized by bed rest with appropriate nursing care directed at logrolling the patient to minimize rotational stresses on the spine.

Medical and neurologic assessment should be performed immediately, and serial neurologic evaluations should follow during the first 24 hours until it is clear that the neurologic injury is not progressive. Appropriate radiographic studies are obtained, and a treatment plan is devised. Patients with mechanically stable injuries may be mobilized when comfortable and started on their rehabilitation programs. Those with unstable spines may require treatment with traction, external immobilization, or internal fixation before they can be safely mobilized for therapy and skills training.

Early decision making should be based on viewing the spinal injury as having two separate components. Mechanical stability should be assessed independent of the quality of neurologic injury. Care of each portion of the injury often overlaps, but we find it useful to consider restoration of stability and potentiation of neurologic recovery individually.

Spinal injuries may be acutely stable or unstable.

Gunshot wounds are typically stable injuries. They may be associated with both complete or incomplete cord injuries. Patients with gunshot wounds can usually be mobilized immediately after their injury with no external immobilization required other than for comfort. Ligamentous dislocations in all areas of the spine, typically flexion-distraction injuries, are generally unstable. Bilateral facet dislocations, notoriously unstable injuries, demand reduction and immobilization before a patient can be placed in a wheelchair or other ambulatory device.

The extent of SCI is determined by clinical neurologic examination after the patient has emerged from the variable period of spinal shock. Complete cord injuries, by definition, do not have potential for neurologic recovery except for root escape. Incomplete injuries have variable recovery and must be treated as having theoretical potential for total return of function.

As a conceptual aid, we recommend formulating a Punnett square with quadrants representing each of the possibilities discussed above.

	Mechanically stable	Mechanically unstable
Neurologically complete	A	B
Neurologically incomplete	C	D

Quadrant A, composed of mechanically stable and complete SCIs, is best represented by gunshot wounds that have traversed the spinal canal but have left enough bony elements intact to confer stability. Patients with this type of injury at any level may be mobilized and their rehabilitation program started as soon as they are medically stable and comfortable. Halo vests or thoracolumbosacral orthoses (TLSOs, body jackets) are not necessary.

In quadrant B, consisting of complete cord injury with an unstable spine, we find the patient with no realistic potential for spinal cord recovery. Injudicious, unprotected mobilization may jeopardize root recovery at or above the level of injury, or may conceivably injure more proximal cord substance by ascending epidural hematoma, or by cord tethering over a traumatic kyphosis. The spine needs to be stabilized before mobilization for rehabilitation. In the cervical spine, bilateral facet dislocation is a good example of this injury type. The dislocation should be reduced, and the spine stabilized by application of a halo vest or by posterior fusion. We recommend the latter treatment for two reasons. Internal fixation allows fuller participation in a rehabilitation program without the restrictions of a halo vest. Secondly, pure ligamentous injuries have a considerably lower healing rate than do surgical fusions, and may necessitate surgery if the initial 12 weeks of halo treatment results in nonunion. For these reasons, we generally recommend internal fixation for our complete, unstable injuries. Only in the thoracic spine do we consider nonoperative treatment, based on a recent review identifying increased morbidity and

mortality with surgical intervention, although these cases are still considered on their individual merits.[8]

Quadrant C represents incomplete SCIs which are mechanically stable. Stab wounds to the spine with Brown-Séquard incomplete SCI, although relatively rare, are an excellent example of this injury type. These patients may be mobilized early, but should have their neurologic progress serially followed. Patients who have plateaued neurologically but demonstrate a persistent anatomic lesion causing cord compression, such as vertebral body or disc fragments, may benefit from late anterior decompression.

Quadrant D, incomplete cord lesions associated with mechanically unstable spines, represents the most challenging subgroup of patients. Their spines must be stabilized not only to facilitate early rehabilitation but also to protect the injured spinal cord from further damage and to allow the zones of edema surrounding the area of actual injury an opportunity to resolve. Critical decision making is essential in this subgroup to minimize the chance of further injury to the already traumatized spinal cord. We recommend spinal immobilization and initial medical stabilization followed by operative internal fixation. Instrumentation involving sublaminar passage of wires should be condemned as it may traumatize the swollen neural tissues. Early internal fixation, we believe, will protect the spinal cord from further injury, and will allow earlier participation in an appropriate rehabilitation program.[9]

When operating on acute cervical spine instability, where the most common mechanism of injury is flexion and compression, the posterior surgical approach is recommended. Posterior ligamentous structures are torn in tension as a result of the injury moment. The anterior structures are generally intact albeit compressed. Anterior surgery, incising these last remaining stabilizers of the spine, may cause circumferential instability which may lead to graft extrusion, nonunion, and progressive kyphosis. Posterior wiring and fusion allows dissection through the already injured tissue planes, and replaces the torn posterior ligaments with a wire tension band.

We recommend a careful, well-planned surgical technique. A large review of patients following posterior fusion has suggested that fusion extension beyond the intended levels may occur in a large percentage of cases.[7] Complete tetraplegics need maximum cervical spine range of motion (ROM) to operate mouthstick devices or to function with upper extremity assistive devices. Fusing potential motion segments may make the patient even more dependent on an aide. The surgeon should consider that any posterior elements exposed by soft tissue stripping may fuse, regardless of where the wire and bone graft are placed. Care should thus be taken to only expose those levels that are intended to be included in the fusion mass. Although many wiring techniques exist for posterior cervical fixation, we have found the simple wire loop to be effective. We drill through the base of the superior spinous process, and pass the wire through the interspinous ligament beneath the inferior spinous process, and hand-tighten the wire (Fig. 34–2). An autogenous

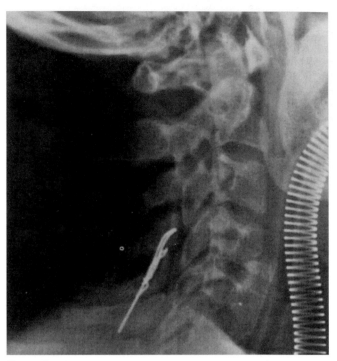

Figure 34–2 ═ The simple wire loop has been demonstrated to be an effective internal tension band. Combined with appropriate external immobilization, the fusion rate with autologous iliac crest bone graft is almost 100%.

iliac crest graft is placed along the exposed laminae. We do not extensively decorticate, and usually use local anesthesia. The fusion rate with this technique, frequently performed under local anesthesia, approaches 100%.[55] Postoperative use of a Philadelphia collar for 6 weeks, followed by a soft collar for 6 weeks, allows upper extremity rehabilitation to proceed unimpaired by a halo vest.

If future corpectomy is being considered, we generally fuse an additional segment posteriorly, so that the posterior fusion will act as a tension band against which an anterior strut graft may be placed. For example, if a patient has a C5 burst fracture with retropulsed bone, we strongly consider a posterior wiring and fusion from C4 to C6 if a later anterior corpectomy of C5 and a bone graft from C4 to C6 are likely.

For injuries at thoracic, thoracolumbar, and lumbar levels that require operative reduction and internal fixation, long-segment rod devices had traditionally been the gold standard of treatment. Major drawbacks to hook-rod constructs have been the need for external immobilization to reduce the risk of hook pullout, and the biomechanical necessity of spanning multiple levels to achieve reduction and fixation goals. Rehabilitation may be impeded by large restrictive orthoses.

Sublaminar or spinous process wiring of rods, use of claw configurations, and hook-screw constructs may allow rehabilitation without the need for external support. Complete thoracic injuries that need open reduction and rodding may be accompanied by sublaminar wiring. We recommend wiring the hooks at the level of laminar insertion to minimize the chances of hook cutout during rehabilitation. We do not recommend sublaminar wire insertion for patients with incomplete injuries where wire passage may cause neural injury. In these cases, use of spinous process wiring (Drummond wires) may allow rehabilitation out of a body jacket. A large review of instrumented patients has demonstrated a significant reduction in rehabilitation time when sublaminar or spinous process wires are used in conjunction with hook-rod constructs.[38] These patients can be rehabilitated without external immobilization, facilitating wheelchair and transfer skills.

Pedicle fixation devices offer a potential advantage by minimizing the number of motion segments involved in fixation. For example, an L1 fracture would require rod fixation from T10 to L3, spanning five motion segments. A construct utilizing pedicle screws could apply reduction and fixation across the L1 injured segment by screw placement into the T12 and L2 pedicles, spanning only two motion segments. Prospective studies are currently under way on the potential benefits of such systems in the traumatic population. Any construct which limits the span of fused segments in the paraplegic patient should be given strong consideration by the surgeon.

PHYSICAL THERAPY IN SPINAL CORD INJURY

Initial rehabilitation for patients with SCI has concentrated on regaining potential function as quickly as possible. This typically includes education about SCI and learning new skills necessary for mobility. Although these skills are important, several critical factors suggest the need to more sharply focus rehabilitation toward a lifetime perspective. These factors include an increased life expectancy for patients with SCI to near normal time frames, shorter lengths of stay available for rehabilitation coupled with difficulty accessing full outpatient services, and a trend toward decreasing societal barriers and legislative progress, as evidenced by the Americans with Disabilities Act.[27] Effective rehabilitation for persons with SCI must now emphasize the capacity to function effectively over the individual's lifetime, rather than just on the immediate gains in functional skills. Long-term health and function rehabilitation must begin during the initial phases, imparted by the clinician and directed by the specific needs of the patient.

The following initially discusses the current data and factors of aging with an SCI. These factors must play a vital role in the development of programs to meet the lifelong health needs of a person with an SCI.

Aging with a Spinal Cord Injury

Cardiovascular System

The current leading causes of death after SCI are cardiopulmonary conditions.[15, 16, 42] The rate of cardiovascular disease in people with SCI has been reported as high as 228% of the rate of the able-bodied population. Additionally, cardiovascular disease is occurring at an earlier age in people with SCIs.[26] The SCI population is susceptible to all known risk factors associated with cardiovascular disease, worsened by (1) a potential for progressive inactivity leading to deconditioning, (2) continued high rates of smoking, (3) susceptibility to hypertension and hypotension, (4) evidence of elevated cholesterol levels, and (5) the potential for a progressive increase in the total body mass with a decreasing lean body or muscle mass.

Respiratory Complications

Respiratory complications, specifically pneumonia, have been identified as a primary cause of death in the first year of life after SCI.[11, 16, 19] Mortality rates are significantly higher during this first year than during subsequent years.[42] Morbidity and mortality in persons with an SCI are related to the neurologic level of the SCI. Patients with tetraplegia and high paraplegia have the greatest risk due to paralysis of intercostal and abdominal muscles resulting in a decreased cough function. Diaphragm weakness or paralysis also occurs with higher-level lesions. Other conditions which have a negative impact on respiratory function include spinal deformity with its increased risk of pulmonary infections. Age-associated changes increase respiratory system risk as well. These include the natural decrease in lung compliance or elasticity and the decreasing vital capacity with age.[16, 51]

Musculoskeletal Dysfunction

As people age with SCI an increased susceptibility to musculoskeletal dysfunction has been reported. This may be a result of increased or abnormal stress placed on the upper extremities while engaging in wheelchair propulsion and transfers, an increased need to engage in overhead activities because of seating height, and in some situations prolonged crutch walking.[25] Data from a large population of patients averaging 12 years post injury demonstrated a 55% incidence of upper extremity pain in tetraplegic subjects, with the shoulder being the primary location. In subjects with paraplegia, 64% had upper extremity pain. The most common site was the wrist, presenting with carpal tunnel symptoms.[41]

Potential causes of the high incidence of upper extremity pain may relate to overuse, underuse, or less than optimal biomechanical use of the arms. For example, increased stress may occur in joints not anatomically suited for a particular activity. Also, the increased life expectancy of people with SCIs results in greater time to accumulate stress and for clinicians to track it. The high incidence of upper extremity pain may also be the result of a musculoskeletal system that is undergoing normal aging changes and poor biomechanics over a long period of time, resulting in muscle strength and flexibility imbalances.[27]

These issues reinforce the need to focus the rehabilitative programs at every phase with a long-term perspective. Tailoring programs to meet specific needs aids in identification of individual areas of vulnerability early in rehabilitation. Clinicians must be educators of patients, family members, and caregivers. Educational interventions should focus on creating lasting knowledge and behavior that encourage and promote the patient as a lifelong manager of his or her own health, wellness, and learning.

Activity for Health

Physical activity and exercise convey substantial benefits for health, fitness, and function in all segments of the population, including people with SCI. Increased physical activity can positively affect a number of cardiovascular risk factors in people with SCI.[45] Links have been identified between activity and physiologic factors. A study of persons with paraplegia found those who were employed to be lighter in weight, leaner, and to possess greater aerobic power than their unemployed counterparts.[30] Short bouts of moderate-intensity activity scattered throughout the day may be sufficient to confer a positive health benefit in the prevention and risk reduction of inactivity-related diseases.

In the area of musculoskeletal dysfunction, therapists can have a substantial impact. Detailed evaluation of an individual with an SCI provides insight into muscle imbalances, joint restrictions, and musculotendinous tightness. The biomechanical analysis of activity performance conducted by clinicians can clearly reveal areas of current vulnerability or potential for future problems. Task analysis provides insight into specific issues such as the muscle energy system used, the type of muscle contraction required, and the position necessary for the function.

Therapy programs should then be tailored to address these issues with patients to target prevention or resolution. A specific strengthening or stretching program to restore muscle strength balance around joints may be possible. Other injuries or conditions existing in conjunction with the SCI have to be factored in to that lifetime equation. Changes in spasticity over time, the development of heterotopic ossification, spinal deformity, or pressure ulcers are conditions that may occur over a lifetime. Also, preexisting conditions such as diabetes and other health-related concerns must be taken into consideration when focusing on the development of a program for the lifetime of the patient.

Evaluation

A comprehensive evaluation of the neurologic status, including the musculoskeletal system, is essential prior to initiating treatment. This evaluation provides the clinician with information necessary to determine the patient's functional level of neurologic injury. This functional level is the basis for development of a treatment plan to achieve long-term goals with the patient. Consideration of premorbid or concomitant medical factors must take place during the treatment planning and goal-setting phases.

Use of the ASIA standards for evaluation is recommended (see Appendix 34-1). These provide consistent data for communication between clinicians and centers

presents in the initial rehabilitation phase with a complete thoracic or higher-level injury, the treatment team must work together with the patient to focus on the body-handling, transfers, and wheelchair skills necessary to maximize independent function. It may be appropriate for a person presenting with an incomplete lesion and potentially functional lower extremities or a spinal injury of the lumbar or cauda equina region to focus on ambulation during initial rehabilitation. In some circumstances, ambulation is a long-term goal and the patient will require intense therapy in an outpatient setting. The functional needs, motivation, and potential must be evaluated individually in each case.

In the spinal cord–injured population, lower extremity orthoses function as a replacement for totally paralyzed muscles or as an assist for weak muscles. This provides both stability and protection for the joints of the lower extremities. The selection of orthotic components influences the potential for successful ambulation. It is critically important to recognize the high physiologic cost of ambulation with paralysis in comparison to wheelchair propulsion. In a study of persons with paraplegia, the average walking speed was less than half of normal, while oxygen consumption increased 50% and the heart rate was elevated by 28%. In comparison, the same persons tested propelling wheelchairs demonstrated a mean heart rate decrease of 22%, while oxygen consumption per minute decreased 44%, and velocity increased by two thirds.[12]

If the level of injury requires walking with bilateral locked KAFOs and a swingthrough gait, it is important to realize what a physically challenging task this is. In the absence of adequate quadriceps strength to stabilize the knee, locked KAFOs or other devices providing knee stability are required. The patient must have the ability to lift and swing the body forward in the swing phase and also maintain balance and lower body stability in the stance phase. Walking using this method is very slow and requires high-energy expenditure. Despite slow velocities, oxygen is consumed at a high rate. Many persons choose this method of walking only as a form of exercise, for limited use on special occasions, or to access inaccessible locations.[44]

A trial with temporary braces and preparation time to achieve the specific physical requirements necessary to walk successfully in the locked KAFOs is recommended before permanent braces are ordered. The more challenging physical demands include sufficient upper extremity strength to repeatedly lift the entire body, adequate cardiorespiratory endurance, and adequate hamstring range to avoid injury if falling and permit the patient the range to get up from the floor. Patients should train to meet these physical requirements while simultaneously learning the basic skills of transfers to and from bed and wheelchair. The capacity to perform 50 to 100 continuous dips in the parallel bars, to achieve a minimum of 20% of predicted maximum oxygen consumption (VO_2max) on an exercise test, and to achieve full ROM in all lower extremity joints is recommended for the patient planning to walk with locked KAFOs.

As technology advances the use of electrical stimulation for ambulation becomes more feasible. Improvements in electrode design, the use of electrodes sewn into lower extremity garments, and compact stimulation units are currently in use. People still find limitations in the functional application of these devices and electrical stimulation is currently not appropriate for all persons with SCI.

Ambulation with unlocked KAFOs, a combination of KAFO and AFO, or bilateral AFOs requires much less of an energy demand. People using bilateral AFOs have energy costs for ambulation approaching near normal values. This has resulted in higher success rates for independent ambulation in patients requiring this form of bracing. Efficiency studies have demonstrated that wheelchair propulsion is still faster and more efficient than walking with a combination AFO and KAFO. Patients with this need should be encouraged to walk, but many may still prefer to use a chair for long-distance mobility.[44]

Bracing with AFOs is necessary for the patient exhibiting plantar flexor or dorsiflexor weakness. The AFO can provide stability and controlled forward progression in persons with calf weakness. Normal muscle strength in the calf is indicated by the ability to perform 20 continuous unilateral toe raises. This functional muscle test closely replicates the demand placed on the gastrocnemius-soleus complex during ambulation. The calf must function repeatedly to meet a high torque demand with each step of the gait cycle. A muscle grade of less than 4 will not provide the endurance needed to maintain stability and controlled forward progression for functional distances.[32] Studies have demonstrated that the use of an AFO will not prevent the calf muscles from contracting during ambulation.[36] Therefore, a muscle group with the capacity to gain strength will not be precluded from doing so by use of the brace. Walking function is enhanced, joint stability is maintained, and functional muscle strengthening occurs simultaneously with use of an appropriately adjusted AFO.[34]

Equipment

Items such as wheelchairs, cushions, braces, assistive ambulation devices, and bathing and toilet devices can significantly enhance a patient's function and increase independence. However, not all people view equipment from a positive perspective. Acceptance, use, or abandonment of equipment is a personal choice made by the individual. A clinician can do several things to reduce the likelihood of ordering inappropriate and costly items of equipment that will not be used. An open discussion with the patient, and if appropriate, the caregiver, furnishes an opportunity to explore attitudes, uncover fears, and provide education about the pros and cons of specific equipment use. Giving the person an opportunity to use equipment, make choices, and provide feedback during the decision-making phase brings that individual into an active role. The more active the patient is in the identification of benefits, drawbacks, uses, and limitations of equipment, the more likely he or she is to feel comfortable with the ultimate choice.

The members of the rehabilitation team can make recommendations for home, school, or work modifications to improve accessibility. It is helpful for team members involved in decision making to visit the sites with the patient to determine actual needs. It is also important that the patient play an active role in the problem-solving process since he or she will ultimately be the one living with, working, and using the equipment. Clinicians must remain current on the latest technology available and gain an understanding of the patient's individual life-style and needs. When necessary and possible, the therapist should make a visit to the home. If this is not possible, a detailed drawing with measurements of doorways and pertinent space, such as the bathroom design showing bathtub, sink, and commode distances, should be made available to the therapist. This is critical to ensure that the equipment will be feasible in the actual home environment.

Wheelchairs

A wheelchair is necessary when full-time walking is not a goal. As a result of technological advances in wheelchair design and wheelchair components, the selection of the most appropriate chair requires knowledge, expertise, and careful study. Wheelchairs vary in price from low-end economy chairs to extremely high-tech, high-priced models. In the era of third-party payment, the therapist must be able to justify the need for the specific chair chosen and its components. The following is a general discussion of the various types of wheelchairs available on the market today.

A manual wheelchair requires the patient to provide the motive power by pushing on the rims of the wheels. If the person does not have good grip strength, the rims can be plastic-coated to increase the friction and substitute for the patient's lack of grip. The type of wheelchair found in general hospitals or pharmacies is inappropriate for most persons with an SCI. It is critical to this population that a chair be lightweight, have a low center of gravity, have maneuverability, and be easily transported in a vehicle. A standard hospital wheelchair may weigh between 45 and 55 lbs, while the ultralight models can weigh as little as 17 lbs. The increase in price to obtain a lightweight chair is justified when potential trauma to the shoulder joint exists from repeated lifting of the wheelchair and full-time propulsion is considered. In addition, the low center of gravity and high maneuverability of these chairs allows the person to handle most architectural barriers with lower energy expenditure than needed in a standard-weight chair.

Power wheelchairs vary from a manual wheelchair with an add-on motor to a computer-operated chair controlled by breath or voice. Owing to the need for continued maintenance of parts for repair and upkeep, a patient must have resources for long-term equipment support. Only the necessary components should be ordered. These include power recline systems that enable the person to obtain ischial pressure relief independently, custom seating systems for maintenance of proper positioning, and environmental control systems that allow independent action in specific surrounds. The most sophisticated and expensive wheelchairs are required by those who are ventilator dependent. The physical limitations in mobility necessitate intricate power-activation methods such as head, breath, or tongue control switches.

Another consideration in selecting the appropriate wheelchair is the ability of the patient to transport the chair. Some models of power wheelchairs weigh more than 350 lbs and are not transported easily without a van and lift or ramp accommodation. Other power models are designed for easier transport, but the patient will require assistance for disassembly, reassembly, loading, and unloading of the chair.

The most important consideration in wheelchair prescription is the functional capability the chair provides. Having a power wheelchair may enable a person with a high-level lesion to return to work. When prescribing a wheelchair all the factors listed previously—injury level, physical requirements, resources for upkeep, and transportability—must be weighed to provide the patient with the most appropriate wheelchair.

Wheelchair Cushions

Of equal importance to the wheelchair is the wheelchair cushion. Skin breakdown over the ischial tuberosities, coccyx, greater trochanter, or sacrum is a frequent cause of rehospitalization in this population. The proper cushion is an important component in the prevention of this totally unnecessary and costly complication. A large variety and price range of cushions are available. Materials also vary. Cushions may be made of foam, air, gel, or other substances. They are available off the shelf or can be customized to provide pressure relief.

Capillary occlusion and tissue necrosis result from 13 to 34 mm of unrelieved pressure. The cushion should serve to prevent the person from bearing excessive weight on the bony prominences through one of two means: total relief of all contact over the high-risk areas, or dispersion of weight over a wider area via total contact with the buttocks and lower extremities. Worn and ineffective cushions must be replaced on a regular basis. Outpatient services should be provided to maintain proper seating throughout the patient's life span. An individual's needs will vary with functional, health, and age-related changes.

Bathroom Equipment

The first and most important bathroom accessory is the padded commode. If the patient is unable to assist in any aspect of the bowel program, or does not have the trunk balance to sit on a toilet, a commode chair should be considered. Many of the models available commercially can be wheeled directly over the toilet and provide more balance support than a toilet alone. While the bowel program can be carried out in bed, the upright position allows gravity to aid in elimina-

can operate a computer. These include using mouth-sticks or other pointing devices on a keyboard, head movement to control the cursor on the screen with an on-screen keyboard, a pneumatic sip-and-puff switch to operate a computer with Morse code or a scanning array, or even voice input. For more detailed information about computer access, a book written specifically for persons with SCI is available from the Bay Areas and Western Paralyzed Veterans' Administration, 3801 Miranda Ave., Palo Alto, CA 94304.[30]

Environmental control units (ECUs) have also had a great impact on the independence of persons with tetraplegia. ECUs allow control of lights, appliances, and other electrical devices when the usual method of operation is difficult or impossible. By pressing a button or switch, or giving voice commands, a person has the ability to answer the telephone, unlock and open a door, change the TV channel, turn a light on and off, activate a call alarm, and much more. Many benefit from simple adaptations and low-cost ECUs. Others may need more sophisticated and complex ECUs.

As technology advances, the number of possible solutions to meet the needs of patients with disabilities increases. These range from low cost–low tech solutions to more sophisticated and complex high tech solutions with their associated higher costs. Multiple technology needs are best met by an interdisciplinary team specializing in assistive technology, including the client and care providers. An evaluation is conducted to determine solutions that will best meet the individual's needs and abilities, and the constraints of costs and environments in which the technology is to be used. When technological recommendations are made, they must be compatible with other equipment used to assist the individual in the performance of necessary and desired activities within his or her environment(s). For example, the technology now exists to operate a power wheelchair, communication device, computer, and ECU with the same power wheelchair controller, the whole a neat and aesthetically pleasing package. Even though this technology exists it may or may not be the most beneficial solution for a particular patient. A team approach is needed to determine if it would actually be beneficial for mobility, communication, and other functional needs.

Some functional use of the upper extremities can be seen in the C4 tetraplegic with some C5 root escape. While for most patients at this functional level, driving a wheelchair with hand controls may be the highest functional goal, stronger patients may be able to engage in light self-care and selected tabletop activities. With deltoid and biceps strength of 2− or better, and with maximum assistance in setting up an activity, the tetraplegic patient may be able to feed, brush teeth, wash the face, shave, and write, type, and perform other desktop activities. These tasks are accomplished with the aid of orthoses. To support the weight of the arm and to enhance proximal strength, a mobile arm support (MAS) is fitted. This excellent mechanical device, which is also called a ball-bearing feeder, "supports the weight of the arm and provides assistance to

shoulder and elbow motions through a linkage of ball-bearing joints."[52]

To achieve prehension, the person with C4 tetraplegia with weak C5 muscles (deltoids and biceps, 2− to 3) requires an additional orthosis because of lack of wrist or hand function. The universal cuff, also known as the utensil holder, is the most common device used for feeding. This cuff fits around the palm of the hand and has a pocket for inserting utensils. To change from feeding to another activity, the patient or an aide changes the tool inserted into the pocket. Other activities which can be achieved with a universal cuff include brushing teeth and performing light hygiene and grooming. The universal cuff is very light and therefore appropriate for patients who have weak deltoids and biceps strength of 2− to 3. Although it is inexpensive and easy to fabricate, it lacks versatility. A more versatile and durable functional metal orthosis is the ratchet wrist-hand orthosis, a mechanical device which enables a person with wrist and hand paralysis to manipulate objects. The ratchet WHO is positioned on the forearm, wrist, thumb, index, and middle fingers. To pick up an object, orthosis closure is achieved by manual pressure on the fingerpieces to approximate the thumb. To release objects, a button is pressed. The ratchet, although versatile and durable, is expensive, heavy, and more noticeable on the patient's hand than the universal cuff.

The patient should experiment with all available orthoses. The therapist assists the patient in selecting the best orthosis to meet his or her functional needs. Thorough training is critical for the patient to derive maximal functional benefit from orthoses. (Orthosis training is discussed later in this chapter.)

Some patients with weak C5 muscles benefit from combining the upper extremity orthosis and a mouthstick. This is especially advantageous when one arm is too weak to assist the more functional upper extremity. In this case, the mouthstick is used to stabilize objects (Fig. 34–4).

To achieve optimal functioning, all working muscles must be strengthened. To increase strength and endurance, the patient participates in a routine strengthening

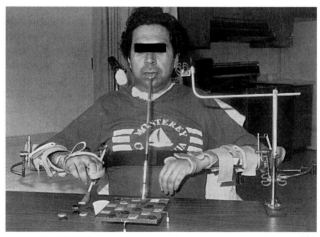

Figure 34–4 ═ A patient participating in occupational therapy using mobile arm supports, upper extremity orthoses, and a mouthstick.

program. Proximal muscles of 2– or 3 strength are exercised on a skateboard table by placing the arm on a skateboard, thus eliminating the effect of gravity and reducing resistance to movement. Weights are gradually added as muscles gain strength. Therapeutic activities that offer repetitive resistive motion, such as sanding or copper tooling, are used to build endurance and improve upper extremity control.

To prepare patients for return to home and community, a home visit is crucial in assuring barrier-free and safe accessibility. Locating and preparing surfaces to house routine equipment such as a computer and mouthstick docking stations eliminate the need for assistance in setting up, thereby providing the patient with greater independence. Training in the community will teach the patient to utilize new skills in real situations and to learn to solve problems as they arise.

The expected functional goals of high-level tetraplegic patients are limited. Thus, a critical element in their rehabilitation process involves enhancing independence through the use of attendants and community resources. Group discussions are designed to enable patients to feel confident in exercising control over their environment. Since all tetraplegic patients with high-level injuries require attendant care, special emphasis is placed on education in the use of attendants. Discussions focus on hiring, training, and optimally utilizing the limited time they may have with their attendants. Assertiveness training in which patients role-play realistic scenarios helps them to focus on effective communication as a means of gaining control of their lives. Other group discussions cover subjects such as returning to school and work, and pursuing leisure activities.

The vocational opportunities of the high-level tetraplegic have expanded markedly with the advent of computer technology. The tetraplegic patient can execute all business activities such as networking, directing employees, and managing office work with an adapted computer terminal. These technological advances are of special significance to a person with tetraplegia who either must or chooses to be homebound, as it enables him or her to work at home. The occupational therapist explores with the patient his or her interests as well as vocational aptitudes. The therapist provides the patient with a simulated work setting in which the patient can become aware of capabilities and limitations. All prevocational data are given both to the patient and to a department of vocational rehabilitation counselor to further prepare the patient for work and to aid in vocational placement. It must be noted, however, that only a few high tetraplegics are able to work. Most lack the education, resources, and the appropriate environment to become employed.

Treatment of Tetraplegics with Lower Cervical Injuries (C5–8)

Persons with tetraplegia functioning at the C5 level (deltoids and biceps 3+ or above and intact pain sensation) may be able independently to don and doff their orthoses. Following assistance in setup, they are able to feed, brush their teeth, wash their face, apply makeup, shave, and comb their hair. In addition, they are expected to be able to write, type, and execute more complex desktop vocational and leisure activities. C5 tetraplegics may also be able to drive a specially equipped van independently (see Appendix E).

To reach these goals, upper extremity management must first be addressed. As with high-level tetraplegics, upper extremity deformity, edema, and pain must be prevented and managed. Functional joint ROM is maintained through bed and wheelchair positioning, daily exercises, and educating the patient and caregivers. While the patient is lying in bed, emphasis is placed on avoiding direct pressure on the glenohumeral joint and on maintaining shoulder external rotation. C5 tetraplegics may develop elbow flexion and forearm supination contractures due to unopposed biceps activity. To avoid such deformities, the elbow must be maintained in extension and the forearm in full pronation. If limitations develop, serial casting with long arm casts is most effective.

As with high-level tetraplegic patients, to maintain the functional position of the hand, the hand and forearm are initially placed in a prefabricated temporary splint, which is later replaced with a custom-made WHO.

Strengthening of the upper extremities begins as soon as the patient's neck is stabilized. Strict precautions are taken to protect the spine from further damage. For the first 4 weeks following neck stabilization with a halo vest, shoulder and elbow exercises are only performed bilaterally with minimal resistance.

With these precautions in mind, it is recommended that strengthening begin as soon after the injury as possible. With the aid of an overhead frame and springs and slings, the patient can begin upper extremity active assistive exercises while still in bed. Neuromuscular electric stimulation (NMES), an electric current which brings about muscle excitation and induces motor response, provides for additional muscle activation when the patient is lying in bed.[5] In the wheelchair, strengthening is achieved through the use of orthotic devices and weights, as well as through therapeutic and functional activities.

The MAS is often used during the initial period following bed rest to support the arms and enhance proximal shoulder movement. The MAS assists patients whose deltoid strength is 2– or better to achieve shoulder flexion, thus enabling them to increase strength and endurance through repetitive motion. Additionally, it allows them to perform functional activities involving the head, such as feeding, hygiene, and grooming. When deltoids and biceps develop 3+ or better strength and when endurance improves, the MAS is no longer needed.

Strengthening is also achieved by a program of progressive exercises which begins with active assistive exercises through the use of the MAS and skateboards. Next, active exercises are performed against gravity. To further strengthen muscles, mechanical resistance is applied through the use of weights and exercise ma-

Capen D, Zigler J, Garland D: Surgical stabilization in cervical spine trauma. Contemp Orthop 14:25–32, 1987.

Cerny K: Energetics of walking and wheelchair propulsion in paraplegic patients. Orthop Clin North Am 9:370–372, 1978.

Ducker TB, Bellegarrigue R, Saleman M, et al: Timing of operative care in cervical spinal cord injury. Spine 9:525–531, 1984.

Fine PR, Kuhlemeier KV, De Vivo MJ, et al: Spinal cord injury: An epidemiologic perspective. Paraplegia 17:237–250, 1979.

Fishman S, et al: Lower-limb orthotics. *In* American Academy of Orthopaedic Surgeons: Atlas of Orthotics. St Louis, Mosby–Year Book, 1985.

Freehafer A: Orthotics in spinal cord injury. *In* American Academy of Orthopaedic Surgeons: Atlas of Orthotics. St Louis, Mosby–Year Book, 1985.

Garfin SR, Shackford SR, Marshall LF, et al: Care of the multiply injured patient with cervical spine injury. Clin Orthop 239:19–29, 1989.

Garland DE, Lilling M, Keenan MA: Percutaneous phenol blocks to motor points or spastic forearm muscles in head-injured adults. Arch Phys Med Rehabil 68:243–245, 1984.

Garland DE, Lucie RS, Waters RL: Current uses of open phenol nerve block for adult acquired spasticity. Clin Orthop 165:217–222, 1982.

Green BA, Callahan RA, Klose KJ, et al: Acute spinal cord injury: current concepts. Clin Orthop 154:125–135, 1981.

Guttman L: Spinal Cord Injuries. Comprehensive Management and Research. Oxford, Blackwell Scientific, 1973, pp 122–157.

Hill JP: Spinal Cord Injury: A Guide to Functional Outcomes in Occupational Therapy. Rockville, Md, Aspen, 1986.

Kaye JJ, Nance EP Jr: Cervical spine trauma. Orthop Clin North Am 21:449–462, 1990.

Kübler-Ross E: On Death and Dying. New York, Collier, 1993.

Parsons T: The Social System. Glencoe, Ill, Free Press, 1951.

Perry J: Gait Analysis: Normal and Pathologic Function. Thorofare, NJ, Slack 1992.

Rizzolo SJ, Cotler JM: Unstable cervical spine injuries: Specific treatment approaches. J Am Acad Orthop Surg 1:57–66, 1993.

Scott BA: Engineering principles and fabrication techniques for the Scott-Craig long leg brace for paraplegics. Orthot Prosthet 25:14.

Sie IH, Waters RL, Adkins RH, et al: Upper extremity pain in the postrehabilitation spinal cord injured patient. Arch Phys Med Rehabil 73:44–48, 1992.

Sontang VK, Douglas RA: Management of cervical spinal cord trauma. J Neurotrauma 9 (suppl 1):S385–S396, 1992.

Stover SL, DeLisa JA, Whiteneck GG: Spinal Cord Injury: Clinical Outcomes from the Model Systems. Gaithersburg, Md: Aspen, 1995.

Stover SL, Fine PR: The epidemiology and economics of spinal cord injury. Paraplegia 25:225–228, 1987.

Verran, AG, Baumgarten, JM, Paris K: Occupational therapy management of tendon transfers in persons with spinal cord injury quadriplegia. Occup Ther Health Care 4:155–169, 1987.

Waters R, Moore KR, Graboff S, et al: The brachioradialis to flexor pollicis longus tendon transfer for active lateral pinch in the quadriplegic. J Hand Surg [AM] 10:385–393, 1985.

Waters RL, Sie IH, Adkins RH: Rehabilitation of the patient with spinal cord injury. Orthop Clin North Am 26:117–122, 1995.

Waters RL, Sie IH, Adkins RH, et al: Motor recovery following spinal cord injury caused by stab wounds: A multicenter study. Paraplegia 33:98–101, 1995.

Waters RL, Sie I, Gellman H, et al: Functional hand surgery following tetraplegia. Arch Phys Med Rehabil 76:440–443, 1995.

Waters RL, Yakura JS, Adkins RH, et al: Effect of injury pattern on motor recovery following traumatic SCI. Arch Phys Med Rehabil 77:86–94, 1996.

White AA, Southwick WO, Panjabi MM: Clinical instability in the lower cervical spine: A review of past and current concepts. Spine 1:15–27, 1976.

Whiteneck G, Adler C, Corter E, et al: The Management of High Quadriplegia. New York, Demos, 1989.

Whiteneck G, Charlifue SW, Gerhart KA, et al: Aging with Spinal Injury. New York, Demos, 1993.

Williamson GG: Children with Spina Bifida—Early Intervention and Preschool Programming. Baltimore, Brookes, 1987.

Zeydlik CP Management of Spinal Cord Injury, ed 2. Boston, Jones & Bartlett, 1992.

Zigler J, Capen D: Management of unstable cervical spine injuries. Complications Orthop July/August 124–128, 1989.

Zigler J, Waters R, Capen D, et al: Posterior cervical fusion under local anesthesia. Spine 12:206–208, 1987.

STANDARD NEUROLOGICAL CLASSIFICATION OF SPINAL CORD INJURY

TREATMENT GUIDELINES FOR PATIENTS WITH QUADRIPLEGIA

These are treatment guidelines only. Alterations in the program may be initiated with physician approval. The dates given below are approximate and the program depends on the medical and physical status of the patient. Pain, decreases in muscle strength, or sensory changes are indications to modify the patient program. Treatment should be initiated only in those patients with stable spines. Patients with gunshot wounds (GSWs) generally have spinal stability; however, this must be confirmed by radiograph. Once stability is confirmed, patients with GSWs may be on an unrestricted program.

Patients with unstable spines or requiring uncommon procedures are progressed on an individual basis. Common procedures are anterior spinal decompression (ASD) with discectomy or corpectomy and posterior spinal fusion (PSF) with wires.

TIME	ORTHOPAEDIC TREATMENT	PROGRAM	CONSIDERATIONS/PRECAUTIONS
Onset or first 3 weeks postoperatively	Radiographs: AP and lateral neck in flexion and extension to determine stability Patient in halo or hard collar Hard collar to remain on at all times	• 3-person turn • Wheelchair (W/C) tolerance • Self-raises • Upper extremity (UE) resistive exercises, bilaterally • Light unilateral UE activities, ie, self-feeding and light hygiene • Light tabletop activities • UE ROM exercises—easy available exercises • Neck strengthening—isometric, symmetrical only • Respiratory program • Dependent sliding board transfers • W/C propulsion • Lower extremity (LE) ROM exercises • Walking only if safe and able without UE aids	Stability MUST be confirmed by physician prior to upright activities All postoperative patients must avoid neck extension and rotation; patients with PSF should avoid neck flexion Minimal resistance only to shoulders during manual muscle testing No reciprocal activities Logroll before stabilization and when patient is out of collar UE resistive exercises, unilaterally, for elbows, wrists, fingers
3–6 weeks	Radiographs: not needed to progress program	• 2-person turn • UE resistive exercises, unilaterally • UE reciprocal pulleys • UE ROM exercises—no limitations • Manual muscle testing—no limitations • Neck strengthening—isometric, unilateral • Assisted sliding board transfers • Active sitting balance • Walking with UE aids for balance only • UE self-ROM exercises bilaterally	Avoid head, neck, and trunk rotation during activities—allow straight depression only Maintain head in neutral
6–12 weeks	**ASD** Radiographs: AP and lateral neck Hard collar to remain on at all times	**ASD** • Turn with patient assist as able • Prone • Pedestal bath with one side of collar on • UE dressing • UE self-ROM exercises • Driver training	**ASD** No change
	PSF Radiographs: AP and lateral neck in flexion and extension to determine stability D/C hard collar if stable Soft collar as needed for patient comfort	**PSF** • Turn with patient assist as able • Prone • Self-bowel program • Self-intermittent catheterization and self-application of external catheter • Self-positioning • Dressing • UE self-ROM exercises • Driving • Home and community skills • Bathing • Neck strengthening—isotonic • All mat activities	**PSF** Program begun only after patient is determined to be stable and hard collar is removed If patient is unstable and hard collar is continued, advance program only as stated for ASD

TIME	ORTHOPAEDIC TREATMENT	PROGRAM	CONSIDERATIONS/PRECAUTIONS
		• LE self-ROM exercises • Independent transfers W/C into car • Advanced W/C skills • Walking with UE aids as needed	
	ASD	**ASD**	**ASD**
12 weeks	Radiographs: AP and lateral neck in flexion and extension to determine stability D/C hard collar if stable	• Refer to PSF 6–12 wk for program	Program begun only after patient is determined to be stable and hard collar is removed

From Rancho Los Amigos Medical Center, spinal injury service, physical therapy, occupational therapy, and nursing departments.

TREATMENT GUIDELINES FOR PATIENTS WITH PARAPLEGIA

These are treatment guidelines only. Alterations in the program may be initiated with physician approval. The dates given below are approximate and the program depends on the medical and physical status of the patient. Pain, decreases in muscle strength, or sensory changes are indications to modify the patient program. Treatment should be initiated only in those patients with stable spines. Patients with gunshot wounds (GSWs) generally have spinal stability; however, this must be confirmed by radiograph. Once stability is confirmed, patients with GSWs may be placed on an unrestricted program.

Patients with unstable spines or requiring uncommon procedures are progressed on an individual basis. Common procedures are posterior spinal fusion (PSF) with rods and anterior decompression with spinal fusion (ASF). PSF may be with or without sublaminar wires.

TIME	ORTHOPAEDIC TREATMENT	PROGRAM	CONSIDERATIONS/PRECAUTIONS
Phase 1 (onset or first 3 wk postoperatively)	Radiographs: AP and lateral spine to determine stability T1–2 fracture (fx): body jacket (BJ) with neck ring T3–4 fx: BJ with shoulder straps T5 fx and below: BJ only	• 2-person turn • Wheelchair (W/C) tolerance • Self-raise • T4 fx and above: upper extremity (UE) resistive exercises bilaterally • T5 fx and below: unrestricted UE activity • Respiratory program • W/C propulsion • Dependent sliding board transfers • L2 fx and above: unrestricted lower extremity (LE) ROM exercises except when hooks are below fx • L3 fx and below or when hooks are used at L3, L4, or L5: hip flexion limited to 90 degrees • UE dressing with BJ	Stability MUST be confirmed by physician prior to upright activities All postoperative patients must avoid back extension and rotation No resistance to trunk and hips during manual muscle testing Logroll before stabilization and when patient is out of BJ
Phase 2 (3–6 wk)	Radiographs: AP and lateral spine 1. CD instrumentation 2. Harrington rods with segmental wires Begin guidelines at 3–6 wk	• Prone • Males: self-application of external catheter side-lying or upright with BJ and self-intermittent catheterization (IC) • UE dressing, LE dress, bathing with BJ • LE resistive exercises, bilaterally • Hamstring stretch • Abdominal and back strengthening—isometric, symmetrical only • Straight depression transfers—assisted with legs • Walking with UE aids for balance only • Active sitting balance activities • Advanced W/C skills if no BJ	Minimal resistance only to trunk and hips during manual muscle testing Avoid excessive torque
Phase 3 (6–12 wk)	Radiographs not needed to progress program	• Turn with patient assistance • Self-bowel program in BJ • Pedestal bath with back of BJ on • LE dressing in BJ • UE activities—unrestricted for all levels of injury including power building • Independent transfers to bed, toilet, and car • LE resistive exercises, unilaterally • Self-ROM exercises • Walking with UE aids as needed • Manual muscle testing—no limitations	No change
Phase 4 (12 wk)	Radiographs: AP and lateral spine in flexion and extension to determine stability Discontinue orthosis if stable	• Unrestricted program • Self-positioning and prone • Self–skin inspection • Self IC—females • Abdominal and back strengthening—isotonic	Program begun only after patient is determined to be stable and orthosis is removed

TIME	ORTHOPAEDIC TREATMENT	PROGRAM	CONSIDERATIONS/PRECAUTIONS
		• All mat activities • All advanced transfers • All advanced W/C skills	

From Rancho Los Amigos Medical Center, spinal injury service, physical therapy, occupational therapy, and nursing departments.

APPENDIX 34-4

FUNCTIONAL GOALS FOR PATIENTS WITH COMPLETE SPINAL CORD INJURY (CONSIDER AGE, SEX, WEIGHT, BODY TYPE, MOTIVATION)

	QUADRIPLEGICS				PARAPLEGICS			
	C1–C4 Neck UPPR Trapezius	C5 Deltoids Biceps	C6 Wrist Extensors	C7–8 Triceps Weak Hand	T1–8 Chest Extension	T9–12 Trunk Extension	L1–2 Hip Extensors	L3–5 Knee Extensors
Relief of skin pressure								
(I) With electric recliner	x	x						
(I) Forward loop or lean		*	*	*				
(I) Depression raises			x	x	x	x	x	x
Wheelchair Propulsion								
Electric	x	*	*	*				
Manual with projection rims		*	*	*				
Manual with friction rims			x	*				
Manual with standard rims			*	x	x	x	x	x
Bed Transfers								
Mechanical/manual lift	x	*						
(A) Sliding board		x	*					
(I) Sliding board			x	*				
(I) Depression			*	x	x	x	x	x
Car Transfers								
Mechanical lift/dependent	x	x	*					
(A) Sliding board		*	*	*	*			
(I) Sliding board			x	*				
(I) Depression			*	x	x	x	x	x
Toilet Transfers								
Mechanical lift to commode	x							

(A) Sliding board to commode	*	*	*				
(I) Sliding board to raised seat		x	x				
(I) Depression to raised seat		*	*	x	x	x	x
Tub Transfers							
(A) Sliding board to tub bench		*	*				
(I) Sliding board to tub bench		x	x				
(I) Depression to tub bench		*	*	x	x	x	x
(I) To bottom of tub					*	*	*
Cough							
Dependent manual	x	x					
Self-manual	*	x	*	*			
Independent		x	x	x	x	x	x
Curb Management							
(I) 2-in. curbs		*	*				
(I) 4- and 6-in. curbs		*	*	x	x	x	x
Wheelchair into Car							
(A) Dependent/unable		*	*				
(I) With loop on wheelchair		*	*				
Independent		x	x	x	x	x	x
Ambulation							
Physiologic		*	*	*	*	*	x
Household						x	
Limited community						*	x
Community						*	x

FUNCTIONAL GOALS FOR PATIENTS WITH QUADRIPLEGIA (CONSIDER AGE, SEX, WEIGHT, BODY TYPE, MOTIVATION)

FUNCTIONAL LEVEL* OF KEY MUSCLES† (MMT GRADE)	WHEELCHAIR	FEEDING	HYGIENE AND GROOMING	BOWEL AND BLADDER CARE	DRESSING SKILLS	DESKTOP	HOME SKILLS	DRIVING
C4 Neck accessories *Diaphragm* *Trapezius*	Electric with chin control	*Dependent*	*Dependent*	*Dependent*	*Dependent*	*Assisted with equipment*	*Dependent*	*Dependent*
C4 with weak C5 muscles Muscles above and *Deltoids* (P-/2-F/3) *Biceps* (P-/2-F/3)	Electric with hand control and MAS*	*Assisted with equipment*	*Assisted with equipment*	*Dependent*	*Dependent*	*Assisted with equipment*	*Dependent*	*Dependent*
	Note that key muscles' strength for this functional level is P-/2-F/3 (below F+).							
C5 Muscles above and *Deltoids Biceps*	Electric with hand control	*Assisted with equipment*	*Assisted with equipment*	*Dependent*	*Dependent*	*Assisted with equipment*	*Dependent*	*Independent* Van with lift and sensitized controls

Level	Manual							
C6 Muscles above and *Wrist extensors* *Clavicular Pectoralis* *Serratus anterior* Other important muscle: Pronator Teres	*Manual*	*Independent* May require equipment	*Independent* May require equipment	*Assisted-independent* with equipment	*Independent* Upper body *Assisted-independent* Lower body	*Independent* May require equipment	*Independent* Light *Assisted* Heavy	*Independent* Hand controls *Dependent* Wheelchair loading
C7 Muscles above and *Triceps* Other important muscle: Latissimus dorsi	*Manual*	*Independent* May require equipment	*Independent* May require equipment	*Assisted-independent* with equipment	*Independent* Both upper and lower body	*Independent* May require equipment	*Independent* Light *Assisted* Heavy	*Independent* Wheelchair loading Hand controls
C8 Muscles above and *Extrinsic finger flexors*	*Manual*	*Independent*	*Independent*	*Independent*	*Independent*	*Independent*	*Independent*	*Independent* Hand controls
T1 Normal hand muscles above and *Intrinsic finger muscles*	*Manual*	*Independent*	*Independent*	*Independent*	*Independent*	*Independent*	*Independent*	*Independent* Hand controls

MAS, mobile arm support.
* The lowest segment at which muscle strength of key motors is F+ or better and pain sensation is intact.
† A muscle which significantly changes functional outcome (*italic*).
From Rancho Los Amigos Medical Center, occupational therapy department.

CHAPTER 35

Post-traumatic Syringomyelia

Parley W. Madsen III ‖ *Steven Falcone* ‖ *Brian C. Bowen*
Barth A. Green

While cavitation of the spinal cord has been recognized for more than three centuries as a pathologic entity, and although spinal cord cavitation was experimentally produced more than a century ago, considerable controversy regarding the terminology, the pathophysiologic basis, and the optimal treatment for this disorder continues.[2, 47, 48, 94, 121] *Syringomyelia* was defined by the *Oxford English Dictionary* as a "dilatation of the central canal of the spinal cord or formation of abnormal tubular cavities in its substance."[108] The classic clinical feature of syringomyelia was described as segmental dissociative loss of sensory function in the upper extremities which most commonly consisted of the loss of distal sensation to pain and temperature and of the preservation of proprioceptive sensation and light touch.

Although the cervical enlargement was the most frequently involved area, clinical presentation was directly related to the involved spinal segments and the affected areas reported range from the conus to the midbrain. The disorder was described as slowly progressive and ultimately involving the loss of lower motor function. If a syrinx extended to the medulla, the pathologic lesion was termed a *syringobulbia;* compromise of brain stem function has been reported with this lesion. Extension of the more frequently encountered cervical syrinx has been implicated in syringobulbia formation.[2, 144, 162]

In the first monograph on syringomyelia, Schlesinger[134] in 1902 stated that this condition ranks among the commonest of spinal diseases, but S.A.K. Wilson[174] cited admission statistics from the National Hospital during the interval 1909 to 1925 to dispute this claim. There were only 115 cases of syringomyelia identified of the 6846 patients admitted. This group represented only 1.6% of the total admissions; the admissions for each of the following diagnoses were more frequent: tabes, syphilitic paraplegia, multiple sclerosis, subacute combined degeneration, and spinal tumor, but no notation was made of syringomyelia secondary to trauma. Barnett and associates[18] reported that syringomyelia was diagnosed only 75 times out of 535,464 admissions over a 24-year period at the Toronto General Hospital. Poser[121] found only 18 cases of syringomyelia during a review of 1600 autopsies performed at the Neurological Institute of New York over a 20-year period. The discrepancy between the early statistics reported in the German literature and the relatively later reports from England and the United States most likely reflected the slow course of the disorder, with the majority of affected patients dying at home and an autopsy not having been obtained.[174]

The most commonly reported ages of clinical presentation of a symptomatic syrinx of the spinal cord were between the years of 25 and 40. There was a slight predominance of males compared with females. Although syringomyelia had been described as a slowly progressive, degenerative disorder of insidious onset and with periods of quiescence, the natural history of the lesion had been reported to be extremely variable.[2, 5, 48] In 1965, Barnett and associates[18] described the onset of neurologic deterioration of patients who had suffered a serious spinal cord injury years prior to the onset of their subsequent neurologic decline; each patient was found to have a syringomyelic cavity. Since this initial description, syringomyelia has been seen with increasing frequency for a variety of reasons, including improved noninvasive diagnostic techniques and increased survival of spinal cord–injured patients.[68]

Cavitation of the gray matter of the spinal cord adjacent to or directly involving the central canal, and an inner layer of gliotic tissue, were the most frequently reported pathologic features of syringomyelia[156, 161] (Fig. 35–1). Tumors, vascular anomalies, infective processes, and extramedullary compressive lesions have been reported in association with syrinx formation.[28, 32, 161] The presence of these associated pathologic lesions contributed to the lively debate over the pathophysiologic basis of this disorder which has continued to the present day.[143] No consensus has emerged and the existent clinical and experimental data suggested that this disorder was not a single disease entity with a solitary cause. The evidence appeared to be more consistent with the hypothesis that syringomyelia represented a syndrome of similar clinical entities with a diversity of pathologic changes which produced cavitation of the substance of the spinal cord. Adams and Victor[2] employed *syringomyelia* to refer directly to a "central cavitation of the spinal cord of undetermined cause" and *syringomyelic syndrome* to denote "the syndrome of segmental sensory dissociation with brachial amyotrophy.

Treatment of syringomyelia has been dependent upon the practitioner's perception of the underlying pathologic derangement, was often modified for each

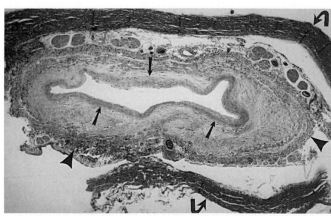

Figure 35–1 = Post-traumatic cord cyst. Low-power (×1.25) microscopic section images of a post-traumatic syringomyelia in a 56-year-old man who died 5 years after an upper thoracic gunshot wound. There is a large centrally located syrinx in the parenchyma of the spinal cord which is surrounded by a thick wall of reactive astrocytes *(arrows)*. The pia is thickened and there are tissue changes which involve the spinal roots *(arrowheads)*. The dura is also thickened *(curved arrows)*.

individual patient, and reflected the practioner's most recent experience. Considerable controversy continued, with no consensus developed regarding the preferred therapy for this disorder. As understanding of the pathophysiologic basis of syrinx formation has evolved, an alteration in therapeutic interventions has occurred to conform to the new information. This process has been impaired, however, by the extremely variable clinical course of patients diagnosed with syringomyelia, which necessitates extended post-treatment follow-up to accurately determine efficacy.[5, 9, 26, 54, 139, 165] Frazier,[51] in 1930, lamented the difficulty in the objective analysis of the late results of surgical treatment of syringomyelia because of the variability and complexity of the cases as well as the lack of detail in the reports in the clinical literature. Aschoff and colleagues,[9] in 1994, reported that although more than 3000 operations had been reported for the treatment of syringes, there continued to be no optimal treatment for this disorder because of the variability in the types of syringes, multiple procedures on individual cases, and the lack of long-term follow-up.

The diagnosis of syringomyelia was a formidable task even as recently as the last two decades because there were no acceptable clinical or radiologic criteria for the disorder.[38] Diagnostic techniques employed before the advent of clinically useful computed tomography (CT) and magnetic resonance imaging (MRI) were unreliable and exposed the patient to a significant risk of morbidity. Fortunately, one no longer must perform pneumoencephalography in the operating suite with the patient prepared to undergo emergent ventriculostomy or craniotomy.[59, 64] Newer MRI techniques promised to facilitate the diagnosis of syringomyelia (Fig. 35–2) and to elucidate the pathophysiologic basis of its formation and progression.[4, 43, 73, 142]

HISTORY

Syringomyelia, or cavitation within the substance of the spinal cord, has been recognized for more than three centuries as a pathologic entity. Finlayson[48] credited Etienne in 1564 with the first published description of the disorder, in *La Dissection du corps humain*. The latter author reported a cystic lesion in the spinal cord which contained a "fluid, reddish, like the fluidity of

Figure 35–2 = Post-traumatic cord cyst. A T1-weighted sagittal image *(A)* of the lower thoracic spinal cord and a T1-weighted axial image *(B)* at the C2 level. There is an expansile septated cyst of the spinal cord. The axial image demonstrates the "double barrel" appearance of the cyst. There have been lower thoracic laminectomies *(A, arrows)*.

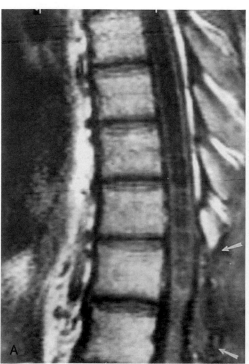
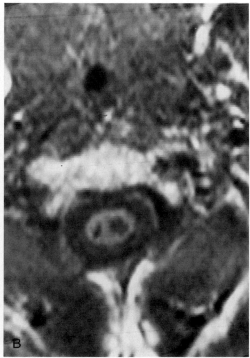

that in the ventricles." Since this initial description, others, including Brunner in 1688, Morgagni in 1740, and Santorini, would publish additional descriptions. Portal, in 1804, was the first to appreciate and report the relationship between clinical signs of motor paralysis and the observed pathologic changes.[174] Two decades later Ollivier conceived the term *syringomyelia*, combining the Greek words *syrinx*, "tube" or "pipe," and *myelos*, "marrow," and applied it to any pathologic cavitation of the substance of the spinal cord, including the persistent central canal.[13, 48, 50]

Tamaki and Lubin,[150] in 1938, credited Bruhl with the first description, during the late 19th century, of sensory dissociation and muscular atrophy with *main en griffe* (clawhand) as being diagnostic of syringomyelia. Schultze in 1887 and Kahler in 1888, also publishing in the German literature, outlined the clinical features of syringomyelia essentially as recognized today. The first American report was by Starr in 1888.[174] Hassin[71] credited Thomas and Quercy with recognizing, in 1913, that syringomyelia was a syndrome of multiple causes. Barnett,[17] in the first English language monograph on syringomyelia published in 1973, proposed a classification based upon a variety of clinical and experimental observations and studies:

1. Communicating syringomyelia (syringo-hydromyelia).
   (a) With associated developmental anomalies at the foramen magnum and of the posterior fossa contents.
   (b) Associated with acquired abnormalities at the skull base.
2. Syringomyelia as a sequel to arachnoiditis confined to the spinal canal.
3. Syringomyelia associated with spinal cord tumors.
4. Syringomyelia as a late sequel to trauma (post-traumatic cystic myelopathy).
5. Idiopathic syringomyelia.

Of these categories, post-traumatic syringomyelia has become the most frequently observed clinical group, but it is difficult to separate this group totally from syringomyelia arising from arachnoiditis as scarring of the meninges is also seen after a traumatic injury[68, 94] (Figs. 35–3 and 35–4). This chapter will consider the historical aspects of efforts to define the pathology and treatment of all types of syringomyelia since efforts directed at the diagnosis and treatment of earlier appreciated types of syringes directly contributed to current understanding of the mechanisms responsible for the formation and therefore to the management of the most recently defined syringes: post-traumatic cystic myelopathy (PTCM). Recent experimental and clinical work, including that by Oldfield and Milhorat and their co-workers, have helped to clarify the pathophysiology and treatment of this syndrome.[101, 102, 104–107, 114]

Pathophysiology of Syringomyelia

The association of syringomyelia and congenital abnormalities was appreciated more than a century ago.

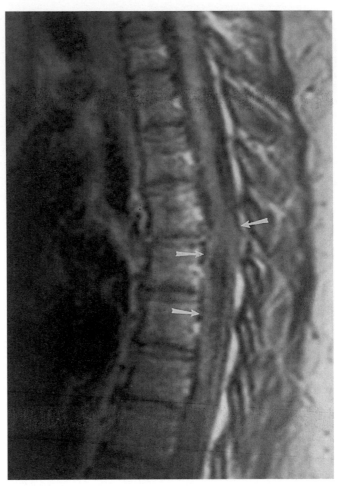

Figure 35–3 = Cystic changes in the post-traumatic cord. Postgadolinium T1-weighted sagittal image demonstrates a kyphotic deformity with apex at T4–5. There is abrupt cord enlargement at T5 and enhancement of the cord surface from T5 to T6–7. At surgery, dural adhesions were identified.

Tamaki and Lubin[150] credited Bäumler in an 1887 paper with establishment of this relationship, and Poser[121] noted that H. Schlesinger (in an 1895 monograph[134]) stated that there was an associated congenital anomaly in fully one third of the cases of syringomyelia he reviewed. MacKay and Favill[90] credited Ollivier d'Angers with the formulation of the developmental theory of syringomyelia formation. Poser[121] cited an 1876 publication by Leyden in which syringomyelia was considered a congenital disorder. The latter believed the syrinx was a result of incomplete occlusion of the primitive fold.

However, the developmental theory was largely ignored until an 1894 report by Gerlach of a teratoma associated with a syrinx and a very similar case reported by Bielschowsky in 1920 revived enthusiasm for the hypothesis. Proponents of this theory argued that improper fusion of the two folds of the primitive medullary groove allowed the groove to become lined with germinal cells and simple hydromyelia was the result. A more significant malformation of the median dorsal septum caused not only proliferation of the glia in the region but resulted in an increase of connective

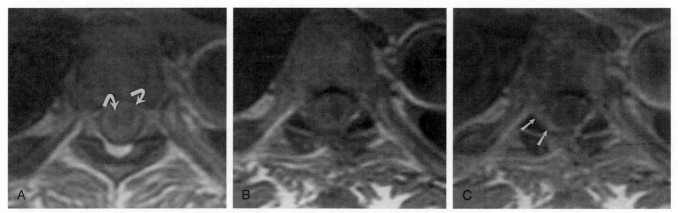

Figure 35–4 = Cystic changes in the post-traumatic cord in the same patient as in Figure 35–3. Preoperative *(A)* and postoperative *(B)* T1-weighted axial images at the T5–6 level were obtained without gadolinium. In *A*, there are poorly defined intramedullary regions *(curved arrows)* of slightly decreased signal. In *B*, the same regions are more sharply defined, have lower signal, and greater cephalocaudad extent. *C*, The postoperative and post-gadolinium T1-weighted image demonstrates linear enhancement *(arrows)* consistent with scarring and probable recurrence of adhesions postoperatively.

tissue in the lining of the cavity. Inclusion of mesodermal tissue trapped during the defective closure was thought to be the causal element; this resulted in the proliferation of blood vessels in the adjacent spinal cord substance. The cases of teratoma reported by Gerlach and Bielschowsky represented the worst-case scenarios according to this theory.[90] Kahler and Pick in 1879 theorized that the aberrant development of the spinal cord which led to syrinx formation was the result of intrauterine chronic inflammation with resultant gliosis.[121]

Haener in 1910 speculated that birth trauma may have aroused neural activity in the abnormally enclosed tissue with resultant syrinx formation, while Oppenheim in 1920 denied the need for a triggering mechanism and stated that this proliferation may occur spontaneously.[121] Hassin[71] argued forcefully that although the patient who developed syringomyelia had a congenital lesion, the lesion was a developmental defect of the glia cells. He termed this defect an "abiotrophy" which caused the glial tissue to break down and the abnormal glial tissue to be separated from the substance of the cord by a connective tissue reaction. Netsky[110] postulated that congenital vascular anomalies were the pathophysiologic basis for syrinx formation. These abnormal vessels become occluded with aging, and the resultant ischemic tissue damage provided the initial cavitation. Reactive gliosis and connective tissue proliferation completed the syrinx formation and caused any observed extension of the mature cavitary lesion.

Chiari, in 1896, published an addition to an earlier (1891) work in which he described anomalies associated with congenital hydrocephalus; included in the latter publication were a number of patients with hydromyelia.[81] Turnbull[153] and Russell and Donald[130] noted the association between hydromyelia and the Chiari malformation, and Gardner and Goodall[64] found that 13 of 17 patients undergoing operation for symptomatic Arnold-Chiari malformation had a concurrent syringomyelia. Gardner and co-workers[59] demonstrated, at operation, communication between the syr-inx of the upper cervical cord and the ventricles in patients undergoing suboccipital craniotomy and cervical laminectomy as treatment for symptomatic Arnold-Chiari malformation. Indigo-carmine was injected into the patient's lateral ventricle via a burr hole craniotomy and then dye-colored fluid was recovered by direct puncture of the cervical syrinx. The authors stated that in their experience "a hydromyelic cyst always communicates with the fourth ventricle by a patent central canal," but acknowledged that this communication was difficult to demonstrate in every case (Figs. 35–5 and 35–6).

In a series of papers, Gardner and co-authors expounded his "hydrodynamic theory" of the pathogenesis of syringomyelia.[55–58, 60, 61, 65] His contention was that syringomyelia resulted from a failure of the embryonic rhombic roof to fenestrate during a critical period of development and Gardner and Angel[61] cited a report by Weed in 1917 of a study conducted on pig embryos as the experimental evidence for this hypothesis. The authors' contention was that the inability of cerebrospinal fluid (CSF) in the fourth ventricle to gain the usual access to the subarachnoid space during the sixth to eighth week of embryogenesis forced the hindbrain through the foramen magnum. A Chiari malformation was thereby created and the failure of the CSF to expand the subarachnoid space also resulted in communicating hydrocephalus. Gardner[57] believed that the effect of the hindbrain malformation was to both increase the obstruction to outflow at the foramen of Magendie and to deflect the pulse wave of CSF described by Bering[22] onto the opening of the central spinal canal at the obex. This action of the CSF gradually either dilated the central canal or dissected the substance of the spinal cord around the canal and formed a syrinx. The experimental and clinical evidence Gardner and Angel cited to support their view of a direct communication from the syrinx to the ventricular system consisted of three important observations[61]:

1. Dye injected into the ventricular system was recovered from the syrinx at operation.[59]

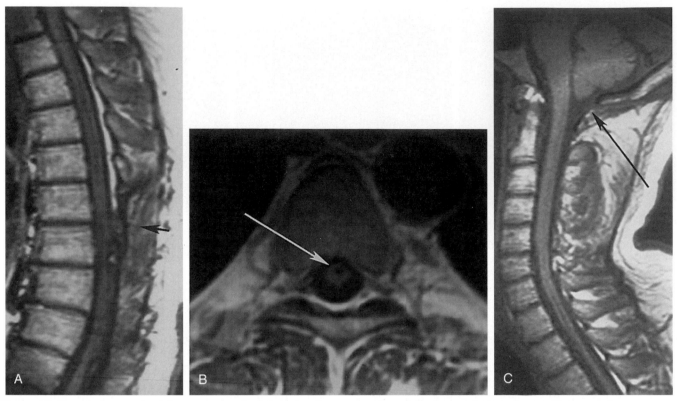

Figure 35–5 = Syringomyelia following removal of thoracic schwannoma. T1-weighted sagittal *(A)* and axial *(B)* images demonstrate an intramedullary cyst which extends cephalad from the laminectomy site at T7 *(arrow)* to the level of C7. The axial image at T6–7 shows the location of the cystic cavity *(arrow)* within the cord. *C,* The T1-weighted sagittal image of the cervical spine demonstrates a normal position for the cerebellar tonsil *(arrow)*.

2. Fluid withdrawn from the syrinx at operation strongly resembled CSF found in the ventricular system.
3. Experimental hydrocephalus produced by obstruction of the normal outflow of CSF from the fourth ventricle resulted in the formation of syringomyelia which was in communication with the ventricular system.[91]

A spinal cord syrinx with a direct connection to the fourth ventricle either via the central canal or through a developmental diverticulum was labeled as "communicating" syringomyelia by Williams in a 1969 publication.[160] However, Gardner and McMurray[65] objected to the use of the term as a "misleading title" which "confuse[d] thinking concerning [this] disease process" because it implied that noncommunicating varieties existed. From their perspective, a congenital hindbrain defect, which obstructed CSF outflow from the fourth ventricle to the subarachnoid space, was the sine qua non of syringomyelia formation; therefore an asymptomatic, congenital anomaly must have existed in all patients who were found to have syringomyelia. This included those cases associated with spinal "arachnoiditis" and trauma. Ellertsson and Greitz[40] were able to demonstrate communication of the syringes with the cerebrospinal spaces after intrathecal injection of fluorescein or of a radioisotope in a series of patients. Others, including West and Williams,[158] and Ball and Dayan,[12] questioned the necessity of a direct

connection to the fourth ventricle for production of a syrinx (see Fig. 35–6A). Milhorat and colleagues[101, 105] demonstrated that the majority of syringes found in a large necropsy series did not communicate with the fourth ventricle and that the central canal was not patent in a majority of normal adult patients reviewed.

Williams[160] proposed an alternative theory to explain syrinx formation and extension, and speculated that a partial block of the spinal subarachnoid space produced a pressure differential between the ventricular system and the spinal subdural space during Valsalva-type maneuvers. He implicated the venous distention associated with these maneuvers as producing an increased intracranial pressure which was not completely distributed to the lumbar subarachnoid space because of the complete or partial block. This pressure difference was labeled craniospinal pressure dissociation, and the lower pressure in the lumbar theca caused fluid to be drawn into the syrinx. This phenomenon was labeled "suck," and the author was able to demonstrate, with simultaneous pressure recordings at the cisterna magna and lumbar subarachnoid space, a particularly prominent effect after a cough or a Valsalva maneuver.[163] This theory was modified and refined in a series of publications after its initial presentation.[138, 139, 158, 160–169] The hypothesis was offered, not to totally obviate the acceptance of that advocated by Gardner, but rather to afford a parsimonious pathophysiologic basis for the development of syringomyelia in patients with either a congenital or acquired foramen magnum

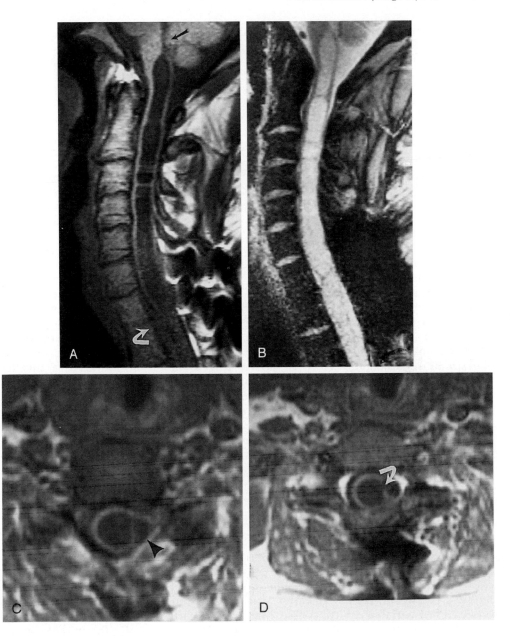

Figure 35–6 = Post-traumatic cord cyst. *A,* A T1-weighted sagittal image of the cervical spine demonstrates a septated syrinx of the spinal cord which extends to the obex *(arrow).* Myelomalacia is seen in the upper thoracic spinal cord *(curved arrow). B,* The gradient echo sagittal image shows the abnormally expanded spinal cord, with increased signal intensity. The septations are less apparent. *C,* The T1-weighted axial image at the C6–7 level demonstrates a fluid loculation *(arrowhead),* which has characteristics of either an extramedullary collection or an intramedullary component of the cyst. *D,* The T1-weighted axial image at C7–T1 more clearly reveals a rent or fissure on the left side of the cord surface communicating with the subarachnoid space *(curved arrow).* Note metallic artifact from prior posterior fusion *(A–D).*

abnormality or a spinal subarachnoid lesion; the latter entity was of importance in the development of post-traumatic syringomyelia.[56]

Williams[162] and Ellertsson and Greitz[41] disagreed with the arterial pulse mechanism proposed by Gardner and Angel[61] to explain extension of the syrinx, especially in the rostral direction, thereby creating syringobulbia. Neither group found evidence for the arterial pulsations in pressure recordings of the syrinx, ventricular, or spinal subarachnoid spaces, and both concluded that venous pressure changes were more important in syringomyelia formation.[168] Williams[162] also felt that the cavity enlarged after its initial formation as the result of several forces, the most important of which was compression of the lower end of the cavity at the rapid filling of the epidural venous plexus during a cough or sneeze. Bertrand[23] also felt that coughing, straining, and postural changes modified the size and extent of syrinxes in the three cases constitut-

ing his report and Williams[166] applied the term "slosh" to this phenomenon as a matter of economy. Martin[98, 99] invoked Laplace's theorem to explain syrinx expansion. Oldfield and associates[114] used MRI with and without cardiac gating, intraoperative ultrasound, and direct intraoperative observation of the exposed hindbrain and documented the downward movement of the cerebellar tonsils during systole. This group interpreted the data collected to obviate the necessity of a direct connection with the fourth ventricle as advocated by Gardner and McMurray[65] and observed that the syringomyelic cord did not enlarge with the Valsalva maneuver unless the subarachnoid space at the hindbrain had been reestablished by a decompressive procedure. The latter observation, coupled with the observation that pulsatile movement of the enlarged cord segment was synchronous with the movement of the cerebellar tonsils and the pulse waves of the abnormal cord ceased when the subarachnoid obstruction was cleared, led to the proposal that venous pressure had little to do with syrinx elongation. The authors proposed that the abnormal pulse waves in the spinal subarachnoid space as a consequence of the partial obstruction by the hindbrain placed "relentless" pressure on the spinal cord and dissected the central canal to cause the cyst to enlarge.

Milhorat and co-workers[107] proposed that normal CSF flow was from the spinal subarachnoid space through the parenchyma of the spinal cord into the central canal. The CSF then flowed into the fourth ventricle outlet at the obex. By injecting kaolin into the central canal of rats, the resulting inflammatory reaction stenosed the proximal central canal and a syrinx was formed. The syrinx was a dilated, yet isolated, segment of the spinal canal. The authors suggested that the disruption of normal CSF flow by the inflammatory stenosis caused the syrinx to form and was a model of syringes associated with the majority of hindbrain malformations which pressed upon the proximal spinal cord obstructing the central canal and blocking communication of the syrinx and the fourth ventricle. Stoodley and associates[148] demonstrated that CSF in the spinal subarachnoid space is rapidly forced into the spinal cord central canal in normal rats and speculated that this one-way flow was a result of arterial pulsations. This work supported the proposal of Milhorat and colleagues[106] that disruption of the central canal outflow could cause an isolated central canal to be dilated into a syrinx without a disruption of the free flow of fluid in the subarachnoid space as proposed by Williams.[166]

Diagnosis of Syringomyelia

Diagnosis of syringomyelia in the late 19th and early 20th centuries was based on clinical presentation and course. This presented a formidable task to the attending physician, as the disorder was of insidious onset and of variable clinical course. Many of the earliest authors would have disputed the statement in a well-known neurology text that the "clinical neurologic picture is so characteristic that diagnosis is seldom in doubt."[2] Netsky[110] commented that at the onset of symptoms, a syrinx may be particularly difficult to diagnose, and Finlayson[48] stated that intramedullary neoplasms were the most troublesome to differentiate from a syringomyelic process. A careful interview and thorough examination of the patient have been, and will continue to be, the initial and most informative elements of any investigation of a patient. Adams and Victor[2] emphasized the existence of certain clinical features of syringomyelia and stated that "the clinical diagnosis can hardly be made without them. These features are segmental weakness and atrophy of the hands and arms with loss of tendon reflexes and segmental anesthesia of the dissociated type." Honan and Williams[75] were able to find dissociated sensory loss in only 49% of the patients with documented syringomyelia and Milhorat and colleagues[101] demonstrated that a significant number of syringes had asymmetrical

involvement of the parenchyma of the spinal cord which could account for this finding.

A lateral radiograph of the upper cervical spine was recommended by Finlayson[48] as an initial ancillary examination to rule out cervical spondylosis and basilar impression of the skull. These conditions have been confused clinically with syringomyelia and have also been reported to coexist with the lesion. Gardner and co-workers[59] employed pneumoencephalography to diagnose syringomyelia and noted that the procedure was done in the operating suite only after preparations for an immediate surgical intervention were completed. This rather dramatically underscores the significance of the risk the diagnostic procedure posed to the patient.

The introduction of myelography allowed the presurgical diagnosis of syringomyelia. With the use of conventional myelography, one could not differentiate a cavitary lesion from an intramedullary tumor or a collapsed lesion from an atrophic cord.[147] Positive contrast myelography was used in the series reported by Foster and Hudgson,[50] and in 14% of the patients with syringomyelia, no evidence of any abnormality could be found with this test. Conway[30] reported that gas myelography was more sensitive in detecting syringomyelia than was contrast myelography. Even though Ellertsson[38, 39] credited gas myelography with being the first significantly useful diagnostic procedure, in his series 4 of 34 patients known to have syringomyelia had a normal gas myelographic study.

Delayed CT following metrizamide myelography was the next significant advance in the radiographic diagnostic technique. Although this test was more sensitive and resulted in less morbidity when compared with earlier techniques, differentiation between a syrinx and an intramedullary tumor remained challenging.[147] Quencer and co-authors[124, 125] demonstrated that percutaneous needle aspiration and endomyelography could be performed safely and that these procedures yielded important diagnostic information in the evaluation of spinal cystic lesions.

By the mid-1980s MRI had assumed the role of the test of choice for the diagnosis of syringomyelia.[120] Although it was both accurate and noninvasive, some intramedullary tumors and areas of myelomalacia were difficult to differentiate from a syrinx.[141] Sherman and co-workers[141] noted a loss of signal in the syrinx thereby lending creditability to Williams's "slosh" theory of cavity extension.[166] Cine MRI has been employed and while the initial experience suggested the possibility of a preoperative determination of the relative benefit of surgical intervention, subsequent clinical experience was not favorable.[122] The introduction of gadolinium-diethylenetriamine pentaacetic acid (Gd-DTPA) decreased the difficulty of differentiation of a syrinx from a tumor.[142] Batzdorf[20] has used MRI to demonstrate a decrease in size of the syrinx postoperatively and this test has been reported as a valuable method of monitoring the effectiveness of surgical decompression.[136] Others have not found a correlation between the postoperative images and clinical outcome.[11, 139]

Treatment of Syringomyelia

Treatment of syringomyelia has been a controversial topic without a universally accepted method of intervention or consensus on the benefit of therapy, and this state has continued to the present time. Wechsler[159] stated "the treatment is symptomatic" and "although syringomyelia may show remissions the prognosis is very unfavorable." S.A.K. Wilson[174] related the use of radiation therapy during his training in 1902 and continued to advocate, in the second edition of his book, the employment of either x-ray or radium radiation before consideration of surgical therapy. Putnam,[123] in a case report, stated that "in every case, as soon as the diagnosis is made, roentgen radiation should be administered," and advocated a "trial" of radiation as a "measure of prevention." This recommendation was voiced despite the acknowledgment that morbidity was associated with radiation therapy and that his personal experience was not as favorable as the 60% improvement reported in the then current medical literature. Wechsler stated that "deep x-ray therapy to the spine at the level of the syrinx may have occasional good effect, if not on the progress, at least on the pains and trophic disturbances."[159] Finlayson[48] related that a total dosage as high as 10,540 rad was recommended. The use of radiation therapy may seem extreme by current treatment standards but was rational therapy for those clinicians who believed disordered gliosis was the underlying pathophysiologic disorder of syringomyelia not associated with an intramedullary neoplasm. The study of Boman and Ilvanainen[26] demonstrated no effect of radiation on the progression of either the signs or symptoms of patients with syringomyelia. Currently, use of radiation therapy should be restricted to the primary therapy or used as an adjunct to surgical excision of a known neoplasm.

The first report of successful surgical therapy of syringomyelia was by Abbe and Coley in 1892.[1] They performed a three-level laminectomy and opened the dura to expose the cyst. The authors described the cord as swollen to twice its normal size by a "lemon"-shaped cystic cavity from which was aspirated a clear fluid. The cyst collapsed with aspiration of the fluid but no CSF escaped upon opening of the dura. This suggested that a subarachnoid block was present, but the authors reported finding only delicate adhesions of the cord to the meninges. This report was significant, not because of any amelioration of the clinical symptoms, but for demonstrating that the spinal cord syrinx could be approached surgically without morbidity. Elsberg[42] recounted his report to the International Congress held in London in 1913, of an operation for drainage of the cystic cavity in cases of syringomyelia via a midline myelotomy. Frazier and Rowe[52] were apparently unaware of these reports when they stated that their case was the first report by an American author. They also performed a laminectomy and, in spite of spontaneous cyst collapse, decided to perform a paramedian myelotomy. Unlike Elsberg, Frazier stented the opening with "a thin strip of the finest percha tissue" in an attempt to maintain patency of the opening to the subarachnoid space.[42, 51] The patient improved neurologically during the convalescent period and the author found "this initial experience with the surgery of syringo-myelia . . . more than pleasing."[51] The author's enthusiasm had not diminished when he presented a review of selected cases of syringomyelia who had several years of postoperative follow-up, even though the patient who was the subject of his previous case report had relapsed. At reoperation, no evidence of the previous myelotomy was initially visible because of dense adhesions. Frazier suggested that the scarring was evidence of the glial proliferation theory and advocated repeated operative intervention when the patient deteriorated. In a later report, however, acknowledgment was made that long-term follow-up was necessary before the effectiveness of a particular treatment could be accessed.[52] Adelstein[3] collected reports of 120 patients who were subjected to laminectomy and myelotomy, and was able to tabulate clinical data on 86 cases. Of these, 65 (76%) were reported improved with 10 patients (12%) declining in neurologic function.[13] Pitts and Groff[119] reported that 67% of patients who underwent laminectomy improved, and Love and Olafson[86] reported 72% of their patients either stabilized or improved. A recent review of the surgical treatment of syringomyelia as reported in the medical literature since the initial reports of Abbe and Cooley established that the reported effectiveness of surgical intervention had not changed with time; more recent series reported the same rates of response to surgery that were reported in the initial 75 cases treated before 1940.[1, 10] Only the mortality rate had decreased from 5% in the initial series to 1% in the most recent report period (1971 to 1989).

Gardner and Angel[60] championed a new approach to the patient with a posterior fossa herniation (Chiari I malformation) based on their theory of syringomyelia formation previously reviewed. The operation advocated was suboccipital craniectomy for decompression of the hernia and closure of the communication between the syrinx and the fourth ventricle by plugging the obex with a piece of muscle. While there have been a number of variations of posterior fossa surgery for decompression of the hindbrain, the necessity or advisability of the use of an obex plug continues to be a matter of controversy.[10, 100, 118] Hoffman and associates[73] presented data that documented an increase in favorable results with use of an obex plug and Pillay and co-workers[118] reported that 182 Gardner procedures had been successfully performed without adverse complication. Sahuquillo and colleagues[131] noted that plugging of the obex has all but been abandoned during the last decade because of increased complications associated with the procedure and a paucity of evidence of therapeutic benefit.

Rhoton[126] also did not plug the obex but rather stented the foramen of Magendie if dense scarring was found and performed a dorsal root entry zone myelotomy in the upper cervical cord. E.B. Schlesinger and associates[133] also reported that plugging of the obex was unnecessary and carried the risk of increased morbidity. They, however, questioned the advisability of cervical myelotomy. Logue and Edwards[85] demonstrated that simple posterior fossa decompression was as effective as the obstruction of the central canal and they argued that clinical improvement following the operation was due to relief of the mechanical compressive effect of the cerebellar tonsils on the medulla. These authors advocated preservation of the arachnoid membrane and the use of syringostomy only if the syrinx did not respond to simple decompression.

Batzdorf[20] outlined an approach to the patient with symptomatic syringomyelia associated with a Chiari I malformation and combined a suboccipital decompression with opening of the foramen of Magendie and a duraplasty to reestablish the subarachnoid path at the skull base. He argued that a plug of the obex was not necessary and potentially blocked a drainage path for the syrinx when the obstruction to CSF flow at the skull base was resolved. Postoperative MRI scan confirmed the drainage of the syringes; the author has now extended his series to more than 20 patients.[21] Included in this series was one patient with coccidioidomycosis meningitis who required a second operation for placement of a shunt. Patients in the 1(a) group of syringomyelia (acquired lesion at the foramen magnum) may not have as favorable a response to suboccipital decompression as the congenital group. The operative mortality in the series reported by Batzdorf[20] was 0% and represented a significant improvement over the 6% reported by Ballantine and associates[13] in a review of operative treatment of syringomyelia. While Batzdorf advocated a limited suboccipital craniectomy to prevent downward herniation of the cerebellar tonsils postoperatively, Milhorat and associates,[103] in a comment which followed the report of Sahuquillo and co-workers,[131] praised the authors for performing a large craniectomy in a subgroup of patients. The cisterna magna was restored in this subgroup and the cerebellar tonsils actually ascended compared to the majority of the tonsils in the subgroup with a smaller craniectomy which descended.[20] Milhorat and co-workers[103] also noted that the syrinx associated with the Chiari malformation did not necessarily resolve with the former procedure and reported a shunting technique to connect the syrinx to the posterior fossa cisterns which was named syrinocisternostomy.

The high incidence of operative morbidity and mortality associated with decompression of the posterior fossa limited initial acceptance of the technique. Even the staunchest supporter of posterior fossa decompression reported a series of patients who had undergone resection of the filum terminale, terminal ventriculostomy, as an alternative therapy for symptomatic syringomyelia.[63] Williams and Fahy,[171] however, had little enthusiasm for the technique and felt that it was used because of a faulty comprehension of the pathophysiologic basis of syrinx formation. The series they reported did not achieve the improvement rate reported by the authors of the earlier series.

Barbaro and Suzuki and their co-authors reported 80% and 86% favorable response rates with syringoperitoneal shunting.[14, 149] Tator and associates[151] demonstrated that laminectomy with midline myelotomy con-

tinued to be a viable alternative to other surgical techniques and used silicone rubber ventricular catheter tubing to stent the myelotomy. Padovani and colleagues reported a 90% favorable response rate with this technique.[116] Milhorat and associates[103] reported good short-term follow-up of patients treated with a syrinx–to–posterior fossa cistern shunt as the primary surgical procedure. Sgouros and Williams[138] reported that drainage procedures alone have a poor long-term prognosis and that only one half of the patients so treated continued to enjoy a favorable outcome at 10 years postoperatively. They therefore recommended that drainage procedures be reserved for patients who do not respond to posterior fossa decompression. Milhorat and co-workers[104] advocated a ventriculoperitoneal shunt for communicating syringes associated with hydrocephalus, as did Sgouros and Williams.[138] Milhorat and co-workers[104] also treated syringes associated with Chiari II malformations with a ventriculoperitoneal shunt if there was an isolated fourth ventriculomegaly.

Reports on the natural history of syringomyelia have tempered some enthusiasm for surgical therapy without obviation of its continued use for amelioration of symptomatic syringomyelia. Boman and Ilvanainen[26] documented the relatively favorable outcome of patients treated conservatively, while Gamache and Ducker[54] and Anderson and co-workers[5] confirmed the earlier observation of Faulhauer and Loew[46] that the long-term results of surgical therapy were less favorable than results reported after a limited postoperative observation period. Gamache and Ducker also documented a significant decrease in the percentage of patients continuing to have the favorable outcome seen in the immediate postoperative period when the patients were reevaluated after a more extended period of observation.[54]

Syringomyelia Associated with Arachnoiditis of the Spinal Canal

The report of Appleby and co-workers[7] established that a "communicating" type of syringomyelia could be acquired from chronic arachnoiditis involving the basal cisterns and obstructing the outflow of CSF from the fourth ventricle. Barnett[15] correctly advised his readers that the use of the term *arachnoiditis* was inaccurate since all meningeal membranes are usually involved, and suggested that a more accurate terminology would be "pachymeningitis with a leptomeningitis." He also noted that use of the term does not implicate an etiology and he cited multiple reviews of the subject. Arachnoiditis has been reported with syphilis, tuberculosis, pyogenic meningitis, nontraumatic hemorrhage into the subarachnoid space, the use of spinal anesthetics, and a variety of intrathecally introduced agents, as well as traumatic spinal cord injury. In a significant number of cases, no etiologic factor was identified.[15]

The association of spinal arachnoiditis and syringomyelia was reported by Vulpian in 1861 and by Charcot and Joffroy in 1869. MacKay[89] reviewed a series of five patients with chronic adhesive spinal arachnoiditis and included two cases where an autopsy was conducted. Syringomyelia was noted in the latter cases and the author implicated occlusion of the blood vessels supplying the cord by the arachnoid scarring as the cause of the cavitation. Nelson[109] also reported a patient with chronic arachnoiditis who subsequently developed an intramedullary cavitation; he also believed that the underlying pathophysiological process was interference with the spinal cord circulatory system. Caplan and associates[27] found occlusion of spinal feeding arteries in one of their reported cases with syringomyelia and chronic arachnoiditis; they suggested this evidence supported ischemic damage as the initial event in the development of a cavitary lesion.

Barnett[16] reviewed the published reports of experimental ischemic spinal cord lesions starting with the initial attempts by Tauber and Langworthy,[152] and including those of Woodard and Freeman[176] and Wilson and co-workers.[173] The experimental evidence supporting a role for ischemia in the formation of cavitary lesions in the spinal cord was unconvincing in Barnett's opinion because the majority of the cavitary lesions produced experimentally were microscopic. When Williams[160] implicated craniospinal pressure dissociation secondary to obstruction of the subarachnoid space, he extended the most plausible explanation for cyst extension, if not its initial formation. Cho and colleagues[29] investigated the role of arachnoiditis in syringomyelia formation and demonstrated that an injury to the spinal cord was necessary for the production of a syrinx. The dense arachnoiditis produced by intrathecal injection of kaolin did not result in a syrinx, while a weight drop lesion of the cord performed before or after the production of the arachnoid adhesions resulted in an enlarging cystic cavity.

After a review of the published reports of syringomyelia, Barnett determined that only seven cases appeared to have been related to arachnoiditis limited to the spinal canal. To these he reported an additional seven cases.[15] In his series all patients were shown to have arachnoiditis with myelography, but only one patient was known to have a cavitary lesion prior to surgical exploration. The author stated that even retrospective review of the myelograms failed to demonstrate the cystic lesion. Arachnoid cysts were demonstrated in 5 of the 14 patients reviewed. The author considered syringomyelia to be of the "non-communicating" type because no connection between the cyst and the fourth ventricle could ever be demonstrated. Milhorat and co-workers[101] found several cases of syrinx associated with arachnoid scarring and documented that there was no communication with the fourth ventricle.

Management of his patients with arachnoiditis was reported by Barnett[15] to be "unrewarding" whether medical or surgical therapy was attempted. He considered both steroids and lysis of adhesions to be ineffective in the treatment of the disorder (see Fig. 35–4). Barnett suggested surgery for exploratory laminectomy if the practitioner faced a "serious progression of the neurological deficit" in a patient known to have arachnoiditis. The recommended procedure was an exploratory laminotomy at the superior limit of the arachnoiditis, with placement of a silastic catheter from the cyst into the superior subarachnoid space. Sgouros and Williams[138, 139] agreed with the view of Barnett that "dissecting adhesions [was] an unrewarding surgical task" and thought that placement of a permanent drain was of "questionable value."[15]

Syringoperitoneal and syringosubarachnoid shunting was reported as an effective therapy for syringomyelia.[14, 116, 149, 151] A small number of patients in each of the series was identified as having spinal arachnoiditis (10 with syringoperitoneal shunts and 4 with subarachnoid shunts). Sgouros and Williams[139] recommended that the management of syringes associated with areas of "meningeal fibrosis, arachnoiditis" concentrated on the reconstruction of an alternative subarachnoid pathway around the area of adhesion. After a wide laminectomy, a surgical meningocele was created and the dissection of adhesions was limited to the establishment of free communication of the meningocele with the inferior and superior subarachnoid space. The total number of patients with spinal arachnoiditis treated was so small that the efficacy of the reported treatments could not be documented. All authors reported that diagnostic work-up included an MRI examination which had revealed the presence of the lesion preoperatively.

Peerless and Durward[117] recommended metrizamide myelography followed by delayed CT scan for evaluation of patients clinically suspected of syringomyelia, but a later paper by Slasky and associates[142] has presented evidence demonstrating the superiority of Gd-DTPA–enhanced MRI for the evaluation. These authors reviewed the advances in MRI techniques and equipment, which have greatly improved the sensitivity of this diagnostic test, and demonstrated the increased diagnostic accuracy of MRI after augmentation with Gd-DTPA. This enhanced diagnostic accuracy also allowed improved differentiation of cystic areas within tumors from associated cavitary cord lesions. Falcone and co-authors[45] have also demonstrated the utility and limitations of Gd-DTPA–enhanced MRI in the diagnosis of a treatable post-traumatic cystic cavity.

Syringomyelia Associated with Trauma

While there were several early case reports of syringomyelia or cavitary lesions of the spinal cord stated to have been preceded by a history of trauma, including those of Bastiam in 1876 and Strumpel in 1880, these publications were tainted by the lack of pathologic data to confirm the presumed diagnosis.[155] The lack of noninvasive diagnostic procedures and the reliance upon exploratory laminectomy precluded the procurement of diagnostic evidence. Patients were accepted as suffering from "syringomyelia" simply on the presence of clinical symptoms and supporting signs.[19] More neurologically sophisticated authors, including Charcot in 1892, Lloyd in 1894, and Cushing in 1898, reported cases where spinal cord injury produced an immediate clinical picture with the symptoms of syringomyelia.[19, 31, 84] Although Tauber and

Langworthy[152] reported a case of syringomyelia which became symptomatic 8 years after an episode of questionable trauma, no evidence (with the exception of clinical signs) was provided to substantiate the claim that a syrinx existed. That trauma was causally linked to formation of cystic lesions in the spinal cord was eventually established and although late deterioration of residual neurologic function following spinal cord trauma was rarely reported prior to the 1950s, the improvement in longevity of paraplegic and quadriplegic patients allowed the complication to develop and to then become symptomatic.[18, 129, 154]

Increased recognition of the disorder and improved diagnostic techniques resulted in clinical reports from a number of institutions which care for spinal cord–injured patients, but a uniform terminology had not been established. Late deterioration of function following spinal cord injury has been reported as progressive myelopathy as a sequela to traumatic paraplegia, post-traumatic syringomyelia, ascending cystic degeneration of the cord, syndrome of chronic injury to the central cervical spinal cord, post-traumatic progressive myelopathy, and post-traumatic cystic myelopathy or progressive post-traumatic cystic myelopathy.* The last term is favored by us.

This descriptive situation has been compounded by the recently described clinical entity, progressive post-traumatic myelomalacic myelopathy (PPMM), which can clinically and radiographically mimic progressive post-traumatic cystic myelopathy[45] (Figs. 35–7 through 35–10). Unlike the latter entity, patients found to have PPMM do not have an associated cavitary lesion in the spinal cord (see Figs. 35–8, 35–9, and 35–11). Rather than a confluent cyst, microcystic changes within a zone of myelomalacia predominate, most often associ-

*References 18, 66, 69, 87, 112, 113, 135, 137, and 157.

ated with widening and posterior or lateral tethering of the spinal cord (see Figs. 35–7 and 35–12). Although MRI examinations can provide clues to the correct diagnosis because areas of myelomalacia have irregular, ill-defined margins and do not follow CSF signal intensity (see Fig. 35–8A and B), intraoperative ultrasound or myelotomy has been required to unequivocally establish the absence of a cyst (see Fig. 35–7A and B). Recognition of this entity can assist the surgeon in planning for the correct surgical therapy.[45]

The reported overall incidence of the development of a post-traumatic cyst has ranged from 1.1% to 3.2% to greater than 50% in more recent studies using MRI.[11, 77] The rate of syringomyelia reported in one of the latter studies was challenged by Sgouros and Williams[139] because included were small cysts at the injury site which they referred to as primary cysts. These were cavities of less than two vertebral segments in length at the injury site and did not constitute an enlarging cyst but rather were the result of spinal cord parenchymal damage that occurred at the time of the initial injury. Sgouros and Williams felt that these lesions did not need to be treated as they were difficult to collapse and did not correlate with clinical signs of delayed neurologic deterioration.[139] A prospective study of 449 spinal cord injury patients followed yearly for a 6-year period found that 4.45% of the patients developed a symptomatic syrinx.[136] Some groups reported that symptomatic syringes developed with an 8% rate in those patients suffering from a complete quadriplegic lesion but with a 9:1 ratio of paraplegia to quadriplegia in incompletely injured spinal cords.[69, 127] Sgouros and Williams[139] and Backe and co-workers[11] found no correlation between the location of severity of spinal cord injury and the development of a cavitary lesion in their series. The former group stated that their series and a review of the literature demonstrated that

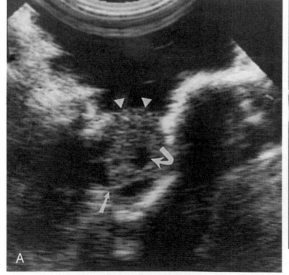
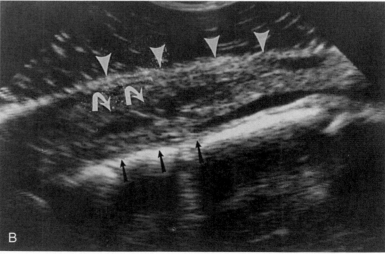

Figure 35–7 = Microcystic myelomalacia in a 56-year-old with radicular pain and a history of spine trauma. Intraoperative sonogram via laminectomy at T6; axial (A) and sagittal (B) images. The spinal cord is tethered both dorsally to the dura (arrowheads), with loss of normal hypoechoic space, and ventrally (arrows). As a result of the tethering, the spinal cord is enlarged. The echo pattern of the spinal cord parenchyma is heterogeneous, with absence of a normal central echo and the presence of microcysts (curved arrows). A confluent cyst is not present and after the spinal cord was surgically untethered, the cysts collapsed.

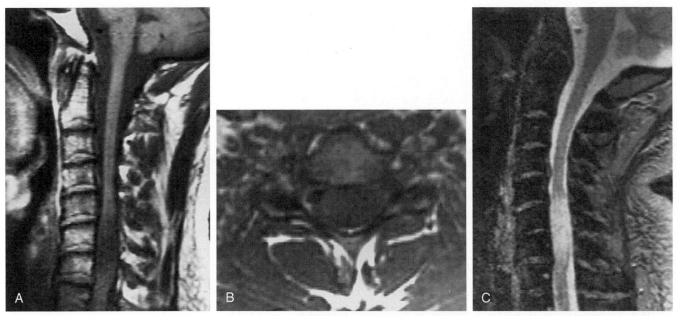

Figure 35–8 ═ Post-traumatic, expansile myelomalacia. T1-weighted sagittal *(A)* and axial *(B)* images of the cervical spine. There is expansion of the spinal cord with an abnormal, decreased signal within the spinal cord parenchyma at C6–7 *(B)*. The signal intensity of the expanded spinal cord is greater than that of cerebrospinal fluid (CSF) and its borders are ill-defined. *C,* On the gradient echo sagittal image, the myelomalaic segment of the spinal cord has increased signal intensity.

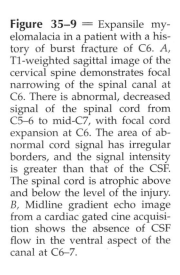

Figure 35–9 ═ Expansile my-elomalacia in a patient with a history of burst fracture of C6. *A,* T1-weighted sagittal image of the cervical spine demonstrates focal narrowing of the spinal canal at C6. There is abnormal, decreased signal of the spinal cord from C5–6 to mid-C7, with focal cord expansion at C6. The area of abnormal cord signal has irregular borders, and the signal intensity is greater than that of the CSF. The spinal cord is atrophic above and below the level of the injury. *B,* Midline gradient echo image from a cardiac gated cine acquisition shows the absence of CSF flow in the ventral aspect of the canal at C6–7.

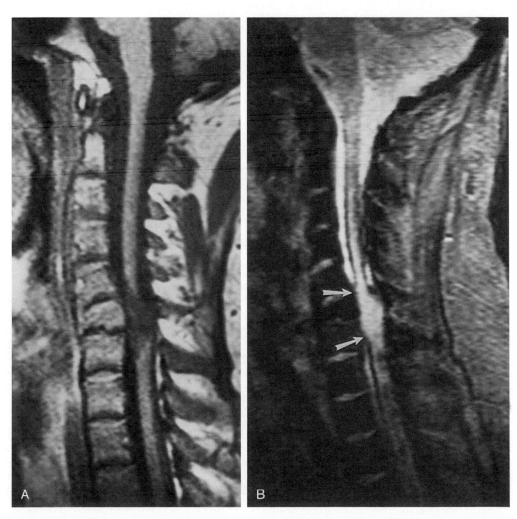

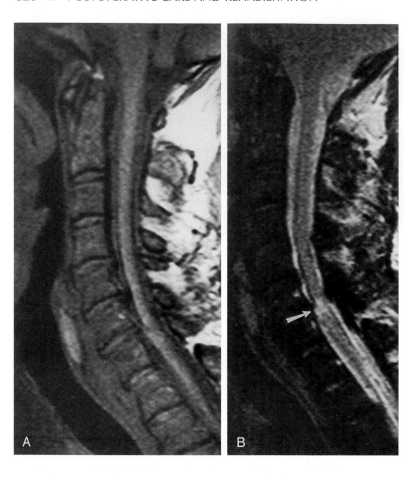

Figure 35–10 ═ Compressive myelomalacia. Proton density *(A)* and T2-weighted *(B)* sagittal images of the cervical spine. Ventral and dorsal osteophytes compress the spinal cord at C6–7. This is associated with a focal area of increased signal *(arrow)* on the T2-weighted image. The proton density image shows that the majority of the abnormal signal is greater than CSF.

any degree of spinal injury, including rather trivial incidences, had been associated with the development of post-traumatic syringomyelia. Two autopsy series found 20% and 17% of spinal cord–injured subjects had syringes identified.[145, 177]

The range for the onset of symptoms post injury has been reported as early as 2 months and as late as 33 years.[72] Rossier and associates[127] reported the most common initial presentation in their series was a complaint of pain, which occurred in 89% of their patients, while Vernon and co-authors[155] documented an occurrence rate of 63% in their series. Pain was well established as the most frequent complaint upon initial presentation, but considerable disagreement existed regarding the frequency of the finding of motor weakness.[157] Although Rossier and Vernon and their co-workers documented increased motor deficit in 63% of symptomatic patients, Watson reported a frequency of occurrence of increased motor weakness of only 20% in his series. Edgar and Quail[38] found dissociated sensory loss in 87% of 600 patients with post-traumatic syringes and motor loss in 80%.

The pathophysiologic basis for the formation and extension of syringes in the injured spinal cord remains the subject of considerable debate and of published speculation. Studies conducted on animal models of syringomyelia have generated considerable information, but progress toward the final definition of the disorder has been impeded by the paucity of truly adequate experimental models of expanding cystic cav-

itation in the spinal cord parenchyma. This deficiency has also slowed formation of a consensus regarding the relative contribution of each of the many factors implicated in the development of symptomatic syringomyelia. The very diversity of these putative factors has also confused efforts to define the disorder and to unravel the conundrum of cyst formation and enlargement. The lack of a scientific method to test a hypothesis derived from a clinical observation has meant that a significant portion of the publications describing syringomyelia in general and specifically those that developed after a traumatic spinal cord injury contain untested and perhaps untestable conclusions regarding the basic pathophysiologic mechanisms underlying the creation of these cavitary lesions in the spinal cord parenchyma. Relevant animal models would obviate this deficiency.

Gardner and McMurray[65] asserted that all cases of syringomyelia were of the "communicating" variety and therefore only those patients with the embryonic substrate would develop the disorder. They cited low incidence figures as evidence to support their conjecture. Oakley and colleagues[113] "unequivocally demonstrated a communication with the fourth ventricle through the cord parenchyma" in the subject of their case report and a similar connection in another case of post-traumatic syringomyelia had earlier been reported by McLean and co-workers.[92] The necropsy study by Milhorat and associates[101] demonstrated that syringes associated with trauma had distinctly differ-

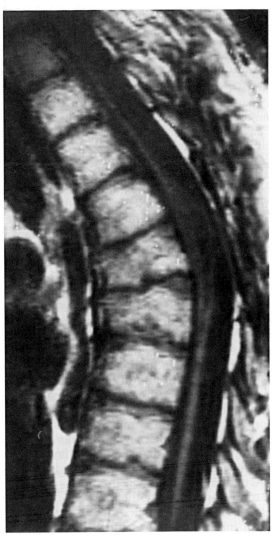

Figure 35–11 ═ Expansile myelomalacia. The T1-weighted sagittal image of the lower thoracic cord demonstrates traumatic wedge deformities in two lower thoracic vertebral bodies, and an associated kyphotic deformity of the bony spinal column. At the level of the bony injury the spinal cord is focally expanded and there is an abnormal, decreased signal in the cord parenchyma which is not as low as the CSF signal intensity. The spinal cord is markedly atrophic above and below the injury level.

evidence of posterior fossa abnormality. Nurick and associates[112] reported the absence of any anomalies of the posterior fossa in the two patients who were the subject of their report. Barnett and co-workers[18] and Williams[161] emphasized the temporal disparity between the onset of symptoms and the initial injury, and the spatial separation of that segment of the spinal cord from which the symptoms of deterioration arose and of the segment affected initially.

The latter group was disposed to view the formation of syringomyelia after trauma as a two-stage process: the creation of the initial cyst and its extension by secondary factors. While a clinically relevant experimental model of syringomyelia associated with trauma had not been successfully developed, many reports of experimental studies of the effects of trauma on the spinal cord have been published.[95] Fehlings and Tator[47] credited Schmasus in 1890 with being the first to demonstrate experimental production of spinal degeneration and cavitation in rabbits by direct application of blows to the backs of the animals and since this initial study many others have confirmed that trauma was a cause of cavitary spinal cord lesions.[25, 35, 111] The possible factors implicated in production of the initial cystic lesions in post-traumatic spinal cords included ischemia secondary to arterial or venous obstruction, lysosomes and other intracellular enzymes, or liquefaction of a prior hematoma or mechanical damage from compression of the substance of the cord at the initial injury.* Yezierski and co-workers[178] observed neuronal degeneration and spinal cavitation following intraspinal injection of the excitatory amino acid (EAA) receptor agonist quisqualic acid. It was proposed that in post-traumatic and postischemic spinal cord injury, excitotoxic cell death occurring secondary to elevated levels of EAAs initiated a pathologic process leading to the formation of spinal cavities. Rossier and associates[127] rejected ischemia as the causal factor because of the paucity of symptoms in the segments remote from the injury site at the time of the initial injury and

---

*References 31, 44, 74, 79, 80, 93, 97, 175, and 176.

ent histopathologic findings and were associated with different clinical symptoms when compared with those lesions which were in communication with the fourth ventricle or those cavities which appeared to be isolated dilations of the spinal cord central canal. The syringes associated with spinal cord injury asymmetrically involved the parenchyma of the cord. They were not associated typically with the central canal and often extended to the pial surface. The authors found a good correlation with the presenting neurologic deficit and the location of the syrinx. Examination of the pathologic specimens revealed nonreversible damage to spinal nuclei and tracts, including focal necrosis, central chromatolysis, and wallerian degeneration.[101]

Williams and co-workers[172] rejected Gardner and McMurray's contention[65] and stressed the fact that the majority of cases of traumatic syringomyelia had no

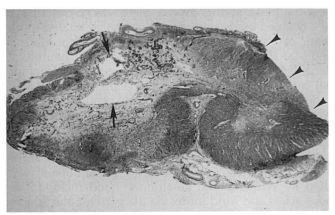

Figure 35–12 ═ Microcystic myelomalacia in a 74-year-old man with ankylosing spondylitis who suffered a midcervical fracture-distraction injury and survived only 4 days postinjury. Low-power (×1.25) microscopic section.

in the cervical and lumbar levels as it affords immediate feedback because it does not require the computer averaging on which SSEP and MEP monitoring depend. The combination of physical and neurologic examination findings plus the imaging studies supplemented by the neurophysiologic assessment battery provides an important database for the clinician to consult when planning therapy.

Presentation of Progressive Post-traumatic Cystic Myelopathy

The syndrome consists of single or multiple spinal cord cysts which may be located intramedullary, subarachnoidally, or in both areas simultaneously, and may be associated with a fissure (see Fig. 35–6D). These cysts, like those associated with neoplasms or congenital lesions, may occur in various locations within or around the spinal cord. Cysts may result from a variety of causes, ranging from a very significant high-velocity injury from a penetrating missile wound causing quadriplegia or paraplegia, to a relatively minor trauma characteristically associated with transient or minimal neurologic deficit. Postsurgical patients form the second most common category of post-traumatic spinal cord cysts (see Fig. 35–5); these patients typically have undergone a spinal procedure which results in local tethering of the spinal cord, subarachnoid space, or both. Most of the senior author's patients in this group presented with a spinal canal mass, either a meningioma or a neurofibroma or, less frequently, an intramedullary neoplasm.[67]

The onset of signs and symptoms of progressive post-traumatic cystic myelopathy have ranged from as early as 2 to 3 months following the initial traumatic event to as long as 30 years post injury and they are listed below in order of decreasing frequency:

1. Motor loss
2. Sensory loss
3. Local or radicular pain (not deafferentated, neurogenic, "burning" pain)
4. Increased spasticity and tone
5. Hyperhidrosis (above the level of lesion)
6. Autonomic dysreflexia
7. Sphincter loss or sexual dysfunction
8. Horner's syndrome (may be alternating)
9. Respiratory insufficiency (usually related to changes in position)

At presentation, the signs and symptoms may be unilateral or bilateral, and may alternate from side to side with changes in position. They may also present as a solitary sign or symptom, or in any combination. The increased utilization of noninvasive MRI has more frequently identified asymptomatic cases compared with the previously employed imaging techniques.[67]

Approximately 5% to 10% of patients suffering a traumatic spinal cord injury experience a progressive spinal cord dysfunction associated with an expanding syrinx. Symptoms are usually accompanied by rostral extension of the cyst from the lesion site, but may also accompany a caudal extension. The majority of these patients have the spinal cord tethered by either a soft tissue scar, a bony gibbus, or a combination of both (see Figs. 35–3, 35–4, and 35–11). The scar tissue tethering is most frequently dorsal because the majority of these patients spend several days in the supine position and the spinal cord assumes a dependent position abutting the dorsal dura. As the blood congeals and scar tissue forms, the pulped spinal cord is tethered to the dura. In the majority of cases where a bony gibbus or herniated disc material tethers the cord locally, the ventral aspect of the spinal column is involved. Although the majority of intramedullary cysts are localized in the dorsal central area of the spinal cord, that is, the dorsal gray matter and adjacent white matter, a significant number present as eccentric unilateral cysts or even double- or triple-barreled complex lesions (see Fig. 35–2B). These cysts may be connected at the rostral or caudal end of the lesion, although they sometimes remain totally independent of each other.

The subarachnoid cysts associated with post-traumatic cysts, in contrast to congenital subarachnoid cysts, have a thinner wall and contain the same clear CSF as found in the adjacent subarachnoid space. They also are more firmly anchored to the adjacent dura and do not present with the same gallbladder or balloon-type configuration characteristic of congenital lesions. A rare variation of this lesion is a traumatic pseudomeningocele which can create an epidural compressive lesion on the spinal cord and may be difficult to identify on routine MRI.

There is little consensus among clinicians regarding the surgical management of post-traumatic syringomyelia, and many neurosurgeons contend that there is no effective surgical treatment. These practitioners believe that patients should ultimately resign themselves to accepting their fate, that is, a progressive neurologic deterioration to complete paralysis or even death. Less controversial is the doctrine that the asymptomatic syringes should not be treated.

Our basic criteria for surgical treatment of post-traumatic cysts has been the presence of one or more signs and symptoms of progressive post-traumatic cystic myelopathy. Normally, cysts less than 1 cm in rostrocaudal extent are not considered to be of an adequate size for successful shunting and are, therefore, followed with serial MRIs and clinical observation. Surgical management of a post-traumatic syrinx requires preoperative assessment of several factors, including the rostrocaudal extent of the cyst or cysts, the exact location in the spinal cord parenchyma, the relationship of associated intramedullary or subarachnoid cysts, and the presence of a fissure. An essential component of the surgery is the untethering of the spinal cord and nerve root adhesions, as well as reduction of any bony gibbus or soft tissue mass at the site of injury. This may first require a posterior approach for intradural exploration and untethering the cord and root adhesions, followed by an anterior approach for removing any bony gibbus or soft tissue mass. The second essential component of a surgical treatment protocol should be shunting of the spinal cord cyst(s) to an extraspinal cavity or fenestration or resection of any associated subarachnoid cyst to allow unrestricted communication with an adjacent patent subarachnoid space. The senior author has abandoned spinal cord cyst–to–subarachnoid space shunts in favor of cyst-to-peritoneal or cyst-to-pleural shunts because of the unacceptably high incidence of distal tube obstruction from subarachnoid placement in his early series (1980 to 1990).[68] This should be accomplished using illumination and magnification either from loupes and headlight or the operating microscope under real-time ultrasonography guidance.

Exploration and shunting of the intramedullary cyst should always proceed from the caudal end, with the tube being directed up toward the rostral extent of the cyst. If the tube will not traverse the entire length of the cyst, the possibility exists that the rostral part of the cyst will become loculated and symptomatic. Some syringes extend from the conus up into the brain stem and one shunt tube may not be adequate to drain the lesion. Passage of the shunt tube may be obstructed by the thoracic kyphosis. In this instance, a single-level laminectomy is performed at the caudal end of the cyst and a second laminectomy is performed just below the innervation of the hands, that is, at approximately T2. Cyst-to-peritoneal or cyst-to-pleural shunts are performed via myelotomies at both levels and the upper shunt is guided into the most rostral extent of the lesion under intraoperative radiographic control to avoid kinking of the tube and to verify proper tube placement.

A small 2-mm vertical myelotomy is usually performed in the midline, avoiding the loops of the dorsal central vein of the spinal cord. The myelotomy is usually performed with a no. 11 blade which has been found in our experience to be more accurate and less destructive than a microlaser. In the case of an eccentrically placed cyst, the myelotomy is placed in the dorsal root entry zone rather than in the midline. In cases with double-barreled or multiloculated cysts, more than one myelotomy and shunt tube may be required. The senior author has designed a series of shunt tubes which are silastic and double-headed (two tips), with holes at each end, but because of difficulties in obtaining Food and Drug Administration (FDA) approval, ventricular or peritoneal hydrocephalus shunt tubing is modified for shunting these spinal cord cysts. Extra holes are cut in the distal and proximal ends to enhance free CSF flow.

The incorporation of a freeze-dried dural allograft or fascia lata autograft is recommended to create a locally enlarged subarachnoid space and an environment less likely to scar and posteriorly retether the spinal cord. Patients should be positioned in the prone position for shunt placement so as to optimize real-time ultrasound assessment which is mandatory to ensure successful cyst collapse and obliteration intraoperatively. Placement of a cyst-to-peritoneal shunt requires repositioning and redraping of the patient and, because of this, the senior author prefers cyst-to-pleural shunting of spinal cysts, thereby obviating the necessity for a two-stage procedure. A percutaneous technique is used to place the distal shunt tubing into the chest cavity, employing a vascular introducer. The trochar is placed

over rib T6–8, 4 cm from the midline and at least 2 cm below the inferior tip of the scapula. The end of the tubing is subcutaneously tunneled and the distal and proximal portions of the shunt are secured to the muscle and fascia to prevent migration.

The maintenance of meticulous intradural hemostasis is important as blood in the surgical site can result in accelerated scarring and retethering of the spinal cord postoperatively. Spinal cord bleeding is best managed with a piece of thrombin-soaked absorbable gelatin sponge (Gelfoam) or microbipolar coagulation, or both. Perioperative intravenous antibiotics and steroids are routinely used in our institution. After the initial shunting procedure, it is essential to repeat real-time ultrasound with sagittal and transverse images to ensure that the entire cystic cavity is collapsed and the shunt tube is in good position. This imaging technique is particularly useful to verify successful treatment of both parts of a confluent double-barrelled cystic lesion when attempting to use a single catheter.

While subarachnoid cysts may be adequately treated by resection and removal of the cyst wall, some cases require a subarachnoid cyst–to–subarachnoid space shunt tube for adequate drainage. Some patients with a combination of subarachnoid and intramedullary cysts connected by a fistula have been adequately treated with a wide removal of the subarachnoid cyst wall. In these cases it is not necessary to stent the fissure, but when the fissure is less apparent, a shunt needs to be placed.

In the future, the best therapy for syringomyelia may be bio-obliteration of the cyst via percutaneous injection of cellular implants. An adequate animal model of progressive post-traumatic cystic myelopathy is needed for the development and evaluation of this and other potentially effective therapies.

CONCLUSION

Although technological advances in noninvasive imaging methods have improved the diagnosis of post-traumatic syringomyelia, and the extent of the lesion can be quite accurately delineated preoperatively in the majority of cases, a universally effective therapy for these lesions has not similarly evolved. The accumulated experience of surgical therapy for these lesions has affirmed that the use of a foreign body (the silastic shunt tube) is not optimal, and that insertion of the shunt or the lysis of adhesions frequently causes the production of additional scar tissue. An increased number of chronic spinal cord injury patients are being identified with spinal cord cysts not only because of improvements in imaging techniques but because of an increased professional and lay awareness of these lesions. The fact that the majority of persons suffering spinal cord injury have a relatively normal life expectancy also has increased the number of patients presenting with these lesions. The research laboratory holds the key to the ultimate solution to the problem of syringomyelia, and only experimental work with animal models offers hope for the final determination of the optimal therapy for spinal cord cysts.

ACKNOWLEDGMENTS

We express our appreciation to Charlaine Rowlette and Alex Marcillo for their expert assistance in the preparation of the manuscript and to William Puckett for the pathology specimens shown in Figures 35–1 and 35–12.

REFERENCES

1. Abbe R, Coley W: Syringo-myelia, operation—exploration of cord—withdrawal of fluid—exhibition of patient. J Nerv Ment Dis 19:512–520, 1892.
2. Adams RD, Victor M: Principles of Neurology, ed 4. New York, McGraw-Hill, 1989, pp 747–754.
3. Adelstein LJ: The surgical treatment of syringomyelia. Am J Surg 40:384–395, 1938.
4. Al-Mefty O, Harkey LH, Middleton TH, et al: Myelopathic cervical spondylitic lesions demonstrated by magnetic resonance imaging. J Neurosurg 68:217–222, 1988.
5. Anderson NE, Willoughby WE, Wrightson P: The natural history and the influence of surgical treatment in syringomyelia. Acta Neurol Scand 71:472–479, 1985.
6. Andrews BT, Weinstein PR, Rosenblum ML, et al: Intradural arachnoid cysts of the spinal canal associated with intramedullary cysts. J Neurosurg 68:544–549, 1988.
7. Appleby A, Bradley WG, Foster JB, et al: Syringomyelia due to chronic arachnoiditis at the foramen magnum. J Neuro Sci 8:451–464, 1969.
8. Arias A, Millan I, Vaquero J: Clinico-morphological correlation in syringomyelia: A statistical study assisted by computer measurement of magnetic resonance images. Acta Neurochir (Wien) 111:33–39, 1991.
9. Aschoff A, Donauer E, Huwel N, et al: Evaluation of syrinx surgery: A critical comment on requirements for reliable follow-up studies. Acta Neurochir (Wien) 123:224–225, 1993.
10. Aschoff A, Kunze S: 100 years of syrinx surgery: A review. Acta Neurochir (Wien) 123:157–159, 1993.
11. Backe HA, Betz RR, Mesgarzadeh M, et al: Post-traumatic spinal cord cysts evaluated by magnetic resonance imaging. Paraplegia 29:607–612, 1991.
12. Ball MJ, Dayan AD: Pathogenesis of syringomyelia. Lancet 2:799–801, 1972.
13. Ballantine HT, Ojemann RG, Drew JH: Syringomyelia. In Kraybuhl H, Maspes PE, Sweet WH (eds): Progress in Neurological Surgery, vol 4. New York, S Karger, 1971, pp 227–245.
14. Barbaro NM, Wilson CB, Gutin PH, et al: Surgical treatment of syringomyelia: Favorable results with syringoperitoneal shunting. J Neurosurg 61:531–538, 1984.
15. Barnett HJM: Syringomyelia associated with spinal arachnoiditis. In Barnett HJM, Foster JB, Hudgson P (eds): Syringomyelia. Philadelphia, WB Saunders, 1973, pp 220–244.
16. Barnett HJM: The pathogenesis of syringomyelic cavitation associated with arachnoiditis localized to the spinal canal. In Barnett HJM, Foster JB, Hudgson P (eds): Syringomyelia. Philadelphia, WB Saunders, 1973, pp 245–260.
17. Barnett HJM: Epilogue. In Barnett HJM, Foster JB, Hudgson P (eds): Syringomyelia. Philadelphia, WB Saunders, 1973, pp 302–313.
18. Barnett HJM, Botterell EH, Jousse AT, et al: Progressive myelopathy as a sequel to traumatic paraplegia. Brain 89:159–178, 1965.
19. Barnett HJM, Jousse AT: Post-traumatic syringomyelia. In Vinken PJ, Bruyn GW (eds): Injuries of the Spine and Spinal Cord, Part II. Handbook of Clinical Neurology, vol 26. Amsterdam, North-Holland, 1976, pp 113–157.
20. Batzdorf U: Chiari I malformation with syringomyelia: Evaluation of surgical therapy by magnetic resonance imaging. J Neurosurg 68:726–730, 1988.
21. Batzdorf U: Personal communication, 1990.
22. Bering EA: Choroid plexus and arterial pulsation of cerebrospinal fluid: Demonstration of the choroid plexuses as a cerebrospinal fluid pump. AMA Arch Neurol Psychiatry 73:165–172, 1955.
23. Bertrand G: Dynamic factors in the evolution of syringomyelia and syringobulbia. In Wilkins RH (ed): Clinical Neurosurgery, vol 20. Baltimore, Williams & Wilkins, 1973, pp 322–333.
24. Biyani A, El Masry WS: Post-traumatic syringomyelia: A review of the literature. Paraplegia 32:723–731, 1994.
25. Blight AR: Cellular morphology of chronic spinal cord injury in the cat: Analysis of myelinated axons by line sampling. Neuroscience 10:521, 1983.
26. Boman K, Ilvanainen M: Prognosis of syringomyelia. Acta Neurol Scand 43:61–68, 1967.
27. Caplan LR, Morohna AB, Amico LL: Syringomyelia and arachnoiditis. J Neurol Neurosurg Psychiatry 53:106–113, 1990.
28. Castillo M, Quencer RM, Green BA, et al: Syringomyelia as a consequence of compressive extramedullary lesions: Postoperative clinical and radiological manifestations. AJR 150:391–396, 1988.
29. Cho KH, Iwasaki Y, Imamura H, et al: Experimental model of posttraumatic syringomyelia: The role of adhesive arachnoiditis in syrinx formation. J Neurosurg 80:133–139, 1994.
30. Conway LW: Hydrodynamic studies in syringomyelia. J Neurosurg 27:501–514, 1967.
31. Cushing HW: Haematomyelia from gunshot wounds of the spine. A report of two cases, with recovery following symptoms of hemilesion of the cord. Am J Med Sci 115:654–683, 1898.
32. Davidson C, Keschner M: Myelitic and myelopathic lesions VI. Cases with marked circulatory interference and a picture of syringomyelia. Arch Neurol Psychiatry 30:1074–1085, 1933.
33. Di Chiro G, Axelbaum SP, Schellinger D, et al: Computerized axial tomography in syringomyelia. N Engl J Med 292:13–16, 1975.
34. Di Chiro G, Schellinger: Computed tomography of spinal cord after lumber intrathecal introduction of metrizamide (computer assisted myelography). Radiology 120:101–104, 1976.
35. Ducker TB: Experimental injury of the spinal cord. In Vinken PJ, Bruyn GW (eds): Injuries of the Spine and Spinal Cord, Part I. Handbook of Clinical Neurology, vol 25. Amsterdam, North-Holland, 1976, pp 9–26.
36. Edgar RE: Surgical management of spinal cord cysts. Paraplegia 14:21–27, 1976.
37. Edgar R, Quail P: Progressive post-traumatic cystic and noncystic myelopathy. Br J Neurosurg 8:7–22, 1994.
38. Ellertsson AB: Semilogic diagnosis of syringomyelia related to roentgenologic findings. Acta Neurol Scand 45:385–402, 1969.
39. Ellertsson AB: Syringomyelia and other cystic spinal cord lesions. Acta Neurol Scand 45:403–417, 1969.
40. Ellertsson AB, Greitz T: Myelocystographic and fluorescein studies to demonstrate communication between intramedullary cysts and the cerebrospinal fluid space. Acta Neurol Scand 45:418–430, 1969.
41. Ellertsson AB, Greitz T: The distending force in the production of communicating syringomyelia. Lancet 1:1234, 1970.
42. Elsberg CA: Surgical Diseases of the Spinal Cord. New York, PB Hoeber, 1941, pp 551–553.
43. Enzmann DR, O'Donohue J, Rubin JB, et al: CSF pulsations within nonneoplastic spinal cord cysts. AJR 149:149–157, 1987.
44. Fairholm DJ, Turnbull IM: Microangiographic study of experimental spinal cork injuries. J Neurosurg 35:277–286, 1971.
45. Falcone S, Quencer RM, Green BA, et al: Progressive post-traumatic myelomalacic myelopathy (PPMM): Imaging and clinical features. AJNR 15:747–754, 1994.
46. Faulhauer K, Loew K: The surgical treatment of syringomyelia. Long-term results. Acta Neurochir 44:215–222, 1978.
47. Fehlings MG, Tator CH: A review of models of acute experimental spinal cord injury. In Illis LS (ed): Spinal Cord Dysfunction: Assessment. Oxford, Oxford University Press, 1988, pp 3–33.
48. Finlayson AI: Syringomyelia and related conditions. In Joynt RJ (ed): Clinical Neurology, vol 3. Philadelphia, JB Lippincott, 1989, pp 1–17.
49. Foo D, Bignami A, Rossier AB: A case of post-traumatic syringomyelia. Neuropathological findings after 1 year of cystic drainage. Paraplegia 27:63–69, 1989.

50. Foster JB, Hudgson P: The radiology of communicating syringomyelia. *In* Barnett HJM, Foster JB, Hudgson P (eds): Syringomyelia. Philadelphia, WB Saunders, 1973, pp 51–63.
51. Frazier CH: Shall syringomyelia be added to the lesions appropriate for surgical intervention? JAMA 95:1911–1912, 1930.
52. Frazier CH, Rowe SN: The surgical treatment of syringomyelia. Ann Surg 103:481–497, 1936.
53. Freeman LW: Ascending spinal paralysis: Case presentation. J Neurosurg 16:120–122, 1959.
54. Gamache FW, Ducker TW: Syringomyelia: A neurological and surgical spectrum. J Spinal Disord 3:293–298, 1990.
55. Gardner WJ: Anatomic anomalies common to myelomeningocele of infancy and syringomyelia of adulthood suggest a common origin. Cleveland Clin Quart 25:118–133, 1959.
56. Gardner WJ: Diastematomyelia and the Klippel-Feil syndrome. Cleve Clin J Med 31:19–44, 1964.
57. Gardner WJ: Hydrodynamic mechanism of syringomyelia: Its relationship to myelocele. J Neurol Neurosurg Psychiatry 28:247–259, 1965.
58. Gardner WJ: Myelocele: Rupture of the neural tube? *In* Ojemann RG (ed): Clinical Neurosurgery, vol 15. Baltimore, Williams & Wilkins, 1968, pp 57–79.
59. Gardner WJ, Abdullah AF, McCormack LJ: The varying expressions of embryonal atresia of the fourth ventricle in adults: Arnold-Chiari malformation, Dandy-Walker syndrome, "arachnoid" cyst of the cerebellum, and syringomyelia. J Neurosurg 14:591–607, 1957.
60. Gardner WJ, Angel J: The cause of syringomyelia and its surgical treatment. Cleve Clin J Med 25:4–8, 1958.
61. Gardner WJ, Angel J: The mechanism of syringomyelia and its surgical correction. *In* Fisher RG (ed): Clinical Neurosurgery, vol 6. Baltimore, Williams & Wilkins, 1959, pp 131–140.
63. Gardner WJ, Bell HS, Poolos PN, et al: Terminal ventriculostomy for syringomyelia. J Neurosurg 46:609–617, 1977.
64. Gardner WJ, Goodall RJ: The surgical treatment of Arnold-Chiari malformation in adults. J Neurosurg 7:199–206, 1950.
65. Gardner WJ, McMurray FG: "Non-communicating" syringomyelia: A non-existent entity. Surg Neurol 6:251–256, 1976.
66. Gebarski SS, Maynard FW, Gabrielsen TO, et al: Posttraumatic progressive myelopathy: Clinical and radiologic correlation employing MR imaging, delayed CT metrizamide myelography, and intraoperative sonography. Radiology 157:379–385, 1985.
67. Green BA: Unpublished observations, 1990.
68. Green BA, Quencer RM, Post MJD, et al: A review of 100 patients surgically treated for progressive post-traumatic cystic myelopathy (abstract). J Neurosurg 72:353A, 1990.
69. Griffiths ER, McCormick CC: Post-traumatic syringomyelia (cystic myelopathy). Paraplegia 19:81–88, 1981.
70. Haney A, Stiller J, Zelnik N, et al: Association of post-traumatic spinal arachnoid cyst and syringomyelia. J Comput Assist Tomogr 9:137–140, 1985.
71. Hassin GB: A contribution to the histopathology and histogenesis of syringomyelia. Arch Neurol Psychiatry 3:130–147, 1920.
72. Hida K, Iwasaki Y, Imamura H, et al: Posttraumatic syringomyelia: Its characteristic magnetic resonance imaging findings and surgical management. Neurosurgery 35:886–891, 1994.
73. Hoffman HJ, Neill J, Crone KR, et al: Hydrosyringomyelia and its management in childhood. Neurosurgery 21:347–351, 1987.
74. Holmes G: The Goulstonian Lectures on spinal injuries of warfare: Part I. The pathology of acute spinal injury. Br Med J 2:769–774, 1915.
75. Honan WP, Williams B: Sensory loss in syringomyelia: Not necessarily dissociated. J R Soc Med 86:519, 1993.
76. Hughes JT: Pathological changes after spinal cord injury. *In* Illis LS (ed): Spinal Cord Dysfunction: Assessment. Oxford, Oxford University Press, 1988, pp 34–40.
77. Hussey RW, Ha CY, Vijay M, et al: Prospective study of the occurrence rate of post-traumatic cystic degeneration of the spinal cord utilizing magnetic resonance imaging (abstract). J Am Paraplegia Soc 13:16, 1990.
78. Jack CR, Kokmen E, Onofrio BM: Spontaneous decompression of syringomyelia: Magnetic resonance imaging findings. Case report. J Neurosurg 74:283–286, 1991.
79. Kao CC, Chang LW: The mechanism of spinal cord cavitation following spinal cord transection: Part 1: A correlated histochemical study. J Neurosurg 46:197–209, 1977.
80. Kao CC, Chang LW, Bloodworth JMB: The mechanism of spinal cord cavitation following spinal cord transection: Part 2: Electron microscope observation. J Neuropathol Exp Neurol 36:140–156, 1977.
81. Koehler PJ: Chiari's description of cerebellar ectopy (1891): With summary of Cleland's and Arnold's contributions and some early observations on neural-tube defects. J Neurosurg 75:823–826, 1991.
82. Koyanagi I, Tator CH, Lea PJ: Three-dimensional analysis of the vascular system in the rat spinal cord with scanning electron microscopy of vascular corrosion casts. Part 2: Acute spinal cord injury. Neurosurgery 33:285–292, 1993.
83. Koyanagi I, Tator CH, Theriault E: Silicone rubber microangiography of acute spinal cord injury in the rat. Neurosurgery 32:260–283, 1993.
84. Lloyd JH: Traumatic affections of the cervical region of the spinal cord, simulating syringomyelia. J Nerv Ment Dis 21:345–358, 1894.
85. Logue V, Edwards MR: Syringomyelia and its surgical treatment: An analysis of 75 patients. J Neurol Neurosurg Psychiatry 44:273–284, 1981.
86. Love GJ, Olafson RA: Syringomyelia: A look at surgical therapy. J Neurosurgy 24:714–718, 1966.
87. Lyons BM, Brown DJ, Calvert JM, et al: The diagnosis and management of post traumatic syringomyelia. Paraplegia 25:340–350, 1987.
88. MacDonald RL, Findlay JM, Tator CH: Microcytic spinal cord degeneration causing post-traumatic myelopathy. J Neurosurg 68:466–471, 1988.
89. MacKay RP: Chronic adhesive spinal arachnoiditis. JAMA 112:802–808, 1939.
90. MacKay RP, Favill J: Syringomyelia and intramedullary tumor of the spinal cord. Arch Neurol Psychiatry 33:1255–1278, 1935.
91. McLaurin RL, Bailey OT, Schurr PH, et al: Myelomalacia and multiple cavitations of spinal cord secondary to adhesive arachnoiditis. Arch Pathol 57:138–146, 1954.
92. McLean DR, Miller JDR, Allen PBR, et al: Posttraumatic syringomyelia. J Neurosurg 39:485–492, 1973.
93. McVeigh JF: Experimental cord crushes: With especial reference to the mechanical factors involved and subsequent changes in the areas of the cord affected. Arch Surg 7:573–600, 1923.
94. Madsen PW, Green BA, Bowen BC: Syringomyelia. *In* Rothman RH, Simeone FA (eds). The Spine, ed 3, vol 2. Philadelphia, WB Saunders, 1991, pp 1575–1604.
95. Madsen PW, Holets V, Yezierske RP: Syringomyelia: Clinical observations and experimental studies. J Neurotrauma 11:241–254, 1994.
96. Madsen PW, Marcillo A: Unpublished data, 1996.
97. Mair WPG, Druckman R: The pathology of spinal cord lesions and their relation to the clinical features in protrusion of cervical intervertebral discs. Brain 76:70–91, 1953.
98. Martin G: Syringomyelia, an hypothesis and proposed method of treatment (letter). J Neurol Neurosurg Psychiatry 46:365, 1983.
99. Martin G: Syringomyelia, an hypothesis and proposed method of treatment (letter). J Neurol Neurosurg Psychiatry 48:193, 1985.
100. Matsumoto T, Symon L: Surgical management of syringomyelia: Current results. Surg Neurol 32:258–265, 1989.
101. Milhorat TH, Capocelli AL, Anzil AP, et al: Pathological basis of spinal cord cavitation in syringomyelia: Analysis of 105 autopsy cases. J Neurosurg 82:802–812, 1995.
102. Milhorat TH, Johnson WD, Milhorat RH, et al: Clinicopathological correlations in syringomyelia using axial magnetic resonance imaging. Neurosurgery 37:206–213, 1995.
103. Milhorat TH, Johnson WD, Miller JI: Syrinx shunt to posterior fossa cisterns (syringocisternostomy) for bypassing obstructions of the upper cervical theca. J Neurosurg 77:871–874, 1992.
104. Milhorat TH, Johnson WD, Miller JI, et al: Surgical treatment of syringomyelia based on magnetic resonance imaging criteria. Neurosurgery 31:231–245, 1992.
105. Milhorat TH, Kotzen RM, Anzil AP: Stenosis of central canal of spinal cord in man: Incidence and pathological findings in 232 autopsy cases. J Neurosurg 80:716–722, 1994.
106. Milhorat TH, Miller JI, Johnson WD, et al: Anatomical basis of

syringomyelia occurring with hindbrain lesions. Neurosurgery 32:748–754, 1993.

107. Milhorat TH, Nobandegani F, Miller JI, et al: Noncommunicating syringomyelia following occlusion of central canal in rats: Experimental model and histological findings. J Neurosurg 78:274–279, 1993.

108. Murray JAH, Bradley H, Craigie WA, et al (eds): The Oxford English Dictionary: Being a Corrected Re-issue with an Introduction, Supplement, and Bibliography of a New English Dictionary on Historical Principles, vol 10. Oxford, Oxford University Press, 1933, p 391.

109. Nelson J: Intramedullary cavitation resulting from adhesive spinal arachnoiditis. AMA Arch Neurol Psychiatry 50:1–7, 1943.

110. Netsky MG: Syringomyelia. A clinicopathologic study. Arch Neurol 70:741–777, 1953.

111. Noble LJ, Wrathall JR: Correlative analysis of lesion development and functional status after graded spinal cord contusive injuries in the rat. Exp Neurol 103:34–40, 1989.

112. Nurick S, Russell JA, Deck MDF: Cystic degeneration of the spinal cord following spinal cord injury. Brain 93:211–222, 1970.

113. Oakley JC, Ojemann GA, Alvord EC: Post-traumatic syringomyelia: Case report. J Neurosurg 55:276–281, 1981.

114. Oldfield EH, Muraszko K, Shawker TH, et al: Pathophysiology of syringomyelia associated with Chiari I malformation of the cerebellar tonsils. J Neurosurg 80:3–15, 1994.

115. Osborne DRS, Vavoulis G, Nashold BS, et al: Late sequelae of spinal cord trauma: Myelographic and surgical correlation. J Neurosurg 57:18–23, 1982.

116. Padovani R, Cavallo M, Gaist G: Surgical treatment of syringomyelia: Favorable results with syringosubarachnoid shunting. Surg Neurol 32:173–180, 1989.

117. Peerless SJ, Durward QJ: Management of syringomyelia: A pathophysiological approach. *In* Weiss MH (ed): Clinical Neurosurgery, vol 3. Baltimore, Williams & Wilkins, 1983, pp 531–576.

118. Pillay PK, Awad IA, Little JR, et al: Symptomatic Chiari malformation in adults: A new classification based on magnetic resonance imaging with clinical and prognostic significance. Neurosurgery 28:639–645, 1991.

119. Pitts FW, Groff, RA: Syringomyelia: Current status of surgical therapy. Surgery 56:806–809, 1964.

120. Pojunas K, Williams AL, Daniels KL, et al: Syringomyelia and hydromyelia: Magnetic resonance evaluation. Radiology 153:679–683, 1984.

121. Poser CM: The Relationship Between Syringomyelia and Neoplasm. Springfield, Ill, Thomas, 1956.

122. Post MJD, Quencer RM, Hinks RS, et al: Spinal CSF flow dynamics: Qualitative and quantitative evaluation by cine MRI. Presented to Annual Meeting of the American Society of Neuroradiology, Orlando, Fla, March 24, 1989.

123. Putnam TJ: Syringomyelia—diagnosis and treatment. Med Clin North Am 19:1571–1582, 1936.

124. Quencer RM: Needle aspiration of intramedullary and intradural extramedullary masses of the spinal canal. Radiology 134:115–126, 1980.

125. Quencer RM, Green BA, Eismont FJ: Post traumatic spinal cysts: Clinical features and characterization with metrizamide computed tomography. Radiology 146:415–423, 1983.

126. Rhoton AL: Microsurgery of Arnold-Chiari malformation in adults with and without hydromyelia. J Neurosurg 45:473–483, 1976.

127. Rossier AB, Foo D, Shillito J, et al: Posttraumatic cervical syringomyelia: Incidence, clinical presentation, electrophysiological studies, syrinx protein and results of conservative and operative treatment. Brain 108:439–461, 1985.

128. Rossier AB, Foo D, Shillito J, et al: Progressive late post-traumatic syringomyelia. Paraplegia 19:96–97, 1981.

129. Rossier AB, Werner A, Wildi E, et al: Contribution to the study of late cervical syringomyelic syndromes after dorsal or lumbar traumatic paraplegia. J Neurol Neurosurg Psychiatry 31:99–105, 1968.

130. Russell DS, Donald C: Mechanism of internal hydrocephalus in spinal bifida. Brain 58:203–215, 1935.

131. Sahuquillo J, Rubio E, Poca M, et al: Posterior fossa reconstruction: A surgical technique for the treatment of Chiari I malformation and Chiari I/syringomyelia complex—preliminary results and magnetic resonance imaging quantitative assessment of hindbrain migration. Neurosurgery 35:874–885, 1994.

132. Savoiardo M: Syringomyelia associated with postmeningitic spinal arachnoiditis. Filling of the syrinx through a communication with the subarachnoid space. Neurology 26:551–554, 1976.

133. Schlesinger EB, Antunes JL, Michelsen WJ, et al: Hydromyelia: Clinical presentation and comparison of modalities of treatment. Neurosurgery 9:356–365, 1981.

134. Schlesinger H: Die Syringomyelie. Leipzig, Deuticke, 1902.

135. Schneider RC, Knighton R: Chronic neurological sequelae of acute trauma to the spine and spinal cord: Part III: The syndrome of chronic injury to the cervical spinal cord in the region of the central canal. J Bone Joint Surg Am 41:905–919, 1954.

136. Schurch B, Wichmann W, Rossier AB: Post-traumatic syringomyelia (cystic myelopathy): A prospective study of 449 patients with spinal cord injury. J Neurol Neurosurg Psychiatry 60:61–67, 1996.

137. Seibert CE, Dreisbach JN, Swanson WB, et al: Progressive post-traumatic cystic myelopathy: Neuroradiologic evaluation. AJR 136:1161–1165, 1981.

138. Sgouros S, Williams B: A critical appraisal of drainage in syringomyelia. J Neurosurg 82:1–10, 1995.

139. Sgouros S, Williams B: Management and outcome of posttraumatic syringomyelia. J Neurosurg 85:197–205, 1996.

140. Shannon N, Symon L, Logue V, et al: Clinical features, investigation and treatment of post-traumatic syringomyelia. J Neurol Neurosurg Psychiatry 44:35–42, 1981.

141. Sherman JL, Farkovich AJ, Citrin CM: The MR appearance of syringomyelia: New observations. AJR 148:381–391, 1987.

142. Slasky BS, Bydder GM, Niendorf HP, et al: MR imaging with gadolinium-DTPA in the differentiation of tumor, syrinx, and cyst of the spinal cord. J Comput Assist Tomogr 11:845–850, 1987.

143. Small JA, Sheridan PH: Research priorities for syringomyelia: A National Institute of Neurological Disorders and Stroke workshop summary. Neurology 46:577–582, 1996.

144. Spiller WG: Syringomyelia. Br Med J 2:1017–1021, 1906.

145. Squier MV, Lehr RP: Post-traumatic syringomyelia. J Neurol Neurosurg Psychiatry 57:1095–1098, 1994.

146. Steinmetz A, Aschoff A, Kunze S: The iatrogenic tethering of the cord. Acta Neurochir (Wien) 123:219–220, 1993.

147. Stoaniemi KA, Pyhtinen J, Myllyla VV: Computed tomography in the diagnosis of syringomyelia. Acta Neurol Scand 68:121–127, 1983.

148. Stoodley MA, Jones NR, Brown CJ: Evidence for rapid fluid flow from the subarachnoid space into the spinal cord central canal in the rat. Brain Res 707:155–164, 1996.

149. Suzuki M, Davis C, Symon L, et al: Syringoperitoneal shunt for treatment of cord cavitation. J Neurol Neurosurg Psychiatry 48:620–627, 1985.

150. Tamaki K, Lubin AJ: Pathogenesis of syringomyelia: Case illustrating the process of cavity formation from embryonic cell rests. Arch Neurol Psychiatry 40:748–761, 1938.

151. Tator CH, Meguro K, Rowed DW: Favorable results with syringosubarachnoid shunts for treatment of syringomyelia. J Neurosurg 56:517–523, 1982.

152. Tauber ES, Langworthy OR: A study of syringomyelia and the formation of cavities in the spinal cord. J Nerv Ment Dis 81:245–264, 1935.

153. Turnbull FA: Syringomyelic complications of spina bifida. Brain 56:304–317, 1933.

154. Van Den Bergh R: Pathogenesis and treatment of delayed post-traumatic syringomyelia. Acta Neurochir (Wien) 123:82–86, 1993.

155. Vernon JD, Silver JR, Ohry A: Post-traumatic syringomyelia. Paraplegia 20:339–364, 1982.

156. Walshe, FMR: Developmental anomalies: Syringomyelia and syringobulbia (status dysraphicus). *In* Diseases of the Nervous System, ed 11. Baltimore, Williams & Wilkins, 1970, pp 267–272.

157. Watson N: Ascending cystic degeneration of the cord after spinal cord injury. Paraplegia 19:89–95, 1981.

158. West RJ, Williams B: Radiographic studies of the ventricles in syringomyelia. Neuroradiology 20:5–16, 1980.

159. Wechsler IS: Syringomyelia (including spinal gliosis). *In* A Text-

book of Clinical Neurology. Philadelphia, WB Saunders, 1927, pp 159–164.

160. Williams B: The distending force in the production of "communicating syringomyelia." Lancet 2:189–193, 1969.
161. Williams B: Current concepts of syringomyelia. Br J Hosp Med 4:331–342, 1970.
162. Williams B: The distending force in the production of communicating syringomyelia. Lancet 2:41–42, 1970.
163. Williams B: Cerebrospinal fluid pressure changes in response to coughing. Brain 99:331–346, 1976.
164. Williams B: Difficult labour as a cause of communicating syringomyelia. Lancet 2:51–53, 1977.
165. Williams B: A critical appraisal of posterior fossa surgery for communicating syringomyelia. Brain 101:223–250, 1978.
166. Williams B: On the pathogenesis of syringomyelia: A review. J R Soc Med 73:798–806, 1980.
167. Williams B: Experimental communicating syringomyelia in dogs after cisternal kaolin injection: Part 1. Pressure studies. J Neurol Sci 48:107–109, 1980.
168. Williams B: Simultaneous cerebral and spinal fluid pressure recordings: 2. Cerebrospinal dissociation with lesions at the foramen magnum. Acta Neurochir 59:123–142, 1981.
169. Williams B: Progress in syringomyelia. Neurol Res 8:130–145, 1986.
170. Williams B: Pathogenesis of syringomyelia. Acta Neurochir (Wien) 123:159, 1993.
171. Williams B, Fahy G: A critical appraisal of "terminal ventriculostomy" for the treatment of syringomyelia. J Neurosurg 58:188–197, 1983.
172. Williams B, Terry AF, Jones HWF, et al: Syringomyelia as a sequel to traumatic paraplegia. Paraplegia 19:67–80, 1981.
173. Wilson CB, Bertan V, Norrell HA, et al: Experimental cervical myelopathy: II. Acute ischemic myelopathy. Arch Neurol 21:571–589, 1969.
174. Wilson SAK: Syringomyelia: Syringobulbia. In Bruce AN (ed): Neurology, vol 2. Baltimore, Williams & Wilkins, 1955, pp 1187–1202.
175. Wolman L: The disturbance of circulation in traumatic paraplegia in acute and late stages: A pathological study. Paraplegia 2:213–226, 1965.
176. Woodard JS, Freeman LW: Ischemia of the spinal cord: An experimental study. J Neurosurg 13:63–72, 1956.
177. Wozniewicz B, Filipowicz K, Swiderska SK, et al: Pathphysiological mechanism of traumatic cavitation of the spinal cord. Paraplegia 21:312–317, 1983.
178. Yezierski RP, Santana M, Park S, et al: Intraspinal injections of quisqualic acid in the adult rat: An experimental model of neurotoxicity and syringomyelia. J Neurotrauma 10:445–456, 1993.

CHAPTER 36

Urologic Complications of Spinal Cord Injury

Edward J. McGuire ‖ *Dana Ohl* ‖ *Steven Wang*
Freidhelm Noll ‖ *Elizabeth Vasher*

HISTORICAL BACKGROUND

The 2-year mortality rate from a spinal cord injury incurred in World War I was 82%.[3] This acute mortality decreased to about 11% following World War II, but cumulative complications still caused a 20-year mortality close to 50%.[11, 32] The acute causes of death included pulmonary insufficiency, pulmonary embolism, and sepsis. More chronic conditions, including urinary infection, amyloidosis, pyelonephritis, stone formation, pressure ulceration, renal failure, hypertension, and bladder malignancy, were the leading causes of death in patients who incurred a spinal cord injury in the period between 1940 and 1965.[38] These conditions were largely related to difficulties with management of the lower urinary tract.

Urologists confronted with spinal cord–injured patients had two major problems. The bladder did not work very well and could not be controlled. It is understandable that catheters were employed in an effort to deal with both problems, but catheters were associated with infection, bladder calculi, penoscrotal angle fistula formation, periurethral abscesses, pyelonephritis, epididymitis, orchitis, and urosepsis. As the time of catheter drainage reached 20 years, renal failure and fatal squamous cell carcinoma of the bladder became more common in persons who had survived that long.[26]

If serious complications of catheter drainage developed, the standard method of management was supravesical diversion. This method, like catheters, was associated with an equally dismal long-term outcome. While this was initially attributed to the bad condition of the urinary tracts of those who came to supravesical diversion, it became obvious, when long-term data became available, that urinary diversion also destroyed normal urinary tracts.[28] Efforts to treat bladder dysfunction in more specific ways began with Emmett,[13] who resected the bladder neck in a spinal cord–injured patient in 1937. For a time such procedures were popular, until the late 1950s, when urologists began to resect the external sphincter in an effort to improve voiding and to create incontinence managed with a condom catheter. It was recognized that catheter drainage was harmful, and condom catheter drainage safer, but not all patients accepted the devices or the incontinence,

and such methods were totally unsuitable for females. Moreover, there was a fairly high rate of failure of sphincterotomy to bring about the desired result: a normally functioning bladder with no residual urine.

There developed, during the period from 1950 through the early 1970s, two basic philosophies of bladder management. One held that recovery of balanced bladder function without surgery or instrumentation was the best possible outcome for a spinal cord–injured patient, and the other, espoused mainly by surgeons, held that drainage of the bladder by any means would best prevent complications. While both groups were basically correct, neither the conservative group nor the surgical group was able to prevent complications, and each could point to obviously bad results engendered by one or the other treatment method as examples of a bad outcome. Guttman and Frankel,[15] members of the conservative group, described the use of sterile, physician-performed, intermittent catheterization to manage the bladder during spinal shock.[5] The technique sharply reduced the incidence of urinary complications in the early stages of spinal cord injury. This method was replaced after 3 months by efforts to induce spontaneous voiding and "balanced bladder function," which had the usual results. When it worked it was fine, but often it did not. Indeed, the problems which led others to use catheters prevented the achievement of a catheter-free state in the majority of patients.[15]

In Ireland, Webb and colleagues[41] used a combination of early intermittent catheterization and sphincterotomy in males and a variety of methods in females, but did not use catheters. Results from the Irish National Center for the period 1965 to 1980 are better than reported series in the United States and Europe for a similar period. The Irish results appear to be the outcome of a "catheterless" management system coupled with a reduction in outlet resistance by urethral surgery where appropriate. In the 1970s, Lapides and co-workers[18] reported the use of clean intermittent catheterization as a long-term method of management of neurogenic vesical dysfunction. This development, which would revolutionize the treatment of patients with neurogenic bladder, did not immediately affect spinal cord injury patients.

THE INFLUENCE OF URODYNAMICS ON SPINAL CORD INJURY

Initially, urodynamics was used to study only bladder activity, but the discoordinate bladder and external sphincter relationship in spinal cord–injured patients required the simultaneous measurement of bladder and urethral pressure, or a pelvic floor electromyogram.[30] When patients with upper motor neuron lesions were studied it became clear that unlike the normal reciprocal, coordinate, bladder and external sphincter relationship, these two structures exhibited antagonistic activity. The sphincter was obstructive to flow, prevented emptying, and led to an elevated bladder pressure (Fig. 36–1). Efforts to improve voiding function were thus concentrated on the external sphincter, usually by sphincterotomy. While an actual increase in external sphincter activity did not accompany bladder filling in lower motor neuron lesions, neither did the sphincter relax when bladder pressure rose with filling. Efforts to improve voiding function in this group of patients also then included sphincterotomy.

While these observations were correct, and sphincterotomy led to improved outcome in spinal cord–injured males, condom catheter drainage and sphincterotomy could not be applied to females, most of whom continued to be treated by catheter drainage or supravesical diversion. Intermittent clean catheterization provided an alternative method of management for females. The technique was first applied to women with lower motor neuron lesions but later was used for those with upper motor neuron injuries. Reflex bladder activity was found relatively easy to control with anticholinergic medication.[22] Given the success in females and the difficulty some male patients had with condom catheter drainage and sphincterotomy, intermittent catheterization was also applied to males as a permanent method of management. Two problems limited the wider application of intermittent catheterization to the spinal cord–injured population: uncontrollable reflex bladder contractility, and limited hand function, which was an impediment to self-catheterization. While both of these are still problems, the relative lack of urologic complications encountered in patients managed by intermittent catheterization led to efforts to control incontinence by augmentation cystoplasty or sacral rhizotomy. To obviate difficulty with intermittent catheterization, continent abdominal stomas were constructed using segments of bowel or the bladder to permit catheterization by the patient or caregiver.[23, 35]

PATHOPHYSIOLOGY OF LOWER URINARY DYSFUNCTION IN SPINAL CORD INJURY

Spinal cord injuries between C1 and the sacral cord segments separate the sacral neural centers involved in lower urinary function from the pontine center responsible for the integration and coordination of lower urinary activity. Immediately after injury, a period of spinal shock occurs, during which time no reflex bladder activity can be elicited. However, the internal sphincter continues to be actively closed so that passive leakage or leakage by abdominal pressure does not occur. The lack of bladder function makes intermittent or continuous catheter drainage necessary. After the period of spinal shock, which lasts longer in higher lesions, bladder reflex activity returns. The activity is abnormal. In spinal cord–injured patients the sphincter fails to respond to bladder filling until reflex bladder contractility occurs, at which time external sphincter activity increases vigorously. There then ensues a kind of repetitive, dysphasic contraction-relaxation response from both bladder and sphincter which is discoordinate, and though some voiding occurs, it is interrupted and of a higher pressure than normal.[20] The bladder contraction is short in duration, being intermittently inhibited by

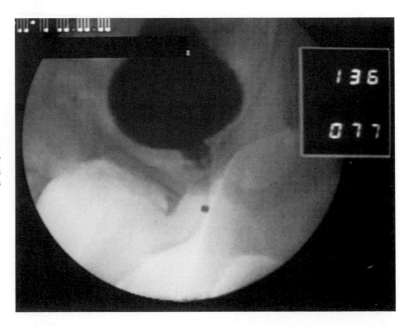

Figure 36–1 = Discoordinate bladder and external sphincter activity in T6 paraplegia. Note the open bladder outlet, and the area of compression of the urethra which corresponds to the external sphincter. Detrusor pressure is 136 cm H_2O. External sphincter pressure is 77 cm H_2O.

external sphincter activity: directly by an obstructive effect, and indirectly by a sacral cord pathway, activated by external sphincter contractility. Urologic treatment was traditionally directed at improving bladder function either by driving the bladder with drugs, increased abdominal pressure, or some kind of triggering maneuver; or by a surgical procedure on the sphincter. These measures, while effective compared to no treatment, resulted neither in complete emptying nor in normal function. Efforts to inhibit the spinal cord bladder are conversely easier, and small doses of anticholinergic agents stop contractility and permit continued intermittent catheterization on a permanent basis if such treatment is begun early.[22]

The recognition that bladder activity in these patients is actually of poor quality, and the pressures attained a reflection of urethral resistance rather than detrusor muscle power, led to use of intermittent catheterization as a method to preserve continence and, in conjunction with anticholinergic agents, to maintain a low-pressure bladder.

Neural lesions involving the sacral cord segments or the sacral roots behave differently from upper motor neuron lesions. Since these injuries involve the motor areas and sensory fibers that serve the lower urinary tract directly, reflex bladder and external sphincter responses are lost to filling of the bladder. Since the motor supply to the internal sphincter is derived from the lower thoracic and upper lumbar cord segments, the internal sphincter functions and stays closed, while bladder reflex responses to filling are lost. This results in a situation where, as the bladder fills, the sphincter maintains pressure until bladder pressure, as a result of filling, becomes high enough to overcome it. The magnitude of urethral resistance determines the intravesical pressure that will cause leakage. If that pressure is high (40 cm H_2O or more) a danger of backpressure effects on the upper urinary tract exists.[25] In the face of high urethral resistance, the bladder undergoes definite changes, so that pressure induced by filling becomes progressively higher at ever smaller volumes. This response, and the danger of backpressure on the upper urinary tract, can be obviated by regular intermittent catheterization and the use of anticholinergic drugs, just as in patients with higher neural lesions.

Recent studies involving pressure measurements in patients with neurogenic bladder dysfunction have shown that control of bladder pressure is the single most important aspect of urologic care. In the end there are two ways to control bladder pressure: decrease bladder activity or destroy the sphincter and induce leakage at low pressure. The method chosen does not appear at this time to make much difference, although one method may be more suitable for a given patient than another.

SPECIFIC COMPLICATIONS OF SPINAL CORD INJURY

Incontinence

Most patients with lesions superior to the sacral cord segments develop incontinence as a result of reflex

bladder activity. If this cannot be controlled by anticholinergic agents and intermittent catheterization, then dorsal root ganglionectomy, percutaneous rhizotomy, or augmentation cystoplasty may be required. If the bladder pressure required to drive urine across the sphincter is low (30 cm H_2O or less), then condom catheter drainage can be used. If the pressure is higher, then sphincterotomy is required as well.

Failure to Empty with High Intravesical Pressures

High residual urine volumes and high storage and micturition pressures (greater than 40 cm H_2O) require treatment. Bladder responses to increased outlet resistance lead to muscular hypertrophy, and finally, fibrosis. Both processes result in increased bladder urine storage and micturition pressures, which are the direct cause of ureteral dilation, vesicoureteral reflux and pyelonephritis, loss of renal parenchyma, stone formation, hypertension, and renal failure (Fig. 36–2). Regardless of the level of injury, increased bladder pressures are related to maintenance of resting or increased outlet resistance.

Complications of Sphincterotomy

Part of the high pressure response to bladder filling in spinal cord–injured patients results directly from the

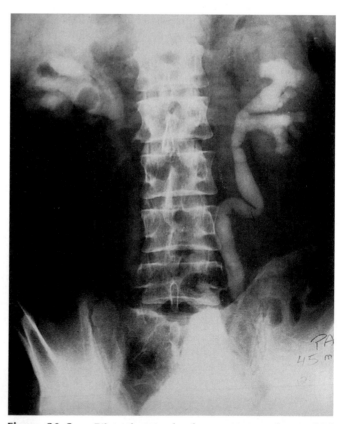

Figure 36–2 = Bilateral ureteral enlargement secondary to high intravesical pressure. The intrarenal collecting system is also dilated, and shows the changes of repeated episodes of acute pyelonephritis.

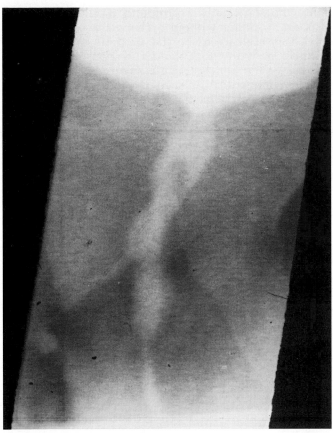

Figure 36–3 ═ Voiding study in a paraplegic patient after sphincterotomy showing no coaptation of the urethra in the active sphincter. Voiding pressure was 18 cm H₂O. This is an adequate sphincterotomy and if there is a high residual urine, it is related to bladder function, not urethral resistance.

Complications of Condom Catheter Drainage

In patients with low outlet resistance, either as a result of sphincterotomy, or spontaneously, condom catheter drainage is safe as far as upper tract function is concerned. There are a number of problems with the method, which include leakage, inability to hold the condom in place, chronic infection, and penile skin breakdown. These difficulties are usually solved by selection of a condom of appropriate design, in conjunction with a penile prosthetic device to prevent loss of penile girth once the condom has been applied. The latter, a problem in quadriplegics with reflex erectile activity excited by application of the condom, can be treated by insertion of a penile prosthesis. A prosthesis of the smallest available diameter should be used to prevent spontaneous erosion by the prosthesis into the urethra or out through the corpora, a common problem in patients with poor sensation. Occasionally, in an effort to prevent leakage, condoms are applied too tightly, creating an obstruction and leading to urethral diverticulum formation, or urethral erosion, with periurethral abscess formation and the development of a urethrocutaneous fistula. The latter complications are especially bad since they prevent further use of a condom. This leaves little in the way of alternative methods of management since sphincter function must be poor to begin with to permit use of condom catheter drainage. The urologist is then faced with a patient incontinent via a fistula, in whom fistula repair is doomed to failure by the same conditions which caused it in the first place (Fig. 36–4). This kind of problem is often complicated by massive perineal skin

effect of increased sphincter pressure. When that is lessened by sphincterotomy, bladder activity may cease, or become ineffective, leading to residual urine, infection, or more of what prompted the operation in the first place (Fig. 36–3). This is more often encountered in quadriplegics, which is why some workers recommend total sphincterotomy for all quadriplegics who need the operation. This converts the urethra to a conduit and permits very low pressure, almost passive leakage.[29] The effect of sphincterotomy in all spinal cord–injured patients is related to a decrease in pressure, and not absence of residual urine. Thus, measurement of the pressure required to drive urine across the resected sphincter is periodically required. In paraplegics a voiding pressure less than 30 cm H₂O is acceptable, while in quadriplegics treated by total sphincterotomy, a voiding pressure of 10 cm H₂O is required.

There are several disadvantages to sphincterotomy, including permanent incontinence, potentially impaired fertility, possible impairment in reflex erectile ability, chronic bacteriuria, as well as a somewhat unpredictable outcome. There is no reported long-term follow-up series of sphincterotomy patients, but our experience would suggest that the procedure has to be repeated at least once in about 30% of patients and in some, more than two times.

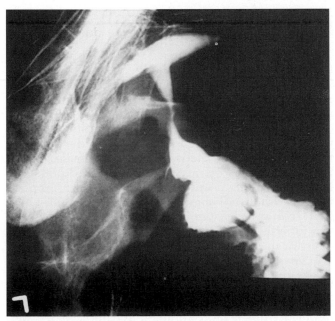

Figure 36–4 ═ Cystourethrogram from a 28-year-old paraplegic man showing a small, trabeculated grossly abnormal bladder, a mildly patent urethra, and a large penile-scrotal angle fistula, communicating freely with a massive perineal and sacral pressure ulceration.

breakdown, and associated osteomyelitis. Most urologists use formal urinary diversion in this circumstance but to stop drainage of infected material, a cystectomy is also required. We prefer to save the bladder, close the urethra at the pelvic floor, and create a continent abdominal stoma for intermittent self-catheterization.

Complications of Intermittent Catheterization

Intermittent catheterization is frequently accompanied by bacteriuria, as is condom catheter drainage. While eradication of bacteriuria would be better, it does not appear that this is possible. No study has reported more than transient success in this regard. The real issue is whether we can prevent renal tissue loss, pyelonephritis, struvite stone formation, and febrile urinary infections. The incidence of febrile urinary infections in patients whose bladder pressures are controlled is very low, as is the development of the other complications associated with symptomatic infection. On average, in those patients with well-controlled, low bladder pressure, a febrile infection occurs only once in 200 patient months. Thus, whether a particular antibiotic routine can control "infection" is almost impossible to establish. It is clearly not enough to establish that the incidence of positive cultures can be diminished, since that can only be done for a short time period, and the problems dealt with in spinal cord–injured patients involve a lifetime of risk. In the short term (1 to 10 years), provided that intravesical pressures are kept low, there does not appear to be any bad effect which can be directly attributed to bacteriuria. Whether the incidence of urothelial carcinoma will be increased in patients treated by intermittent catheterization or low-pressure condom catheter drainage, as it is in patients treated by catheters, remains to be seen.

"Silent hydronephrosis" has been described as a complication in patients treated by intermittent catheterization, but this is clearly a direct result of increased intravesical pressure. The relationship between bladder pressure and ureteral function is linear. When intravesical pressures reach 40 cm H_2O, ureteral dilation and decompensation begin to occur. In males such elevated intravesical pressure need not be associated with incontinence between catheterizations but in females, incontinence almost always accompanies elevated pressures. Hence, the term "silent hydronephrosis" was applied to males who were not incontinent and thus presumed to have a low-pressure bladder when in fact they did not. In this regard pressures must be measured in patients managed by intermittent catheterization or condom catheter drainage. Incontinence between catheterizations is almost always related to detrusor activity, but if measured intravesical pressures are low, then urethral sphincter weakness is the underlying problem. In practice this is more common in paraplegic females, but it does occur in males and is particularly likely in patients whose spinal cord loss involves more than one or two cord segments. Very occasionally we see male patients incontinent between intermittent catheterizations who show only a profound urethral relaxation response to filling without a change in bladder pressure. This appears to be the urethral component of micturition, without a bladder response, apparently because of the anticholinergic agents used to control bladder contractility. As such, the incontinence is very difficult to treat effectively, and even augmentation cystoplasty does not always cure the condition.

Complications of Chronic Catheter Drainage

Males treated by catheter drainage may develop penile scrotal angle fistulas, bladder calculi, chronic urethritis, and ultimately, over a period of 15 to 20 years, end-stage bladder dysfunction with reflux, pyelonephritis, and damaged ureters.[6, 17] With the development of an end-stage bladder, or a fibrotic, noncompliant, nondistensible bladder, upper tract deterioration begins to occur. With ureteral fibrosis, peristalsis is impaired and subsequent treatment compromised by altered urinary transport, so that even if the bladder is bypassed and a supravesical diversion performed, the process of upper tract deterioration will not be halted. Patients with catheters have a much higher incidence over time of upper tract deterioration.[1] While it is true that not all patients will develop such complications, the occurrence of major upper tract difficulties leading to a risk of renal failure is at least 50% over a 20-year period and the incidence of squamous cell carcinoma, a fatal disease, has been estimated to be 460 times the expected incidence in patients treated with catheters as compared to an age-matched normal population. Females are said to fare better with catheter drainage than male patients and in the short term they probably do. In one reported series, however, the incidence of incontinence around the catheter in a 5-year period after placement (and such devices are placed for control of incontinence) was 95%. Moreover, the incidence of upper tract deterioration was greater than 50%, as were the incidence of urethral erosion and bladder calculi development. In short, the same complications reported in males occur in females but require a slightly longer time to develop.[24] It should be emphasized that the complications of catheter drainage are serious, cumulative, and once established there may be little that corrective surgical treatment can do to reverse or stabilize the upper tract disease associated with their use. Suprapubic tubes were initially thought less troublesome than urethral catheters and in the short term that is the case. These devices avoid the urethral and periurethral complications associated with urethral catheters, but the long-term results are equally dismal with regard to bladder carcinoma and upper tract disease, including the formation of staghorn calculi of really impressive dimensions (Fig. 36–5). These stones reflect chronic upper tract infection, ureteral failure, and renal damage. None of these processes is resolved by stone removal, no matter how complete. Most centers now restrict the use of suprapubic tubes to quadriplegics, where they provide a convenient method of drainage, which promotes early rehabilitation. The cost

some magnitude. These stones, untreated, are associated with the development of renal failure (or vice versa) and spontaneous erosion out of the collecting system and kidney and xanthogranulomatous pyelonephritis. In patients with spinal cord injury, the conditions which lead to the development of such stones are often untreatable, as in the case of persons with ileal loop diversion, suprapubic tubes, or catheters, where ureteral function and urinary drainage are compromised and stone removal, no matter how skillful, only prolongs an inevitable recurrence (Fig. 36–6).

The advent of extracorporeal shock wave lithotripsy (ESWL) has had a good effect on struvite stones since, prior to the use of these machines (and the parallel use of percutaneous lithotripsy), open stone removal was the only practicable treatment. This method, while initially successful, led to nephrectomy when repetitive surgery was necessitated by recurrent stone formation, a disaster in a patient with recurrent stone formation related to untreatable lower urinary tract dysfunction. While both electrohydraulic and percutaneous lithotripsy are renal-sparing when compared to open surgery, percutaneous surgery has a lower retained stone fragment rate than ESWL. Perhaps the most efficient method to treat large infection stones is a combination of the two procedures.

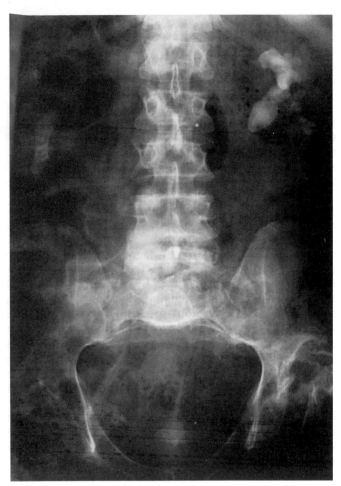

Figure 36–5 ═ Large bilateral staghorn calculi in a quadriplegic patient treated with a suprapubic tube visible just above the pubic symphysis. Even if these stones are removed, the processes which lead to their development will remain active and recurrence is inevitable.

in terms of the upper urinary tract is, however, insupportably high. The convenience of these lethal devices and the length of time required to produce life-threatening complications makes them difficult to remove, once placed, since patients tend to like them. It is better to avoid them entirely so that the problem of removal never comes up.

Urinary Stone Formation

In the first few months after spinal cord injury, when patients are largely immobilized and calcium loss is related to bone demineralization, calcium oxalate stones are relatively common. These generally cause little difficulty and are usually found in the bladder. After the first 1 to 2 years stone formation almost always is related to urinary infection associated with urea-splitting organisms, and a poorly managed lower urinary tract. Once upper tract struvite stone formation begins, stones formed in the caliceal system or renal pelvis tend to grow in situ rather than to be passed. The development of large staghorn calculi forming a cast of the entire collecting system is a problem of

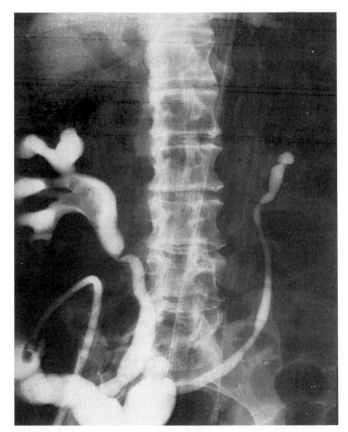

Figure 36–6 ═ A 28-year-old man with a high spinal cord injury and an ileal loop diversion. Note the absent left kidney, removed for stones and pyelonephritis, and a large filling defect in the right renal pelvis indicating progressive, nonremediable disease in the remaining kidney.

Comarr AE (eds): Neurological Urology. Baltimore, University Park Press, 1971, pp 223–261.

7. Bors E, Engle ET, Rosenquist RC, et al: Fertility in paraplegic males—A preliminary report of endocrine studies. J Clin Endocrinol 10:381–398, 1950.
8. Brindley GS: The fertility of men with spinal injuries. Paraplegia 22:337–348, 1984.
9. Chapelle PA, Blanquart F, Peuch AJ, et al: Treatment of anejaculation in the total paraplegic by subcutaneous injection of physostigmine. Paraplegia 21:30–36, 1983.
10. Comarr AE: Observations on menstruation and pregnancy among female spinal cord injury patients. Paraplegia 3:263–271, 1966.
11. Damanski M, Gibbon NOR: The upper urinary tract in the paraplegic: A long term study. Br J Urol 28:24, 1956.
12. Dominque GJ, Roberts JA, Lauciriea R, et al: Pathogenic significance of P-fimbriated E. coli in urinary tract infections. J Urol 133:983, 1985.
13. Emmett JL: Transurethral resection in treatment of true and pseudo cord bladder. J Urol 53:4, 1945.
14. François N, Lichtenberger JM, Jouannet P, et al: L'Éjaculation par le vibromassage chez le paraplégique à propos de 50 cas avec 7 grossesses. Ann Med Phys 23:24–36, 1980.
15. Guttman L, Frankel H: The value of intermittent catheterization in the early management of traumatic tetraplegia and paraplegia. Paraplegia 4:63, 1966.
16. Guttman L, Walsh JJ: Prostigmin assessment of fertility in spinal man. Paraplegia 9:39–51, 1971.
17. Herr HW: Intermittent catheterization in neurogenic bladder dysfunction. J Urol 113:477, 1975.
18. Lapides J, Diokno AC, Silber SJ, et al: Clean intermittent catheterization in the treatment of urinary tract disease. J Urol 107:458, 1972.
19. Leviche A, Berard E, Vanzelle JL, et al: Histological and hormonal testicular changes in spinal cord patients. Paraplegia 15:274–279, 1977.
20. McGuire EJ, Brady S: Detrusor-sphincter dyssynergia. J Urol 121:774, 1979.
21. McGuire EJ, Rossier AB: Treatment of acute autonomic dysreflexia. J Urol 129:1185, 1983.
22. McGuire EJ, Savastano JA: Long term followup of spinal cord injury patients managed by intermittent catheterization. J Urol 129:775, 1983.
23. McGuire EJ, Savastano JA: Urodynamic findings and clinical status following vesical denervation procedures for control of incontinence. J Urol 132:87, 1984.
24. McGuire EJ, Savastano JA: Comparative urological outcome in females with spinal cord injury. J Urol 135:730, 1986.
25. McGuire EJ, Woodside JR, Borden TA: Upper urinary tract deterioration in patients with myelodysplasia and detrusor hypertonia: A follow up study. J Urol 129:823, 1983.
26. Melzak J: The incidence of bladder cancer in paraplegia. Paraplegia 4:85, 1966.
27. Nilsson S, Obrant KO, Persson PS: Changes in the testis parenchyma caused by acute nonspecific epididymitis. Fertil Steril 19:748–757, 1968.
28. Parkhurst EC, Leadbetter WF: A report on 93 ileal loop urinary diversions. J Urol 83:398, 1960.
29. Perkash I: Modified approach to sphincterectomy in spinal cord injured patients: Indications, techniques and results. Paraplegia 13:247, 1976.
30. Perkash I: Detrusor-sphincter dyssynergic responses. J Urol 120:469, 1978.
31. Reid G, Sobel JD: Bacterial adherence in the pathogenesis of urinary tract infection: A review. Rev of Infect Dis 9:3, 1987.
32. Riches EW: The methods and results of treatment of cases of paralysis of the bladder following spinal cord injury. Br J Urol 31:135, 1943.
33. Schaeffer AJ: Bladder defense mechanism. Semin Urol Oncol 1:106–113, 1983.
34. Schaeffer AJ, Chmiel J: Urethral meatal colonization in the pathogenesis of catheter associated bacteriuria. J Urol 130:1096, 1983.
35. Steinberg R, Bennett CJ, Konnak J, et al: Construction of a low pressure reservoir and achievement of continence after diversion and in end stage bladder dysfunction. J Urol 138:39, 1987.
36. Talbot HS: The sexual function in paraplegia. J Urol 73:91–100, 1955.
37. Thomas RJS, McLeich G, McDonald IA: Electroejaculation of the paraplegic male followed by pregnancy. Med J Aust 2:798–799, 1975.
38. Tribe CR: Causes of death in early and late stages of paraplegia. Int J Paraplegia 1:19, 1963.
39. Tsuji I, Nakajima F, Morimoto J, et al: The sexual function in patients with spinal cord injury. Urol Int 12:270–280, 1961.
40. Van Arsdalen KN, Klein FA, Hackler RH, et al: Penile implants in spinal cord injury patients for maintaining external appliances. J Urol 126:331–332, 1981.
41. Webb DR, Fitzpatrick JM, O'Flynn JD: A 15 year followup of 406 consecutive spinal cord injuries. Br J Urol 56:614, 1984.

CHAPTER 37

Complications of the Musculoskeletal System Following Spinal Cord Injury

Michael J. Botte

The disabling nature of acute spinal cord injury and the resultant loss of function are well recognized. However, beyond the *acute* effects on the musculoskeletal system, chronic problems and subsequent complications can further impede functional and emotional recovery. Though many of these extremity problems are unavoidable or are the result of the initial spinal cord injury, many complications may be preventable or minimized with prompt diagnosis and proper management. In this chapter, musculoskeletal complications in the patient with spinal cord injury are discussed. These complications have been divided into four sections: (1) complications involving bone, (2) complications involving muscle, (3) complications associated with upper extremity weight bearing in the paraplegic patient, and (4) miscellaneous complications.

COMPLICATIONS INVOLVING BONE

Two common complications involving bone are (1) fractures in the extremities and (2) neurogenic heterotopic ossification.

Extremity Fractures

Fractures in the extremities of the spinal cord injury patient present unique problems with both diagnosis and treatment. These fractures can be divided into two main types: (1) acute fractures sustained in *normal* bone at the time of spinal cord injury and (2) subsequent pathologic fractures sustained in *osteoporotic* bone in the patient with a long-standing paretic extremity. In addition, a third type of fracture will be briefly discussed; a fracture sustained in a normal limb above the level of paralysis in a patient with long-standing spinal cord injury.[11, 15, 57]

Acute Fractures Sustained at the Time of Spinal Cord Injury

Acute fractures sustained at the time of spinal cord injury occur in previously normal bone and usually involve high-speed injuries.[11, 15, 57] The pathomechanics, configuration, and anatomic location of the fractures are similar to those seen in patients without spinal cord injury. The reported incidence of extremity fractures occurring in the multiple trauma spinal cord injury patient is between 9% and 20%,[15, 57, 78] with long bone fractures accounting for 26% to 44% of these. Eleven percent to 19% of long bone fractures occur in the upper extremity and 19% to 47% occur in the lower extremity. Pelvic fractures occur in up to 28% of these patients.[11, 26, 57] Malunion and delayed union are common.[11, 15, 26] The incidence of reported nonunion varies between 4% and 16%.[15, 26]

Diagnosis. The clinical diagnosis of extremity fracture in the paretic extremity may not be apparent initially, especially when pain is absent because of impaired sensibility, when deformity is lacking, or when patient cognition is decreased. The examiner is often misdirected toward more obvious injuries. Fractures in the carpus and tarsus often show little limb deformity, and swelling may be minimal. The presence of swelling, ecchymosis, increased warmth, lacerations, abrasions, and crepitus requires careful examination and appropriate radiographic evaluation. In addition, the multiple trauma patient deserves routine pelvis radiographs. A high degree of suspicion will help diagnose these difficult fractures.

Treatment. Treatment of acute fractures in the spinal cord injury patient is directed toward early fracture stabilization to allow patient mobilization, early rehabilitation, and to minimize complications associated with prolonged bed rest. Operative stabilization and early mobilization have been shown to decrease the frequency of deep venous thromboses and decubitus ulcers.[23] Besides allowing early mobilization, internal fixation of fractures obviates the need for casts, splints, and traction, all of which are poorly tolerated in the neurologically involved extremity. Impaired sensibility increases the chances of skin ulceration with casts or splints. Spastic limbs with increased muscle tone or clonus are difficult to manage in traction or with splints. In addition, plaster immobilization prevents joint mobilization, interferes with self-care, and hinders wheelchair transfers. The physical weight of these de-

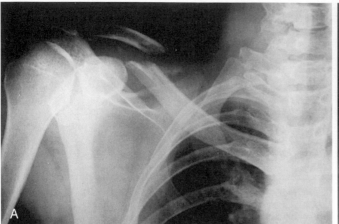
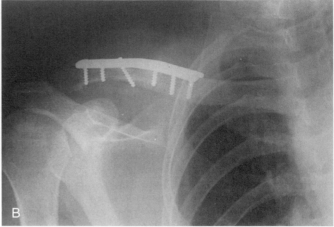

Figure 37–1 = In the spinal cord injury patient, many fractures that might normally be treated with closed methods (such as isolated clavicle, humerus, metacarpal, or tibial fractures) can be more optimally treated with operative stabilization (if the patient's overall medical condition permits). In the radiograph presented here, open reduction and internal fixation of the clavicle were performed on a patient with an incomplete C4 functional level lesion to allow early shoulder motion and facilitate rehabilitation of the spastic paretic limb. This aggressive approach to fracture stabilization in the multiple trauma patient with spinal cord injury usually permits earlier and more aggressive limb mobilization and avoids the use of splints, casts, and traction devices that may cause secondary problems in a limb with spasticity, paralysis, and poor sensibility. *A,* Fracture of clavicle. *B,* After open reduction–internal fixation.

vices can be difficult to manage by the patient with a paretic limb.

If the patient is medically stable and there are no contraindications, early open reduction and internal fixation of major long bone fractures are desirable.[22, 57] These procedures can often be performed at the time of initial spine stabilization. Most fractures are treated according to standard orthopaedic principles. Some fractures that might otherwise be treated with closed methods (such as the clavicle, humerus, metacarpals, tibia, and metatarsals) may be difficult to manage if spasticity or paralytic muscle imbalance is present (Fig. 37–1).[8] Open reduction and internal fixation should be considered if closed methods fail with these fractures. Intramedullary nailing of humerus fractures may allow early upper extremity weight bearing for wheelchair transfers. If operative surgery for extremity fractures is contraindicated, the use of well-padded splints or bivalved casts may provide a reasonable alternative,[57] with consideration given to performing internal fixation at a later date when the patient becomes medically stable. Any external immobilization devices must be well padded and checked frequently for skin irritation or ischemia.

Pathologic Fractures in Long-Standing Spinal Cord Injury

Pathologic fractures occur in osteoporotic bone in the patient with long-standing spinal cord injury. These fractures are usually low-energy injuries and result from minimal trauma to the osteoporotic paralytic limb. Falls from wheelchairs or during transfers, positioning in bed, or manual mobilization of a joint have sufficient energy to result in fractures and are common modes of injury. Fractures in long bones occur more often in paraplegic patients than in quadriplegics, owing to the paraplegic's increased activity level and participation in physical activities. Most fractures are sus-

tained in metaphyseal areas of the lower extremity, commonly near the knee. Other common sites of fracture include the distal tibia, intertrochanteric region of the femur, femoral neck, and diaphysis of the femur or tibia.[70] Because of impaired sensibility and the minimal trauma required to fracture an osteoporotic bone, the fracture often goes initially unrecognized. If deformity is minimal, swelling, ecchymosis, and warmth may be the only signs. Fractures occurring near joints can clinically mimic infection, heterotopic ossification, or phlebitis. A high index of suspicion will enhance radiographic evaluation and confirmation.

Etiology. Osteoporosis in the spinal cord injury patient develops from stress deprivation in the paralytic limbs, due to both lack of muscular forces acting on the bone and to lack of weight bearing. The loss of bone mass commences following spinal cord injury and is accompanied initially by a negative calcium balance. Though calcium balance usually becomes positive by the sixth month post injury, the degree of osteoporosis may not change significantly if normal muscular forces are not acting on bone.[70] The degree of osteoporosis is variable, and in some patients a year may be required before osteoporosis is sufficiently advanced before pathologic fractures will occur.[74]

Treatment. Treatment of these pathologic fractures depends on the type of fracture and the degree of limb paresis or spasticity. In the paralytic nonfunctional extremity with little or no spasticity, pathologic fractures can usually be managed nonoperatively, utilizing well-padded splints or bivalved casts.[20, 70, 74] Operative stabilization is avoided because fixation is often difficult to achieve or easily lost in the osteoporotic bone. There is also an increased incidence of infection due to the atrophy of the surrounding muscle and skin. Fortunately, most of these pathologic fractures heal without surgery. In these nonambulatory patients, moderate degrees of fracture deformity may be acceptable, as long as previous functions are preserved and fracture deformity or callus does not result in areas of increased pressure on the skin. Ease of positioning, sitting, and transfers must be maintained. Fractures of the femoral neck treated nonoperatively often form a pseudarthrosis. Pseudarthrosis of the femoral neck may cause no additional disability to the nonambulatory patient, provided there are no major rotational deformities. In some patients, pseudarthrosis of the hip may actually allow an increased range of motion.[74] Nonambulatory patients with fractures in paralytic limbs usually have little or no discomfort, so the fracture can usually be easily reduced and maintained in well-padded splints or bivalved casts.[74] Nonunion may occur in severely displaced fractures or those with soft tissue interposition. Management of these fractures may require operative stabilization.

In the paraparetic patient who has residual function of the lower extremities or who was ambulatory before the fracture, treatment is directed toward restoring function. Open reduction and internal fixation of displaced femoral neck fractures minimizes the chances of pseudarthrosis of the neck and avascular necrosis of the femoral head. Open reduction and internal fixation of displaced intertrochanteric fractures or subtrochanteric fractures can prevent shortening or varus malunion. Internal fixation of severely shortened diaphyseal femur fractures will minimize limb length discrepancy. Displaced intra-articular fractures in the ambulatory patient require operative restoration of the articular surface. In severely displaced fractures or those with soft tissue interposition, surgery may be required to achieve union.

In the quadriparetic patient with an upper extremity fracture, goals of fracture care are to maintain pre-existing function of the extremities. Fractures must be satisfactorily reduced, utilizing internal fixation as necessary. If internal fixation is required in severely osteoporotic bone, additional external immobilization with splints may be necessary. Postoperative therapy for mobilization of the limb is individualized.

In any limb with severe spasticity, it may be difficult or impossible to manage a fracture with closed methods.[9, 26, 30, 31] If adequate bone stock exists, open reduction and internal fixation should be considered. Alternatively, a phenol nerve block to the involved muscles may allow closed treatment of the fracture. The phenol block will decrease spasticity, and lasts 3 to 6 months,[8, 44, 47, 48] usually enough time to allow fracture healing. Phenol blocks are discussed under Spasticity.

Fracture Sustained in a Normal Extremity in the Long-Standing Paraplegic Patient

Fractures of this type consist of traumatic injuries that occur in normal bone above the level of long-standing paralysis. These injuries are often high-energy fractures, and are sustained in a group of patients who are vigorous and motivated to remain active.[57] Many of these patients drive motor vehicles. In the treatment of these fractures, an effort must be made to maintain the patients' independence. Most fractures can be

treated in a fashion similar to those in the non–spinal cord injury patient, with similar indications for operative stabilization. An aggressive operative approach avoids the use of casts or splints, and thus allows earlier limb mobilization to promote rapid rehabilitation. In fractures of the diaphysis of the humerus, intramedullary nailing usually allows earlier weight bearing during wheelchair transfers.

Neurogenic Heterotopic Ossification

Neurogenic heterotopic ossification is a spontaneous formation of bone that usually occurs near major synovial joints in a patient who has sustained an injury to the central nervous system (CNS). It most commonly develops in the vicinity of the hip (Fig. 37–2). Heterotopic ossification was first described as a complication following spinal cord injury by Riedel in 1883.[23] The exact cause of this bone formation remains unknown. It is not a response to or result of local soft tissue trauma or joint injury. Since the deposited bone in neurogenic heterotopic ossification usually occurs near or around joints, it is sometimes termed *periarticular ossification*.[58, 59]

Associated Problems. The bone formation can result in mechanical restriction of motion or frank ankylosis. Secondary contractures of the soft tissues may form if mobilization of the joint is not maintained or is prevented by the heterotopic bone. Pain or discomfort may be initially present if limb sensibility is intact. The resultant loss of motion can severely impede function. Sitting, transfers, dressing, and hygiene may be prevented. Restricted positioning can secondarily lead to pressure sore formation and subsequent infection.[16, 17, 42, 76, 77] Lack of joint motion can increase the likelihood of pathologic fracture of the osteoporotic bone during positioning or lifting.

Incidence and Joints Involved. The reported inci-

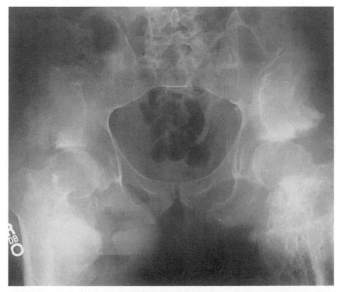

Figure 37–2 = Anteroposterior radiograph of pelvis of spinal cord injury patient with heterotopic ossification. Restricted motion leads to difficulty with wheelchair transfers and positioning.

dence of neurogenic heterotopic ossification in patients with spinal cord injuries is between 10% and 25%. Loss of motion occurs in about one third of these.[23, 28, 83, 84] In about 5%, complete ankylosis develops.[23, 28] Heterotopic ossification is more common in quadriplegics than paraplegics, and forms in neurologically impaired limbs. Both spastic and flaccid extremities may be affected, and ossification may occur in patients with incomplete or complete spinal cord lesions.[83] Large amounts of bone can be formed adjacent to joints. The bone is usually deposited between the muscle planes; it is not placed within muscles or within joints. The bone can, however, distort or displace neighboring muscles or neurovascular structures. The ossification may completely encase nerves or vessels. The hip is the most common joint affected, followed by the knee. When the hip is involved, bone is usually deposited anterior to the joint, extending from the anteriorsuperior iliac crest, anterior to the capsule, to the region of the lesser trochanter or anterior aspect of the proximal femur. It occasionally develops posteriorly, from the ischium to the posterior aspect of the lesser trochanter. When the knee is involved, heterotopic bone usually forms medial to the medial condyle and extends up the femur for variable lengths.[23] The shoulder and elbow are only occasionally involved. Involvement of wrists, hands, ankles, and feet is rare.

Time of Development. The time of initial occurrence of heterotopic bone is variable, and can occur from 2 weeks to 12 months post spinal cord injury. It is usually detected at approximately 2 months post injury.[23] Once diagnosed, its time of *maturation* is even more variable and often difficult to assess. "Maturation" generally refers to the time of cessation of bone growth, and is usually based on radiographic appearance (discussed later), stabilization of levels of serum alkaline phosphatase (though not always reliable), and decreasing or static activity on repeated technetium bone scans and sulfur colloid scans. The bone usually increases in size over a 6-month period, then shows progressive signs of maturation thereafter. Garland[23] has described two classes of heterotopic ossification based on clinical presentations and behavior: Class I (comprising about 90%) has its initial occurrence at about 2 months post spinal cord injury, has a peak of activity over the next 5 or 6 months, and is followed by maturation where ossification becomes relatively inert. In class II (comprising about 10%), the initial occurrence and peak of activity take place at similar times as class I, but the potential to form heterotopic ossification remains for months or years. Chances of recurrence following excision are higher in class II.[23]

Clinical Findings. An inflammatory response usually precedes or coincides with the formation of heterotopic bone formation. Clinical findings during the development of neurogenic heterotopic ossification include tenderness (if sensibility is intact), swelling, warmth, redness, and stiffness or ankylosis of the involved joint. Infection or thrombophlebitis can be mimicked. Occasionally a palpable mass is initially detectable. Once mature, the swelling, warmth, and redness may subside, leaving only joint stiffness and a possible palpable bone mass. Secondary soft tissue contractures of the joint can occur if the limb is not mobilized.

Radiographic and Laboratory Evaluation. Radiographs may be difficult to interpret. Initial radiographs often fail to demonstrate the bone formation, despite positive clinical findings. The technetium bone scan, however, will usually show evidence of bone formation activity. It may take an additional few days to several weeks before the bone formation becomes apparent on standard radiographs. In the early period of bone formation, the heterotopic ossification may appear radiographically as an indistinct, fluffy shadow of ossification around the joint, with poorly defined margins. It increases in size on subsequent radiographs and as it matures the bone becomes well defined with distinct margins and linear trabeculations, and the size of the bone mass stabilizes. Because both mature heterotopic ossification and immature heterotopic ossification may coexist, and since the mature ossification can obscure the immature ossification, radiograph determination of maturity is not always reliable.[83] During active bone formation, serum alkaline phosphatase is usually elevated. It may remain elevated for years, reaching elevations as high as 500 units/L.[22, 23, 66, 83, 84]

Microscopic Findings. Histologically, heterotopic ossification resembles that of woven bone formation, with areas of concurrent inflammation. Initially, it may appear as disorganized lamellar bone with osteoblastic activity (within the first 8 months). The immature bone demonstrates hypervascularity.[83] Eventually, the bone takes on the appearance of mature cortical bone, with a decrease in osteoblastic activity, a decrease in hypervascularity, and a more organized lamellar pattern. It may take 18 months before the bone appears histologically as mature bone.[83]

Treatment. Treatment includes management of associated pain, maintenance of joint motion, use of medications to decrease inflammation and bone production, and surgical resection of bone and release of associated contractures. Use of radiation is under investigation, and ultimately may prove to be useful.

Maintenance of motion by passive mobilization is the initial treatment of neurogenic heterotopic ossification. Maintenance of joint motion helps maximize function, and aids in positioning, dressing, hygiene, and prevention of pressure sores. Mobilization of the affected joint is instituted early, and should be administered as soon as the diagnosis is made. Mobilization does not seem to alter the formation of heterotopic ossification, but can prevent secondary soft tissue contractures and maintain or increase motion by producing microfractures or pseudarthrosis through an ankylosing mass of bone.[29, 83, 84] Aggressive passive motion does not seem to aggravate the inflammatory response or adversely affect bone production. However, in the patient with spared sensibility, mobilization may be difficult because of associated discomfort. Analgesics and anti-inflammatory medications may help. Allowing the joint to undergo prolonged immobilization must be avoided, since secondary soft tissue fixed contractures develop. *Forceful* manipulation of the joint (under anesthesia if needed), is somewhat controversial, but has been shown to increase motion with some types of neurogenic heterotopic ossification.[29] Increased motion usually occurs by causing fracture or microfracture through the forming heterotopic bone. The indications for and role of forceful manipulation in the spinal cord injury patient have not been well established, but this method may prove to be effective. All manipulations must be done with caution to prevent pathologic fracture of osteoporotic long bones.

Disodium etidronate has been shown to be effective in preventing the occurrence of heterotopic ossification or in reducing its extension once it is clinically evident.[23, 24, 30, 73, 76] Disodium etidronate works by inhibition of the formation and growth of hydroxyapatite crystals. The recommended dose is 20 mg/per kilogram per day, for prophylaxis, initiated prior to clinical or radiographic evidence of heterotopic ossification and continued for 3 months. For established heterotopic ossification, treatment is continued for 6 months. Garland[28] has noted recurrence or rebound of heterotopic ossification in class II patients even after 6 months of treatment. It is sometimes felt that disodium etidronate does not prevent heterotopic ossification, but only delays its formation.

Surgical resection of heterotopic ossification can be performed in severe or refractory cases. Indications include limitation of motion with function loss, difficulty in positioning, sitting, dressing, transfers, or hygiene.[23, 25, 28, 83, 84] Resection needs to be planned carefully, as this surgery is associated with high morbidity, including hemorrhage, sepsis, and re-ankylosis.[28] Neurovascular structures may be displaced or encased in the bone mass, thus cautious dissection, good visibility, and adequate exposure are required for resection. Computed tomography (CT) or standard polytomography will help access the three-dimensional structure of the bone mass. The timing of resection of heterotopic ossification is controversial. It is generally accepted that early resection of "immature" bone has a higher incidence of recurrence and hemorrhage than resection of mature bone. The immature bone is usually highly vascular. However, delaying surgery until bone is "mature" may take years and result in problems associated with prolonged joint immobilization (such as fixed soft tissue contracture and cartilage erosions).[2, 10] Evaluating the maturity of bone is difficult, and is usually based on the appearance on plain radiographs, stabilizing alkaline phosphatase levels, and decreasing activity on technetium bone scans. These indicators are not always reliable.[23] Therefore, specific recommendations for time of resection of heterotopic bone are difficult to determine. It has been recommended to wait a minimum of 14 months following diagnosis to achieve adequate bone maturity to minimize hemorrhage and reduce the chance of recurrence. Resection should only involve removal of adequate bone to acquire desired motion. The entire mass does not always need to be resected, and often only a wedge of bone needs to be removed. Because of the dead space created and open bone ends from resection, placement of wound drains is recommended. Substantial postsurgical blood loss can occur through drains, and should be carefully monitored.[83] Blood must be available for transfusion if needed.

Following resection, close follow-up and continued mobilization should be reinstituted early to maintain motion. Physical therapy for 6 months may be required to maintain gains in motion. In patients undergoing resection of heterotopic ossification at the hip to increase motion for sitting, 74% have been shown to gain satisfactory motion to allow sitting, achieving an average gain of 30 degrees in the arc of motion.[28] Preoperative range of motion seems to be an important predictor of final postoperative motion. Patients with ankylosed hips usually gain the least motion following resection. As noted earlier, complication rates are often high (infection or operative blood loss occurring in up to 79%) and bony recurrence common (occurring in 92%). However, surgical resection remains an effective means of increasing motion, and with proper planning and realistic expectations, it offers a reasonable method for management of this difficult problem.

COMPLICATIONS INVOLVING MUSCLE

Correlating Type of Injury with Effects on Muscle

Injury to the spinal cord can produce different effects on muscle, including paralysis (which indicates no volitional muscle function), paresis (weak muscle function), or spasticity (which includes increased tone, hyperactive reflexes, clonus). The effect on muscle depends on the type and level of cord injury, the involvement of nerve roots, and the time elapsed from injury. Immediately following a severe spinal cord injury, flaccid paralysis develops below the level of the lesion. Flaccidity usually lasts less than 24 hours, and is followed by development of spasticity.[74] Spasticity develops as a result of disruption of the upper motor neuron inhibitory pathways from the brain to the anterior horn cells of the spinal cord. Muscle control from the brain is impaired or eliminated. Primitive reflex action predominates from the uninjured cord below the level of injury. Thus, the period of flaccidity is followed by a period of increasing muscle tone, return of stretch reflexes, and a progression to hyperactive reflexes. In addition, sudden muscle contractions or "spasms" may become frequent and occur with minimal stimulus to the muscle or overlying skin. Clonus, rigidity, and the clasp-knife reflex often develop. At this point of increased tone and hyperactivity, the muscles are considered to be spastic.[10]

Spasticity develops in the muscles distal to the level of cord damage, mediated by primitive reflex activity from the intact cord distal to the injury. However, spasticity does not develop at the level of cord injury, since the spinal reflex arc is disrupted at this level. Instead, flaccid paralysis (no function) or paresis (weakness) occurs at the level of injury. Nerve root injury may also contribute to or account for weakness at the level of injury, and is discussed later. If there is an incomplete spinal cord injury, some neurologic recovery may occur. Muscles that are spastic may improve with time and return to a less hyperreflexic state. Gradual recovery of volitional control can occur as well (in the incomplete lesion), and contributes to improved extremity function. This "recovery period" is variable, and usually occurs over a 6- to 12-month period following the initial spinal cord injury. At approximately 1 year post injury, most patients with an incomplete spinal cord injury will have approached or reached the end of the period when spontaneous neurologic recovery usually occurs, and little or no further neurologic recovery can be expected.

In addition to injury to the spinal cord, nerve roots or anterior horn cells in the vicinity of the cord lesion may be injured. Trauma that injures the cervical cord often injures the neighboring nerve root, especially roots in the foramen between dislocated or fractured vertebrae. The nerve root may originate from the normal cord proximal to the injured cord and be damaged as it leaves the foramen,[74] thus resulting in some muscle function loss that is above the level of cord injury. When a nerve root is damaged, the injury is a lower motor neuron lesion. Paralysis or weakness (but not spasticity) of the corresponding muscles results. Therefore, there may be a group of flaccid or weak muscles (from nerve root injury) that are proximal to the level of spastic muscles (from cord injury). If the nerve root is only partially injured and remains structurally intact (neuropraxia or axonotmesis), the impaired function of the corresponding muscle may gradually return. This may explain why some patients with a complete spinal cord injury subsequently gain the function of one or two root levels over time (it is a peripheral nerve that is recovering, not the spinal cord). If the continuity of the nerve root is disrupted (neurotmesis), function will not spontaneously recover, and the affected muscles will remain weak or flaccid.

To summarize, depending on the type of injury to the spinal cord and nerve roots, different types of muscle impairment may ultimately occur at or below the level of injury: (1) paralysis, (2) paresis, and (3) spasticity. At the level of injury, muscles will be weak or flaccid, due to either damage to the cord at this level (thus disrupting both volitional control and spinal reflex activity) or nerve root injury (resulting in peripheral nerve injury and paresis). Below the level of spinal cord injury, the muscles will be paralyzed or paretic (depending on completeness of the cord injury), and spasticity will usually be present due to loss of upper motor neuron inhibitory control.

In many complete cervical spinal cord injuries that involve the cord between the C5 and T1 root levels, muscles in the upper extremity are often predominantly weak or flaccid, with little or no spasticity. This occurs because the cord or nerve roots have been segmentally damaged over a few levels, and thus, as mentioned above, spinal reflex arcs at these levels are disrupted and spasticity cannot occur. Since spasticity only occurs in areas where the spinal reflex is intact, upper extremity spasticity, if present, usually develops at the more distally innervated muscles (innervated by

roots C7, C8, or T1), since these levels are more apt to be distal to the injured segment of cord (and thus the spinal reflex arc is intact). Spasticity does, however, rarely occur in the more proximally innervated muscles in the upper extremity (such as C5 or C4) if the cord lesion is proximal to these levels. Many of these patients, however, do not survive because of paralysis of the diaphragm and resulting respiratory failure. Therefore, spasticity is seen less often in the upper extremity than in the lower extremity, and paralysis or paresis becomes the predominant upper extremity problem.

Injuries to the lumbar spine can produce either upper motor neuron or lower motor neuron injuries. The cauda equina begins at about the L2 level. Injuries proximal to this produce mostly upper motor neuron lesions (with varying degrees of lower motor neuron involvement if nerve roots are injured). These injuries usually result in muscle spasticity distal to the injury. Distal to the conus medullaris, only lower motor neurons exist, and injuries in these areas produce peripheral nerve injuries manifest by paralysis or paresis, without spasticity. In reality, many injuries in the vicinity of L2 injure both the cord above the conus and associated nerve roots or parts of the cauda equina, and therefore clinical presentations with both spasticity and flaccidity are possible.

In spinal cord injuries, the degree of spasticity is variable. In the incomplete cord lesion, some volitional control may be superimposed on either spastic or paretic muscles below the level of injury. Volitional control does not return in the true complete spinal cord injury.

Muscle strength in the spinal cord injury patient should not progressively decrease. Ascending or progressive loss of muscle function is worrisome. In the acute stages of spinal injury it may indicate progressive nerve or cord compression (i.e., from disc protrusion, hematoma, edema, loss of spine reduction). Loss of muscle function that occurs at a later time may indicate ascending syrinx formation within the cord or loss of spine stability. Progressive muscle loss in any of these settings requires immediate investigation.

In the following section, problems associated with spasticity and paralysis and their management are discussed. Though these two topics are discussed separately, it must be kept in mind that they often occur in the same extremity simultaneously, hence the term *spastic paralysis*.

As explained above, weakness is often predominant in the upper extremity and spasticity often predominant in the lower extremities. Management of these problems has evolved so that efforts in the upper extremity are usually directed mainly toward restoring function of weak muscles, utilizing reconstructive procedures such as tendon transfers and tenodeses. In the lower extremity, however, efforts are directed more toward the control of noxious spasticity, utilizing muscle or tendon releases or lengthenings.

Spasticity

Following the initial period of flaccidity immediately following spinal cord injury, spasticity develops to varying degrees.[35] It occurs in both complete and incomplete spinal cord injury. In some patients spasticity is mild, and the muscles remain predominantly weak or flaccid. In others, spasticity is so severe that minimal stimulation of muscle produces sudden violent muscle contractions. Severe increased muscle tone can prohibit adequate joint mobilization.

Nature of Spasticity and Muscle Patterning

The spasticity in the spinal cord injury patient differs in character from that in the brain injury, stroke, and cerebral palsy patient. In brain injury, stroke, and cerebral palsy, chronic increased tone or continuous static muscle contractions are usually seen. In the spinal cord injury patient, however, spasticity is often manifest by periodic distinct sudden muscle contractions triggered by minimal stretch or cutaneous stimulation. Two patterns of muscle contraction often occur: (1) those in which the major limb flexors contract, thus withdrawing the limb toward the body (known as *flexor patterning*); and (2) those in which the extensor muscles contract, resulting in the limb extending away from the body (known as *extensor patterning*). Patients often have alternating flexor and extensor patterning. The type of patterning may be in part dependent on the type of stimulation initiating the response or on the position of the limb at the time of stimulation.

Associated Problems

Joint mobilization in the spastic limb can be difficult. It can be painful, potentially harmful to the limbs, and is time-consuming. If spasticity prevents or impairs limb mobilization, difficulty with positioning the extremity occurs. The feet may not be able to be positioned on the wheelchair platform. Sitting, transfers, and positioning in bed can be difficult. Dressing the patient becomes time-consuming. Proper hygiene may be prevented, especially in the axilla, groin, and antecubital fossa. Mobilization of the joint for articular cartilage and soft tissue nutrition is prevented. Spasticity can interfere with joint mobilization used in the management of heterotopic ossification formation. If the joints cannot be adequately mobilized, stiffness of soft tissues can lead to fixed joint contracture.[9, 43]

Occasionally, severely spastic muscles will produce sudden violent muscle contractions that are hazardous to the patient. These sudden contractions are able to propel a patient out of a wheelchair or bed and make operation of a car or machinery dangerous. Wheelchair transfers are sometimes prevented.

In the patient with an incomplete spinal cord injury, spasticity may be superimposed on a limb with retained motor and sensory function. The spasticity can severely impair what residual function remains. If sensibility is intact, chronic increased muscle tone and sudden muscle contractions can be painful.

Spasticity As an Aid to the Patient

Occasionally, the hyperactive reflexes or increased muscle tone can be of use to the spinal cord injury patient, and this must be kept in mind prior to the surgical ablation of spasticity. By changing muscle position or touching the overlying skin, some patients are able to trigger an extension spinal reflex of the lower extremity, thereby facilitating standing or wheelchair transfers. Pinching the calf of the leg can cause a flexor reflex and thus can help in dressing the lower part of the body.[17] Reflex activity can also be used to provoke desired reflexes to assist with functional electrical stimulation during gait.[53]

Assessment of Spasticity

Assessment of degree of spasticity can be difficult, since other conditions cause stiffness or loss of joint motion. These include soft tissue contracture, heterotopic ossification, undetected fracture or dislocation, and extremity pain.[44] Fracture or dislocation can be evaluated radiographically. Heterotopic ossification, as discussed earlier, is accompanied by an inflammatory reaction, increased alkaline phosphatase, increased activity on technetium bone scan, and radiographic changes. Differentiating between the relative contributions of pain, increased muscle tone, and contracture can be more difficult. Diagnostic lidocaine nerve blocks can help differentiate these by temporarily eliminating pain and muscle tone, thereby allowing the relative contributions of fixed soft tissue contracture to be evaluated. Extremity nerve blocks in the evaluation of spasticity are outlined by Keenan.[44] These include blocks to the brachial plexus, musculocutaneous nerve, median nerve at the elbow, median and ulnar nerve blocks at the wrist, sciatic nerve, femoral nerve, obturator, and posterior tibial nerve block (Figs. 37–3 and 37–4).

It should be noted that a sudden increase in spasticity in the limbs may be a signal that an occult pathologic process is occurring, one that the patient is not aware of because of impaired sensibility. Possible problems include urinary tract infection, renal calculi, blockage of a catheter, or infected decubitus.[17] In the patient with a sudden increase of spasticity, these other problems should be suspected and appropriately evaluated.

Goals in Management

The main goals in the management of spasticity are to decrease muscle tone that interferes with function, retain limb motion to prevent contractures, and relieve pain that is often associated with spasticity. These are best accomplished by a multidisciplinary approach with a well-coordinated rehabilitation team. Management includes manual joint mobilization, limb splinting in a desirable position between therapy sessions, use of a standing frame, electrical stimulation of antagonist muscles to facilitate relaxation of the agonists, oral pharmacologic medications, serial lidocaine nerve blocks, phenol nerve blocks, surgical neurectomy, and surgical reconstruction. In the initial 12-month period of neurologic recovery (when spasticity may be decreasing), irreversible procedures such as neurectomy or tendon lengthenings should be avoided, since spontaneous recovery may obviate the need for these proce-

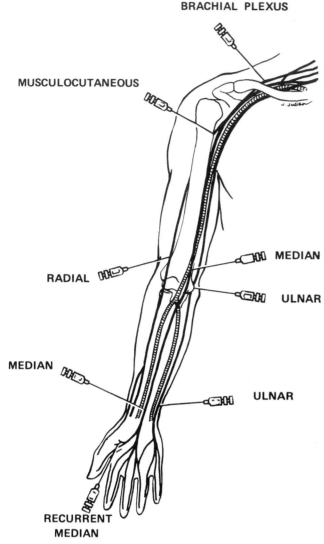

Figure 37–3 ═ Common sites of diagnostic nerve blocks to evaluate spasticity in the upper extremity. (From Keenan MAE: Orthopaedic management of spasticity. J Head Trauma Rehabil 2:62–71, 1987.)

dures, or result in an "overcorrection" deformity. In this 12-month period, mobilization, medications, and lidocaine or phenol nerve blocks should be utilized to their utmost effectiveness to avoid joint contractures.

Mobilization

Mobilization is performed by passive joint manipulation with proper splinting between mobilization sessions. The multiple benefits of joint mobilization include maintenance of lubrication efficiency of the joint, maintenance of the normal patterns of the soft tissue matrix, assistance of orientation of new collagen fibers according to stresses, and prevention of increased cross-links in the collagen matrix, thereby avoiding fixed contractures. Electrical stimulation can be used as an important adjuvant. Electrical stimulation of an agonist muscle not only provides a method of moving the joint but also assists in the relaxation of the antagonist.

Medications

Muscle tone can be reduced with systemic pharmacologic agents. Baclofen, diazepam, and dantrolene are useful for controlling sudden muscle contractions and reducing increased tone.[9] Baclofen blocks release of excitatory transmitters, thereby decreasing the severity of sudden muscle spasms. Given in divided doses of 10 to 60 mg per day, it is well tolerated, has few side effects, and is less sedating than other medications used to reduce muscle tone. Diazepam enhances presynaptic inhibition, also resulting in reduction of painful spasms. It can be given in divided doses of 4 to 30 mg per day. Major side effects are sedation. It is also potentially habit-forming. Dantrolene sodium exerts an inhibitory effect directly on muscle within the cell membrane and has no CNS depressant effect.[17] Side effects are minimal and there is no known tolerance. Hepatotoxicity is a potential side effect of all of these medications. Medications under investigation for treatment of spasticity include propranolol, thymoxamine, and tizanidine.[53]

Lidocaine or Bupivacaine Nerve Blocks

Lidocaine or bupivacaine (Marcaine) nerve blocks are effective temporary means of controlling or temporizing spasticity. As discussed above, regional lidocaine nerve blocks are helpful diagnostically to distinguish deformity caused by spasticity or by fixed contracture. Lidocaine nerve blocks can also be given in a serial fashion, prior to mobilization therapy. In some cases, daily nerve blocks will help elevate spasticity. Lido-

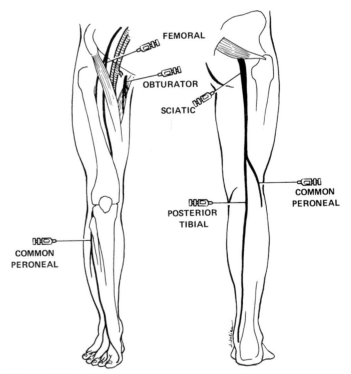

Figure 37–4 ═ Common sites of diagnostic nerve blocks to evaluate spasticity in the lower extremity. (From Keenan MAE: Orthopaedic management of spasticity. J Head Trauma Rehabil 2:62–71, 1987.)

caine nerve block prior to serial casting will ease joint mobilization and cast application. Bupivacaine is much longer-acting than lidocaine, and can be used when a prolonged block is desired.

Phenol Nerve Blocks

Phenol nerve blocks have proved to be useful in the management of spasticity.[7–9, 13, 27, 47, 48, 62] Phenol denatures the protein in a peripheral nerve, causing axonal degeneration. Since the continuity of the nerve sheath is not disrupted, the axons regenerate and nerve function returns.[44, 62] These nerve injections, therefore, provide a much longer nerve block than lidocaine. A dilute solution can be injected in a closed or open (surgical) fashion. Five percent aqueous solutions are used with closed blocks, and 3% to 5% solutions in glycerin are used with open blocks. Glycerin helps provide continued slow release of the phenol.[44] Phenol injection into a "mixed nerve" (containing both motor and sensory components) should not be performed in the patient with intact sensibility, since painful paresthesias may result. If sensibility is present, the phenol blocks should be reserved for nerves or nerve branches that carry predominantly motor fibers (such as pure motor nerves, the motor branches of the mixed nerve, or the motor points of the muscle). Injection into the motor branches are most accurately and safely performed by open block with direct visualization. When injected in a closed fashion, a Teflon-insulated needle with exposed tip guided by a nerve stimulator will assist with accurate placement of the phenol (Fig. 37–5). Closed phenol nerve blocks often provide relief from spasticity for up to 3 months. Open blocks, utilizing a 5% solution in glycerin injected directly into the motor branches of the nerve, will provide longer relief, often up to 6 months. Phenol is not currently a Food and Drug Administration (FDA)–approved substance, and proper patient consent is required. Phenol should not be autoclaved, as it can be denatured. Phenol is most optimally used in the period of neurologic recovery. It is hoped that as the nerve regenerates, the spasticity will decrease (if spontaneous recovery continues). If excessive spasticity remains when neurologic recovery has reached a plateau, then definitive surgery can be planned.[7, 44]

Motor Neurectomy

If a patient has persistent noxious spasticity and no further neurologic recovery is occurring or expected (i.e., the patient is beyond the 12-month period of spontaneous recovery), open motor neurectomy can be performed. Prior to neurectomy, the effects of the neurectomy can be simulated with a lidocaine or phenol block. If the block produces the desired results, neurectomy may be feasible. It must be realized that neurectomy alone will not correct a fixed contracture; it will only address the spastic component of the muscle. Prior lidocaine block will help differentiate the relative contributions of spasticity and fixed contracture causing the deformity. The spastic component will be obliterated with the block; the fixed contracture will remain.

Common neurectomies performed include musculocutaneous (for elbow flexion), motor branch to the brachioradialis (for elbow flexion), deep motor branch of the ulnar nerve (intrinsic plus deformity of the hand), superficial branch of the obturator nerve (adduction deformity of the thighs), motor branches of the femoral nerve (hip flexor or knee extensor spasticity), motor branches of the sciatic nerve (knee flexion spasticity), and motor branches of the posterior tibial nerve (equinovarus deformity). In performing a neurectomy, it is desirable to remove a segment of nerve to prevent spontaneous repair from axonal regeneration.

Intrathecal Injection

Intrathecal injections to control noxious spasticity have been reported, but they are mentioned here only to discourage their use. Intrathecal injections should not be performed. These injections, using either alcohol or phenol, can produce permanent lower motor neuron lesions. This results in a flaccid paralysis. The loss of all spasticity allows severe atrophy to occur, placing the lower extremities at higher risk for pressure sores. Any functionally useful extensor patterning is lost, such as that used for wheelchair transfers. The spastic bowel and bladder are converted to a flaccid bowel and bladder, resulting in loss of reflex evacuation and subsequent incontinence. There should never be a need or indication for intrathecal injection. The peripheral nerves or muscles should be addressed instead of the intrathecal space. Peripheral phenol nerve blocks, motor neurectomies, or muscle lengthening or release will control even the most noxious spastic muscles.

Rhizotomy, Cordotomy, and Cordectomy

Severance of the nerve roots or part or all of the cord has been performed to disrupt the reflex arc and convert a severely spastic extremity into a flaccid extremity. Similar complications as mentioned above with intrathecal injection may occur. Therefore, these procedures should not be performed. Severe spasticity should be treated at the level of the peripheral nerve or muscle, as described above.

Contracture

One of the most disastrous and often preventable complications of spasticity is the formation of a fixed contracture. If a joint is not mobilized, either actively or passively, a contracture will develop. Contractures develop following immobilization from spasticity, pa-

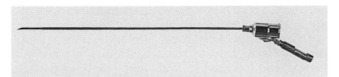

Figure 37–5 ═ Insulated needle with exposed tip is used in closed phenol nerve injections to control spasticity. The needle is connected to a nerve stimulator and guides accurate placement of the phenol.

ralysis, heterotopic ossification, or following injury. A joint moved once daily through its full range of motion will not develop a contracture. Contractures occur from loss of elasticity or fixed shortening of soft tissues. Tissues involved include the joint capsule, ligaments, muscle-tendon units, skin, nerves, and vascular structures. A fixed contracture often prevents any joint motion, and causes subsequent irreversible joint changes. Articular cartilage erosions, fatty infiltration, and intra-articular adhesion formation develop.[1, 2, 86, 87] Contractures interfere with function and hygiene. A joint contracture restricts limb position, causes problems with wheelchair transfers, interferes with dressing and sitting, and secondarily increases the potential for pressure sore formation. Proper hygiene may be difficult to maintain, especially in the groin, axilla, antecubital fossa, and popliteal fossa. Skin maceration can lead to ulceration and infection. In addition, the contractures themselves are often painful, especially when the limb is forcibly manipulated or positioned. Therefore, one of the most important goals in the management of spasticity is to maintain joint motion to prevent fixed contracture.

Treatment. Contractures are difficult to treat, requiring considerable time, discomfort to the patient, and often requiring surgical intervention. The most important aspect in the treatment of contractures is prevention. Joint mobilization and proper splinting should be initiated early following spinal cord injury, commencing when the patient is still in the intensive care unit as soon as medical stability permits. Once established, treatment of a contracture includes manual mobilization followed by well-padded serial casting as needed. Casts are changed weekly to inspect skin, allow further limb mobilization, and achieve further correction in a new cast. Serial dropout casts are effective in the management of contracture. Dynamic splints may be attempted, but these will not work if considerable spasticity coexists, especially if clonus is present.

Management of Specific Deformities

Shoulder. Involvement of the shoulder with spasticity is uncommon in the spinal cord injury patient, since injuries that occur proximal to the C5 root level can result in paralysis of the diaphragm (C4), often resulting in respiratory failure. In the survivors of these proximal cervical spinal cord injuries, spasticity can be severe. Function is usually minimal, and reconstruction difficult because of lack of available donor muscles and the presence of limb spasticity throughout. Deformity of the shoulder with spasticity is usually manifest by adduction and internal rotation. Muscles responsible for the deformity include the pectoralis major, subscapularis, teres major, and latissimus dorsi. Problems with hygiene, positioning, and dressing can arise. Rehabilitation efforts are initially directed toward mobilization to prevent contracture. Orthoses are not practical in correcting this deformity. Phenol nerve blocks to the motor points of the pectoralis can be performed if the patient is in the period of neurologic recovery of spasticity.[8] If the patient has reached a plateau in

improvement and no further neurologic recovery is expected, surgical release of spastic muscles can be performed to aid positioning and hygiene. Releases of the pectoralis major and subscapularis are performed first, followed by the teres major and latissimus dorsi as needed.[13]

Elbow. Severe spasticity of the elbow is rare, since these muscles are innervated primarily by nerve roots from the C5 level, and for spasticity to occur, the lesion must be proximal to this level. Many patients with more proximal lesions do not survive, as discussed earlier. If spasticity is present, initial treatment is mobilization to prevent contracture, and well-padded splints between therapy sessions to maintain correction. During the period of neurologic recovery, closed phenol nerve block to the musculocutaneous nerve can aid with mobilization. If spasticity is severe, and there is no volitional control in the extremity of a patient who is beyond the period of spontaneous recovery, motor neurectomy or surgical release of the biceps, brachialis, and brachioradialis can be performed. These will facilitate hygiene, positioning, and dressing. If there is preservation of volitional control, then selective lengthening of the elbow flexors can be performed to augment function.[45]

Hand and Wrist. Spasticity of the hand and wrist can occur in the spinal cord injury patient, but is usually associated with proximal cord lesions with spasticity throughout the upper extremity. In the severely affected patient, there is usually a flexion deformity at the wrist and hand (combined with flexor patterning of the upper extremity, i.e., elbow flexion, shoulder adduction and flexion). The hand can assume an intrinsic plus position if the intrinsic muscles are spastic and the extrinsic muscles paretic or paralytic.[48] If contracture develops, fixed shortening of the flexor tendons of the wrist or digits can be treated with mobilization, serial casting, or tendon lengthening as needed. If lengthening is necessary, fractional lengthening is preferred when volitional control is present.[46] Fixed intrinsic contracture can be treated with intrinsic lengthening of the intrinsic hood.[7, 45]

In the more distal cervical cord injuries, (i.e., C8–T1 root levels), an intrinsic minus hand deformity may develop. This is due to loss of nerve root or cord disruption at the C8–T1 level, resulting in paralysis of the intrinsic muscles of the hand. If the extrinsic flexors and extensors are intact (these are innervated by a more proximal spinal cord level), the imbalance will produce the intrinsic minus or clawhand deformity." This problem is discussed under Paralysis: Upper Extremity.

Hip. Flexor patterning of the lower extremity results in hip flexion and adduction. Hip flexion is usually caused by spasticity of the rectus femoris and the iliopsoas. The anterior portion of the tensor fascia lata may contribute to hip flexion. Hip adduction is usually caused by spasticity of the adductors longus, brevis, magnus, and the gracilis. Problems with hygiene in the groin are common. Difficulty in transfers, standing, and dressing also occurs. There is no feasible orthosis to treat flexion and adduction deformities of the hip.

Mobilization may be initiated and prone positioning to attempt to prevent contracture. Serial femoral and obturator lidocaine nerve blocks or closed phenol nerve blocks can be given. Open phenol blocks to the motor branches of the obturator nerve or femoral nerve can be given if closed phenol blocks are not adequate. Nerve blocks to the quadriceps muscles will also decrease knee extension, which may or may not be desirable. It is difficult to block the motor nerve to the iliopsoas muscle. If the patient has reached a plateau in a physical therapy program providing mobilization, and is beyond the period of expected neurologic recovery, muscle lengthenings or release can be performed. If the patient is a nonambulator, the adduction deformity can be addressed with tenotomy of the adductor longus and brevis, the gracilis, and possibly a portion of the adductor magnus. Alternatively, obturator neurectomy can be performed, but this may not alleviate a deformity caused by fixed muscle-tendon contracture. If the patient is an ambulator, the adductor magnus should be preserved to provide some adduction of the hip and prevent undesirable overcorrection manifested by hip abduction. In the nonambulator, a chronic refractory hip flexion deformity can be managed with release of the rectus femoris, iliopsoas, sartorius, and anterior portion of the tensor fascia lata.

Whenever surgical lengthenings or releases are considered, care must be given to assessing the residual functional status of the limb. If the patient has functional lower extremities, muscle lengthenings should be performed in place of releases. At the hip, this might include Z lengthening of the iliopsoas tendon, fractional lengthening or release of the rectus femoris, and partial release of the adductor muscles (release of the adductor longus and brevis, and the gracilis, while preserving the adductor magnus). Fixed contractures of these muscles can be treated by lengthening or release, depending on functional status. Residual contracture of the joint capsule can usually be corrected with mobilization or prone positioning once the deforming spastic or contracted muscle forces are eliminated.

Knee. Knee flexion deformity is common in the spinal cord injury patient and is caused by spasticity of the medial and lateral hamstring muscles. This deformity increases the potential for pressure sore development on the hindfoot, makes transfers difficult, and causes hygiene problems in the popliteal fossa. If sudden muscle spasms occur, the patient can be propelled from the wheelchair. Initial treatment of chronic knee flexion deformity from spasticity includes mobilization to prevent contracture and medications to control spasticity. Serial lidocaine nerve blocks to the sciatic nerve in the proximal thigh may help alleviate hamstring spasticity. Closed phenol nerve block to the sciatic nerve can be performed in the patient without sensibility. The sciatic nerve is blocked in a closed fashion by percutaneous injection at the distal margin of the gluteus maximus, guided with the nerve stimulator and insulated needle. If sensibility in the lower extremity is present, closed phenol block to the sciatic nerve should not be done, since painful paresthesias can occur from the phenol injection into a nerve containing sensory

fibers. In these patients, open phenol block to the motor branches of the sciatic nerve can be performed, thus avoiding phenol injection into sensory fibers. This requires a large surgical exposure to adequately identify and inject the motor branches to the hamstrings. It is difficult to inject many of the more distal branches in the thigh. In the ambulatory patient with knee flexor spasticity that interferes with function, and who has reached a plateau in neurologic recovery, surgical lengthening of the hamstrings can be performed. In the nonambulatory patient with noxious knee flexor spasticity that interferes with transfers, positioning, or hygiene, and who has reached a plateau in neurologic recovery, release of the distal hamstrings can be performed.

Occasionally, knee extensor spasticity is present. This can be troublesome or beneficial. Sudden muscle spasms can propel the patient from bed or chair. However, the patient may use knee extensor patterning to stabilize the limb during wheelchair transfers. When knee extensor spasticity is difficult to control or unsafe for the patient, phenol block to the femoral nerve in the proximal thigh will help to temporarily control quadriceps spasms. If the patient is beyond the recovery period (1 year post spinal cord injury), selective release of the distal quadriceps or neurectomy of the motor branches of the femoral nerve may be performed. However, these procedures may accentuate knee flexion spasticity, and should be avoided or performed cautiously in the patient who also has alternating knee flexor spasticity or patterning.

Foot and Ankle. Equinus deformity of the foot is common, caused by spasticity of the gastrocnemius and soleus muscles. Severe deformity causes difficulty with standing, transfers, wearing shoes, and placement of the feet on the wheelchair platform. Manual mobilization, splinting, and pharmacologic control of spasticity are initiated first. Serial lidocaine nerve blocks to the posterior tibial nerve in the popliteal fossa can help alleviate spasticity. Serial casting with well-padded casts can be performed for fixed contracture, but frequent cast replacement is necessary to allow skin inspection. If the patient is no longer improving in a therapy program and is beyond the period of expected neurologic recovery, Achilles tendon lengthening can be performed. If hindfoot varus is present, this can be addressed with lengthening of the tibialis posterior or tibialis anterior tendons. The split tibialis anterior tendon transfer (SPLATT procedure) is only rarely performed in the spinal cord injury patient, since this procedure does not address the commonly spastic tibialis posterior.[81]

Toes. Clawing of the toes (hyperextension at the metatarsophalangeal joint, flexion at the proximal interphalangeal joint) can cause skin irritation on the dorsum of the toes from pressure against the shoes. Clawing can be caused by intrinsic weakness, muscle imbalance, or by spasticity of the extrinsic extensors and flexors. Correction can be performed with lengthening or release of the extensor tendons (and flexors as necessary). These can be combined with resection arthroplasty or arthrodesis of the proximal interphalangeal joint if a fixed joint deformity exists. Phalangectomy should generally be avoided, since the loss of bony and ligamentous stability can result in lateral deviation of the toes if spasticity is present.

Occasionally, only flexion deformities are present, manifest by flexion at the metatarsophalangeal and interphalangeal joints. Painful skin irritation on the distal tip of the toe can result as the toes are flexed into the shoe or floor. Release of both the long and short flexors can be performed. Release of the toe flexors can be performed through incisions on the plantar aspect of the toes. Loss of active toe flexion is usually not a problem.[81]

If flexion deformity is present only at the proximal interphalangeal joint, without flexion at the distal phalangeal joint, the short toe flexors may be responsible. Involvement of these muscles can be verified with a posterior tibial nerve block at the ankle. This selectively blocks the intrinsic flexors, leaving the extrinsic flexors functioning. If the deformity is corrected with this block, then the short toe flexors are responsible, and these can be selectively released.[81]

Paralysis

Upper Extremity

Loss of upper limb function constitutes one of the most severe problems the quadriplegic patient faces. From the results of a survey, many quadriplegic patients indicated they would prefer restoration of hand function over restoration of walking capacity, bladder or bowel function, or sexual function.[36] Orthoses and surgical reconstruction play an important role in the rehabilitation of the upper extremity. Recently, new techniques in functional electrical stimulation of the upper extremity have been shown to be promising in the restoration of function.

Principal Functions to Restore

It has been estimated that 70% of traumatic tetraplegic patients can be helped by surgical reconstruction.[61] Two of the most desirable functions to aim to restore are (1) active elbow extension, and (2) single handgrip (usually provided by lateral pinch).[54, 60, 61, 89] In addition, reconstruction of finger flexion has been emphasized.[20] Other desirable functions include forearm pronation and intrinsic augmentation (for claw hand deformity), but these should be considered only after restoration of elbow extension and single handgrip, provided donor muscles are available.

Elbow extension can be reconstructed if a functional deltoid is present, using a deltoid-to-triceps tendon transfer. Restoration of elbow extension allows a patient to stabilize himself or herself in the wheelchair and improves control of self-help devices. Patients may gain the ability to hang up clothes or to take objects down from an overhead shelf. In rare cases, a patient may gain the ability to move from bed to wheelchair or to pivot without help (even though these bed-to-chair functions depend more on muscles that forwardly flex and depress the humerus such as the pectoralis).

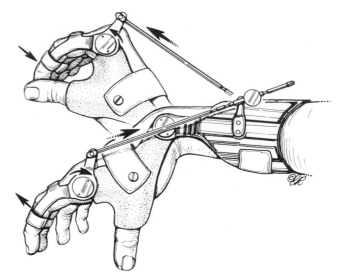

Figure 37–6 $=$ Wrist-driven orthosis. Active wrist extension with the orthosis in place provides a means of single-hand grasp. This device is dependent on adequate wrist extensor strength. As the wrist is dorsiflexed, the fingers are flexed to bring them into contact with the thumb, which is fixed. As the wrist is palmar-flexed, the fingers are extended. If wrist extensor strength is not adequate, tendon transfer to provide extensor strength can be considered. The brachioradialis is commonly used as a donor for this transfer. A similar but static ratchet type of orthosis is available that will hold the fingers in pinch position if the wrist is passively extended into a locked mode. (From McDowell CL: Tetraplegia. *In* Green DP (ed): Operative Hand Surgery. New York, Churchill Livingston, 1988.)

These motions allow locking of the elbow in extension, providing adequate elbow stability for transfers.

Single handgrip can be accomplished by different methods: (1) use of a wrist-driven flexor hinge orthosis, powered by volitional wrist extension to provide pinch (Fig. 37–6); and (2) tendon transfer (brachioradialis to extensor carpi radialis brevis) to provide or augment weak wrist extension to power a wrist-driven flexor hinged orthosis and provide pinch; (3) the Moberg tenodesis procedure to provide lateral pinch, and (4) opponensplasties to provide thumb-to-finger pinch.[21] These will be discussed individually.

Patient Selection and Classification

Patient selection for any type of surgical reconstruction in the tetraplegic patient can be difficult because of the complexity of the physical examination, the possibility of changing neurologic status over the first 12 months, and the multiple subjective factors that should be considered (patient's age, occupation, interests, and expectations). Surgical reconstruction of each of the different functional levels will be discussed separately. However, general considerations are considered first.

Selection for surgical reconstruction is dependent on existing motor and sensory function. In the past, quadriplegic patients were classified by the cervical spine segment injured, assuming that the level of paralysis and sensory loss coincided with the bone injury[89] (Fig. 37–7). However, this classification was not consistently accurate, since the level of bone injured may not coincide with the actual level of cord injury. In addition,

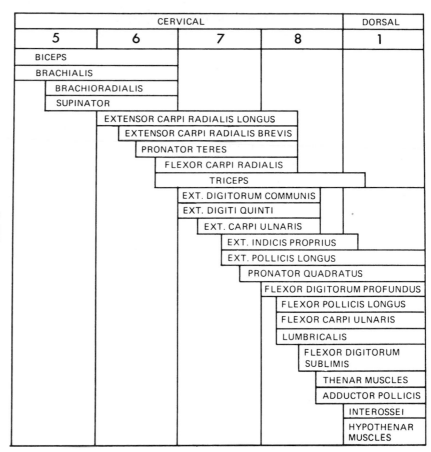

	CERVICAL			DORSAL
5	**6**	**7**	**8**	**1**

(chart content: segmental innervation table)

BICEPS
BRACHIALIS
BRACHIORADIALIS
SUPINATOR
EXTENSOR CARPI RADIALIS LONGUS
EXTENSOR CARPI RADIALIS BREVIS
PRONATOR TERES
FLEXOR CARPI RADIALIS
TRICEPS
EXT. DIGITORUM COMMUNIS
EXT. DIGITI QUINTI
EXT. CARPI ULNARIS
EXT. INDICIS PROPRIUS
EXT. POLLICIS LONGUS
PRONATOR QUADRATUS
FLEXOR DIGITORUM PROFUNDUS
FLEXOR POLLICIS LONGUS
FLEXOR CARPI ULNARIS
LUMBRICALIS
FLEXOR DIGITORUM SUBLIMIS
THENAR MUSCLES
ADDUCTOR POLLICIS
INTEROSSEI
HYPOTHENAR MUSCLES

Figure 37–7 = Segmental innervation of muscles of the elbow, forearm, and hand. (From Zancolli EA: Structural and Dynamic Bases of Hand Surgery, ed 2. Philadelphia, JB Lippincott, 1979, p 231.)

spinal injury may not be symmetrical and there may be unusual patterns of sparing of sensory or motor function. Nerve root injury from a higher spinal level may coexist with the cord lesion. Therefore, a more useful classification was developed by McDowell and associates[55, 56] and approved by an international group of surgeons working with tetraplegics. This classification is based on the most distal muscle available for transfer and patients are grouped into nine groups. The groups are further subdivided according to sensibility (Table 37–1). In group 0 (the most severely affected group), only the deltoid is available for transfer; the rest of the upper extremity is paralytic or paretic. In group 9 (the least involved group in this classification), the only weak muscles are the hand intrinsics, and multiple muscles are available for transfer. Specific transfers will be discussed.

Sensory Evaluation

Successful surgical reconstruction of the upper limbs is dependent on the presence of adequate sensibility. Sensory evaluation should include stereognosis and two-point discrimination. In most patients, stereognosis and two-point discrimination of at least 10 mm is required for pinch or grip to be useful.[60, 61] If two-point discrimination of 10 mm or more is not present, the grip needs to be guided or regulated by direct vision. Using direct vision to regulate grip can usually guide only one hand at a time.[72] Therefore, a prerequisite for

surgical reconstruction of grip is the presence of two-point discrimination and stereognosis in at least one hand.

As mentioned above, the motor group classifications are subdivided according to sensibility. When sensibility is adequate to regulate grip, the classification of Cu (cutaneous) is given, which indicates cutaneous afferents good enough to lead the grip. If sensibility is not adequate to lead grip, direct vision is required to regulate grip, and the sensory classification is 0. For example, a patient with the brachioradialis available for transfer and adequate sensibility in both hands is classified as CuCu 9.

Timing of Surgical Reconstruction

Surgical reconstruction in the quadriplegic upper extremity is usually not performed prior to 1 year post injury. This usually provides adequate time for neurologic recovery to reach a plateau and to allow the patient sufficient time to adjust psychologically to the paralysis and to realize that there will be no further recovery. In addition, recovery from spasticity usually becomes static by 1 year post injury, thus providing a static clinical picture of limb function. If there is any evidence of continuing neurologic recovery or improvement in function in a therapy program, surgical reconstruction should be delayed until there is no longer any motor or sensory improvement.

Table 37–1 = **INTERNATIONAL CLASSIFICATION FOR SURGERY OF THE HAND IN TETRAPLEGIA***

SENSIBILITY	MOTOR GROUP	CHARACTERISTICS	FUNCTION
O or Cu	0	No muscle below elbow suitable for transfer	Flexion and supination of elbow
	1	BR	
	2	ECRL	Extension of wrist (weak or strong)
	3	ECRB†	Extension of wrist
	4	PT	Extension and pronation of wrist
	5	FCR	Flexion of wrist
	6	Finger extensors	Extrinsic extension of fingers (partial or complete)
	7	Thumb extensor	Extrinsic extension of thumb
	8	Partial digital flexors	Extrinsic flexion of fingers (weak)
	9	Lacks only intrinsics	Extrinsic flexion of fingers
	X	Exceptions	

BR, brachioradialis; ECRL, extensor carpi radialis longus; ECRB, extensor carpi radialis brevis; PT, pronator teres; FCR, flexor carpi radialis.

*(1) The classification does not include the shoulder. It is a guide to the forearm and hand only. Determination of patient suitability for posterior deltoid-to-triceps transfer or biceps-to-triceps transfer is considered separately. (2) The need for triceps reconstruction is stated separately. It may be required in order to make brachioradialis transfers function properly. (3) There is a sensory component to the classification. Afferent input is recorded using the method described by Moberg[60, 61] and precedes the motor classification. Both ocular and cutaneous input should be documented. When vision is the only afferent available, the designation is "Occulo" (abbreviated O). Assuming there is 10 mm or less two-point discrimination in the thumb and index finger, the correct classification would be Cu, indicating that the patient has adequate cutaneous sensibility. If two-point discrimination is greater than 10 mm (meaning inadequate cutaneous sensibilty), the designation O would precede the motor group (example O 2). (4) Motor grouping assumes that all listed muscles are grade 4 (Medical Research Council [MRC]) or better and a new muscle is added for each group; for example, a group 3 patient will have BR, ECRL, and ECRB rated at least grade 4 (MRC).

†It is not possible to determine the strength of the ECRB without surgical exposure.

From McDowell CL: Tetraplegia. *In* Green DP (ed): Operative Hand Surgery, ed 2. New York, Churchill Livingstone, 1988, pp 1597–1618, modified by McDowell CL, Moberg EA, House JH: The Second International Conference on Surgical Rehabilitation of the Upper Limb in Tetraplegia (Quadriplegia). J Hand Surg Am 11:604–608, 1986.

Basic Principles in Limb Reconstruction

Principles of limb reconstruction have been outlined by Moberg,[60, 61] Zancolli,[88, 89] McDowell,[54] and others[64] and the reader is referred to these references. The least affected limb should undergo reconstruction first. Surgery should be performed on the dominant extremity first (if both are similarly impaired). If adequate cutaneous sensibility is not present, surgery should be done only on the side with the better residual motor function (using vision to guide the grip in this extremity). Only one surgical procedure should be performed at a time. Restoration of elbow extension should precede other procedures that restore pinch or grasp to the hand. Simplicity in surgery is the safest, utilizing available muscles of the extremity to strive for one or two simple functions. True opposition in pinch is usually not necessary; lateral pinch (key pinch) is more useful. Severe spasticity or fixed contracture needs to be controlled or corrected prior to tendon transfers.

Surgical Procedures

Surgical procedures will be discussed according to motor classification. It must be reiterated, that two-point discrimination of less that 10 mm and intact stereognosis should be present for useful hand function without guidance by direct vision, and that a person can visually guide only one hand at a time. Therefore, at least one hand should have adequate cutaneous sensibility. Direct vision can guide the other.

For further information on reconstruction of the patient with tetraplegia, including details of surgical procedures, the reader is referred to McDowell,[54–56] Moberg,[60, 61] Freehafer and co-workers,[20, 21] House and colleagues,[39–41] Waters and associates,[82] Zancolli,[88, 89] Kelly and co-workers,[50] and Lamb and Chan.[52]

Group 0. In general, patients in group 0 have deltoids functioning but no muscle function below the elbow suitable for transfer (see Table 37–1). This corresponds roughly to a C5 functional level. If elbow flexion itself is lacking, this can be restored provided the deltoid is functional. The posterior portion of the deltoid is transferred to the triceps, using an intercalary tendon graft harvested from the fascia lata, toe extensor, or tibialis anterior (Fig. 37–8). Patients in group 0 may be candidates for an externally powered orthosis. Most of these patients can use some assistive devices attached to one hand.

Group 1. Patients in this group have a strong brachioradialis, but poor function distally, including poor wrist extensors. Transfer of the brachioradialis into the extensor carpi radialis brevis or longus, or both can provide sufficient wrist extension to power a wrist-driven flexor hinged orthosis. This can provide a type of single handgrip (Fig. 37–9). In addition, lateral pinch can be augmented or reconstructed as needed with either the Moberg reconstruction for key pinch[60, 61] or the wrist-driven flexor hinged hand described by Nickel and co-authors.[64] The Moberg reconstruction requires strong wrist extension as a prerequisite. Reconstruction of lateral pinch consists of (1) tenodesis of the flexor pollicis longus to the distal palmar radius, to provide thumb flexion and create lateral pinch when the wrist is actively extended; (2) resection of the proximal annular pulley of the thumb to permit the tendon to bowstring and increase the strength of the key pinch; (3) internal fixation of the interphalangeal joint of the thumb to prevent flexion at the interphalangeal joint and maintain a broad contact surface; and (4) tenodesis of the extensor hood mechanism to the metacarpal of the thumb to prevent hyperflexion of the metacarpophalangeal joint (Fig. 37–10). Many modifications of

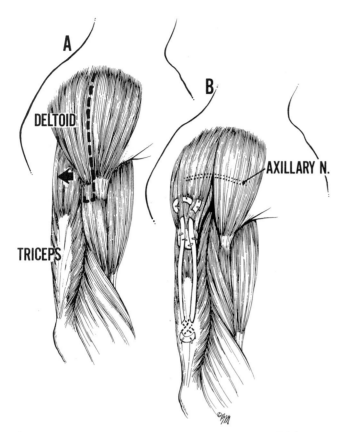

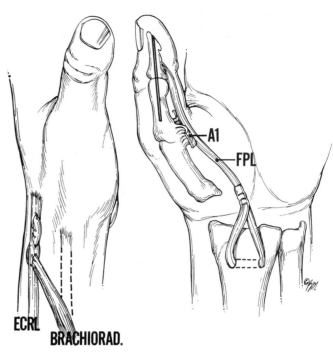

Figure 37–8 = Posterior deltoid-to-triceps transfer (Moberg) can provide active elbow extension. *A,* The posterior border of the muscle belly is isolated, preserving as much of the tendinous insertion as possible. *B,* An intercalary tendon graft is required, usually obtained from toe extensors. The tendon grafts are laced into the distal end of the deltoid muscle belly and triceps aponeurosis. (From McDowell CL: Tetraplegia. *In* Green DP (ed): Operative Hand Surgery. New York, Churchill Livingstone, 1988.)

Figure 37–10 = Moberg reconstruction to provide key pinch. Strong wrist extension is a prerequisite. If wrist extension is weak, the brachioradialis can be transferred to the extensor carpi radialis brevis to provide wrist extension. Salient features of this reconstruction include (1) tenodesis of the flexor pollicis longus *(FPL)* to the distal palmar radius, to provide thumb flexion and create key pinch when the wrist is actively extended; (2) resection of the proximal annular pulley of the thumb to permit the tendon to bowstring and increase the strength of the key grip; (3) internal fixation of the interphalangeal joint of the thumb to prevent interphalangeal joint flexion and maintain a broad contact surface; (4) tenodesis of the extensor hood mechanism to the metacarpal of the thumb to prevent hyperflexion of the metacarpophalangeal joint. (From Moberg E: The Upper Limb in Tetraplegia. New York, Stratton Intercontinental, 1978.)

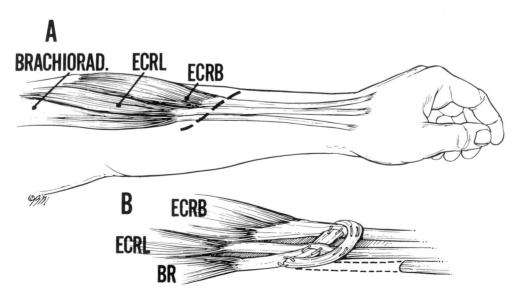

Figure 37–9 = Brachioradialis *(BR)* to extensor carpi radialis brevis *(ECRB)* and longus *(ECRL)* can be used to provide wrist extension so that either a wrist-driven orthosis for grip or the Moberg tenodesis becomes feasible. (From McDowell CL: Tetraplegia. *In* Green DP (ed): Operative Hand Surgery. New York, Churchill Livingstone, 1988.)

contraction can assist mobilization of the joint to prevent contractures, can help relax spastic antagonist muscles, and if timed or controlled carefully, can augment function of the limb. In addition, there is evidence that electrical stimulation of muscle strengthens the muscle and improves endurance.[69] If the muscle is stimulated to provide a specific movement or function of the extremity (e.g., digital flexion for grasp, ankle dorsiflexion during gait), the stimulation is called *functional electrical stimulation*. The muscles can be stimulated by surface electrodes placed on the skin, or by surgically implanted electrodes placed either on the epimysium or near the respective motor nerve.[49, 51, 67, 68, 80]

In the tetraplegic upper extremity, functional control by electrical stimulation has been studied by Peckham, Keith, and Freehafer and their co-workers.[20, 21, 49, 67, 68] Restoration of key pinch, grasp, and release has been studied using a percutaneous electrode system. Patients have included those in groups 0 and 1 (functional C5 or C6), with cutaneous sensibility that was usually intact. At these levels of cord injury, there are few adequate muscles available for tendon transfer. Prerequisites for successful use include control of spasticity, adequate seated balance, and nearly full range of movement of the shoulder, elbow, and fingers. Intact lower motor neurons are required, and the muscle must be electrically excitable by stimulation of its peripheral nerve. The electrodes are strategically placed in the forearm to stimulate the digital and thumb flexors and extensor muscles. The electrodes are connected to a controller which in turn is connected to a transducer placed on the contralateral shoulder (Fig. 37–11). Firing the electrodes is controlled volitionally by the patient via contralateral shoulder movements through the transducer. The electrodes usually remain in place over a year. This system requires no voluntary control below the level of the elbow, yet yields adequate key grip or lateral pinch to handle small objects and palmar prehension to handle large objects. Many alternative methods of volitional control of muscle excitation have been developed, including potentiometers mounted on a fixed surface and moved by the patient's opposite extremity; potentiometers attached to an orthosis that measure the position of the wrist; on/off switches that select a slowly increasing or decreasing command; and voice control.[67, 68] Using two grasp patterns, the user can hold objects such as eating utensils and writing implements, and position the hand for functions such as the use of a keyboard or control of switches and knobs.[49, 68]

Functional Electrical Stimulation in the Paraplegic Lower Extremity

Function in the lower extremity can be augmented by electrical stimulation. In paraplegic patients (and usually with preservation of some lower extremity function), functional electrical stimulation is able to improve standing or walking. These systems are promising to provide significant gains in function. However, the systems are not always practical. Patients must be carefully selected, goals must be realistic, and obstacles

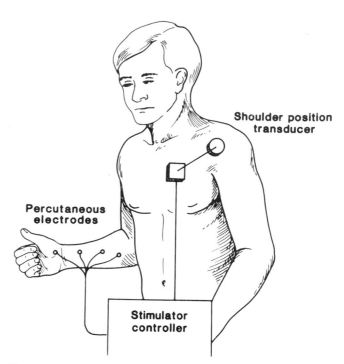

Figure 37–11 = Diagram of percutaneous electrical stimulation system. Percutaneous electrodes are placed in the forearm to stimulate digital and thumb flexor and extensor muscles. Stimulation of these muscles is volitionally controlled by the patient via the transducer placed on the contralateral shoulder. Specific movements of the shoulder are processed by the stimulator controller, and the muscles are stimulated to produce the desired function. (From Keith MW, Peckham PH, Thrope GB, et al: Functional neuromuscular stimulation neuroprosthesis for the tetraplegic hand. Clin Orthop 223:25–33, 1988.)

such as adapting to and maintaining the equipment need to be overcome.

Kralj and co-workers[51] have developed a successful system to augment standing and walking in the paraparetic patient. In their system, the patient utilizes and incorporates as much preserved function as possible into the restoration of ambulation. Patient capabilities are utilized to the maximal extent, including remaining motor skills and preserved reflexes. A four-channel stimulation unit is utilized. The four-channel gait pattern is controlled by the patient via trigger switches built into the handles of walkers or crutches. Standing is accomplished by stimulation of the quadriceps, enabling the patient to stand with an exaggerated lordotic posture. Gravity is used to stabilize the extended hips. Limb advancement is accomplished by stimulating a reflex synergistic flexion in the extremity, combined with the patient's shifting body weight using the upper extremities and the walker or crutches. In the authors' series, only 15% of all admitted patients were selected as candidates. Of these selected, 75% of patients with T4–5 lesions were able to utilize the four-channel walking system. Only 60% continued to use the system at home because of the time required to put on the equipment.[51]

Though relatively few well-documented studies in functional electrical stimulation have been performed, investigations by Kralj and others seem to support several conclusions: functional electrical stimulation for standing is an important function enabling patients to perform tasks in an upright position. Such standing may extend the transfer capabilities for patients and may be considered a therapeutic modality. Functional electrical stimulation used to augment walking seems to be able to provide useful but limited household ambulation. Its importance and role in the daily life of spinal cord injury patients needs to be determined. For long-term use, the time for putting on and removing the device is an important consideration. In addition, cosmesis and availability of the functional electrical stimulation (FES)–assisted devices are of prime importance. Surgically implantable systems have advantages over the surface-applied systems, and may prove to be superior for long-term use. Surface systems are useful for short-term use, such as therapeutic, training, and evaluation purposes to prepare and select patients for implantation.[51]

COMPLICATIONS ASSOCIATED WITH UPPER EXTREMITY WEIGHT BEARING IN THE PARAPLEGIC PATIENT

The paraplegic patient relies on the upper extremities for activities of daily living, locomotion, and wheelchair transfers. These activities result in higher stresses on the shoulders, elbows, wrists, and hands, which can precipitate problems associated with overuse. Frequent problems include extremity pain (especially at the shoulder) and peripheral neuropathies.[3, 5, 6, 19, 34, 63, 75, 85]

Upper Extremity Pain: Rotator Cuff Tears, Tendinitis, Bursitis

Multiple studies have shown that a high percentage (51% to 100%) of spinal cord injury patients eventually develop pain in their upper extremities. The pain is usually associated with or aggravated by wheelchair use or crutch walking. The reported incidence of extremity pain increases with time, from 52% during the first 5 years to 100% after 20 years.[6, 34, 63, 85]

The shoulder joint has the highest incidence of pain, with one third to one half of all patients developing shoulder pain during wheelchair transfers within the first 5 years. This incidence of pain increases to 70% at 10 years. Implicated causes of chronic shoulder pain include rotator cuff tears, bicipital tendinitis, and bursitis. Arthrography performed in paraplegic patients with persistent shoulder pain revealed a 45% incidence of rotator cuff tears. Intra-articular pressures of the shoulder joint are elevated during active transfers, reaching pressures greater than 250 mm Hg. Though increased stresses and activity at the shoulder seem to contribute to soft tissue injury, degenerative arthritis does not universally develop, even in long-standing paraplegic patients or those who have used crutches for swingthrough gait for many years. Gait studies in paraplegic crutch walkers implicate occurrence of increased loads through the glenohumeral and acromiohumeral joints during upper extremity weight bearing.[85]

Subdeltoid (subacromial) bursitis of the shoulder is manifest by pain under the acromion. The pain is increased with activity and sometimes increased with abduction (as in rotator cuff injury). Diagnosis of bursitis is usually made by exclusion of other causes. Chronic rotator cuff attritional injuries can be excluded by arthrography or magnetic resonance imaging (MRI). Tendinitis of the rotator cuff may be difficult to exclude. Radiographs may show calcifications in the supraspinatus tendon. Bicipital tendinitis causes pain along the biceps tendon in the bicipital groove on the anterior surface of the humeral head. Pain is well localized and increased with elbow flexion against resistance. Bursitis and tendinitis are usually self-limiting, and can often be controlled by rest, decreasing activity, and anti-inflammatory medications. Since the wheelchair patient requires use of the upper extremities for activities of daily living, decreasing activity may be difficult. Occasional and limited lidocaine and steroid injections can be useful in the treatment of bursitis and tendinitis. Treatment of rotator cuff tears depends on the extent of injury and limitations of the patient. Rarely have chronic attritional tears of the cuff been of sufficient magnitude to require surgical repair. In general, indications for surgical repair are the same as for patients in the general population.

Besides the shoulder, the hand is also commonly involved with pain. About 9% of patients complain of hand pain, usually in the palm. Pain in the palm is usually due to direct soft tissue irritation from repeated trauma during wheelchair propulsion. A second source of hand pain is the development of carpal tunnel syndrome (discussed next). Pain also occurs in the elbow and forearm, involving approximately 5% of patients.[6, 33, 85] Bone density in the forearm has been noted to be increased in paraparetic patients who rely on swing-through crutch walking.[85]

Carpal Tunnel Syndrome

Carpal tunnel syndrome has been associated with wheelchair use and transfers.[3, 6, 32] Up to 64% of paraplegic patients studied were noted to have signs or symptoms consistent with carpal tunnel syndrome, and the prevalence was noted to increase with the length of time from spinal cord injury. The high incidence has been attributed to both the frequent use of the wrist in an extended position during lifting and transfers, and to the repetitive trauma sustained to the palmar aspect of the wrist while propelling a wheelchair. Concurrent ulnar neuropathy at the elbow was noted in 40% of those with carpal tunnel syndrome.[3]

In the paraplegic patient with symptoms, signs, and electrodiagnostic confirmation of carpal tunnel syndrome, treatment should include standard initial treatment measures of rest, splinting, and anti-inflammatory medications. Splinting may not be practical in this population and persistent or severe symptoms usually require surgical decompression. Prolonged recovery of grip strength and persistent incisional discomfort are common, probably related to these patients being dependent on upper extremity function for activities of daily living.

Cubital Tunnel Syndrome

Besides carpal tunnel syndrome, an increased incidence of ulnar neuropathy has been associated with upper extremity use in paraplegic patients.[3, 75] Of those with carpal tunnel syndrome, concurrent cubital tunnel syndrome was noted in 40%.[3] An awareness of this problem and appropriate evaluation of nerve function will allow prompt detection and appropriate management.

MISCELLANEOUS COMPLICATIONS

Additional problems in the musculoskeletal system that face the patient with spinal cord injury include reflex sympathetic dystrophy, thrombophlebitis, gravitational edema, and pressure sores.

Reflex Sympathetic Dystrophy

Reflex sympathetic dystrophy is a recognized cause of upper extremity pain in the tetraplegic patient, with a reported incidence in spinal cord injury as high as 10%.[4, 33, 34, 65, 79] Common findings include diffuse hand or extremity pain, swelling, and stiffness. Less frequently, trophic changes of skin and hyperhydrosis are present. Radiographs often show macular and periarticular osteopenia. Three-phase radionuclide scintigraphy is a sensitive and specific diagnostic study to confirm the diagnosis. Management of this problem includes mobilization and splinting to prevent contractures, peripheral nerve or stellate ganglion block, systemic medication (sympatholytic medications such as α blockers, or calcium channel blockers) and surgical sympathectomy.

Venous Thrombosis

Venous thrombosis usually occurs within the first 40 days of hospitalization, and appears to be more common in spinal cord injury patients than in other hospitalized patients. Contributing factors include immobilization and the loss of pump action from active muscle contraction. If sensibility is not intact, diagnosis may be difficult. Findings include edema, warmth, and an increase in calf circumference. Minor edema may be the only presenting sign. Differential diagnosis includes heterotopic ossification, infection, tumor, gravitational edema, and pathologic fracture. Venography is usually diagnostic. Treatment is anticoagulation, usually beginning with intravenous heparin followed by oral long-term anticoagulant drugs such as warfarin. Physical therapy should cease temporarily during the acute stage. Late venous thrombosis can also occur, presenting in the second or third month post injury.

Gravitational Edema

Gravitational edema is caused by extravascular fluid pooling from dependence of the limb and lack of active muscle action. It occurs mostly in the lower extremities. Gravitational edema usually subsides within a few hours with extremity elevation. It is mentioned here briefly because it can mimic or mask other more serious disorders, such as thrombophlebitis, infection, occult fracture, or heterotopic bone formation.

Pressure Sores

Pressure sores are one of the most preventable complications in the spinal cord injury patient. Proper care should completely eliminate this problem. However, pressure sores continue to be a common problem in the spinal cord injury patient. A single indiscretion in care can lead to persistent, repeated ulceration with resultant hospitalization, loss of independence, and disruption of social adjustment. Areas where subcutaneous tissue is thin and skin overlies a bony prominence are at high risk for ulceration. Common areas include the ischial tuberosities, sacrum, greater tro-

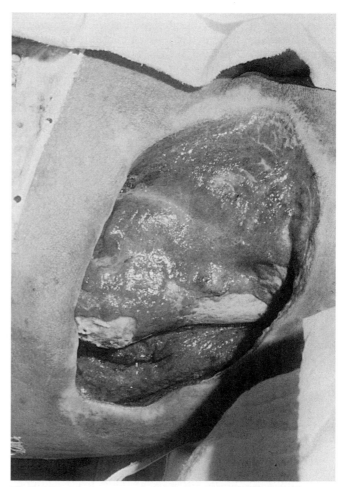

Figure 37–12 = Pressure sore in hip region with exposed greater trochanter. Osteomyelitis commonly develops when bone is exposed. In the management of pressure sores, it must be emphasized that the most important aspect of treatment is prevention.

chanter, malleoli, and the os calcis. Flexion contractures increase the risk because of limited or prolonged positioning. Continuous pressure leads to ischemia of all tissues between the skin and underlying bone. Lack of sensibility and paralysis prevent the patient from shifting position to relieve the ischemic area. Necrosis follows, usually in the subcutaneous fat (which has a lesser blood supply than the dermis). Healing may occur, and the ulcer fills with dense nonresilient scar tissue covered with thin epithelial tissue. A thick cicatrix covered with thin epithelium has poor resistance to repeated breakdown, and repeated or chronic ulcers may result. Chronic ulcers are also at high risk for infection. Osteomyelitis can develop in a bony prominence, such as the greater trochanter, that becomes exposed in the ulcer (Fig. 37–12).

Treatment of pressure sores is prevention. Proper padding, frequent positioning, and constant surveillance for early evidence of skin ischemia need to be instituted. Established ulcers require unloading of the pressure, local wound care, control of infection, correction of nutritional deficiencies, correction of contractures or spasticity that may be contributing to pressure areas, and surgical reconstruction, if needed.[71] Surgery often involves resection of infected bone, soft tissue debridement, and coverage using skin grafting, and local pedicle or distant tissue flaps.

CONCLUSION

The many possible complications of the musculoskeletal system in the patient with spinal cord injury have been outlined. The vast array of problems, and the consequences of delay in diagnosis or improper management emphasize the need for a constant high index of suspicion for complications and an aggressive treatment approach in the management of these patients. Though some of the problems presented here are unavoidable or are an unchangeable consequence of spinal cord injury, many can be prevented or minimized with an awareness of the potential problems, the use of proper preventive measures, and a thorough evaluation when a problem is suspected.

REFERENCES

1. Akeson WH, Amiel D, Abel MF, et al: Effects of immobilization on joints. Clin Orthop 219:28, 1987.
2. Akeson WH, Amiel D, Woo SL-Y: Immobility effects on synovial joints: The pathomechanics of joint contracture. Biorheology 17:95, 1980.
3. Aljure J, Eltorai I, Bradley WE, et al: Carpal tunnel syndrome in paraplegics. Paraplegia 23:182, 1985.
4. Andrews LG, Armitage KJ: Sudek's atrophy in traumatic quadriplegia. Paraplegia 9:159, 1971.
5. Bayley JC, Cochran TP, Sledge CB: The weight-bearing shoulder: The impingement syndrome in paraplegics. J Bone Joint Surg Am 69:182, 1987.
6. Blankstein A, Shmueli R, Weingarten I, et al: Hand problems due to prolonged use of crutches and wheelchairs. Orthop Rev 14:29–34, 1985.
7. Botte MJ, Keenan MAE: Reconstructive surgery of the upper extremity in the patient with head trauma. J Head Trauma Rehabil, 2:34–45, 1987.
8. Botte MJ, Keenan MAE: Percutaneous phenol blocks of the pectoralis major muscle to treat spastic deformities. J Hand Surg Am 13:147–149, 1988.
9. Botte MJ, Moore TJ: The orthopaedic management of extremity injuries in head trauma. J Head Trauma Rehabil 2:13–27, 1987.
10. Botte MJ, Nickel VL, Akeson WH: Spasticity and contracture: Physiologic aspects of formation. Clin Orthop 233:7–18, 1988.
11. Botte MJ: Extremity problems in spinal cord injury. In Nickel VL, Botte MJ: Orthopaedic Rehabilitation. New York, Churchill Livingstone, 1992, pp 427–452.
12. Brand PW: Clinical Mechanics of the Hand. St Louis, Mosby–Year Book, 1985.
13. Braun RM, Hoffer MM, Mooney V: Phenol nerve block in the treatment of acquired spastic hemiplegia in the upper limb. J Bone Joint Surg Am 55:580–585, 1973.
14. Braun RM, West F, Mooney V: Surgical treatment of the painful shoulder contracture in the stroke patient. J Bone Joint Surg Am 53:1307–1312, 1971.
15. Comarr AE, Hutchinson RH, Bors E: Extremity fractures of patients with spinal cord injuries. Am J Surg 103:732, 1962.
16. Couvee LMJ: Heterotopic ossification in the surgical treatment of serious contractures. Paraplegia 19:89, 1981.
17. Damanske M: Heterotopic ossification in paraplegia. J Bone Joint Surg Br 43:286, 1961.
18. Davis R: Spasticity following spinal cord injury. Orthop Clin 112:66–75, 1975.
19. Davis R: Pain and suffering following spinal cord injury. Orthop Clin 112:76–80, 1975.
20. Freehafer AA: Long-term management of lumbar paraplegia. In Pierce DA, Nickel VL (eds): The Total Care of the Spinal Cord Injuries. Boston, Little, Brown, 1977.
21. Freehafer AA, Vonhaam E, Allen V: Tendon transfers to improve grasp after injuries of the cervical spinal cord. J Hand Surg Am 56:951–959, 1974.
22. Furman R, Nicholas JJ, Jivoff L: Elevation of serum alkaline phosphatase coincident with ectopic bone formation in paraplegic patients. J Bone Joint Surg Am 52:1131, 1970.
23. Garland DE: Clinical observations on fractures and heterotopic ossification in the spinal cord and traumatic brain injured populations. Clin Orthop 233:86–101, 1988.
24. Garland DE, Alday B, Venos KG, et al: Diphosphonate treatment for heterotopic ossification in spinal cord injury patients. Clin Orthop 176:197, 1983.
25. Garland DE, Blum CE, Waters RL: Periarticular heterotopic ossification in head injured adults: Incidence and location. J Bone Joint Surg Am 62:1143, 1980.
26. Garland DE, Jones RC, Kuncle RWI: Upper extremity fractures in the acute spinal cord injured patient. Clin Orthop 233:110–115, 1988.
27. Garland DE, Lilling M, Keenan MA: Percutaneous phenol blocks to motor points of spastic forearm muscles in head-injured adults. Arch Phys Med Rehabil 65:243–245, 1984.
28. Garland DE, Orwin JF: Resection of heterotopic ossification in patients with spinal cord injuries. Clin Orthop 242:169, 1989.
29. Garland DE, Razza BE, Waters RL: Forceful joint manipulation in head-injured adults with heterotopic ossification. Clin Orthop 169:133, 1982.
30. Garland DE, Reiser TVC, Singer DI: Treatment of femoral shaft fractures associated with acute spinal cord injuries. Clin Orthop 197:191, 1985.
31. Garland DE, Saucedo T, Reiser TV: The management of tibial fractures in acute spinal cord injury patients. Clin Orthop 213:237, 1986.
32. Gellman H, Chandler D, Sie I, et al: Carpal tunnel syndrome in paraplegic patients. J Bone Joint Surg Am 70:517–519, 1988.
33. Gellman H, Eckert RR, Botte MJ, et al: Reflex sympathetic dystrophy in cervical spinal cord injury patients. Clin Orthop 233:126–131, 1988.
34. Gellman H, Sie I, Waters RL: Late complications of the weight-bearing upper extremity in the paraplegic patient. Clin Orthop 233:132–135, 1988.
35. Guttman L: Spinal shock and reflex behavior in man. Paraplegia 8:100, 1970.
36. Hansson RW, Franklin WR: Sexual loss in relation to other functional losses for spinal cord injured males. Arch Phys Med Rehabil 57:291, 1976.

37. Hentz VR, Brown M, Keoshian LA: Upper limb reconstruction in quadriplegia: Functional assessment and proposed treatment modifications. J Hand Surg 8:119–131, 1983.

38. Hiersche DL, Waters RL: Interphalangeal fixation of the thumb in Moberg's key grip procedure. J Hand Surg Am 10:30–32, 1985.

39. House JH: Reconstruction of the thumb in tetraplegia following spinal cord injury. Clin Orthop 195:117–128, 1985.

40. House JH, Gwathmey FW, Lundsgaard DK: Restoration of strong grasp and lateral pinch in tetraplegia due to cervical spinal cord injury. J Hand Surg 1:152–159, 1976.

41. House JH, Shannon MA: Restoration of strong grasp and lateral pinch in tetraplegia: A comparison of two methods of thumb control in each patient. J Hand Surg Am 10:22–29, 1985.

42. Hsu BD, Sakimura I, Stauffer ES: Heterotopic ossification around the hip joint in spinal cord injured patients. Clin Orthop 112:165, 1975.

43. Jordan C: Current status of functional lower extremity surgery in adult spastic patients. Clin Orthop 233:102, 1988.

44. Keenan MAE: The orthopaedic management of spasticity. J Head Trauma Rehabil 2:62–71, 1987.

45. Keenan MAE: Management of the spastic upper extremity in the neurologically impaired adult. Clin Orthop 233:116, 1988.

46. Keenan MAE, Abrams RA, Garland DE, et al: Results of fractional lengthening of the finger flexors in adults with upper extremity spasticity. J Hand Surg Am 12:575–581, 1987.

47. Keenan MAE, Botte MJ: Technique of percutaneous phenol block to the recurrent motor branch of the median nerve. J Hand Surg [Am] 12:806–807, 1987.

48. Keenan MAE, Todderud EP, Henderson R, et al: Management of intrinsic spasticity in the hand with phenol injection or neurectomy of the motor branch of the ulnar nerve. J Hand Surg Am 12:734–739, 1987.

49. Keith MW, Peckham PH, Thrope GB, et al: Functional neuromuscular stimulation neuroprostheses for the tetraplegic hand. Clin Orthop 233:25–33, 1988.

50. Kelly CM, Freehafer AA, Peckham PH, et al: Postoperative results of opponensplasty and flexor tendon transfer in patients with spinal cord injuries. J Hand Surg Am 10:890–894, 1985.

51. Kralj A, Bajd T, Turk R: Enhancement of gait restoration in spinal injured patients by functional electrical stimulation. Clin Orthop 233:34–43, 1988.

52. Lamb DW, Chan KM: Surgical reconstruction of the upper limb in traumatic tetraplegia: A review of 41 patients. J Bone Joint Surg Br 65:291–298, 1983.

53. Marsolais EB, Kobetic R: Development of a practical electrical stimulation system for restoring gait in the paralyzed patient. Clin Orthop 233:64–74, 1988.

54. McDowell CL: Tetraplegia. In Green DP (ed): Operative Hand Surgery, ed 2. New York, Churchill Livingstone, 1988, pp 1597–1618.

55. McDowell CL, Moberg EA, Graham-Smith A: International conference on surgical rehabilitation of the upper limb in tetraplegia. J Hand Surg 4:387–390, 1979.

56. McDowell CL, Moberg EA, House JH: The second international conference on surgical rehabilitation of the upper limb in tetraplegia (quadriplegia). J Hand Surg Am 11:604–608, 1986.

57. McMaster WC, Stauffer ES: The management of long bone fracture in the spinal cord injured patient. Clin Orthop 112:44, 1975.

58. Mendelson L, Grosswasser Z, Najenson T, et al: Periarticular new bone formation in patients suffering from severe head injuries. Scand J Rehabil Med 7:141, 1975.

59. Mielants H, Vanhove E, Deneels J, et al: Clinical survey of and pathogenic approach to para-articular ossifications in long-term coma. Acta Orthop Scand 46:190, 1975.

60. Moberg E: The Upper Limb in Tetraplegia. Stuttgart, Thieme, 1978.

61. Moberg EA: Upper limb surgical rehabilitation in tetraplegia. In Evarts CM (ed): Surgery of the Musculoskeletal System. New York, Churchill Livingstone, 1983.

62. Mooney V, Frykman G, McLamb J: Current status of intraneural phenol injections. Clin Orthop 63:132–141, 1969.

63. Nichols PJR, Normal PA, Ennis JR: Wheelchair user's shoulder? Shoulder pain in patients with spinal cord injuries. Scand J Rehabil Med 11:29, 1979.

64. Nickel VL, Perry J, Garrett AL: Development of useful function in the severely paralyzed hand. J Bone Joint Surg Am 45:933–952, 1963.

65. Ohry A, Brooks ME, Steinbach TV, et al: Shoulder complication as a cause of delay in rehabilitation of spinal cord injured patients. Paraplegia 16:310, 1978.

66. Orzel JA, Rudd TG: Heterotopic bone formation: Clinical, laboratory, and imaging correlation. J Nucl Med 26:125, 1985.

67. Peckham PH: Functional electrical stimulation: Current status and future prospects of applications to the neuromuscular system in spinal cord injury. Paraplegia 25:279–288, 1987.

68. Peckham PH, Keith MW, Freehafer AA: Restoration of functional control by electrical stimulation in the upper extremity of the quadriplegic patient. J Bone Joint Surg Am 70-A:144–148, 1988.

69. Ragnarsson KT: Physiologic effects of functional electrical stimulation-induced exercises in spinal cord–injured individuals. Clin Orthop 233:53–63, 1988.

70. Ragnarsson KT, Sell GH: Lower extremity fractures after spinal cord injury: A retrospective study. Arch Phys Med Rehabil 62:418–423, 1981.

71. Shea JD: Pressure sores: Classification and management. Orthop Clin 112:89–100, 1975.

72. Smith AG: Early complications of key grip hand surgery for tetraplegia. Paraplegia 19:123–126, 1981.

73. Spielman G, Gennarelli TA, Rogers CR: Disodium etidronate: Its role in preventing heterotopic ossification in severe head injury. Arch Phys Med Rehabil 64:539, 1983.

74. Stauffer ES: Long-term management of traumatic quadriplegia. In Pierce DS, Nickel VL (eds): The Total Care of Spinal Cord Injuries. Boston, Little, Brown, 1977.

75. Stephaniwsky L, Bilowitt DS, Prasad SS: Reduced motor conduction velocity of the ulnar nerve in spinal cord injured patients. Paraplegia 18:21–24, 1980.

76. Stover SL, Hataway CJ, Ziegler HE: Heterotopic ossification in spinal cord injured patients. Arch Phys Med Rehabil 56:199, 1975.

77. Tibone J, Sakimura I, Nickel VL, et al: Heterotopic ossification around the hip in spinal cord injured patients. A long term follow-up study. J Bone Joint Surg Am 60:769, 1978.

78. Tricot A, Hallot R: Traumatic paraplegia and associated fractures, Paraplegia 5:211, 1968.

79. Wainapel SR, Freed MM: Reflex sympathetic dystrophy in quadriplegia: Case report. Arch Phys Med Rehabil 65:35, 1984.

80. Waters RL, Campbell JM, Nakai R: Therapeutic electrical stimulation of the lower limb by epimysial electrodes. Clin Orthop 233:44–52, 1988.

81. Waters RL, Garland DE: Acquired neurologic disorders of the adult foot. In Mann RA (ed): Surgery of the Foot. St Louis, Mosby–Year Book, 1986.

82. Waters RL, Moore KR, Graboff SR, et al: Brachioradialis to flexor pollicis longus tendon transfer for active lateral pinch in the tetraplegic. J Hand Surg [Am] 10:385–391, 1985.

83. Wharton GW: Heterotopic ossification. Clin Orthop 112:142–150, 1975.

84. Wharton GW, Morgan TH: Ankylosis in the paralyzed patient. J Bone Joint Surg Am 52:105, 1970.

85. Wing PC, Treadwell SJ: The weight-bearing shoulder. Paraplegia 21:107, 1983.

86. Woo SL-Y, Gomez MA, Young-Knyn W, et al: Mechanical properties of tendons and ligaments. II. The relationships of immobilization and exercise on tissue remodeling. Biorheology 19:397, 1982.

87. Woo SL-Y, Matthews JV, Akeson WH, et al: Connective tissue response to immobility: Correlative study of biomechanical measurements of normal and immobilized rabbit knees. Arthritis Rheum 18:257, 1975.

88. Zancolli E: Surgery for the quadriplegic hand with active strong wrist extension preserved. A study of 97 cases. Clin Orthop 112:101–113, 1975.

89. Zancolli EI: Structural and Dynamic Basis of Hand Surgery. Philadelphia, JB Lippincott, 1979, p 231.

Index

Note: Page numbers in *italics* refer to illustrations; page numbers followed by t refer to tables.

ISBN 0-7216-2957-1